Explore more essential resources in the
NETTER BASIC SCIENCE COLLECTION!

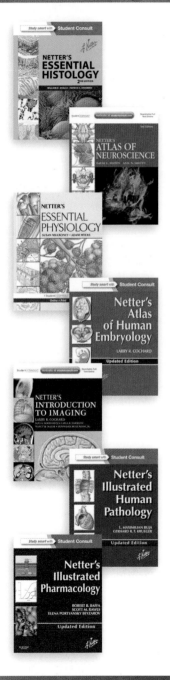

Netter's Essential Histology
With **Student Consult** Access

By William K. Ovalle, PhD and Patrick C. Nahirney, PhD

Bring histologic concepts to life through beautiful Netter illustrations!

Netter's Atlas of Neuroscience
With **Student Consult** Access

By David L. Felten, MD, PhD and Anil Shetty, PhD

Master the neuroscience fundamentals needed
for the classroom and beyond.

Netter's Essential Physiology
With **Student Consult** Access

By Susan Mulroney and Adam Myers, MD

Enhance your understanding of physiology the Netter way!

Netter's Atlas of Human Embryology
With **Student Consult** Access

By Larry R. Cochard, PhD

A rich pictorial review of normal and abnormal human prenatal development.

Netter's Introduction to Imaging
With **Student Consult** Access

By Larry R. Cochard, PhD et al.

Finally...an accessible introduction to diagnostic imaging!

Netter's Illustrated Human Pathology
With **Student Consult** Access

By Maximilian L. Buja, MD and Gerhard R. F. Krueger

Gain critical insight into the structure-function relationships
and the pathological basis of human disease!

Netter's Illustrated Pharmacology
With **Student Consult** Access

*By Robert B. Raffa, PhD, Scott M. Rawls
and Elena Portyansky Beyzarov*

Take a distinct visual approach to understanding both
the basic science and clinical applications of pharmacology.

Learn more at MyNetter.com!

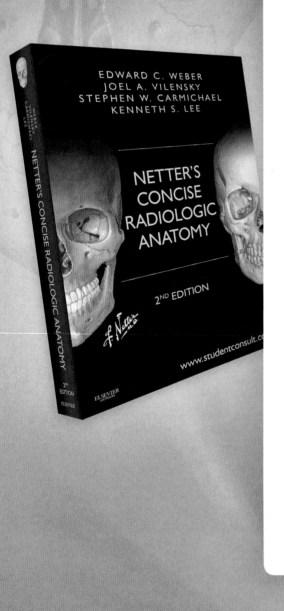

Netter's
Clinical Anatomy

3rd Edition

John T. Hansen, PhD

Professor of Neurobiology and Anatomy
Associate Dean for Admissions
University of Rochester School of Medicine and Dentistry
Rochester, New York

Illustrations by

Frank H. Netter, MD

Contributing Illustrators

Carlos A.G. Machado, MD
John A. Craig, MD
James A. Perkins, MS, MFA
Kristen Wienandt Marzejon, MS, MFA
Tiffany S. DaVanzo,MA, CMI

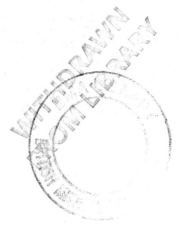

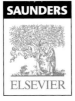

SAUNDERS

ELSEVIER

SAUNDERS

1600 John F. Kennedy Blvd.
Ste. 1800
Philadelphia, PA 19103-2899

NETTER'S CLINICAL ANATOMY, THIRD EDITION   ISBN: 978-1-4557-7008-3

ISBN: 978-1-4557-7008-3

Senior Content Strategist: Elyse O'Grady
Content Development Manager: Marybeth Thiel
Publishing Services Manager: Patricia Tannian
Senior Project Manager: John Casey
Senior Design Manager: Lou Forgione
Illustration Buyer: Karen Giacomucci

Printed in China

Last digit is the print number: 9 8 7 6 5 4 3 2

I dedicate this book to my wife
Paula,

and to my children
Amy and Sean,

and to my grandchildren
Abigail, Benjamin and Jonathan.

Without their unconditional love, presence, and encouragement, little would have been accomplished either personally or professionally. Because we've shared so much, this effort, like all the others, was multiauthored.

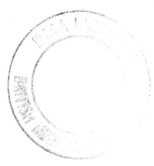

About the Artists

Frank H. Netter, MD

Frank H. Netter was born in 1906, in New York City. He studied art at the Art Students' League and the National Academy of Design before entering medical school at New York University, where he received his medical degree in 1931. During his student years, Dr. Netter's notebook sketches attracted the attention of the medical faculty and other physicians, allowing him to augment his income by illustrating articles and textbooks. He continued illustrating as a sideline after establishing a surgical practice in 1933, but he ultimately opted to give up his practice in favor of a full-time commitment to art. After service in the United States Army during World War II, Dr. Netter began his long collaboration with the CIBA Pharmaceutical Company (now Novartis Pharmaceuticals). This 45-year partnership resulted in the production of the extraordinary collection of medical art so familiar to physicians and other medical professionals worldwide.

In 2005, Elsevier, Inc., purchased the Netter Collection and all publications from Icon Learning Systems. More than 50 publications featuring the art of Dr. Netter are available through Elsevier, Inc. (in the US: www.us.elsevierhealth.com/Netter and outside the US: www.elsevierhealth.com).

Dr. Netter's works are among the finest examples of the use of illustration in the teaching of medical concepts. The 13-book *Netter Collection of Medical Illustrations*, which includes the greater part of the more than 20,000 paintings created by Dr. Netter, became and remains one of the most famous medical works ever published. *The Netter Atlas of Human Anatomy*, first published in 1989, presents the anatomic paintings from the Netter Collection. Now translated into 16 languages, it is the anatomy atlas of choice among medical and health professions students the world over.

The Netter illustrations are appreciated not only for their aesthetic qualities, but, more important, for their intellectual content. As Dr. Netter wrote in 1949, ". . . clarification of a subject is the aim and goal of illustration. No matter how beautifully painted, how delicately and subtly rendered a subject may be, it is of little value as a *medical illustration* if it does not serve to make clear some medical point." Dr. Netter's planning, conception, point of view, and approach are what inform his paintings and what make them so intellectually valuable.

Frank H. Netter, MD, physician and artist, died in 1991.

Learn more about the physician-artist whose work has inspired the Netter Reference collection: http://www.netterimages.com/artist/netter.htm.

Carlos Machado, MD

Carlos Machado was chosen by Novartis to be Dr. Netter's successor. He continues to be the main artist who contributes to the Netter collection of medical illustrations.

Self-taught in medical illustration, cardiologist Carlos Machado has contributed meticulous updates to some of Dr. Netter's original plates and has created many paintings of his own in the style of Netter as an extension of the Netter collection. Dr. Machado's photorealistic expertise and his keen insight into the physician/patient relationship informs his vivid and unforgettable visual style. His dedication to researching each topic and subject he paints places him among the premier medical illustrators at work today.

Learn more about his background and see more of his art at: http://www.netterimages.com/artist/machado.htm.

About the Author

John T. Hansen, PhD, is Professor of Neurobiology and Anatomy, and Associate Dean for Admissions at the University of Rochester School of Medicine and Dentistry. Dr. Hansen served as Chair of the Department of Neurobiology and Anatomy before becoming Associate Dean. Dr. Hansen is the recipient of numerous teaching awards from students at three different medical schools. In 1999, he was the recipient of the Alpha Omega Alpha Robert J. Glaser Distinguished Teacher Award given annually by the Association of American Medical Colleges to nationally recognized medical educators. Dr. Hansen's investigative career encompassed the study of the peripheral and central dopaminergic systems, neural plasticity, and neural inflammation. In addition to about 100 research publications, he is co-author of *Netter's Atlas of Human Physiology;* the lead consulting editor of Netter's *Atlas of Human Anatomy;* author of *Netter's Anatomy Flash Cards, Essential Anatomy Dissector*, and *Netter's Anatomy Coloring Book;* and co-author of the *TNM Staging Atlas with Oncoanatomy.*

Acknowledgments

Compiling the illustrations for, researching, and writing *Netter's Clinical Anatomy*, third edition, has been both enjoyable and educational, confirming again the importance of lifelong learning in the health professions.

Netter's Clinical Anatomy is for all my students, and I am indebted to all of them who, like many others, yearn for a better view to help them learn the relevant essential anatomy that informs the practice of medicine. Anatomy is a visual science, and Netter's illustrations are the gold standard of medical illustration.

Thanks and appreciation belong to my colleagues and reviewers who provided encouragement and constructive comments that clarified many aspects of the book. Especially, I wish to acknowledge David Lambert, MD, Senior Associate Dean for Undergraduate Medical Education at Rochester, who co-authored the first edition of this book with me and remains a treasured colleague and friend.

At Elsevier, it has been a distinct pleasure to work with dedicated, professional people who massaged, molded, and ultimately nourished the dream beyond even my wildest imagination. I owe much to the efforts of Marybeth Thiel, Senior Content Development Editor, and John Casey, Senior Project Manager, both of whom kept me organized, focused, and on time. Without them, little would have been accomplished. Thanks and appreciation also to Lou Forgione, Design Direction and Karen Giacomucci, Illustration Manager. A special thank you to Madelene Hyde, Publishing Director, and Elyse O'Grady, Senior Content Strategist, for believing in the idea and always supporting my efforts. This competent team defines the word "professionalism," and it has been an honor to work with all of them.

Special thanks to Carlos Machado, MD, for his beautiful artistic renderings that superbly complemented, updated, and extended the Netter anatomy collection. Also, I wish to express my thanks to my faculty colleagues at Rochester for their generous and constructive feedback.

Finally, I remain indebted to Frank H. Netter, MD, whose creative genius lives on in generations of biomedical professionals who have learned clinical anatomy from his rich collection of medical illustrations.

To all of these remarkable people, and others, "Thank you."

JOHN T. HANSEN, PHD

Preface

Human anatomy is the foundation upon which the education of our medical, dental, and allied health science students is built. However, today's biomedical science curriculum must cover an ever-increasing body of scientific knowledge, often in fewer hours, as competing disciplines and new technologies emerge. Many of these same technologies, especially those in the imaging science fields, have made understanding the anatomy even more important and have moved our discipline firmly into the realm of clinical medicine. It is fair to say that competent clinicians and allied health professionals can no longer simply view their anatomical training in isolation from the clinical implications related to that anatomy.

In this context, I am proud to introduce the third edition of *Netter's Clinical Anatomy*. Generations of students have used Dr. Frank H. Netter's elegant anatomical illustrations to learn anatomy, and this book combines his beautiful anatomical and embryological renderings with numerous clinical illustrations to help students bridge the gap between normal anatomy and its clinical application across each region of the human body.

This third edition provides succinct text, key bulleted points, and ample summary tables, which offer students a concise textbook description of normal human anatomy, as well as a quick reference and review guide for clinical practitioners. Additionally, some of the more commonly encountered clinical conditions seen in medical practice are integrated within the textbook as *Clinical Focus* boxes. These clinical correlations are drawn from a wide variety of medical fields including emergency medicine, radiology, orthopedics, and surgery, but also include relevant clinical anatomy related to the fields of cardiology, endocrinology, infectious diseases, neurology, oncology, reproductive biology, and urology. By design, the text and clinical correlations are not exhaustive but are meant to help students focus on the essential

elements of anatomy and begin to appreciate some of the clinical manifestations related to that anatomy. Other features of this edition include:

- An introductory chapter designed to orient students to the body's organ systems
- A set of end-of-chapter clinically oriented multiple choice review questions to help reinforce student learning of key concepts
- Basic embryology of each system that provides a contextual framework for human postnatal anatomy and several common congenital defects
- Online access with additional *Clinical Focus* boxes

My intent in writing this updated third edition of *Netter's Clinical Anatomy* was to provide a concise and focused introduction to clinical anatomy as a viable alternative to the more comprehensive anatomy textbooks, which few students read and often find difficult to navigate when looking for essential anatomical details. Moreover, this textbook serves as an excellent essential review text for students beginning their clinical clerkships or elective programs, and as a reference text that clinicians will find useful for review and patient education.

The text is by no means comprehensive but does provide the essential anatomy needed by the generalist physician-in-training that is commonly encountered in the first year of medical school. I have intentionally focused on the anatomy that a first-year student might be expected to grasp and carry forward into his or her clerkship training, especially in this day and age when anatomy courses are often streamlined and dissection exercises abbreviated. Those students, who by choice, choose to enter specialties where advanced anatomical training is required (e.g., surgical specialties, radiology, physical therapy, etc.) may encounter a need for additional anatomical expertise that will be provided by their graduate medical or allied health education. By meeting the needs of the beginning student and providing ample detail for subsequent review or handy reference, my hope is that *Netter's Clinical Anatomy* will be the anatomy textbook of choice that will actually be read and used by students throughout their undergraduate medical or allied health careers.

I hope that you, the health science student-in-training or the physician-in-practice, will find *Netter's Clinical Anatomy*, third edition, the valuable link you've searched for to enhance your understanding of clinical anatomy as only Frank Netter can present it.

JOHN T. HANSEN, PhD

Contents

Clinical Focus Boxes

chapter 4   **Abdomen**

chapter 5   ## Pelvis and Perineum

chapter 6 ## Lower Limb

chapter 7

Upper Limb

Introduction to the Human Body

1. TERMINOLOGY

Anatomical Position

The study of anatomy requires a clinical vocabulary that defines position, movements, relationships, and planes of reference, as well as the systems of the human body. The study of anatomy can be by **body region** or by **body organ systems**. Generally, courses of anatomy in the United States approach anatomical study by regions, integrating all applicable body systems into the study of a particular region. This textbook therefore is arranged regionally, and for those studying anatomy for the first time, this initial chapter introduces you to the major body systems that you will encounter in your study of anatomy. You will find it extremely helpful to refer back to this introduction as you encounter various body systems in your study of regional anatomy.

By convention, anatomical descriptions of the human body are based on a person in the **anatomical position** (Fig. 1-1), as follows:

- Standing erect and facing forward
- Arms hanging at the sides with palms facing forward
- Legs placed together with feet facing forward

Terms of Relationship and Body Planes

Anatomical descriptions often are referenced to one or more of three distinct body planes (Fig. 1-2 and Table 1-1), as follows:

- **Sagittal plane:** vertical plane that divides the body into equal right and left halves (median or midsagittal plane) or a plane parallel to the median sagittal plane (parasagittal) that divides the body into unequal right and left portions.
- **Frontal (coronal) plane:** vertical plane that divides the body into anterior and posterior portions (equal or unequal); this plane is at right angles to the median sagittal plane.
- **Transverse (axial) plane:** horizontal plane that divides the body into superior and inferior portions (equal or unequal) and is at right angles to both the median sagittal and the frontal planes (sometimes called *cross sections*).

Key terms of relationship used in anatomy and the clinic are summarized in Table 1-1. A structure or feature closer to the front of the body is considered *anterior* (ventral), and one closer to the back is termed *posterior* (dorsal). The terms *medial* and *lateral* are used to distinguish a structure or feature in relationship to the midline; the nose is medial to the ear, and in anatomical position, the nose also is anterior to the ear. Sometimes these terms of relationship are used in combination (e.g., *superomedial,* meaning closer to the head and nearer the median sagittal plane).

Movements

Body movements usually occur at the joints where two or more bones or cartilages articulate with one another. Muscles act on joints to accomplish these movements and may be described as follows: "The biceps muscle flexes the forearm at the elbow." Figure 1-3 summarizes the terms of movement.

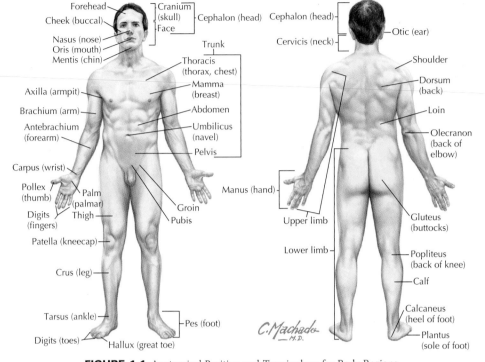

FIGURE 1-1 Anatomical Position and Terminology for Body Regions.

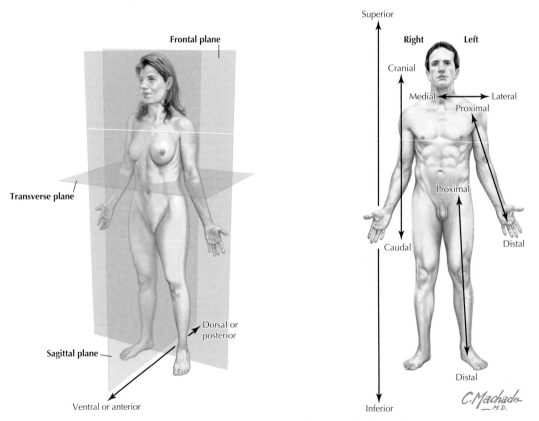

FIGURE 1-2 Body Planes and Terms of Anatomical Relationship.

TABLE 1-1 General Terms of Anatomical Relationship

TERM	DEFINITION	TERM	DEFINITION
Anterior (ventral)	Near the front	Median plane	Divides body into equal right and left parts
Posterior (dorsal)	Near the back		
Superior (cranial)	Upward, or near the head	Midsagittal plane	Median plane
Inferior (caudal)	Downward, or near the feet	Sagittal plane	Divides body into unequal right and left parts
Medial	Toward the midline or median plane		
		Frontal (coronal) plane	Divides body into equal or unequal anterior and posterior parts
Lateral	Farther from the midline or median plane		
Proximal	Near a reference point	Transverse plane	Divides body into equal or unequal superior and inferior parts (cross sections)
Distal	Away from a reference point		
Superficial	Closer to the surface		
Deep	Farther from the surface		

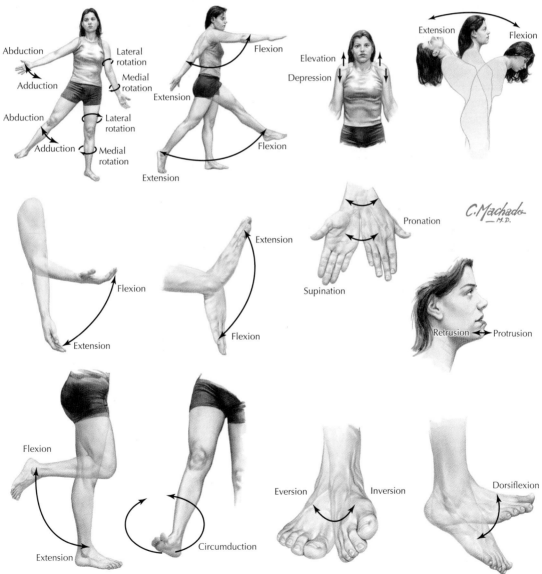

FIGURE 1-3 Terms of Movement.

Anatomical Variability

The human body is remarkably complex and remarkably consistent anatomically, but normal variations do exist, often related to size, gender, age, number, shape, and attachment. Variations are particularly common in the following structures:

- **Bones:** fine features of bones (processes, spines, articular surfaces) may be variable depending on the forces working on a bone.
- **Muscles:** vary with size and fine details of their attachments (it is better to learn their actions and general attachments rather than focus on detailed exceptions).
- **Organs:** the size and shape of some organs will vary depending on their normal physiology or pathophysiologic changes that have occurred previously.
- **Arteries:** surprisingly consistent, although some variation is seen in the branching patterns, especially in the lower neck (subclavian branches) and in the pelvis (internal iliac branches).
- **Veins:** consistent, although variations, especially in size and number of veins, can occur and often can be traced to their complex embryologic development; veins generally are more numerous than arteries, larger, and more variable.

2. SKIN

The skin is the largest organ in the body, accounting for about 15% to 20% of the total body mass, and has the following functions:

- *Protection:* against mechanical abrasion and in immune responses, as well as prevention of dehydration
- *Temperature regulation:* largely through vasodilation, vasoconstriction, fat storage, or activation of sweat glands
- *Sensations:* to touch by specialized mechanoreceptors such as pacinian and Meissner's corpuscles; to pain by nociceptors; and to temperature by thermoreceptors
- *Endocrine regulation:* by secretion of hormones, cytokines, and growth factors, and by synthesis and storage of vitamin D
- *Exocrine secretions:* by secretion of sweat and oily sebum from sebaceous glands

The skin consists of two layers (Fig. 1-4):

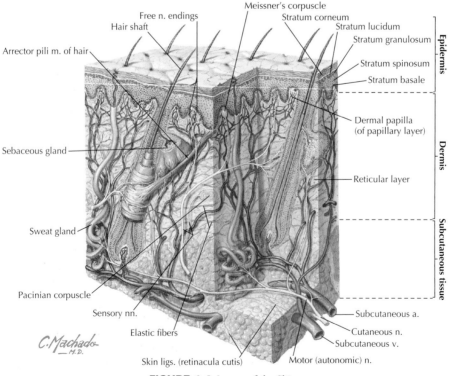

FIGURE 1-4 Layers of the Skin.

Clinical Focus 1-1

Psoriasis

Psoriasis is a chronic inflammatory skin disorder that affects approximately 1% to 3% of the population (women and men equally). It is characterized by defined red plaques capped with a surface scale of desquamated epidermis. Although the pathogenesis is unknown, psoriasis seems to involve a genetic predisposition.

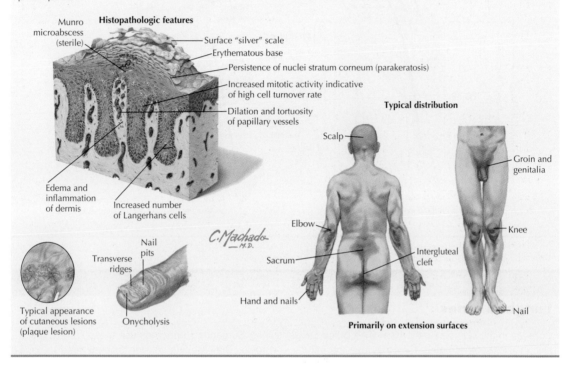

- **Epidermis:** outer protective layer consisting of a keratinized stratified squamous epithelium derived from the embryonic ectoderm.
- **Dermis:** dense connective tissue layer that gives skin most of its thickness and support, and is derived from the embryonic mesoderm.

Fascia is a connective tissue sheet that may contain variable amounts of fat. It can interconnect structures, provide a conduit for vessels and nerves (termed **neurovascular bundles**), and provide a sheath around structures (e.g., muscles) that permits them to slide over one another easily. **Superficial fascia** is attached to and lies just beneath the dermis of the skin and can vary in thickness and density; it acts as a cushion, contains variable amounts of fat, and allows the skin to glide over its surface. **Deep fascia** usually consists of a dense connective tissue, is attached to the deep surface of the superficial fascia, and often ensheathes muscles and divides them into functional groupings. Extensions of the deep fascia encasing muscles also may course inward and attach to the skeleton, dividing groups of muscles with **intermuscular septa.**

- **First-degree:** burn damage is limited to the superficial layers of the epidermis; termed a *superficial* burn, clinically it causes erythema.
- **Second-degree:** burn damage includes all the epidermis and extends into the superficial dermis; termed a *partial-thickness* burn, it causes blisters but spares the hair follicles and sweat glands.
- **Third-degree:** burn damage includes all the epidermis and dermis and may even involve the subcutaneous tissue and underlying deep fascia and muscle; termed a *full-thickness* burn, it causes charring.

Burns

Burns to the skin are classified into three degrees of severity based on the depth of the burn:

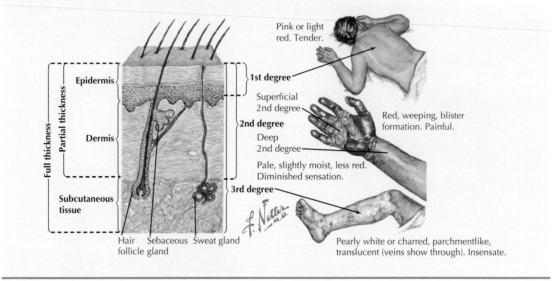

Pink or light red. Tender.

1st degree

Superficial 2nd degree

2nd degree

Deep 2nd degree

Red, weeping, blister formation. Painful.

Pale, slightly moist, less red. Diminished sensation.

3rd degree

Pearly white or charred, parchmentlike, translucent (veins show through). Insensate.

Epidermis

Dermis

Subcutaneous tissue

Full thickness

Partial thickness

Hair follicle   Sebaceous gland   Sweat gland

Langer's Lines

Collagen in the skin creates tension lines called *Langer's lines.* Surgeons sometimes use these lines to make skin incisions; other times, they may use the natural skin folds. The resulting incision wounds tend to gape less when the incision is parallel to Langer's lines, resulting in a smaller scar after healing. However, skin fold incisions also may conceal the scar following healing of the incision.

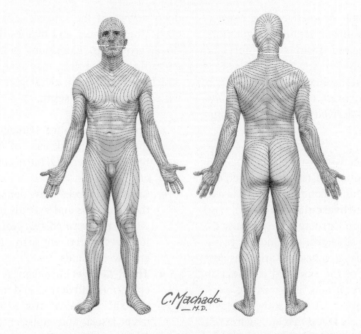

3. SKELETAL SYSTEM

Descriptive Regions

The human skeleton is divided into two descriptive regions (Fig. 1-5):

- **Axial skeleton:** bones of the skull, vertebral column (spine), ribs, and sternum, which form the "axis" or central line of the body (80 bones).
- **Appendicular skeleton:** bones of the limbs, including the pectoral and pelvic girdles, which attach the limbs to the body's axis (134 bones).

Shapes and Function of Bones

The skeleton is composed of a living, dynamic, rigid connective tissue that forms the bones and cartilages. Generally, humans have about 214 bones, although this number varies, particularly in the number of small sesamoid bones that may be present. (Many resources claim we have only 206 bones but have not counted the eight sesamoid bones of the hands and feet.) Cartilage is attached to some bones, especially where flexibility is important, or covers the surfaces of bones at points of articulation. About 99% of the body's calcium is stored in bone, and many bones possess a central cavity that contains bone marrow—a

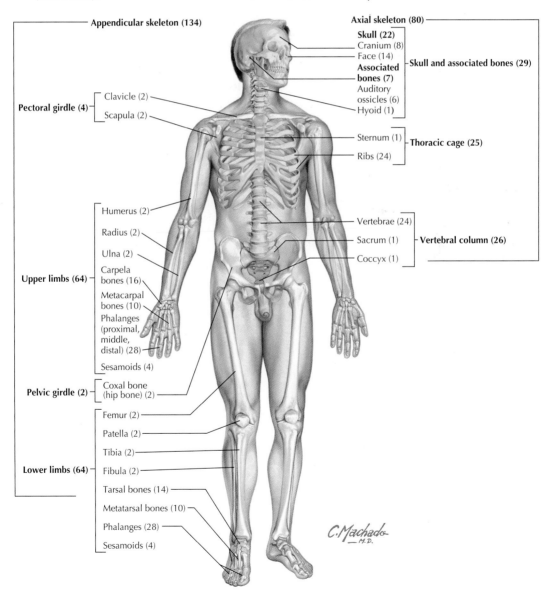

FIGURE 1-5 Axial and Appendicular Regions of Skeleton.

collection of hemopoietic (blood-forming) cells. Most of the bones can be classified into one of the following five shapes (Fig. 1-6):

- Long
- Short
- Flat
- Irregular
- Sesamoid

The functions of the skeletal system include:

- Support
- Protection of vital organs
- A mechanism, along with muscles, for movement
- Storage of calcium and other salts
- A source of blood cells

There are two types of bone:

- **Compact:** a relatively solid mass of bone, commonly seen as a superficial layer of bone, that provides strength.
- **Spongy** (trabecular or cancellous): a less dense trabeculated network of bone spicules making up the substance of most bones and surrounding an inner marrow cavity.

Long bones also are divided into the following descriptive regions (Fig. 1-7):

- **Epiphysis:** the ends of long bones, which develop from secondary ossification centers.
- **Epiphysial plate:** site of growth in length; contains cartilage in actively growing bones.
- **Metaphysis:** site where the bone's shaft joins the epiphysis and epiphysial plate.
- **Diaphysis:** the shaft of a long bone, which represents the primary ossification center and the site where growth in width occurs.

As a living, dynamic tissue, bone receives a rich blood supply from:

- *Nutrient arteries:* usually one or several larger arteries that pass through the diaphysis and supply the compact and spongy bone, as well as the bone marrow.
- *Metaphysial and epiphysial arteries:* usually from articular branches supplying the joint.

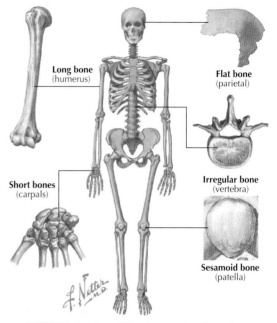

FIGURE 1-6 Bone Classification Based on Shape.

- *Periosteal arteries:* numerous small arteries from adjacent vessels that supply the compact bone.

Markings on the Bones

Various surface features of bones (ridges, grooves, and bumps) result from the tension placed on them by the attachment of tendons, ligaments, and fascia, as well as by vessels or other structures that pass along the bone. Descriptively, these features include the following:

- **Condyle:** rounded articular surface covered with articular (hyaline) cartilage
- **Crest:** a ridge (narrow or wide) of bone
- **Epicondyle:** prominent ridge or eminence superior to a condyle
- **Facet:** flat, smooth articular surface, usually covered with articular (hyaline) cartilage
- **Fissure:** very narrow "slitlike" opening in a bone
- **Foramen:** round or oval "hole" in the bone for passage of another structure (nerve or vessel)
- **Fossa:** a "cuplike" depression in the bone, usually for articulation with another bone
- **Groove:** a furrow in the bone
- **Line:** fine linear ridge of bone, but less prominent than a crest
- **Malleolus:** a rounded eminence
- **Meatus:** a passageway or canal in a bone

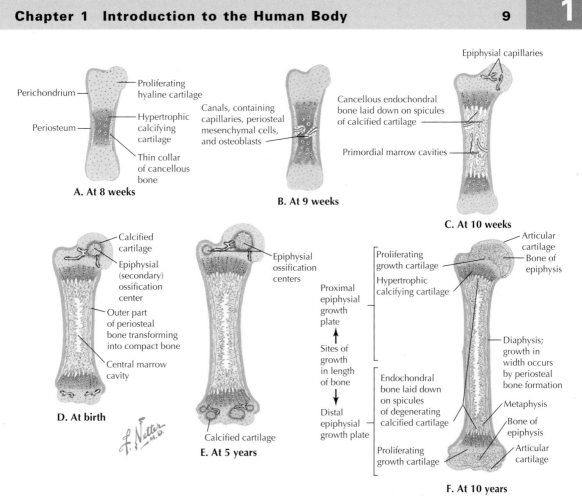

FIGURE 1-7 Growth and Ossification of Long Bones (Midfrontal Sections).

- **Process:** bony prominence that may be sharp or blunt
- **Protuberance:** protruding eminence on an otherwise smooth surface
- **Ramus:** thin part of a bone that joins a thicker process of the same bone
- **Spine:** sharp process projecting from a bone
- **Trochanter:** large, blunt process for muscle tendon or ligament attachment
- **Tubercle:** small, elevated process
- **Tuberosity:** large, rounded eminence that may be coarse or rough

Bone Development

Bones develop in one of the following two ways:

- **Intramembranous formation:** most flat bones develop in this way by direct calcium deposition into a mesenchymal (primitive mesoderm) precursor or model of the bone.
- **Endochondral formation:** most long and irregularly shaped bones develop by calcium deposition into a cartilaginous model of the bone that provides a scaffold for the future bone.

The following sequence of events defines endochondral bone formation (Fig. 1-7, *A-F*):

- Formation of a thin collar of bone around a hyaline cartilage model
- Cavitation of the primary ossification center and invasion of vessels, nerves, lymphatics, red marrow elements, and osteoblasts
- Formation of spongy (cancellous) endochondral bone on calcified spicules
- Diaphysis elongation, formation of the central marrow cavity, and appearance of the secondary ossification centers in the epiphyses
- Long bone growth during childhood
- Epiphysial fusion occurring from puberty into maturity (early to mid-20s)

Types of Joints

Joints are the sites of union or articulation of two or more bones or cartilages and are classified into one of the following three types (Fig. 1-8):

- **Fibrous** (synarthroses): bones joined by fibrous connective tissue.
- **Cartilaginous** (amphiarthroses): bones joined by cartilage, or by cartilage and fibrous tissue.
- **Synovial** (diarthroses): bones joined by a joint cavity filled with a small amount of synovial fluid and surrounded by a capsule; the bony articular surfaces are covered with hyaline cartilage.

Fibrous joints include **sutures** (flat bones of the skull), **syndesmoses** (two bones connected by a fibrous membrane), and **gomphoses** (teeth fitting into fibrous tissue-lined sockets).

Cartilaginous joints include **primary** (synchondrosis) joints between surfaces lined by hyaline cartilage (epiphysial plate connecting the diaphysis with the epiphysis), and **secondary** (symphysis) joints between hyaline-lined articular surfaces and an intervening fibrocartilaginous disc. Primary joints allow for growth and some bending, whereas secondary joints allow for strength and some flexibility.

Synovial joints generally allow for considerable movement and are classified according to their shape and the type of movement that they permit (uni-, bi-, or multiaxial movement) (Fig. 1-9), as follows:

- **Hinge** (ginglymus): uniaxial joints for flexion and extension
- **Pivot** (trochoid): uniaxial joints for rotation
- **Saddle:** biaxial joints for flexion, extension, abduction, adduction, and circumduction
- **Condyloid** (ellipsoid; sometimes classified separately): biaxial joints for flexion, extension, abduction, adduction, and circumduction
- **Plane** (gliding): joints that only allow simple gliding movements
- **Ball-and-socket** (spheroid): multiaxial joints for flexion, extension, abduction, adduction, mediolateral rotation, and circumduction

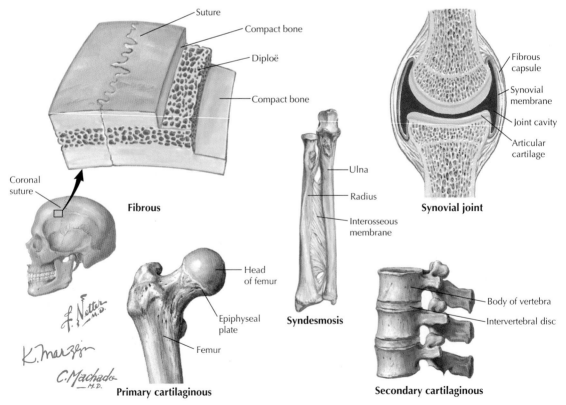

FIGURE 1-8 Types of Joints.

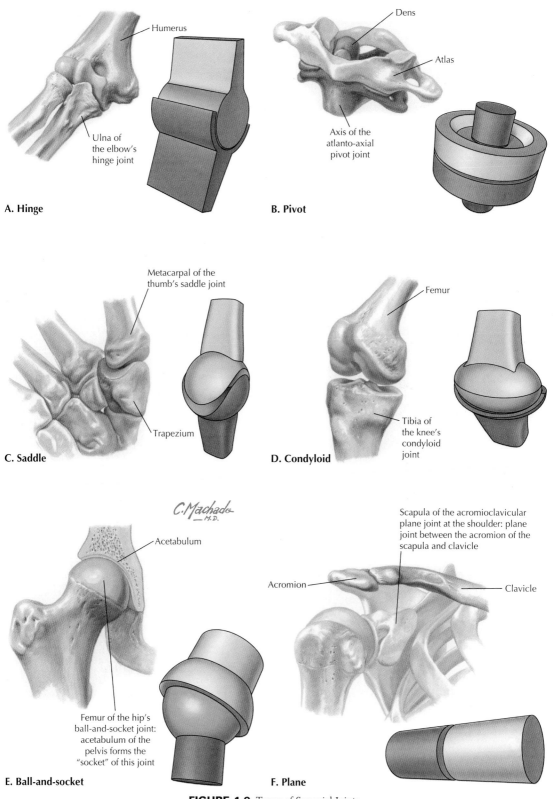

FIGURE 1-9 Types of Synovial Joints.

Fractures

Fractures are classified as either **closed** (the skin is intact) or **open** (the skin is perforated; often referred to as a *compound fracture*). Additionally, the fracture may be classified with respect to its anatomical appearance (e.g., transverse, spiral).

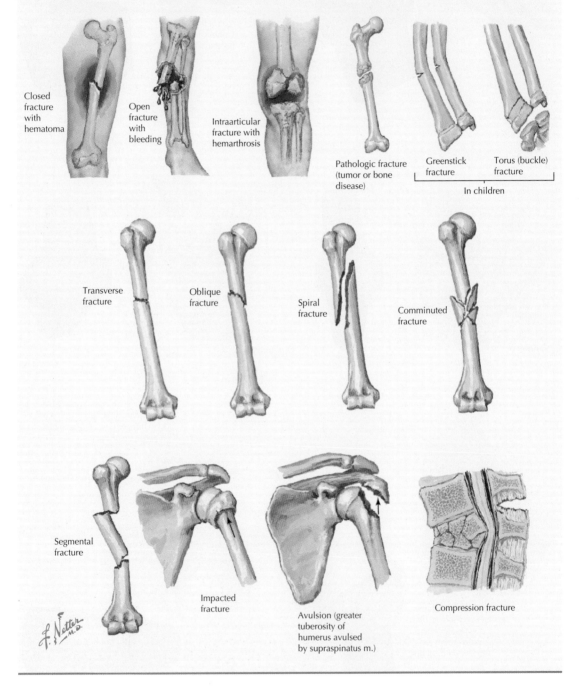

Closed fracture with hematoma

Open fracture with bleeding

Intraarticular fracture with hemarthrosis

Pathologic fracture (tumor or bone disease)

Greenstick fracture

Torus (buckle) fracture

In children

Transverse fracture

Oblique fracture

Spiral fracture

Comminuted fracture

Segmental fracture

Impacted fracture

Avulsion (greater tuberosity of humerus avulsed by supraspinatus m.)

Compression fracture

Degenerative Joint Disease

Degenerative joint disease is a catch-all term for osteoarthritis, degenerative arthritis, osteoarthrosis, or hypertrophic arthritis; it is characterized by progressive loss of articular cartilage and failure of repair. **Osteoarthritis** can affect any synovial joint but most often involves the foot, knee, hip, spine, and hand. As the articular cartilage is lost, the joint space (the space between the two articulating bones) becomes narrowed, and the exposed bony surfaces rub against each other, causing significant pain.

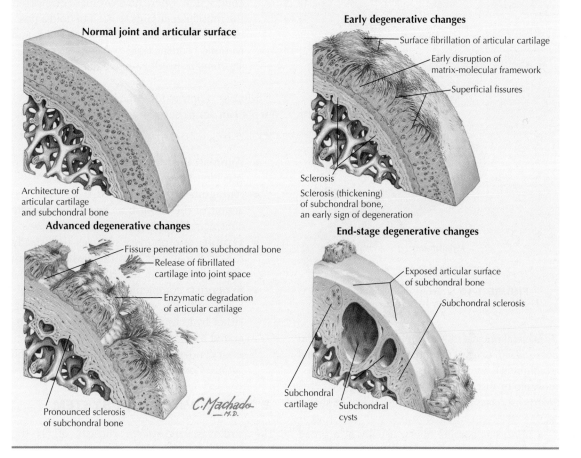

Normal joint and articular surface

Architecture of articular cartilage and subchondral bone

Early degenerative changes

Surface fibrillation of articular cartilage

Early disruption of matrix-molecular framework

Superficial fissures

Sclerosis

Sclerosis (thickening) of subchondral bone, an early sign of degeneration

Advanced degenerative changes

Fissure penetration to subchondral bone

Release of fibrillated cartilage into joint space

Enzymatic degradation of articular cartilage

Pronounced sclerosis of subchondral bone

C. Machado
—M.D.

End-stage degenerative changes

Exposed articular surface of subchondral bone

Subchondral sclerosis

Subchondral cartilage

Subchondral cysts

4. MUSCULAR SYSTEM

Muscle cells (fibers) produce contractions (shortenings in length) that result in movement, maintenance of posture, changes in shape, or the propulsion of fluids through hollow tissues or organs. There are three different types of muscle:

- **Skeletal:** striated muscle fibers that are attached to bone and are responsible for movements of the skeleton (sometimes simplistically referred to as *voluntary muscle*)
- **Cardiac:** striated muscle fibers that make up the walls of the heart and proximal portions of the great vessels

- **Smooth:** nonstriated muscle fibers that line various organs, attach to hair follicles, and line the walls of most blood vessels (sometimes simplistically referred to as *involuntary muscle*)

Skeletal muscle is divided into **fascicles** (bundles), which are composed of muscle fibers (muscle cells) (Fig. 1-10). The muscle fiber cells contain longitudinally oriented **myofibrils** that run the full length of the cell. Each myofibril is composed of many **myofilaments,** which are composed of individual **myosin** (thick filaments) and **actin** (thin filaments) that slide over one another during muscle contraction.

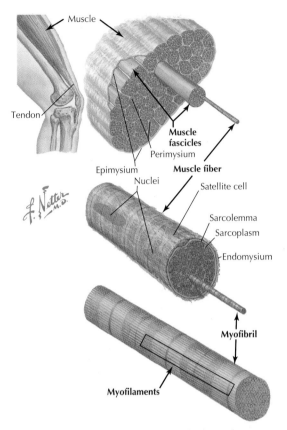

FIGURE 1-10 Structure of Skeletal Muscle.

Skeletal muscle moves bones at their joints and possesses an **origin** (the muscle's fixed or proximal attachment) and an **insertion** (the muscle's movable or distal attachment). At the gross level, anatomists classify muscle on the basis of its shape:

- *Flat:* has parallel fibers, usually in a broad flat sheet with a broad tendon of attachment called an *aponeurosis.*
- *Quadrate:* has a four-sided appearance.
- *Circular:* forms sphincters that close off tubes or openings.
- *Fusiform:* has a wide center and tapered ends.
- *Pennate:* has a feathered appearance (uni-, bi-, or multipennate forms).

Muscle contraction shortens the muscle. Generally, skeletal muscle contracts in one of three ways:

- *Reflexive:* involuntary or automatic contraction; seen in the diaphragm during respiration or in the reflex contraction elicited by tapping a muscle's tendon with a reflex hammer.
- *Tonic:* maintains "muscle tone," a slight contraction that may not cause movement but allows the muscle to maintain firmness necessary for stability of a joint and important in maintaining posture.
- *Phasic:* two types of contraction; isometric contraction, where no movement occurs but the muscle maintains tension to hold a position (stronger than tonic contraction), and isotonic contraction, where the muscle shortens to produce movement.

Muscle contraction that produces movements can act in several ways, depending on the conditions:

- **Agonist:** the main muscle responsible for a specific movement (the "prime mover").
- **Antagonist:** the muscle that opposes the action of the agonist; as an agonist muscle contracts, the antagonistic muscle relaxes.
- **Fixator:** one or more muscles that steady the proximal part of a limb when a more distal part is being moved.
- **Synergist:** complements (works synergistically with) the contraction of the agonist, either by assisting with the movement generated by the agonist or by reducing unnecessary movements that would occur as the agonist contracts.

5. CARDIOVASCULAR SYSTEM

The cardiovascular system consists of (1) the heart, which pumps blood into the pulmonary circulation for gas exchange and into the systemic circulation to supply the body tissues; and (2) the vessels that carry the blood, including the arteries, arterioles, capillaries, venules, and veins. The blood passing through the cardiovascular system consists of the following formed elements (Fig. 1-11):

- Platelets
- White blood cells (WBCs)
- Red blood cells (RBCs)
- Plasma

Blood is a fluid connective tissue that circulates through the arteries to reach the body's tissues and then returns to the heart through the

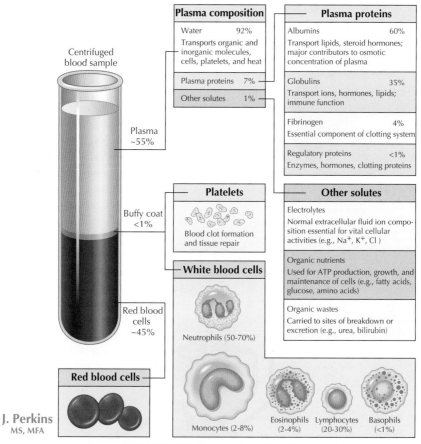

FIGURE 1-11 Composition of Blood.

veins. When blood is "spun down" in a centrifuge tube, the RBCs precipitate to the bottom of the tube, where they account for about 45% of the blood volume. This is called the **hematocrit** and normally ranges from 40% to 50% in males and 35% to 45% in females. The next layer is a **"buffy coat,"** which makes up slightly less than 1% of the blood volume and includes WBCs (leukocytes) and platelets. The remaining 55% of the blood volume is the **plasma** (**serum** is plasma with the clotting factors removed and includes water, plasma proteins, and various solutes). The functions of blood include:

- Transport of dissolved gases, nutrients, metabolic waste products, and hormones to and from tissues
- Prevention of fluid loss via clotting mechanisms
- Immune defense
- Regulation of pH and electrolyte balance
- Thermoregulation through blood vessel constriction and dilation

Blood Vessels

Blood circulates through the blood vessels (Fig. 1-12). **Arteries** carry blood away from the heart, and **veins** carry blood back to the heart. Arteries generally have more smooth muscle in their walls than veins and are responsible for most of the vascular resistance, especially the small muscular arteries and arterioles. Alternatively, at any point in time, most of the blood resides in the veins (about 64%) and is returned to the right side of the heart; thus veins are the capacitance vessels, capable of holding most of the blood, and are more variable and numerous than their corresponding arteries.

The major arteries are illustrated in Figure 1-13. At certain points along the pathway of the systemic arterial circulation, large and medium-sized arteries lie near the body's surface and can be used to take a **pulse** by compressing the artery against a hard underlying structure (usually a bone). The most distal pulse from the heart is usually taken over the dorsalis pedis artery on the dorsum of the foot.

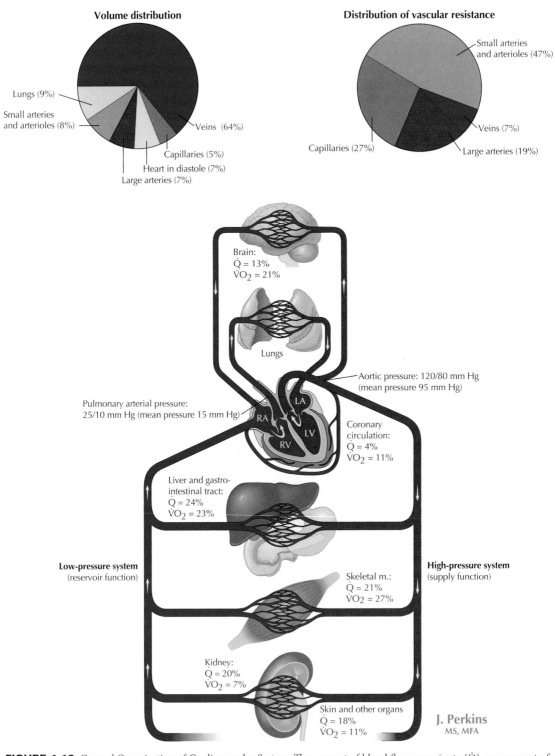

Volume distribution

Lungs (9%)

Small arteries
and arterioles (8%)

Veins (64%)

Capillaries (5%)

Heart in diastole (7%)

Large arteries (7%)

Distribution of vascular resistance

Small arteries
and arterioles (47%)

Veins (7%)

Large arteries (19%)

Capillaries (27%)

Brain:
$\dot{Q}$ = 13%
$\dot{V}O_2$ = 21%

Lungs

Aortic pressure: 120/80 mm Hg
(mean pressure 95 mm Hg)

Pulmonary arterial pressure:
25/10 mm Hg (mean pressure 15 mm Hg)

LA

RA

LV

RV

Coronary
circulation:
$\dot{Q}$ = 4%
$\dot{V}O_2$ = 11%

Liver and gastro-
intestinal tract:
$\dot{Q}$ = 24%
$\dot{V}O_2$ = 23%

Low-pressure system
(reservoir function)

High-pressure system
(supply function)

Skeletal m.:
$\dot{Q}$ = 21%
$\dot{V}O_2$ = 27%

Kidney:
$\dot{Q}$ = 20%
$\dot{V}O_2$ = 7%

Skin and other organs
$\dot{Q}$ = 18%
$\dot{V}O_2$ = 11%

J. Perkins
MS, MFA

FIGURE 1-12 General Organization of Cardiovascular System. The amount of blood flow per minute ($\dot{Q}$), as a percent of the cardiac output, and the relative percent of oxygen used per minute ($\dot{V}O_2$) by the various organ systems are noted.

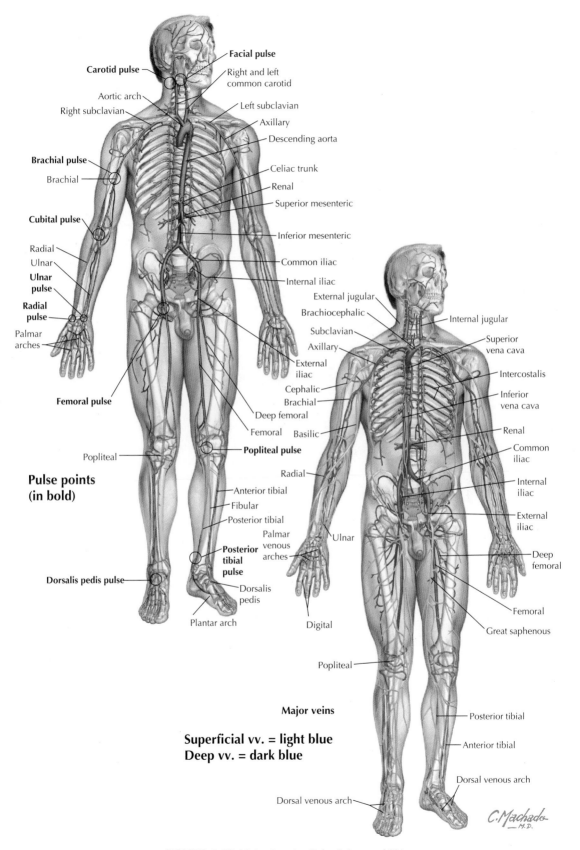

FIGURE 1-13 Major Arteries, Pulse Points, and Veins.

Atherogenesis

Thickening and narrowing of the arterial wall and eventual deposition of lipid into the wall can lead to one form of **atherosclerosis.** The narrowed artery may not be able to meet the metabolic needs of the adjacent tissues, which may become ischemic. Multiple factors, including focal inflammation of the arterial wall, may result in this condition. When development of a plaque is such that it is likely to rupture and lead to thrombosis and arterial occlusion, the atherogenic process is termed **unstable plaque formation.**

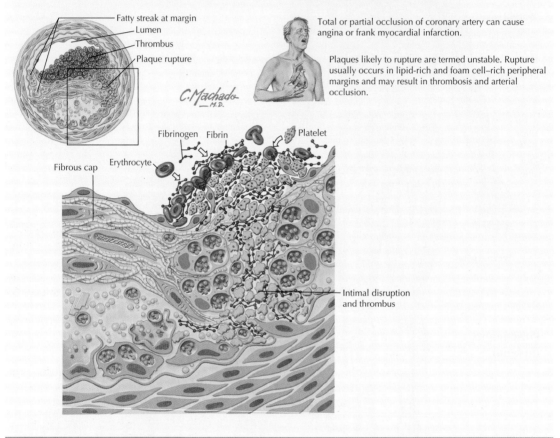

Fatty streak at margin
Lumen
Thrombus
Plaque rupture

Total or partial occlusion of coronary artery can cause angina or frank myocardial infarction.

Plaques likely to rupture are termed unstable. Rupture usually occurs in lipid-rich and foam cell–rich peripheral margins and may result in thrombosis and arterial occlusion.

C. Machado
—M.D.

Fibrinogen   Fibrin   Platelet

Fibrous cap   Erythrocyte

Intimal disruption and thrombus

The major veins are also illustrated in Figure 1-13. Veins are capacitance vessels because they are distensible and numerous and can serve as reservoirs for the blood. Because veins carry blood at low pressure and often against gravity, larger veins of the limbs and lower neck region have numerous valves that aid in venous return to the heart (several other veins throughout the body may also contain valves). Both the presence of valves and the contractions of adjacent skeletal muscles help to "pump" the venous blood against gravity and toward the heart. In most of the body, the veins occur as a superficial set of veins in the subcutaneous tissue that connects with a deeper set of veins that parallel the arteries. Types of veins include:

- *Venules:* very small veins that collect blood from the capillary beds
- *Veins:* small, medium, and large veins that contain some smooth muscle in their walls, but not as much as their corresponding arteries
- *Portal venous systems:* veins that transport blood between two capillary beds (e.g., the hepatic portal system)

Heart

The heart is a hollow muscular (cardiac muscle) organ that is divided into four chambers (Fig. 1-14):

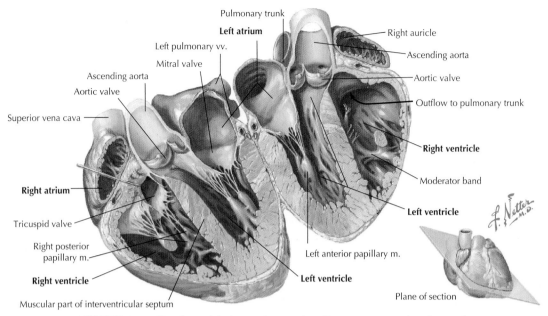

Pulmonary trunk
Left atrium
Left pulmonary vv.
Mitral valve
Ascending aorta
Aortic valve
Superior vena cava
Right auricle
Ascending aorta
Aortic valve
Outflow to pulmonary trunk
Right ventricle
Moderator band
Right atrium
Tricuspid valve
Right posterior papillary m.
Right ventricle
Muscular part of interventricular septum
Left anterior papillary m.
Left ventricle
Left ventricle
Plane of section

FIGURE 1-14 Chambers of the Heart. (From *Atlas of human anatomy,* ed 6, Plate 221.)

- **Right atrium:** receives the blood from the systemic circulation via the superior and inferior venae cavae.
- **Right ventricle:** receives the blood from the right atrium and pumps it into the pulmonary circulation via the pulmonary trunk and pulmonary arteries.
- **Left atrium:** receives the blood from the lungs via pulmonary veins.
- **Left ventricle:** receives the blood from the left atrium and pumps it into the systemic circulation via the aorta.

The atria and ventricles are separated by atrio-ventricular valves (**tricuspid** on the right side and **mitral** on the left side) that prevent the blood from refluxing into the atria when the ventricles contract. Likewise, the two major outflow vessels, the pulmonary trunk from the right ventricle and the ascending aorta from the left ventricle, possess the **pulmonic** valve and the **aortic** valve (semilunar valves), respectively.

6. LYMPHATIC SYSTEM

General Organization

The lymphatic system is intimately associated with the cardiovascular system, both in the development of its lymphatic vessels and in its immune function. The lymphatic system functions to:

- Protect the body against infection by activating defense mechanisms of the immune system.
- Collect tissue fluids, solutes, hormones, and plasma proteins and return them to the circulatory system (bloodstream).
- Absorb fat (chylomicrons) from the small intestine.

Components of the lymphatic system include the following:

- **Lymph:** watery fluid that resembles plasma but contains fewer proteins and may contain fat, together with cells (mainly lymphocytes and a few RBCs).
- **Lymphocytes:** the cellular components of lymph, including T cells and B cells.
- **Lymph vessels:** extensive network of vessels and capillaries in the peripheral tissues that transport lymph and lymphocytes.
- **Lymphoid organs:** collections of lymphoid tissue, including lymph nodes, aggregates of lymphoid tissue along the respiratory and gastrointestinal passageways, tonsils, thymus, spleen, and bone marrow.

Lymphatic Drainage

The body is about 60% fluid by weight, with 40% located in the intracellular fluid (ICF) compartment (inside the cells) and the remaining 20% in the extracellular fluid (ECF) compartment. The lymphatics are essential for returning ECF, solutes, and protein (lost via the capillaries into the ECF compartment) back to the bloodstream, thus helping to maintain a normal blood volume. On average, the lymphatics return about 3.5 to 4.0 liters of fluid per day back to the bloodstream. The lymphatics also distribute various hormones, nutrients (fats from the bowel and proteins from the interstitium), and waste products from the ECF to the bloodstream.

Lymphatic vessels transport lymph from everywhere in the body (except the central nervous system) to major lymphatic channels. The majority of lymph ultimately collects in the **thoracic duct** for delivery back to the venous system (joins the veins at the union of the left internal jugular and left subclavian veins) (Fig. 1-15). A much smaller **right lymphatic duct** drains the right upper quadrant of the body lymphatics to a similar site on the right side. Along the route of these lymphatic vessels, encapsulated lymph nodes are strategically placed to "filter" the lymph as it moves toward the venous system. Lymph nodes form a key site for phagocytosis of microorganisms and other particulate matter, and they initiate the body's immune responses.

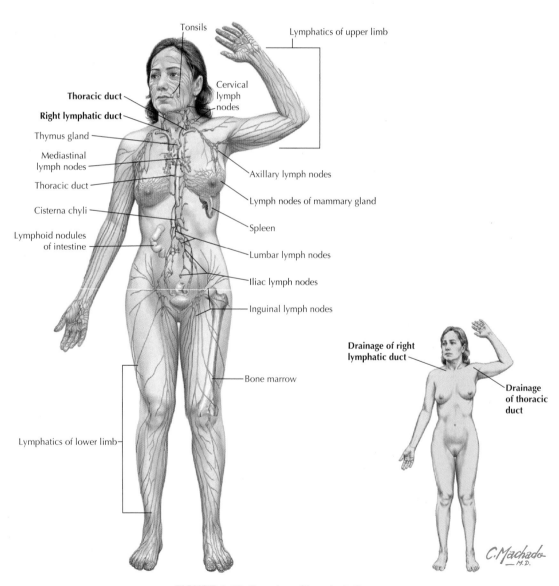

FIGURE 1-15 Overview of Lymphatic System.

Immune Response

When a foreign microorganism, virus-infected cell, or cancer cell is detected within the body, the lymphatic system mounts what is called an *immune response.* The detected pathogens are distinguished from the body's own normal cells, and then a response is initiated to neutralize the pathogen. The human body has evolved three major responses to protect against foreign invaders:

- **Nonspecific barriers:** first line of defense is composed of physical barriers to invasion. These include the skin and mucous membranes that line the body's exterior (skin) or its respiratory, gastrointestinal, urinary, and reproductive systems (mucosa and its secretions, which may include enzymes, acidic secretions, flushing mechanisms such as tear secretion or the voiding of urine, sticky mucus to sequester pathogens, and physical coughing and sneezing to remove pathogens and irritants).
- **Innate immunity:** second line of defense (if the nonspecific barrier is breached) is composed of a variety of cells and antimicrobial secretions, and manifests with inflammation and fever.

- **Adaptive immunity:** third line of defense is characterized by specific pathogen recognition, immunologic memory, amplification of immune responses, and rapid response against pathogens that reinvade the body.

7. RESPIRATORY SYSTEM

The respiratory system provides oxygen to the body for its metabolic needs and eliminates carbon dioxide. Structurally, the respiratory system includes the following (Fig. 1-16):

- Nose and paranasal sinuses
- Pharynx and its subdivisions (naso-, oro-, and laryngopharynx)
- Larynx
- Trachea
- Bronchi, bronchioles, alveolar ducts/sacs, and alveoli
- Lungs

Functionally, the respiratory system performs five basic functions:

- Filters and humidifies the air and moves it in and out of the lungs

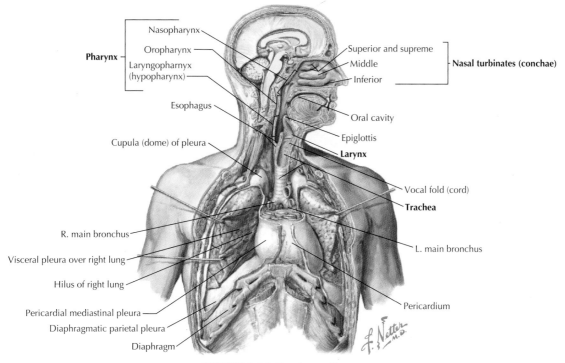

FIGURE 1-16 Respiratory System.

Asthma

Asthma can be *intrinsic* (no clearly defined environmental trigger) or *extrinsic* (has a defined trigger). Asthma usually results from a hypersensitivity reaction to an allergen (dust, pollen, mold), which leads to irritation of the respiratory passages and smooth muscle contraction (narrowing of the passages), swelling (edema) of the epithelium, and increased production of mucus. Presenting symptoms are often wheezing, shortness of breath, coughing, tachycardia, and feelings of chest tightness. Asthma is a pathologic inflammation of the airways and occurs in both children and adults.

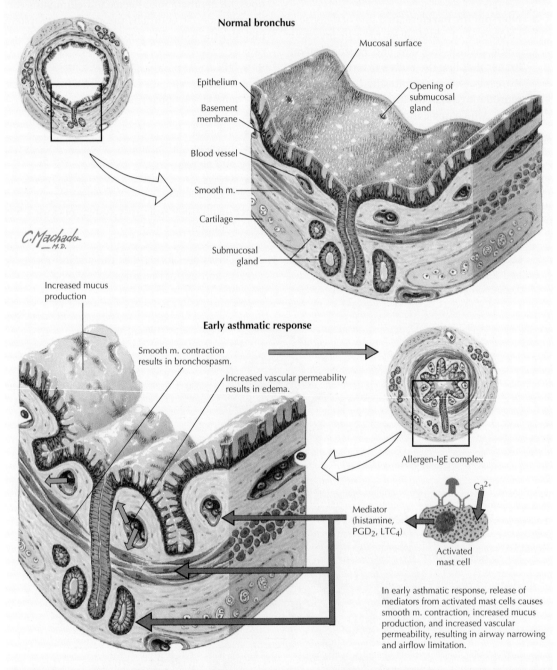

Normal bronchus

Mucosal surface

Epithelium

Opening of submucosal gland

Basement membrane

Blood vessel

Smooth m.

Cartilage

C. Machado
M.D.

Submucosal gland

Increased mucus production

Early asthmatic response

Smooth m. contraction results in bronchospasm.

Increased vascular permeability results in edema.

Allergen-IgE complex

Ca^{2+}

Mediator (histamine, PGD_2, LTC_4)

Activated mast cell

In early asthmatic response, release of mediators from activated mast cells causes smooth m. contraction, increased mucus production, and increased vascular permeability, resulting in airway narrowing and airflow limitation.

- Provides a large surface area for gas exchange with the blood
- Helps to regulate the pH of body fluids
- Participates in vocalization
- Assists the olfactory system with the detection of smells

8. NERVOUS SYSTEM

General Organization

The nervous system integrates and regulates many body activities, sometimes at discrete locations (specific targets) and sometimes more globally. The nervous system usually acts quite rapidly and

can also modulate effects of the endocrine and immune systems. The nervous system is separated into two structural divisions (Fig. 1-17):

- **Central nervous system** (CNS): brain and spinal cord
- **Peripheral nervous system** (PNS): somatic, autonomic, and enteric nerves in the periphery and outside the CNS

Neurons

Nerve cells are called **neurons,** and their structure reflects the functional characteristics of an individual neuron (Fig. 1-18). Information comes to the neuron largely through treelike processes

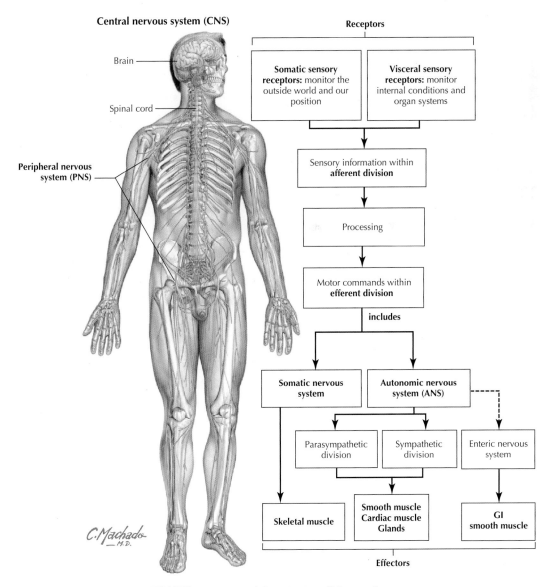

FIGURE 1-17 General Organization of Nervous System.

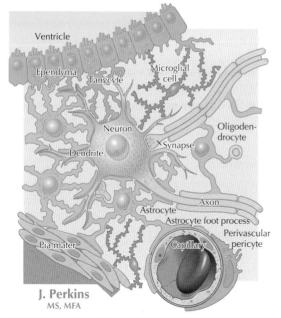

FIGURE 1-18 Cell Types Found in Central Nervous System.

called **axons**, which terminate on the neuron at specialized junctions called **synapses.** Synapses can occur on neuronal processes called **dendrites** or on the neuronal cell body, called a **soma** or *perikaryon.*

Neurons convey efferent information via action potentials that course along a single axon arising from the soma that then synapses on a selective target, usually another neuron or target cell, such as muscle cells. Common types of neurons include the following:

- *Unipolar* (often called *pseudounipolar*): one axon that divides into two long processes (sensory neurons found in the dorsal root ganglion of a spinal nerve)
- *Bipolar:* possesses one axon and one dendrite (rare but found in the retina and olfactory epithelium)
- *Multipolar:* possesses one axon and two or more dendrites (most common type)

Although the human nervous system contains billions, neurons can be classified largely into one of three functional types:

- **Motor neurons:** convey **efferent** impulses from the CNS or ganglia (collections of neurons outside the CNS) to target (effector) cells; somatic efferent axons target skeletal

muscle, and visceral efferent axons target smooth muscle, cardiac muscle, and glands.
- **Sensory neurons:** convey **afferent** impulses from peripheral receptors to the CNS; somatic afferent axons convey pain, temperature, touch, pressure, and proprioception (nonconscious) sensations; visceral afferent axons convey pain and other sensations (e.g., nausea) from organs, glands, and blood vessels to the CNS.
- **Interneurons:** convey impulses between sensory and motor neurons in the CNS, thus forming integrated networks between cells; interneurons probably account for more than 99% of all neurons in the body.

Neurons can vary considerably in size, ranging from several micrometers to more than 100 μm in diameter. Neurons may possess numerous branching dendrites, studded with dendritic spines that increase the receptive area of the neuron manyfold. The neuron's axon may be quite short or over 1 meter long. The axonal diameter may vary. Axons that are larger than 1 to 2 μm in diameter are insulated by **myelin** sheaths. In the CNS, axons are myelinated by a special glial cell called an **oligodendrocyte,** whereas in the PNS they are surrounded by a glial cell called a **Schwann cell**. Schwann cells also myelinate many of the PNS axons they surround.

Glia

Glia are the cells that support neurons, within both the CNS (the neuroglia) and the PNS. Glial cells far outnumber the neurons in the nervous system and contribute to most of the postnatal growth, along with axonal myelination, seen in the CNS. Functionally, glia:

- Provide structural isolation of neurons and their synapses.
- Sequester ions in the extracellular compartment.
- Provide trophic support to the neurons and their processes.
- Support growth and secrete growth factors.
- Support some of the signaling functions of neurons.
- Myelinate axons.
- Phagocytize debris and participate in inflammatory responses.
- Participate in the formation of the blood-brain barrier.

The different types of glial cells include the following (see Fig. 1-18):

- **Astrocytes:** the most numerous of the glial cells; provide physical and metabolic support for CNS neurons and contribute to the formation of the blood-brain barrier.
- **Oligodendrocytes:** smaller glial cells; responsible for the formation and maintenance of myelin in the CNS.
- **Microglia:** smallest and rarest of CNS glia, although more numerous than neurons in CNS; these phagocytic cells participate in inflammatory reactions.
- **Ependymal cells:** line the ventricles of the brain and the central canal of the spinal cord, which contains cerebrospinal fluid.
- **Schwann cells:** glial cells of the PNS; surround all axons (myelinating many of them) and provide trophic support, facilitate regrowth of PNS axons, and clean away cellular debris.

Peripheral Nerves

The peripheral nerves observed grossly in the human body are composed of bundles of thousands of nerve fibers enclosed within a connective tissue covering and supplied by small blood vessels. The nerve "fibers" consist of axons (efferent and afferent) individually separated from each other by the cytoplasmic processes of Schwann cells or myelinated by a multilayered wrapping of continuous Schwann cell membrane (the myelin sheath).

The peripheral nerve resembles an electrical cable of axons that is further supported by three connective tissue sleeves or coverings (Fig. 1-19):

- **Endoneurium:** thin connective tissue sleeve that surrounds the axons and Schwann cells.
- **Perineurium:** dense layer of connective tissue that encircles a bundle (fascicle) of nerve fibers.
- **Epineurium:** outer thick connective tissue sheath that encircles bundles of fascicles; this is the "nerve" typically seen grossly coursing in the human body.

Peripheral nerves include the 12 pairs of **cranial nerves** arising from the brain and the 31 pairs of **spinal nerves** arising from the spinal cord.

Meninges

The brain and spinal cord are surrounded by three membranous connective tissue layers called the *meninges.* These three layers include the following (Fig. 1-20):

- **Dura mater:** the thick, outermost meningeal layer, richly innervated by sensory nerve fibers
- **Arachnoid mater:** the fine, weblike avascular membrane directly beneath the dural surface

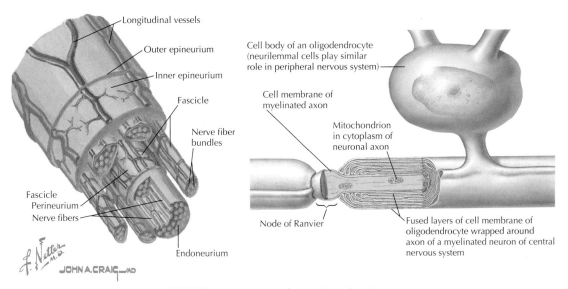

FIGURE 1-19 Features of Typical Peripheral Nerve.

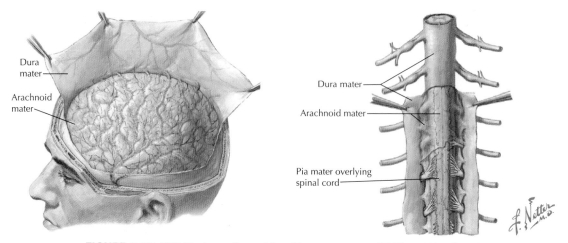

FIGURE 1-20 CNS Meninges. (From *Atlas of human anatomy*, ed 6, Plates 103 and 165.)

- **Pia mater:** the delicate membrane of connective tissue that intimately envelops the brain and spinal cord

The space between the arachnoid and the underlying pia is called the **subarachnoid space** and contains **cerebrospinal fluid** (CSF), which bathes and protects the CNS.

Cranial Nerves

Twelve pairs of cranial nerves arise from the brain, and they are identified both by their names and by Roman numerals I to XII (Fig. 1-21). The cranial nerves are somewhat unique and can contain multiple functional components:

- **General:** same general functions as spinal nerves
- **Special:** functions found only in cranial nerves
- **Afferent** and **efferent:** sensory and motor functions, respectively
- **Somatic** and **visceral:** related to skin and skeletal muscle (somatic) or to smooth muscle, cardiac muscle, and glands (visceral)

Therefore, each cranial nerve (CN) may possess multiple functional components, such as the following:

- *General somatic afferents* (GSAs): contain nerve fibers that are sensory from the skin, such as those of a spinal nerve.
- *General visceral efferents* (GVEs): contain motor fibers to visceral structures (smooth muscle and/or glands), such as a

parasympathetic fiber from the sacral spinal cord (S2 to S4 gives rise to parasympathetics).
- *Special somatic afferents* (SSAs): contain special sensory fibers, such as those for vision and hearing.

In general, CN I and CN II arise from the forebrain and are really tracts of the brain for the special senses of smell and sight. Cranial nerves III, IV, and VI move the extra-ocular skeletal muscles of the eyeball. CN V has three divisions: V_1 and V_2 are sensory, and V_3 is both motor to skeletal muscle and sensory. Cranial nerves VII, IX, and X are both motor and sensory. CN VIII is the special sense of hearing and balance. CN XI and CN XII are motor to skeletal muscle. Cranial nerves III, VII, IX, and X also contain parasympathetic fibers of origin (visceral), although many of the autonomic fibers will "jump" onto the branches of CN V to reach their targets. Table 1-2 summarizes the types of fibers in each cranial nerve.

Spinal Nerves

The spinal cord gives rise to 31 pairs of spinal nerves (Figs. 1-22 and 1-23), which then form two major branches (rami):

- **Dorsal (posterior) ramus:** small ramus that courses dorsally to the back; conveys motor and sensory information to and from the skin and intrinsic back skeletal muscles (erector spinae, transversospinales).
- **Ventral (anterior) ramus:** much larger ramus that courses laterally and ventrally; innervates all the remaining skin and skeletal muscles of the neck, limbs, and trunk.

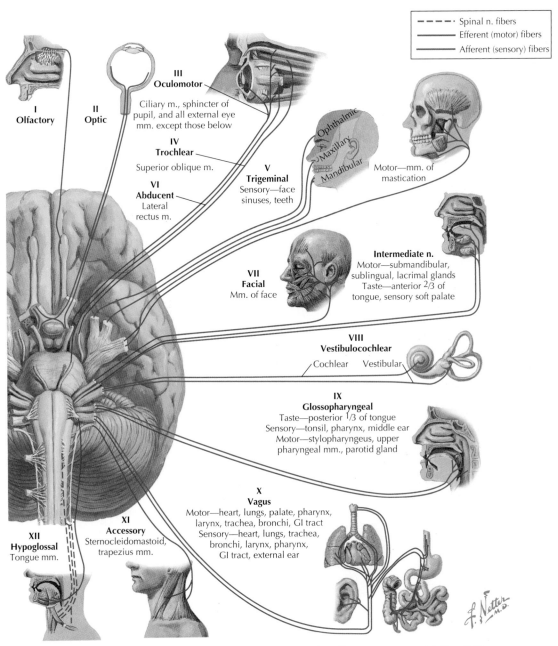

- - - - - Spinal n. fibers
——————— Efferent (motor) fibers
——————— Afferent (sensory) fibers

I
Olfactory

II
Optic

III
Oculomotor
Ciliary m., sphincter of pupil, and all external eye mm. except those below

IV
Trochlear
Superior oblique m.

VI
Abducent
Lateral rectus m.

V
Trigeminal
Sensory—face sinuses, teeth

Ophthalmic
Maxillary
Mandibular

Motor—mm. of mastication

VII
Facial
Mm. of face

Intermediate n.
Motor—submandibular, sublingual, lacrimal glands
Taste—anterior 2/3 of tongue, sensory soft palate

VIII
Vestibulocochlear
Cochlear   Vestibular

IX
Glossopharyngeal
Taste—posterior 1/3 of tongue
Sensory—tonsil, pharynx, middle ear
Motor—stylopharyngeus, upper pharyngeal mm., parotid gland

X
Vagus
Motor—heart, lungs, palate, pharynx, larynx, trachea, bronchi, GI tract
Sensory—heart, lungs, trachea, bronchi, larynx, pharynx, GI tract, external ear

XI
Accessory
Sternocleidomastoid, trapezius mm.

XII
Hypoglossal
Tongue mm.

FIGURE 1-21 Overview of Cranial Nerves. (From *Atlas of human anatomy*, ed 6, Plate 119.)

Once nerve fibers (sensory or motor) are beyond, or peripheral to, the spinal cord proper, the fibers (axons) then reside in nerves of the PNS. Components of the PNS include the following (Fig. 1-23):

- **Somatic nervous system:** sensory and motor fibers to skin, skeletal muscle, and joints (Fig. 1-23, left side)

- **Autonomic nervous system** (ANS): sensory and motor fibers to all smooth muscle (viscera, vasculature), cardiac muscle (heart), and glands (Fig. 1-23, right side)
- **Enteric nervous system:** plexuses and ganglia of the gastrointestinal (GI) tract that regulate bowel secretion, absorption, and motility (originally considered part of ANS); linked to the ANS for optimal regulation

TABLE 1-2 Cranial Nerve Fibers

CRANIAL NERVE		FUNCTIONAL COMPONENT*
I	Olfactory	SVA (Special sense of smell)
II	Optic	SSA (Special sense of sight)
III	Oculomotor	GSE (Motor to extra-ocular muscles)
		GVE (Parasympathetic to smooth muscle in eye)
IV	Trochlear	GSE (Motor to one extra-ocular muscle)
V	Trigeminal	GSA (Sensory to face, orbit, nose, anterior tongue)
		SVE (Motor to skeletal muscles)
VI	Abducent	GSE (Motor to one extra-ocular muscle)
VII	Facial	GSA (Sensory to skin of ear)
		SVA (Special sense of taste to anterior tongue)
		GVE (Motor to glands—salivary, nasal, lacrimal)
		SVE (Motor to facial muscles)
VIII	Vestibulocochlear	SSA (Special sense of hearing and balance)
IX	Glossopharyngeal	GSA (Sensory to posterior tongue)
		SVA (Special sense of taste—posterior tongue)
		GVA (Sensory from middle ear, pharynx, carotid body, sinus)
		GVE (Motor to parotid gland)
		SVE (Motor to one muscle of pharynx)
X	Vagus	GSA (Sensory external ear)
		SVA (Special sense of taste—epiglottis)
		GVA (Sensory from pharynx, larynx, thoracoabdominal organs)
		GVE (Motor to thoracoabdominal organs)
		SVE (Motor to muscles of pharynx/larynx)
XI	Accessory	GSE (Motor to two muscles)
XII	Hypoglossal	GSE (Motor to tongue muscles)

*GSA, General somatic afferent; GSE, general somatic efferent; GVA, general visceral afferent; GVE, general visceral efferent; SSA, special somatic afferent; SVA, special visceral afferent; SVE, special visceral efferent.

Spinal cord and ventral rami in situ

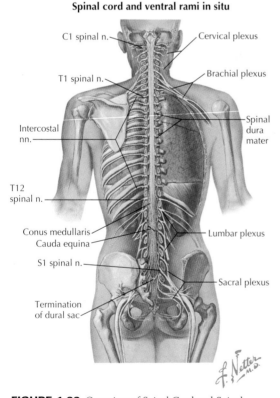

FIGURE 1-22 Overview of Spinal Cord and Spinal Nerves. (From *Atlas of human anatomy*, ed 6, Plate 160.)

Features of the somatic nervous system include the following:

- It is a one-neuron motor system.
- The motor (efferent) neuron is in the CNS, and an axon projects to a peripheral target (e.g., skeletal muscle).
- The sensory (afferent) neuron (pseudounipolar) resides in a peripheral ganglion called the *dorsal root ganglion* (DRG) and conveys sensory information from the skin, muscle, or joint to the CNS (in this case the spinal cord).

The unilateral area of skin innervated by the somatic sensory fibers from a single spinal cord level is called a **dermatome**. Clinically, dermatome maps of the body can be helpful in localizing spinal cord or peripheral nerve lesions (see Chapter 2).

Features of the ANS division of the PNS include the following:

- It is a two-neuron motor system; the first neuron resides in the CNS and the second neuron in a peripheral autonomic ganglion.

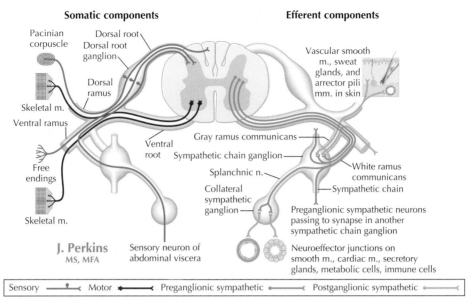

Somatic components   **Efferent components**

FIGURE 1-23 Elements of Peripheral Nervous System. For clarity, this schematic shows the arrangement of the efferent and afferent somatic nerve components of a typical spinal nerve on the left side and the efferent components of the ANS of a typical spinal nerve on the right side.

- The axon of the first neuron is termed *preganglionic* and of the second neuron, *postganglionic.*
- The ANS has two divisions, sympathetic and parasympathetic.
- The sensory neuron (pseudounipolar) resides in a DRG (similar to the somatic system) and conveys sensory information from the viscera to the CNS.

Autonomic Nervous System

The ANS is divided into sympathetic and parasympathetic divisions. In contrast to the somatic division of the PNS, the ANS is a two-neuron system with a **preganglionic neuron** in the CNS that sends its axon into a peripheral nerve to synapse on a **postganglionic neuron** in a peripheral autonomic ganglion (Fig. 1-24). The postganglionic neuron then sends its axon to the target (smooth muscle, cardiac muscle, and glands). The ANS is a visceral system, since many of the body's organs are composed of smooth muscle walls or contain secretory glandular tissue.

Sympathetic Division

The **sympathetic division** of the ANS is also known as the *thoracolumbar division* because:

- Its preganglionic neurons are found only in the T1-L2 spinal cord levels.

- Its preganglionic neurons lie within the intermediolateral gray matter of the spinal cord, in the 14 spinal cord segments previously defined.

Preganglionic axons exit the T1-L2 spinal cord in a ventral root, then enter a spinal nerve via a white **ramus communicans** to enter the **sympathetic chain.** The sympathetic chain is a bilateral chain of ganglia just lateral to the vertebral bodies that runs from the base of the skull to the coccyx. Once in the sympathetic chain, the preganglionic axon may take one of three synaptic routes:

1. Synapse on a postganglionic sympathetic neuron at the T1-L2 level, or ascend or descend to synapse on a sympathetic chain neuron at any of the 31 spinal nerve levels.
2. Pass through the sympathetic chain, enter a splanchnic (visceral) nerve, and synapse in a collateral ganglion in the abdominopelvic cavity.
3. Pass through the sympathetic chain, enter a splanchnic nerve, pass through a collateral ganglion, and synapse on the cells of the adrenal medulla.

Axons of the postganglionic sympathetic neurons may act in one of four ways:

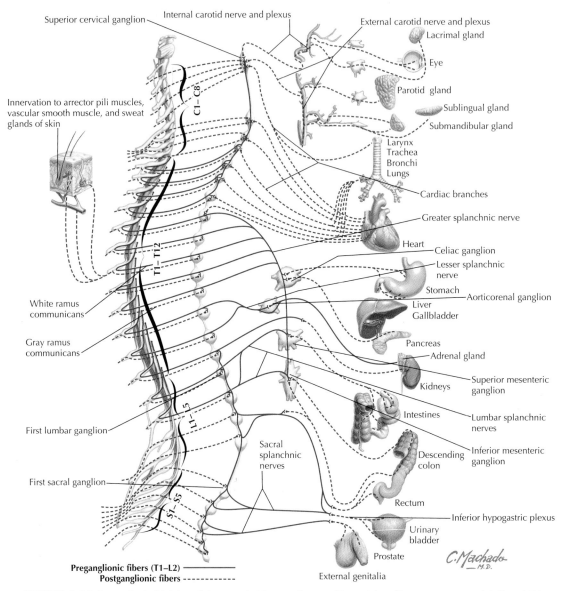

FIGURE 1-24 Sympathetic Division of Autonomic Nervous System. (From *Atlas of human anatomy,* ed 6, Plate 163.)

1. Reenter the spinal nerve via a **gray ramus communicans** and join any one of the 31 spinal nerves as they distribute widely throughout the body.
2. Reenter the spinal nerve but course along blood vessels in the head, or join cardiopulmonary or hypogastric plexuses of nerves to distribute to the head, thorax, and pelvic viscera.
3. Arise from postganglionic neurons in collateral ganglia and course with blood vessels to abdominopelvic viscera.
4. Cells of the adrenal medulla are differentiated endocrine cells (paraneurons) that do not have

axons but release hormones directly into the bloodstream.

Preganglionic axons release acetylcholine (ACh) at their synapses, and norepinephrine (NE) is the transmitter released by postganglionic axons (except ACh released on sweat glands). The cells of the adrenal medulla (modified postganglionic sympathetic neurons) release epinephrine and some NE into the blood, not as neurotransmitters but as hormones. The sympathetic system acts globally throughout the body to mobilize it in "fright-flight-fight" situations (Table 1-3).

TABLE 1-3 Effects of Sympathetic Stimulation on Various Structures

STRUCTURE	EFFECTS	STRUCTURE	EFFECTS
Eye	Dilates the pupil	Liver	Causes glycogen breakdown, glucose synthesis and release
Lacrimal glands	Reduces secretion slightly (vasoconstriction)	Salivary glands	Reduces and thickens secretion via vasoconstriction
Skin	Causes goose bumps (arrector pili muscle contraction)	Genital system	Causes ejaculation and orgasm, and remission of erection
Sweat glands	Increases secretion		Constricts male internal urethral sphincter muscle
Peripheral vessels	Causes vasoconstriction		
Heart	Increases heart rate and force of contraction	Urinary system	Decreases urine production via vasoconstriction
Coronary arteries	Vasoconstriction (metabolic vasodilation override)		Constricts male internal urethral sphincter muscle
Lungs	Assists in bronchodilation and reduced secretion	Adrenal medulla	Increases secretion of epinephrine or norepinephrine
Digestive tract	Decreases peristalsis, contracts internal anal sphincter muscle, causes vasoconstriction to shunt blood elsewhere		

Parasympathetic Division

The parasympathetic division of the ANS also is a two-neuron system with its preganglionic neuron in the CNS and postganglionic neuron in a peripheral ganglion (Fig. 1-25). The **parasympathetic division** also is known as the *craniosacral division* because:

- Its preganglionic neurons are found in cranial nerves III, VII, IX, and X and in the sacral spinal cord at levels S2-S4.
- Its preganglionic neurons reside in the four cranial nuclei associated with the four cranial nerves listed earlier or in the lateral gray matter of the sacral spinal cord at levels S2-S4.

Preganglionic parasympathetic axons exit in one of two ways:

- Exit the brainstem in the cranial nerve (except CN X) and pass to a peripheral ganglion in the head (ciliary, pterygopalatine, submandibular, and otic ganglia) to synapse on the parasympathetic postganglionic neurons residing in these ganglion.
- Exit the sacral spinal cord via a ventral root and then enter the pelvic splanchnic nerves, to synapse on postganglionic neurons in terminal ganglia located in or near the viscera to be innervated.

Axons of the postganglionic parasympathetic neurons take one of two courses:

- Pass from the parasympathetic ganglion in the head on existing nerves or blood vessels, to innervate smooth muscle and glands of the head.
- Pass from terminal ganglia in or near the viscera innervated and synapse on smooth muscle, cardiac muscle, or glands in the neck, thorax, and abdominopelvic cavity.

The vagus nerve (CN X) is unique. Its preganglionic axons exit the brainstem and synapse on terminal ganglia in or near the targets in the neck, thorax (heart, lungs, glands, smooth muscle), and abdominal cavity (proximal two thirds of GI tract and its accessory organs). Axons of the terminal ganglia neurons then synapse on their targets.

Parasympathetic axons do not pass into the limbs as do sympathetic axons. Therefore, the vascular smooth muscle, arrector pili muscles of the skin (attached to hair follicles), and sweat glands are all innervated only by the sympathetic system. ACh is the neurotransmitter at all parasympathetic synapses.

The parasympathetic system is involved in feeding and sexual arousal functions and acts more slowly and focally than the sympathetic system. For example, CN X can slow the heart rate without affecting input to the stomach. In general, the sympathetic and parasympathetic systems maintain homeostasis, although as a protective measure, the body maintains a low level of "sympathetic tone" and can activate this division on a moment's notice. ANS function is regulated ultimately by the hypothalamus. Table 1-4 summarizes the specific functions of the parasympathetic division of the ANS.

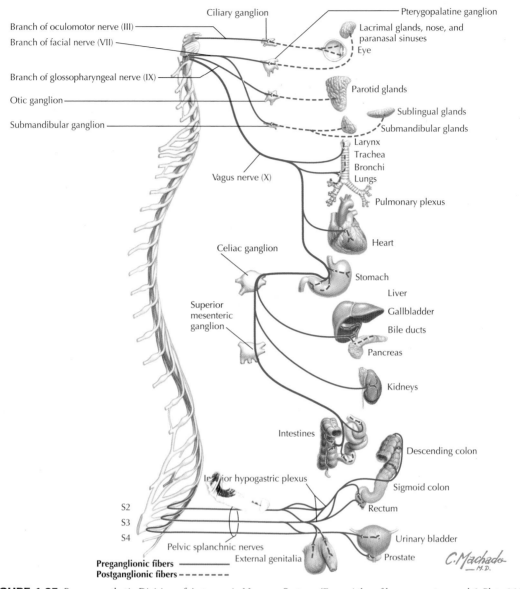

Ciliary ganglion

Pterygopalatine ganglion

Branch of oculomotor nerve (III)

Branch of facial nerve (VII)

Lacrimal glands, nose, and paranasal sinuses

Eye

Branch of glossopharyngeal nerve (IX)

Otic ganglion

Parotid glands

Sublingual glands

Submandibular ganglion

Submandibular glands

Larynx

Trachea

Bronchi

Lungs

Vagus nerve (X)

Pulmonary plexus

Heart

Celiac ganglion

Stomach

Liver

Superior mesenteric ganglion

Gallbladder

Bile ducts

Pancreas

Kidneys

Intestines

Descending colon

Sigmoid colon

Inferior hypogastric plexus

Rectum

S2

S3

S4

Urinary bladder

Prostate

Pelvic splanchnic nerves

External genitalia

Preganglionic fibers ——————
Postganglionic fibers - - - - - - - -

FIGURE 1-25 Parasympathetic Division of Autonomic Nervous System. (From *Atlas of human anatomy*, ed 6, Plate 164.)

TABLE 1-4 Effects of Parasympathetic Stimulation on Various Structures

STRUCTURE	EFFECTS	STRUCTURE	EFFECTS
Eye	Constricts pupil	Digestive tract	Increases peristalsis, increases secretion, inhibits internal anal sphincter for defecation
Ciliary body	Constricts muscle for accommodation (near vision)		
Lacrimal glands	Increase secretion	Liver	Aids glycogen synthesis and storage
Heart	Decreases heart rate and force of contraction	Salivary glands	Increase secretion
		Genital system	Promotes engorgement of erectile tissues
Coronary arteries	Vasodilation (of little importance)		
Lungs	Cause bronchoconstriction and increased secretion	Urinary system	Contracts bladder (detrusor muscle) for urination, inhibits contraction of internal urethral sphincter, increases urine production

Enteric Nervous System

The enteric nervous system was formally considered the third division of the ANS. The word *enteric* refers to ⟨obscured⟩ PNS consists of ⟨obscured⟩ walls of the GI tr⟨obscured⟩ networks includ⟨obscured⟩

- **Myenteri**⟨obscured⟩ and nerve⟨obscured⟩ longitudin⟨obscured⟩ musculari⟨obscured⟩
- **Submuco**⟨obscured⟩ ganglia an⟨obscured⟩ of the bo⟨obscured⟩

The enteric n⟨obscured⟩ to both division⟨obscured⟩ optimal regulat⟨obscured⟩ and motility. M⟨obscured⟩ substances hav⟨obscured⟩ neurons of the enteric nervous system, pointing to the fine degree of regulation that occurs at the level of the bowel wall. Optimal GI functioning requires coordinated interactions of the ANS, the enteric nervous system, and the endocrine system.

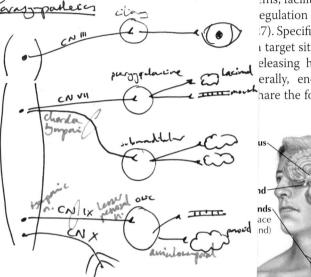

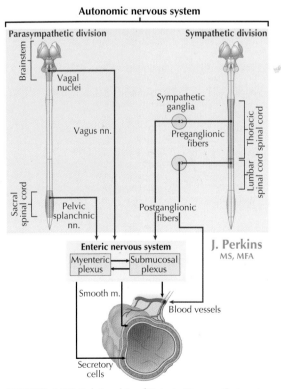

FIGURE 1-26 Relationship of Enteric Nervous System to Sympathetic and Parasympathetic ANS Divisions.

9. ENDOCRINE SYSTEM

The endocrine system, along with the nervous and ⟨obscured⟩ems, facilitates communication, integ⟨obscured⟩egulation of many of the body's func-⟨obscured⟩7). Specifically, the endocrine system ⟨obscured⟩ target sites (cells and tissues), many ⟨obscured⟩eleasing hormones into the blood-⟨obscured⟩erally, endocrine glands and hor-⟨obscured⟩hare the following features:

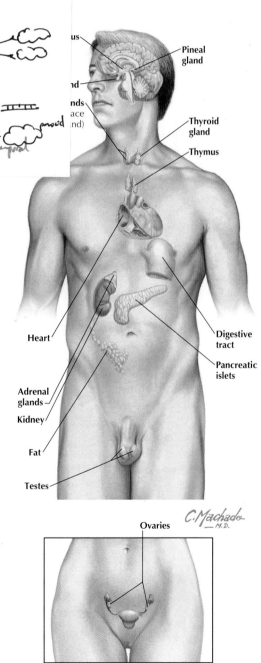

FIGURE 1-27 Major Endocrine Organs.

- Secretion is controlled by feedback mechanisms.
- Hormones bind target receptors on cell membranes or within the cells (cytoplasmic or nuclear).
- Hormone action may be slow to appear but may have long-lasting effects.
- Hormones are chemically diverse molecules (amines, peptides/proteins, steroids).

Hormones can communicate through a variety of cell-to-cell interactions, including:

- *Autocrine:* on another cell as well as on itself.
- *Paracrine:* directly on an adjacent or nearby cell.
- *Endocrine:* at a great distance by the bloodstream.
- *Neurocrine:* similar to a neurotransmitter, except released into the bloodstream.

Table 1-5 summarizes the major hormones and the tissues responsible for their release.

Additionally, the **placenta** releases human chorionic gonadotropin (hCG), estrogens, progesterone, and human placental lactogen (hPL), whereas other cells release a variety of growth factors. Again, the endocrine system is widespread and critically important in regulating functions.

10. GASTROINTESTINAL SYSTEM

The GI system includes the epithelial-lined tube that begins with the oral cavity and extends to the anal canal, as well as GI-associated glands, including the following:

- **Salivary glands:** three major glands and hundreds of microscopic minor salivary glands scattered throughout the oral mucosa
- **Liver:** the largest solid gland in the body
- **Gallbladder:** function is to store and concentrate bile needed for fat digestion
- **Pancreas:** an exocrine (digestive enzymes) and endocrine organ

The epithelial-lined tube that is the GI tract measures about 25 feet (7.5 m) in length (from mouth to anal canal) and includes the following cavities and visceral structures (Fig. 1-28):

- **Oral cavity:** tongue, teeth, and salivary glands

TABLE 1-5 Major Hormones

TISSUE/ORGAN	HORMONE
Hypothalamus	Antidiuretic hormone (ADH), oxytocin, thyrotropin-releasing hormone (TRH), corticotropin-releasing hormone (CRH), growth hormone–releasing hormone (GHRH), gonadotropin-releasing hormone (GnRH), somatostatin (SS), dopamine (DA)
Pineal gland	Melatonin
Anterior pituitary gland	Adrenocorticotropic hormone (ACTH), thyroid-stimulating hormone (TSH), growth hormone (GH), prolactin, follicle-stimulating hormone (FSH), luteinizing hormone (LH), melanocyte-stimulating hormone (MSH)
Posterior pituitary gland	Oxytocin, vasopressin (ADH)
Thyroid gland	Thyroxine (T_4), triiodothyronine (T_3), calcitonin
Parathyroid glands	Parathyroid hormone (PTH, parathormone)
Thymus gland	Thymopoietin, thymulin, thymosin, thymic humoral factor, interleukins, interferons
Heart	Atrial natriuretic peptide (ANP)
Digestive tract	Gastrin, secretin, cholecystokinin (CCK), motilin, gastric inhibitory peptide (GIP), glucagon, SS, vasoactive intestinal peptide (VIP), ghrelin
Liver	Insulin-like growth factors (IGFs)
Adrenal glands	Cortisol, aldosterone, androgens, epinephrine (E), norepinephrine (NE)
Pancreatic islets	Insulin, glucagon, SS, VIP, pancreatic polypeptide
Kidneys	Erythropoietin (EPO), calcitriol, renin, urodilatin
Fat	Leptin
Ovaries	Estrogens, progestins, inhibin, relaxin
Testes	Testosterone, inhibin
White blood cells and some connective tissue cells	Various cytokines; interleukins, colony-stimulating factors, interferons, tumor necrosis factor (TNF)

- **Pharynx:** throat, subdivided into the naso-, oro-, and laryngopharynx
- **Esophagus**
- **Stomach**
- **Small intestine:** subdivided into the duodenum, jejunum, and ileum
- **Large intestine:** subdivided into the cecum, ascending colon, transverse colon, descending colon, sigmoid colon, rectum, and anal canal

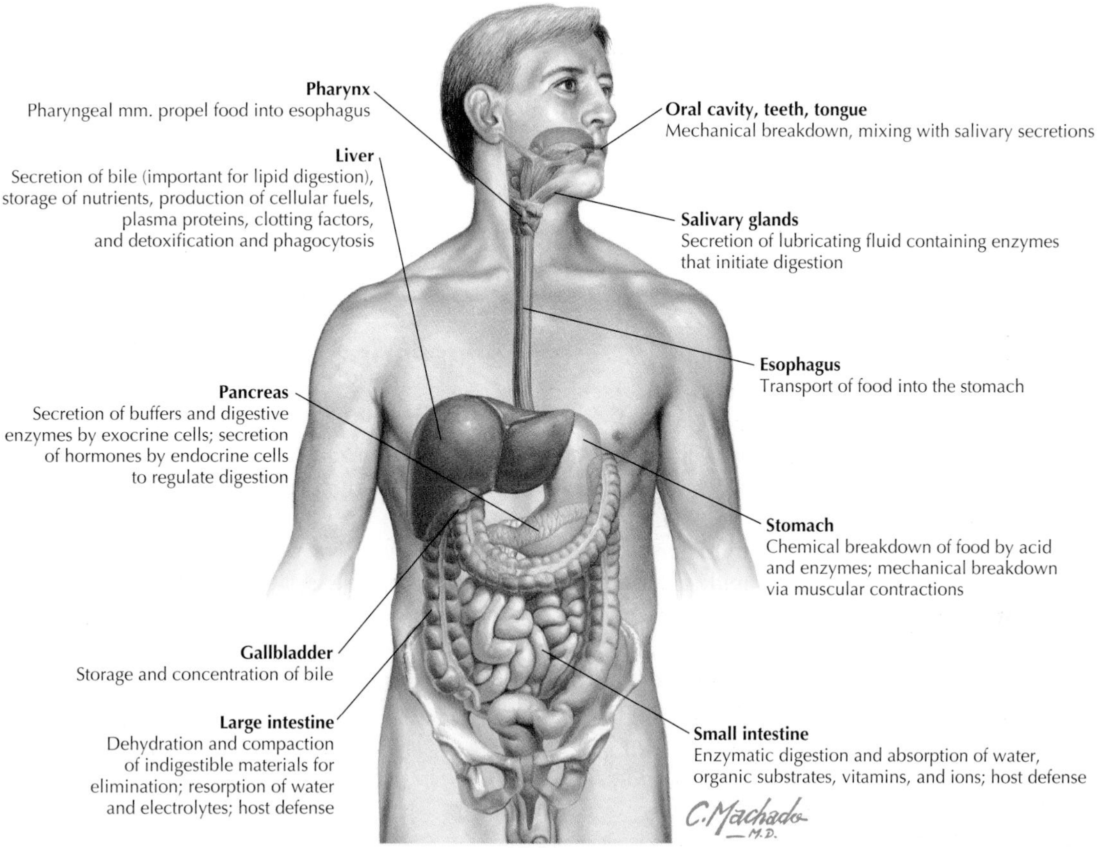

Pharynx
Pharyngeal mm. propel food into esophagus

Liver
Secretion of bile (important for lipid digestion),
storage of nutrients, production of cellular fuels,
plasma proteins, clotting factors,
and detoxification and phagocytosis

Pancreas
Secretion of buffers and digestive
enzymes by exocrine cells; secretion
of hormones by endocrine cells
to regulate digestion

Gallbladder
Storage and concentration of bile

Large intestine
Dehydration and compaction
of indigestible materials for
elimination; resorption of water
and electrolytes; host defense

Oral cavity, teeth, tongue
Mechanical breakdown, mixing with salivary secretions

Salivary glands
Secretion of lubricating fluid containing enzymes
that initiate digestion

Esophagus
Transport of food into the stomach

Stomach
Chemical breakdown of food by acid
and enzymes; mechanical breakdown
via muscular contractions

Small intestine
Enzymatic digestion and absorption of water,
organic substrates, vitamins, and ions; host defense

C.Machado
—M.D.

FIGURE 1-28 Overview of Gastrointestinal System.

11. URINARY SYSTEM

The urinary system includes the following components (Fig. 1-29):

- **Kidneys:** paired retroperitoneal organs that
  filter the plasma and produce urine; located
  high in the posterior abdominal wall just
  anterior to the muscles of the posterior wall.
- **Ureters:** course retroperitoneally from the
  kidneys to the pelvis and convey urine from
  the kidneys to the urinary bladder.
- **Urinary bladder:** lies subperitoneally in the
  anterior pelvis, stores urine, and when
  appropriate, discharges the urine through
  the urethra.
- **Urethra:** courses from the urinary bladder
  to the exterior.

The kidneys function to:

- Filter plasma and begin the process of urine
  formation.

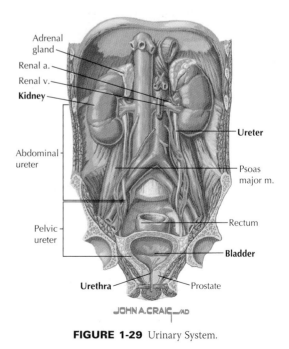

Adrenal
gland

Renal a.

Renal v.

Kidney

Abdominal
ureter

Pelvic
ureter

Urethra

Ureter

Psoas
major m.

Rectum

Bladder

Prostate

JOHN A.CRAIG—AD

FIGURE 1-29 Urinary System.

- Reabsorb important electrolytes, organic molecules, vitamins, and water from the filtrate.
- Excrete metabolic wastes, metabolites, and foreign chemicals (e.g., drugs).
- Regulate fluid volume, composition, and pH.
- Secrete hormones that regulate blood pressure, erythropoiesis, and calcium metabolism.
- Convey urine to the ureters, which then pass the urine to the bladder.

The kidneys filter about 180 liters of fluid each day. Grossly, each kidney measures about 12 cm long × 6 cm wide × 3 cm thick and weighs about 150 grams, although variability is common. Approximately 20% of the blood pumped by the heart passes to the kidney each minute for plasma filtration, although most of the fluid and important plasma constituents are returned to the blood as the filtrate courses down the tubules of the kidney's nephrons (kidney's filtration units).

Each ureter is about 24 to 34 cm long, lies in a retroperitoneal position, and contains a thick smooth muscle wall. The urinary bladder serves as a reservoir for the urine and is a muscular "bag" that expels the urine when appropriate. The female urethra is short (3-5 cm), whereas the male urethra is long (~20 cm), coursing through the prostate gland, external urethral sphincter, and corpus spongiosum of the penis.

12. REPRODUCTIVE SYSTEM

Female Reproductive System

The female reproductive system is composed of the following structures (Fig. 1-30):

- **Ovaries:** the paired gonads of the female reproductive system; produce the female germ cells called *ova* (oocytes, eggs) and secrete the hormones estrogen and progesterone.

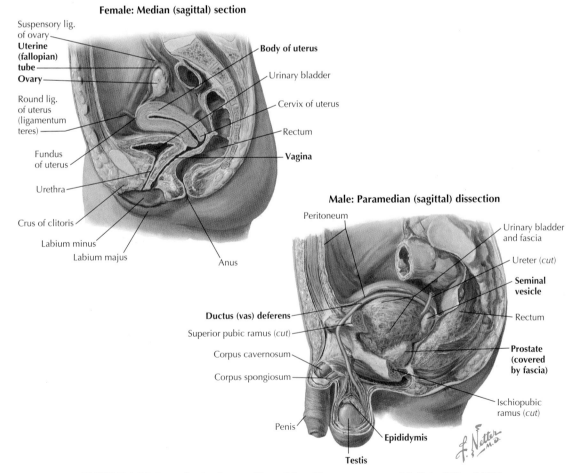

FIGURE 1-30 Reproductive System. (From *Atlas of human anatomy*, ed 6, Plates 340 and 344.)

- **Uterine tubes** (fallopian tubes): paired tubes that extend from the superolateral walls of the uterus and open as fimbriated funnels into the pelvic cavity adjacent to the ovary, to "capture" the oocyte as it is ovulated.
- **Uterus:** hollow, pear-shaped muscular (smooth muscle) organ that protects and nourishes a developing fetus.
- **Vagina:** distensible fibromuscular tube (also called *birth canal*) approximately 8 to 9 cm long that extends from the uterine cervix (neck) to the vestibule.

Male Reproductive System

The male reproductive system is composed of the following structures (see Fig. 1-30):

- **Testes:** the paired gonads of the male reproductive system, egg shaped and about the size of a chestnut; produce the male germ cells, *spermatozoa,* and reside in the scrotum (externalized from the abdominopelvic cavity).
- **Epididymis:** convoluted tubule that receives the spermatozoa and stores them as they mature.
- **Ductus (vas) deferens:** a muscular (smooth muscle) tube about 40 to 45 cm long that conveys sperm from the epididymis to the ejaculatory duct (seminal vesicle).

- **Seminal vesicles:** paired tubular glands that lie posterior to the prostate, about 15 cm long; produce seminal fluid and join the ductus deferens at the ejaculatory duct.
- **Prostate gland:** walnut-sized gland that surrounds the urethra as it leaves the urinary bladder; produces prostatic fluid, which is added to semen (sperm suspended in glandular secretions).
- **Urethra:** a canal that passes through the prostate gland, enters the penis, and conveys the semen for expulsion from the body during ejaculation.

13. BODY CAVITIES

Organ systems and other visceral structures are often segregated into body cavities. These cavities can protect the viscera and also may allow for some expansion and contraction in size. Two major collections of body cavities are recognized (Fig. 1-31):

- **Dorsal cavities:** include the brain, surrounded by the meninges and bony cranium, and the spinal cord, surrounded by the same meninges as the brain and the vertebral column.
- **Ventral cavities:** include the thoracic and abdominopelvic cavities, separated by the abdominal diaphragm (skeletal muscle important in respiration).

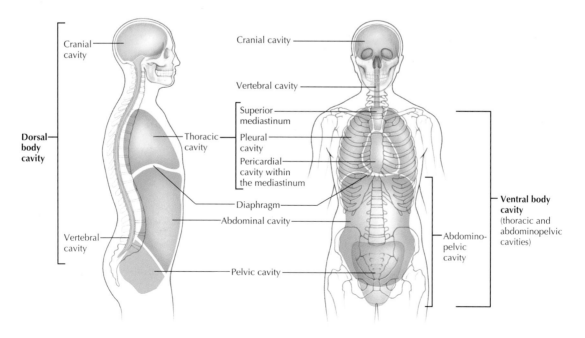

FIGURE 1-31 Major Body Cavities.

The CNS (brain and spinal cord) is surrounded by three membranes (see Fig. 1-20):

- Pia mater
- Arachnoid mater
- Dura mater

The thoracic cavity contains two **pleural cavities** (right and left) and a single midline space called the **mediastinum** (middle space) that contains the heart and structures lying posterior to it, including the thoracic descending aorta and esophagus. The heart itself resides in the **pericardial sac,** which has a parietal and a visceral layer.

The abdominopelvic cavity also is lined by a serous membrane, the **peritoneum,** which also has parietal and visceral layers.

14. OVERVIEW OF EARLY DEVELOPMENT

Week 1: Fertilization and Implantation

Fertilization occurs in the ampulla of the uterine tube (fallopian tube) usually within 24 hours after ovulation (Fig. 1-32). The fertilized ovum (the union of sperm and egg nuclei, with a diploid number of chromosomes) is termed a **zygote.** Subsequent cell division (cleavage) occurs at the two-, four-, eight-, and 16-cell stages and results in formation of a ball of cells that travels down the uterine tube toward the uterine cavity. When the cell mass reaches days 3 to 4 of development,

it resembles a mulberry and is called a **morula** (16-cell stage). As the morula enters the uterine cavity at about day 5, it develops a fluid-filled cyst in its interior and is then known as a **blastocyst.** At about days 5 to 6, implantation occurs as the blastocyst literally erodes or burrows its way into the uterine wall (endometrium).

Clinical Focus 1-8
Potential Spaces

Each of these spaces—pleural, pericardial, and peritoneal—is considered a "potential" space, because between the parietal and visceral layers, there is usually only a small amount of serous lubricating fluid, to keep organ surfaces moist and slick and thus reduce friction from movements such as respiration, heartbeat, and peristalsis. However, during inflammation or trauma (accumulation of pus or blood), fluids can collect in these spaces and restrict movement of the viscera. In this case, these "potential" spaces become real spaces and may necessitate removal of the offending fluid so as not to compromise organ function or exacerbate an ongoing infection.

Week 2: Formation of the Bilaminar Embryonic Disc

As the blastocyst implants, it forms an inner cell mass (future embryo, **embryoblast**) and a larger fluid-filled cavity surrounded by an outer cell

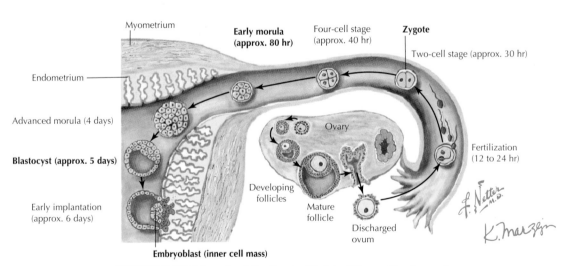

FIGURE 1-32 Schematic of Key Events: Week 1 of Human Development.

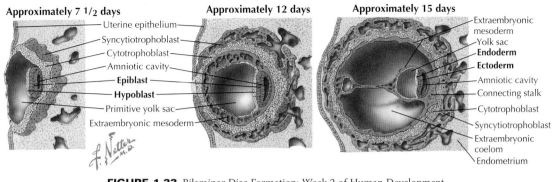

FIGURE 1-33 Bilaminar Disc Formation: Week 2 of Human Development.

layer called the **trophoblast** (Fig. 1-33). The tro-phoblast undergoes differentiation and complex cellular interactions with maternal tissues to initiate formation of uteroplacental circulation. Simultaneously, the inner cell mass develops into the following two cell types (bilaminar disc):

- **Epiblast:** columnar cells on the dorsal surface of the embryoblast
- **Hypoblast:** cuboidal cells on the ventral surface of the embryoblast

The epiblast forms a cavity on the dorsal side that gives rise to the amniotic cavity. The blastocyst cavity on the ventral side becomes the primitive yolk sac, which is lined by simple squamous epithelium derived from the hypoblast. About day 12, further hypoblast cell migration forms the true yolk sac, and the old blastocyst cavity becomes coated with extraembryonic mesoderm.

Week 3: Gastrulation

Gastrulation (development of trilaminar embryonic disc) begins with appearance of the **primitive streak** on the dorsal surface of the epiblast (Fig. 1-34). This streak forms a groove demarcated at its cephalic end (head) by the **primitive node**. The node forms a midline cord of mesoderm that becomes the **notochord**. Migrating epiblast cells move toward the primitive streak, invaginate, and replace the underlying hypoblast cells to become the **endoderm** germ layer. Other invaginating epiblast cells develop between the endoderm and overlying epiblast and become the **mesoderm.** Finally, the surface epiblast cells form the **ectoderm**, the third germ layer. All body tissues are derived from one of these three embryonic germ layers.

Embryonic Germ Layer Derivatives

Figures 1-35 to 1-37 and the accompanying tables provide a general overview of the adult derivatives of the three embryonic germ layers that are formed during gastrulation. As you study each region of the body, refer to these summary pages to review the embryonic origins of the various tissues. Many clinical problems arise during the development *in utero* of these germ layer derivatives.

In general, **ectodermal** derivatives include the following (Fig. 1-35):

- Epidermis and various appendages associated with the skin (hair, nails, glands)
- Components of the central and peripheral nervous systems
- Some bones, muscles, and connective tissues of the head and neck (neural crest)

In general, **mesodermal** derivatives include the following (Fig. 1-36):

- Notochord
- Skeletal, smooth, and cardiac muscle
- Parenchyma or reticular structures and connective tissues of many organ systems
- Reproductive and urinary systems
- Most skeletal structures
- Dermis of the skin

In general, **endodermal** derivatives include the following (Fig. 1-37):

- Lining of GI tract and accessory GI organs
- Lining of the airway
- Various structures derived from the pharyngeal pouches
- Embryonic blood cells
- Derivatives associated with development of the cloaca

Formation of intraembryonic mesoderm from the primitive streak and node (knot)

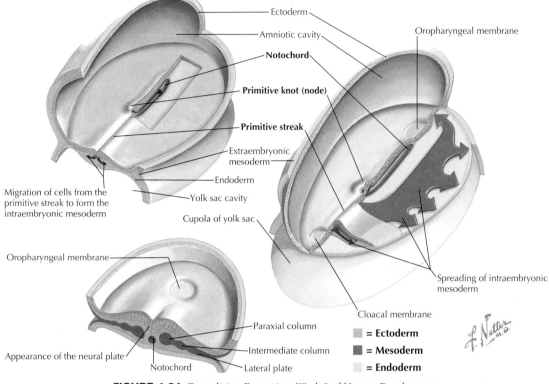

Ectoderm

Amniotic cavity

Notochord

Primitive knot (node)

Primitive streak

Extraembryonic mesoderm

Endoderm

Migration of cells from the primitive streak to form the intraembryonic mesoderm

Yolk sac cavity

Cupola of yolk sac

Oropharyngeal membrane

Oropharyngeal membrane

Spreading of intraembryonic mesoderm

Cloacal membrane

Appearance of the neural plate

Paraxial column

Intermediate column

Notochord

Lateral plate

☐ = **Ectoderm**

■ = **Mesoderm**

☐ = **Endoderm**

FIGURE 1-34 Gastrulation Formation: Week 3 of Human Development.

Ectoderm of the gastrula

Neural plate

Hair

Nails

Epidermis of skin

Neural tube

Surface ectoderm

Amnion

Central and peripheral nervous system

Primordia	Derivatives or fate
Surface ectoderm	Epidermis of the skin
	Sweat, sebaceous, and mammary glands
	Nails and hair
	Tooth enamel
	Lacrimal glands
	Conjunctiva
	External auditory meatus
(Stomodeum and nasal placodes)	Oral and nasal epithelium Anterior pituitary
(Otic placodes)	Inner ear
(Lens placodes)	Lens of eye
Neural tube	Central nervous system
	Somatomotor neurons
	Branchiomotor neurons
	Presynaptic autonomic neurons
	Retina/optic nerves
	Posterior pituitary
Neural crest	Peripheral sensory neurons
	Postsynaptic autonomic neurons
	All ganglia
	Adrenal medulla cells
	Melanocytes
	Bone, muscle, and connective tissue in the head and neck
Amnion	Protective bag (with chorion) around fetus

FIGURE 1-35 Ectodermal Derivatives.

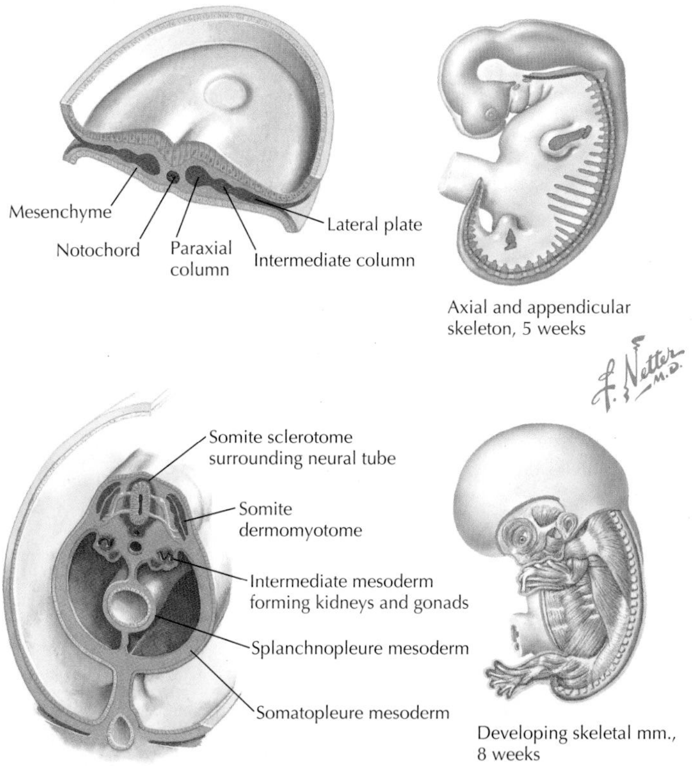

Mesenchyme

Notochord   Paraxial   Intermediate column
            column

Lateral plate

Axial and appendicular
skeleton, 5 weeks

Somite sclerotome
surrounding neural tube

Somite
dermomyotome

Intermediate mesoderm
forming kidneys and gonads

Splanchnopleure mesoderm

Somatopleure mesoderm

Developing skeletal mm.,
8 weeks

Primordia	Derivatives or fate
Notochord	Nucleus pulposus of an intervertebral disc Induces neurulation
Paraxial columns (somites)	Skeletal muscle Bone Connective tissue (e.g., dorsal dermis, meninges)
Intermediate mesoderm	Gonads Kidneys and ureters Uterus and uterine tubes Upper vagina Ductus deferens, epididymis, and related tubules Seminal vesicles and ejaculatory ducts
Lateral plate mesoderm	Dermis (ventral) Superficial fascia and related tissues (ventral) Bones and connective tissues of limbs Pleura and peritoneum GI tract connective tissue stroma
Cardiogenic mesoderm	Heart Pericardium

FIGURE 1-36 Mesodermal Derivatives.

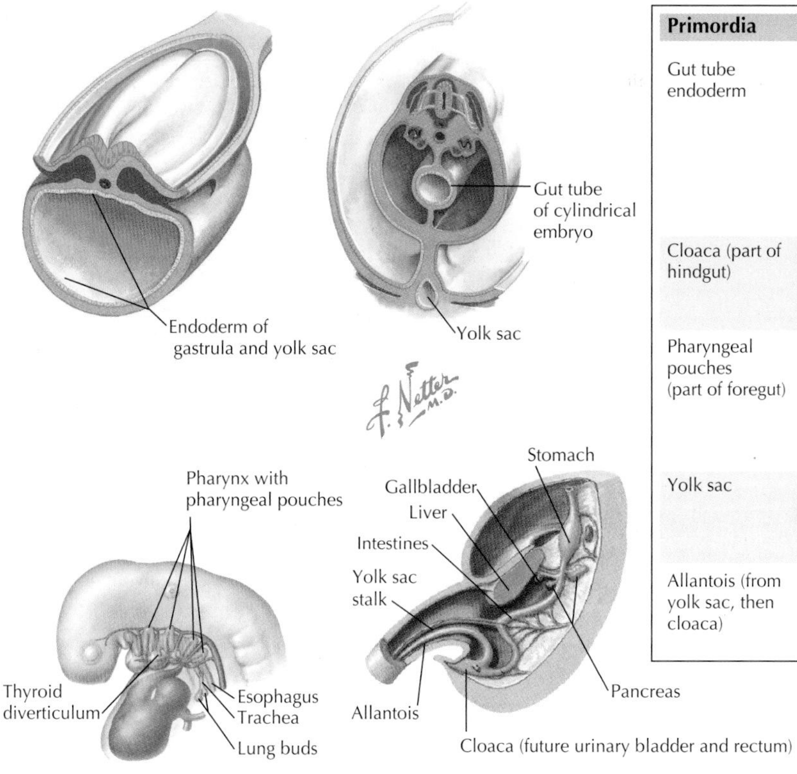

Endoderm of
gastrula and yolk sac

Gut tube
of cylindrical
embryo

Yolk sac

Pharynx with
pharyngeal pouches

Gallbladder
Liver
Intestines
Yolk sac
stalk

Stomach

Thyroid
diverticulum

Esophagus
Trachea

Lung buds

Allantois

Pancreas

Cloaca (future urinary bladder and rectum)

Primordia	Epithelial derivatives or fate
Gut tube endoderm	GI tract (enterocytes) Mucosal glands of GI tract Parenchyma of GI organs (liver, pancreas) Airway lining (larynx, trachea, bronchial tree) Thyroid gland Tonsils
Cloaca (part of hindgut)	Rectum and anal canal Bladder, urethra, and related glands Vestibule Lower vagina
Pharyngeal pouches (part of foregut)	Auditory tube and middle ear epithelium Palatine tonsil crypts Thymus gland Parathyroid glands C cells of thyroid gland
Yolk sac	Embryonic blood cell production (mesoderm) Pressed into umbilical cord, then disappears
Allantois (from yolk sac, then cloaca)	Embryonic blood cell production (mesoderm) Vestigial, fibrous urachus Umbilical cord part disappears

FIGURE 1-37 Endodermal Derivatives.

15. IMAGING THE INTERNAL ANATOMY

General Introduction

In 1895, Wilhelm Roentgen (Würzburg, Germany) used x-rays generated from a cathode ray tube to make the first radiographic image, for which he ultimately was awarded the first Nobel Prize in Physics in 1901. As the x-rays (a form of electromagnetic radiation) pass through the body, they lose energy to the tissues, and only the photons with sufficient energy to penetrate then expose a sheet of photographic film. Radiographic images are now largely collected as digital information (Table 1-6).

Plain (Conventional) Radiographs

A plain radiograph, also known as conventional or plain film radiography, provides an image in which the patient is positioned either anterior (anteroposterior, AP) to or posterior (posteroanterior, PA) to the x-ray source (Fig. 1-38, *A*). The x-ray tube also may be placed in a lateral or oblique position in reference to the patient. Contrast media (radiopaque fluids such as barium sulfate or iodine compounds) can be administered to study tubular structures such as the bowel or vessels. A *double contrast* study uses barium and air to image the lumen of structures such as the distal colon (Fig. 1-38, *B*). X-rays now are collected digitally in real time by producing a stream of x-rays. Techniques are now available that can even image moving structures in the body using angiography (contrast medium in the heart and larger vessels) and fluoroscopy.

Computed Tomography

Computed tomography (CT) was invented in 1972 by Sir Godfrey Hounsfield (at EMI Labs, Hayes, England), who received the Nobel Prize in Medicine or Physiology in 1979 (shared with

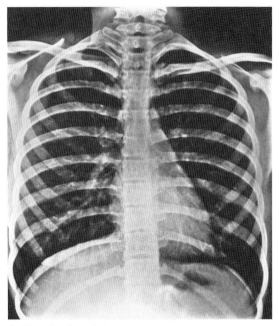

A. PA projection of chest.

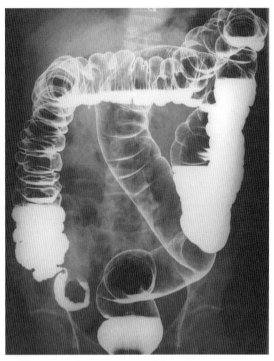

B. Double contrast radiograph of the colon.

FIGURE 1-38 Plain (Conventional) Radiographs. *PA*, Posteroanterior. (**A** from Wicke L: *Atlas of radiologic anatomy*, ed 7, Philadelphia, 2004, Saunders; **B** from Major NM: *A practical approach to radiology*, Philadelphia, 2006, Saunders.)

TABLE 1-6 Attenuation of X-rays Passing through the Body*	
MEDIUM	**GRAY SCALE**
Bone	White
Soft tissue	Light gray
Water (reference)	Gray
Fat	Dark gray
Lung	Very dark gray
Air	Black

*Greatest to least attenuation.

Allen McLeod Cormack of Tufts). A CT scanner uses x-rays generated by a tube that passes around the body and collects a series of images in the axial (transverse slices) plane. A sophisticated computer program then transforms the multiple images into a single slice (Fig. 1-39).

In the 1980s, multislice (multidetector) CT scanners were developed that capture many slices as the tube rotates in a helical pattern around the patient, who is moving through the scanner on a table. Three-dimensional (3-D) images can be re-created by the computer from these slices. Bone is well imaged by CT, and contrast media may be employed to enhance the imaging of hollow viscera (e.g., GI tract). Additionally, CT angiography (CTA) can image larger blood vessels in 2-D and 3-D after intravascular administration of contrast material (Fig. 1-39, *B*).

Advantages of CT include lower costs than magnetic resonance imaging (MRI), availability, 3-D capabilities, ability to image bony features,

and faster speed than MRI. Disadvantages of CT include the high dose of x-rays compared to plain films, artifacts (motion, scattering), and relatively poor tissue definition compared to MRI.

Positron Emission Tomography/ Computed Tomography

Glucose uptake in tissues (following 18-fluorodeoxy-D-glucose administration) can be imaged by positron emission tomography (PET)/ CT, an especially useful technique for detecting tissues or structures with a higher metabolic rate, such as malignant tumors and inflammatory lesions.

Magnetic Resonance Imaging

Paul Lauterbur (Illinois) and Sir Peter Mansfield (Nottingham, England) were awarded the Nobel Prize in Medicine or Physiology in 2003 for their contributions to the development of MRI. Since the first MR image of a human subject in 1977,

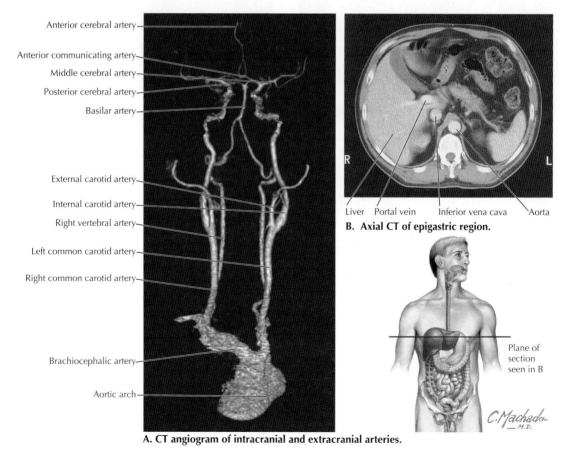

Anterior cerebral artery
Anterior communicating artery
Middle cerebral artery
Posterior cerebral artery
Basilar artery
External carotid artery
Internal carotid artery
Right vertebral artery
Left common carotid artery
Right common carotid artery
Brachiocephalic artery
Aortic arch

Liver   Portal vein   Inferior vena cava   Aorta

B. Axial CT of epigastric region.

Plane of section seen in B

A. CT angiogram of intracranial and extracranial arteries.

FIGURE 1-39 Computed Tomography (CT). (From Kelley LL, Petersen C: *Sectional anatomy for imaging professionals,* St Louis, 2007, Mosby.)

this process has become a versatile and safe diagnostic tool. Strong magnets align hydrogen's free protons (the hydrogen in molecules of water present in almost all biologic tissues). Then a radio wave pulse passes through the patient and deflects the protons, which return to their aligned state but emit small radio pulses whose strength, frequency, and time produce distinct signals. Computers then analyze these signals and create axial, coronal, and sagittal images (Fig. 1-40).

Advantages of MRI include the lack of ionizing radiation, the ability to image all planes, and the capability to image soft tissues at very high resolution compared to CT. Disadvantages include high cost, inability to image patients with metallic implants or foreign bodies, inability to image bone well, longer procedure time than CT, potential for patients to become claustrophobic in the scanner, and the tendency for artifacts (movement).

Ultrasound

Ultrasound uses very-high-frequency longitudinal sound waves that are generated by a transducer. The waves produced by the transducer are reflected or refracted as they collide with the soft tissue interfaces. The proportion of sound reflected is measured as acoustic impedance and represents different densities of soft tissue. A computer then interprets these signals and produces a real-time image (Fig. 1-41).

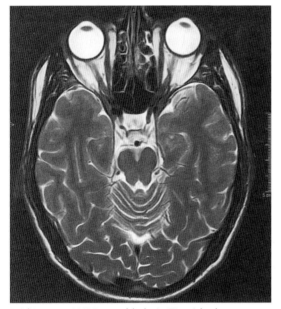

Axial (transverse) MR image of the brain, T2-weighted

FIGURE 1-40 Magnetic Resonance Imaging (MRI). (From Wicke L: *Atlas of radiologic anatomy*, ed 7, Philadelphia, 2004, Saunders.)

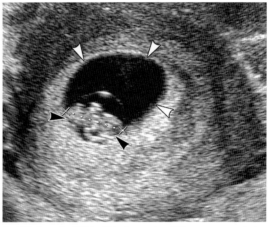

A viable 9-week-old fetus (*black arrowheads*) is seen, surrounded by the gestational sac (*white arrowheads*)

FIGURE 1-41 Ultrasound. (Reprinted with permission from Jackson S, Thomas R: *Cross-sectional imaging made easy*, Philadelphia, 2004, Churchill Livingstone.)

Clinical Focus

Available Online

1-9 Myasthenia Gravis

Additional figures available online (see inside front cover for details).

Challenge Yourself Questions

1. A radiologist is examining a computer-generated series of MR scans in the frontal plane. Which of the following terms is synonymous with the frontal plane?

   A. Axial
   B. Coronal
   C. Cross section
   D. Sagittal
   E. Transverse

2. Clinically, the bones can be classified by their shape. Which of the following shapes is used to define the patella (kneecap)?

   A. Flat
   B. Irregular
   C. Long
   D. Sesamoid
   E. Short

3. Long bones are responsible for most of our height. Which of the following portions of the long bone is most important in lengthening the bone?

   A. Diaphysis
   B. Epiphysis
   C. Epiphysial plate
   D. Metaphysis
   E. Shaft

4. An elderly woman falls and fractures her femoral neck ("breaks her hip"). Which of the following type of synovial joints was involved in the fracture?

   A. Ball-and-socket (spheroid)
   B. Condyloid (ellipsoid)
   C. Hinge (ginglymus)
   D. Plane (gliding)
   E. Saddle (biaxial)

5. When examining your musculoskeletal system, the orthopedist may check the strength of a contracting muscle at a joint. As this is done, another muscle relaxes and would be designated by which of the following terms?

   A. Agonist
   B. Antagonist
   C. Extensor
   D. Fixator
   E. Synergist

6. During cardiac catheterization, the physician watches the blood flow from the right ventricle into which of the following vessels?

   A. Aorta
   B. Coronary arteries
   C. Inferior vena cava
   D. Pulmonary trunk
   E. Superior vena cava

7. The lymphatic and immune systems are vitally important in defense of the body. Most of the lymph ultimately drains back into the venous system by which of the following structures?

   A. Arachnoid granulations
   B. Choroid plexus
   C. Cisterna chyli
   D. Right lymphatic duct
   E. Thoracic duct

8. A patient experiencing a central nervous system (CNS) inflammatory process will be activating which of the following phagocytic glial cells?

   A. Astrocytes
   B. Ependymal cells
   C. Microglia
   D. Oligodendrocytes
   E. Schwann cells

9. The brain and spinal cord are surrounded by membranous connective tissue layers. The pain associated with most CNS inflammatory processes is mediated by sensory nerves in which of these tissue layers?

    A. Arachnoid mater
    B. Dura mater
    C. Endoneurium
    D. Ependyma
    E. Pia mater

10. A neurologist is concerned about a patient's inability to walk without a distinct limp (movement disorder). Which of the following portions of the peripheral nervous system (PNS) will the neurologist examine first?

    A. Autonomic
    B. Enteric
    C. Myenteric
    D. Somatic
    E. Submucosal

11. In response to a perceived threat of danger, which of the following PNS components will be globally activated?

    A. Enteric
    B. Parasympathetic
    C. Postganglionic
    D. Preganglionic
    E. Sympathetic

12. In designing a novel pharmaceutical agonist for use in controlling blood pressure, the scientists must be cognizant of which of the following distinguishing features of the autonomic nervous system?

    A. It is a one-neuron efferent system.
    B. It is a two-neuron efferent system.
    C. It is associated with 10 cranial nerves.
    D. It releases only neuropeptides as transmitters.
    E. It releases only norepinephrine as a transmitter.

13. A kidney stone becomes lodged in the portion of the urinary system between the kidney and bladder. In which of the following structures will the stone be found?

    A. Bile duct
    B. Oviduct
    C. Thoracic duct
    D. Ureter
    E. Urethra

14. A patient has difficulty digesting fats (e.g., french fries) and experiences pain after a heavy meal, which then subsides. Of the following organs of the gastrointestinal tract, which would most likely be the culprit?

    A. Colon
    B. Gallbladder
    C. Pancreas
    D. Salivary glands
    E. Stomach

15. A patient who presents with an autoimmune disease characterized by loss of weight, rapid pulse, sweating, shortness of breath, bulging eyes (exophthalmos), and muscle wasting likely has oversecretion of a hormone produced and stored by which endocrine organ?

    A. Ovary
    B. Pancreas
    C. Pineal gland
    D. Posterior pituitary gland
    E. Thyroid gland

16. Bleeding into the pericardial sac would also suggest that blood would be present in which cavity?

    A. Abdominal
    B. Left pleural
    C. Mediastinum
    D. Right pleural
    E. Vertebral

17. A congenital defect of the spinal cord occurs during the third week of embryonic development. Which of the following events characterizes this critical period of embryonic development?

    A. Blastocyst formation
    B. Embryoblast formation
    C. Gastrulation
    D. Morula formation
    E. Zygote formation

18. Malformation of the primitive heart would most likely point to a problem with the development of which embryonic tissue?

    A. Amnion
    B. Chorion
    C. Ectoderm
    D. Endoderm
    E. Mesoderm

19. Of the following types of medical imaging approaches, which is the least invasive and least expensive?

    A. Computed tomography
    B. Magnetic resonance imaging
    C. Plain radiograph
    D. Positron emission tomography
    E. Ultrasound

20. As an x-ray beam passes through the human body, which of the following is the correct order of attenuation of the photons, from greatest to least attenuation?

    A. Bone-fat-lung–soft tissue–water-air
    B. Bone-fat–soft tissue–lung-water-air
    C. Bone-lung–soft tissue–fat-water-air
    D. Bone–soft tissue–lung-fat-water-air
    E. Bone–soft tissue–water-fat-lung-air

Answers to Challenge Yourself Questions

1. **B.** The coronal plane is named for the coronal suture on the skull and is a plane that is parallel to that suture and synonymous with frontal plane. Axial, transverse, and cross section also are synonymous terms and divide the body into superior and inferior portions.

2. **D.** The patella is a round bone and the largest of the sesamoid bones. Two sesamoid bones also usually exist at the base of each thumb and base of each large toe.

3. **C.** Bone growth in length occurs at the epiphysial plate, where hyaline cartilage undergoes proliferation and ossification. Growth in width occurs at the diaphysis.

4. **A.** The hip is a perfect example of a ball-and-socket joint and is one of the more stable synovial joints in the body. The shoulder joint also is a ball-and-socket joint but is more mobile and less stable than the hip joint.

5. **B.** The antagonist is the muscle that opposes the action of the agonist, the muscle that is contracting and in this case the muscle being tested by the orthopedist.

6. **D.** Venous blood from the body passes through the right side of the heart (right atrium and ventricle) and then passes into the pulmonary trunk, which divides into a right and left pulmonary artery carrying blood away from the heart and to the lungs for gas exchange.

7. **E.** The thoracic duct drains lymph from about three quarters of the body and returns it to the venous system at the junction of the left internal jugular and left subclavian veins. The cisterna chyli is the beginning of the thoracic duct in the upper abdomen.

8. **C.** Microglia are the endogenous glial cells in the CNS that are phagocytic and respond to any breach in the blood-brain barrier or to infection.

9. **B.** The dura mater is heavily innervated by sensory nerve fibers, whereas the arachnoid and pia mater are not innervated.

10. **D.** The neurologist will examine the somatic division of the PNS first to determine if the problem is associated with a peripheral nerve and/or skeletal muscle. Skeletal muscle is innervated by the somatic nervous system.

11. **E.** The sympathetic division of the ANS is functionally the "fight or flight" responder to any threat, perceived or real, and mobilizes the body globally.

12. **B.** This is the only answer that accurately reflects the ANS. It is a two-neuron efferent system, and different transmitters are co-localized and released. Because of this, ACh, NE, and neuropeptides can be targeted at different synaptic sites pharmacologically to alter the response of the system.

13. **D.** The ureter is the duct connecting the kidney (renal pelvis) to the urinary bladder.

14. **B.** The gallbladder stores and concentrates bile, which is necessary for the emulsification of fats in our diet. When fats enter the GI tract, the gallbladder is stimulated, contracts, and releases concentrated bile into the second portion of the duodenum.

15. **E.** These signs and symptoms are characteristic of Graves' disease (hyperthyroidism), an excess synthesis and release of thyroid hormone, which upregulates metabolism.

16. **C.** The pericardium and the heart reside in the mediastinum (middle space), the region between the two pleural cavities, all of which are in the thoracic cavity.

17. **C.** Gastrulation is the defining event of the third week of embryonic development. This is when the trilaminar disc (ectoderm, mesoderm, endoderm) develops and when the ectoderm begins to migrate medially and fold along the midline axis to form the future neural tube and spinal cord.

18. E. The heart (cardiac muscle) is a derivative of the mesoderm. Later in its development, the neural crest also plays an important role.

19. E. Ultrasound uses very-high-frequency longitudinal sound waves, is relatively safe, and is cost effective compared to the other imaging modalities. Unfortunately, it is not suitable for all imaging; its resolution is limited and it cannot penetrate bone.

20. E. The densest structure in the body is bone with the greatest attenuation of photons, followed by soft tissues, water (the reference medium), fat, lung (mostly air), and then air itself. On a plain radiograph, a very dense tissue like bone appears white, while air appears black.

Back

chapter **2**

1. INTRODUCTION

The back forms the axis (central line) of the human body and consists of the vertebral column, spinal cord, supporting muscles, and associated tissues (skin, connective tissues, vasculature, and nerves). A hallmark of human anatomy is the concept of "segmentation," and the back is a prime example. **Segmentation** and **bilateral symmetry** of the back will become obvious as you study the vertebral column, the distribution of the spinal nerves, the muscles of the back, and its vascular supply. Functionally, the back is involved in three primary tasks, as follows:

- *Support.* The vertebral column forms the axis of the body and is critical for upright posture (standing or sitting), as a support for the head, as an attachment point and brace for movements of the upper limbs, and as a support for transferring the weight of the trunk to the lower limbs.
- *Protection.* The vertebral column protects the spinal cord and proximal portions of the spinal nerves before they distribute throughout the body.
- *Movements.* Muscles of the back function in movements of the head and upper limbs and in support and movements of the vertebral column.

2. SURFACE ANATOMY

Figure 2-1 shows key surface landmarks of the back, including the following bony landmarks:

- **Vertebrae prominens:** the spinous process of the C7 vertebra, usually the most prominent process in the midline at the posterior base of the neck.

- **Scapula:** part of the pectoral girdle that supports the upper limb; note its spine, inferior angle, and medial border.
- **Iliac crests:** felt best when you place your hands "on your hips." An imaginary horizontal line connecting the iliac crests passes through the spinous process of the vertebra L4 and the intervertebral disc of L4-L5, providing a useful landmark for lumbar puncture or epidural block (see Clinical Focus 2-11).
- **Posterior superior iliac spines:** an imaginary horizontal line connecting these two points passes through the spinous process of S2 (second sacral segment).

3. VERTEBRAL COLUMN

The vertebral column (spine) forms the central axis of the human body, highlighting the segmental nature of all vertebrates, and usually is composed of 33 vertebrae distributed as follows (Fig. 2-2):

- **Cervical:** seven total; first two called the atlas (C1) and axis (C2).
- **Thoracic:** 12 total; each articulates with a pair of ribs.
- **Lumbar:** five total; large vertebrae for support of the body's weight.
- **Sacral:** five fused vertebrae for stability in the transfer of weight from the trunk to the lower limbs.
- **Coccyx:** four total; Co1 often is not fused, but Co2-Co4 are fused (a remnant of embryonic tail).

The actual number of vertebrae can vary, especially the number of coccygeal vertebrae.

49

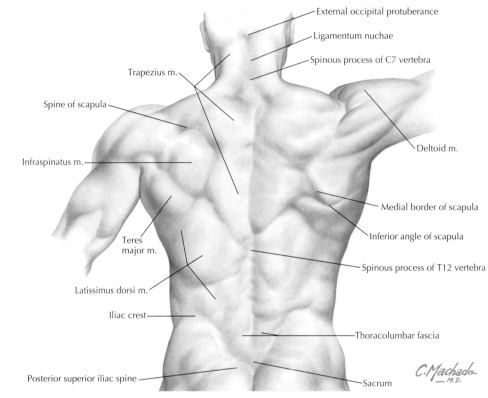

FIGURE 2-1 Key Bony and Muscular Landmarks of the Back. (From *Atlas of human anatomy,* ed 6, Plate 152.)

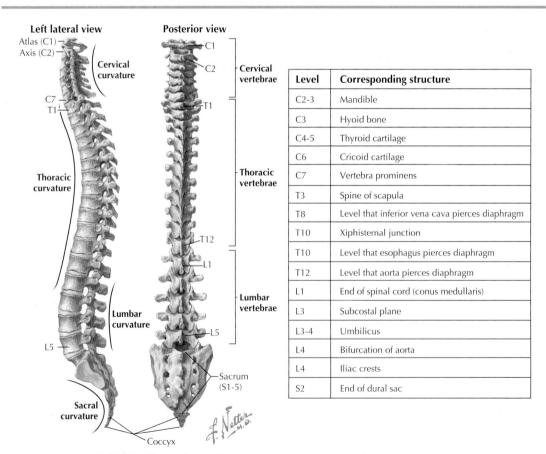

Level	Corresponding structure
C2-3	Mandible
C3	Hyoid bone
C4-5	Thyroid cartilage
C6	Cricoid cartilage
C7	Vertebra prominens
T3	Spine of scapula
T8	Level that inferior vena cava pierces diaphragm
T10	Xiphisternal junction
T10	Level that esophagus pierces diaphragm
T12	Level that aorta pierces diaphragm
L1	End of spinal cord (conus medullaris)
L3	Subcostal plane
L3-4	Umbilicus
L4	Bifurcation of aorta
L4	Iliac crests
S2	End of dural sac

FIGURE 2-2 Vertebral Column. (From *Atlas of human anatomy,* ed 6, Plate 153.)

Scoliosis

Scoliosis is abnormal lateral curvature of the spine, which also includes an abnormal rotation of one vertebra upon another. In addition to scoliosis, accentuated curvatures of the spine include **kyphosis** (hunchback) and **lordosis** (swayback).

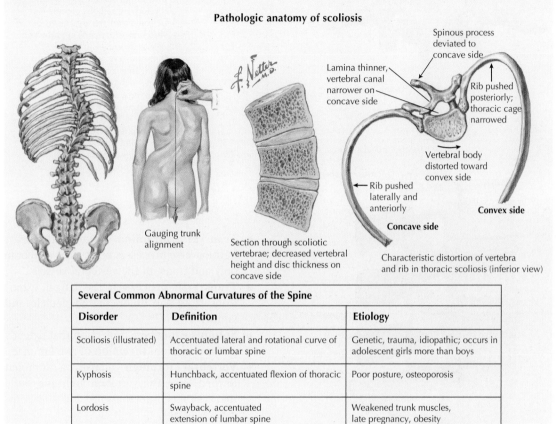

Pathologic anatomy of scoliosis

Spinous process deviated to concave side

Lamina thinner, vertebral canal narrower on concave side

Rib pushed posteriorly; thoracic cage narrowed

Vertebral body distorted toward convex side

Rib pushed laterally and anteriorly

Convex side

Concave side

Gauging trunk alignment

Section through scoliotic vertebrae; decreased vertebral height and disc thickness on concave side

Characteristic distortion of vertebra and rib in thoracic scoliosis (inferior view)

Several Common Abnormal Curvatures of the Spine		
Disorder	**Definition**	**Etiology**
Scoliosis (illustrated)	Accentuated lateral and rotational curve of thoracic or lumbar spine	Genetic, trauma, idiopathic; occurs in adolescent girls more than boys
Kyphosis	Hunchback, accentuated flexion of thoracic spine	Poor posture, osteoporosis
Lordosis	Swayback, accentuated extension of lumbar spine	Weakened trunk muscles, late pregnancy, obesity

Viewed from the lateral aspect (Fig. 2-2), one can identify the following:

- **Cervical curvature** (cervical lordosis): a secondary curvature acquired when the infant can support the weight of the head.
- **Thoracic curvature** (thoracic kyphosis): a primary curvature present in the fetus (imagine the spine in the "fetal position").
- **Lumbar curvature** (lumbar lordosis): a secondary curvature acquired when the infant assumes an upright posture and supports its own weight.
- **Sacral curvature**: a primary curvature present in the fetus.

Typical Vertebra

A "typical" vertebra has the following features (Fig. 2-3):

- **Arch:** a projection formed by paired pedicles and laminae.
- **Articular processes** (facets): two superior and two inferior facets for articulation with adjacent vertebrae.
- **Body:** the weight-bearing portion of a vertebra that tends to increase in size as one descends the spine.
- **Intervertebral foramen** (foramina): the opening formed by the vertebral notches that is traversed by spinal nerve roots and associated vessels.

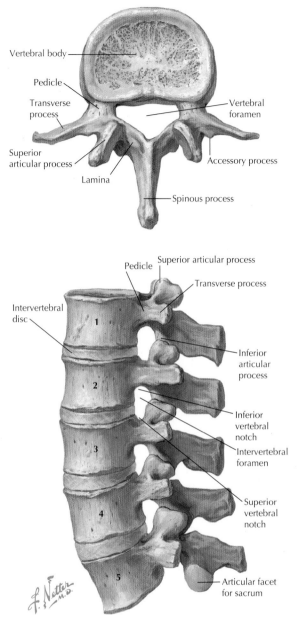

Vertebral body

Pedicle

Transverse process

Vertebral foramen

Superior articular process

Accessory process

Lamina

Spinous process

Pedicle

Superior articular process

Transverse process

Intervertebral disc

Inferior articular process

Inferior vertebral notch

Intervertebral foramen

Superior vertebral notch

Articular facet for sacrum

FIGURE 2-3 Features of Typical Vertebra, as Represented by L2 Vertebra (superior view) and Articulated Lumbar Vertebrae (L!-L5). (From *Atlas of human anatomy*, ed 6, Plate 155.)

TABLE 2-1 Key Features of the Cervical Vertebrae (C1-C7)	
VERTEBRAE	**DISTINGUISHING CHARACTERISTICS**
Atlas (C1)	Ringlike bone; superior facet articulates with occipital bone. Two lateral masses with facets No body or spinous process C1 rotates on articular facets of C2. Vertebral artery runs in groove on posterior arch.
Axis (C2)	Dens projects superiorly. Strongest cervical vertebra
C3 to C7	Large, triangular vertebral foramen Transverse foramen through which vertebral artery passes (except C7) Narrow intervertebral foramina Nerve roots at risk of compression
C3 to C5	Short, bifid spinous process
C6 to C7	Long spinous process
C7	Vertebra prominens; nonbifid

- **Transverse foramina:** apertures that exist in transverse processes of cervical vertebrae only and transmit the vertebral vessels.
- **Transverse processes:** the lateral extensions from the union of the pedicle and lamina.
- **Spinous process:** a projection that extends posteriorly from the union of two laminae.
- **Vertebral foramen** (canal): a foramen formed from the vertebral arch and body that contains the spinal cord and its meningeal coverings.
- **Vertebral notches:** superior and inferior semicircular features that in articulated vertebrae form an intervertebral foramen (two semicircular notches form a circle).

Regional Vertebrae

Cervical Vertebrae

The cervical spine is composed of seven cervical vertebrae. The first two cervical vertebrae are unique and called the atlas and axis (Fig. 2-4). The **atlas** (C1) holds the head on the neck (the titan Atlas of Greek mythology held the heavens on his shoulders as punishment by Zeus). The **axis** (C2) is the point of articulation where the head turns on the neck, providing an "axis of rotation."

Table 2-1 summarizes key features of the cervical vertebrae. The cervical region is a fairly mobile portion of the spine, allowing for flexion and extension as well as rotation and lateral bending.

- **Lamina** (laminae): paired portions of the vertebral arch that connect the transverse processes to the spinous process.
- **Pedicle:** paired portions of the vertebral arch that attach the transverse processes to the body.

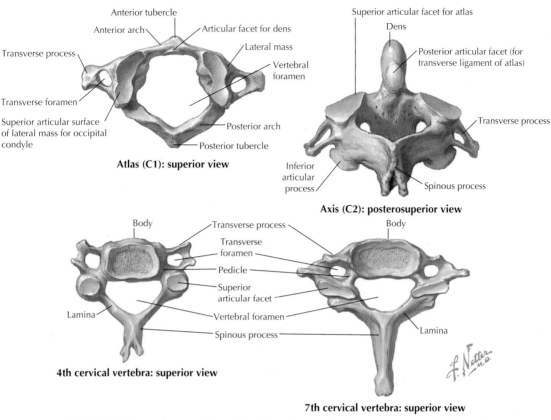

FIGURE 2-4 Representative Cervical Vertebrae. (From *Atlas of human anatomy*, ed 6, Plate 19.)

Clinical Focus 2-2

Cervical Fractures

Fractures of the axis (C2) often involve the dens and are classified as types I, II, and III. Type I fractures are usually stable, type II fractures are unstable, and type III fractures, which extend into the body, usually reunite well when immobilized. The **hangman fracture,** a pedicle fracture of the axis, can be stabilized, if survived, with or without spinal cord damage. A **Jefferson fracture** is a burst fracture of the atlas (C1), often caused by a blow to the top of the head.

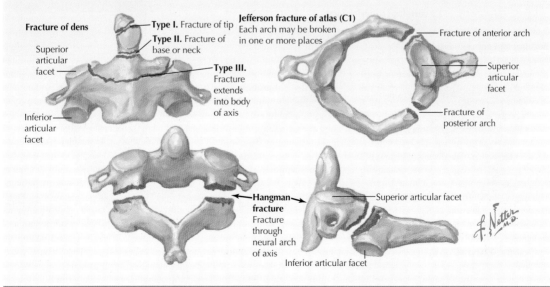

Thoracic and Lumbar Vertebrae

The thoracic spine is composed of 12 thoracic vertebrae (Fig. 2-5 and Table 2-2). The 12 pairs of ribs articulate with the thoracic vertebrae. This region of the spine is more rigid and inflexible than the cervical region.

The lumbar spine is composed of five lumbar vertebrae (see Figs. 2-3 and 2-5 and Table 2-2). The lumbar vertebrae are comparatively large for bearing the weight of the trunk and are fairly mobile, but not nearly as mobile as the cervical vertebrae.

Sacrum and Coccyx

The sacrum is composed of five fused vertebrae that form a single, wedge-shaped bone (Fig. 2-5 and Table 2-2). The sacrum provides support for the pelvis. The coccyx is a remnant of the embryonic tail and usually consists of four vertebrae, with the last three often fused into a single bone. The coccyx lacks vertebral arches and has no vertebral canal.

The features and number of vertebrae can vary, and clinicians must always be aware of subtle differences, especially on radiographic imaging, that may be variants within a normal range.

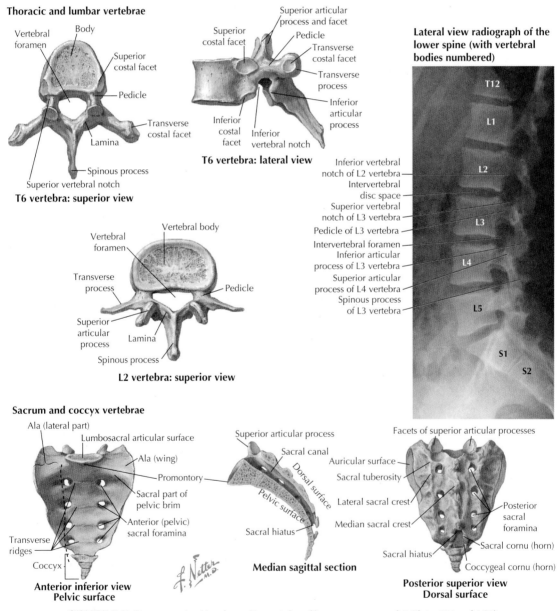

FIGURE 2-5 Representative Vertebrae. (From *Atlas of human anatomy*, ed 6, Plates 154 and 157.)

TABLE 2-2 Key Features of Thoracic, Lumbar, Sacral, and Coccygeal Vertebrae

VERTEBRAE	DISTINGUISHING CHARACTERISTICS	VERTEBRAE	DISTINGUISHING CHARACTERISTICS
Thoracic (T1-T12)	Heart-shaped body, with facets for rib articulation Small circular vertebral foramen Long transverse processes, with facets for rib articulation in T1-T10 Long spinous processes, which slope posteriorly and overlap next vertebra		Spinous process is short, strong, and horizontal. L5: largest vertebra with massive transverse processes
		Sacrum (S1-S5)	Large, wedge-shaped bone that transmits body weight to pelvis Five fused vertebrae, with fusion complete by puberty
Lumbar (L1-L5)	Kidney-shaped body, massive for support Midsized triangular vertebral foramen Facets face medial or lateral direction, which permits good flexion and extension		Four pairs of sacral foramina on dorsal and ventral (pelvic) side Sacral hiatus, the opening of sacral vertebral foramen
		Coccyx (Co1-Co4)	Co1 often is not fused. Co2 to Co4 are fused. No pedicles, laminae, or spines Remnant of embryonic tail

Clinical Focus 2-3

Osteoarthritis

Osteoarthritis is the most common form of arthritis and often involves erosion of the articular cartilage of weight-bearing joints, such as those of the vertebral column.

Cervical spine involvement

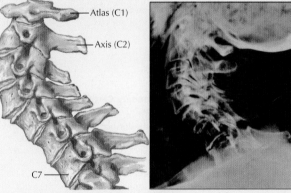

Atlas (C1)

Axis (C2)

C7

Extensive thinning of cervical discs and hyperextension deformity. Narrowing of intervertebral foramina. Lateral radiograph reveals similar changes.

Lumbar spine involvement

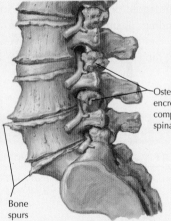

Osteophytic encroachment compressing spinal nn.

Bone spurs

Degeneration of lumbar intervertebral discs and hypertrophic changes at vertebral margins with spur formation. Osteophytic encroachment on intervertebral foramina compresses spinal nerves.

Characteristics of Osteoarthritis	
Characteristic	**Description**
Etiology	Progressive erosion of cartilage in joints of spine, fingers, knee, and hip most commonly
Prevalence	Significant after age 65 years
Risk factors	Age, female sex, joint trauma, repetitive stress, obesity, genetic, race, previous inflammatory joint disease
Complications	In spine, involves intervertebral disc and facet joints, leading to hyperextension deformity and spinal nerve impingement

Joints and Ligaments of Craniovertebral Spine

The craniovertebral joints include the **atlanto-occipital** (atlas and occipital bone of the skull) and **atlanto-axial** (atlas and axis) joints. Both are synovial joints that provide a relatively wide range of motion compared with other joints of the vertebral column. The atlanto-occipital joint permits one to nod the head up and down (flexion and extension), whereas the atlanto-axial joint is a pivot joint that permits one to rotate the head from side to side, as if to indicate "no" (Fig. 2-6 and Table 2-3).

Joints and Ligaments of Vertebral Arches and Bodies

The joints of the vertebral arches (zygapophysial joints) occur between the superior and inferior articular processes (facets) of adjacent vertebrae and allow for some gliding or sliding movement (Fig. 2-7 and Table 2-4). These joints slope inferiorly in the cervical spine (facilitate flexion and extension), are more vertically oriented in the thoracic region (limit flexion and extension but allow for rotation), and are interlocking in the lumbar spine (but do allow flexion and extension, but not to the degree present in the cervical spine). Corresponding ligaments connect the spinous processes, laminae, and bodies of adjacent vertebrae (see Tables 2-2 and 2-3). Strong anterior and posterior longitudinal ligaments run along most of the length of the vertebral column. Of these two ligaments, the anterior longitudinal ligament is stronger and prevents hyperextension (see Table 2-4).

The joints of the vertebral bodies (intervertebral joints) occur between the adjacent vertebral bodies (see Fig. 2-7 and Table 2-4). The intervertebral joints are lined by a thin layer of hyaline cartilage with an intervening intervertebral disc (except between first two cervical vertebrae). These stable, weight-bearing joints also absorb pressure because the intervertebral disc is between the bodies. Intervertebral discs are composed of a central nuclear zone of collagen and hydrated proteoglycans called the **nucleus pulposus,** which is surrounded by concentric lamellae of collagen fibers that compose the **anulus fibrosus.** The inner gelatinous nucleus pulposus (remnant of embryonic notochord) is hydrated and acts

TABLE 2-3 Key Features of Atlanto-occipital and Atlanto-axial Joints

LIGAMENT	ATTACHMENT	COMMENT
Atlanto-occipital (Biaxial Condyloid Synovial) Joint		
Articular capsule	Surrounds facets and occipital condyles	Allows flexion and extension
Anterior and posterior membranes	Anterior and posterior arches of C1 to foramen magnum	Limit movement of joint
Atlanto-axial (Uniaxial Synovial) Joint		
Tectorial membrane	Axis body to margin of foramen magnum	Is continuation of posterior longitudinal ligament
Apical	Dens to occipital bone	Is very small
Alar	Dens to occipital condyles	Limits rotation
Cruciate	Dens to lateral masses	Resembles a cross; allows rotation

TABLE 2-4 Features of the Zygapophysial and Intervertebral Joints

LIGAMENT	ATTACHMENT	COMMENT
Zygapophysial (Plane Synovial) Joints		
Articular capsule	Surrounds facets	Allows gliding motion. C5-C6 is most mobile. L4-L5 permits most flexion.
Intervertebral (Secondary Cartilaginous [Symphyses]) Joints		
Anterior longitudinal (AL)	Anterior bodies and intervertebral discs	Is strong and prevents hyperextension
Posterior longitudinal (PL)	Posterior bodies and intervertebral discs	Is weaker than AL and prevents hyperflexion
Ligamenta flava	Connect adjacent laminae of vertebrae	Limit flexion and are more elastic
Interspinous	Connect spines	Are weak
Supraspinous	Connect spinous tips	Are stronger and limit flexion
Ligamentum nuchae	C7 to occipital bone	Is cervical extension of supraspinous ligament and is strong
Intertransverse	Connect transverse processes	Are weak ligaments
Intervertebral discs	Between adjacent bodies	Are secured by AL and PL ligaments

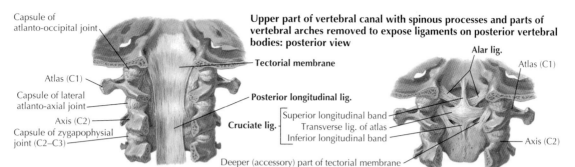

Capsule of
atlanto-occipital joint

**Upper part of vertebral canal with spinous processes and parts of
vertebral arches removed to expose ligaments on posterior vertebral
bodies: posterior view**

Atlas (C1)

Capsule of lateral
atlanto-axial joint

Axis (C2)

Capsule of zygapophysial
joint (C2–C3)

Tectorial membrane

Posterior longitudinal lig.

Cruciate lig.

Superior longitudinal band
Transverse lig. of atlas
Inferior longitudinal band

Deeper (accessory) part of tectorial membrane

Alar lig.

Atlas (C1)

Axis (C2)

Principal part of tectorial membrane removed to expose deeper lig.: posterior view

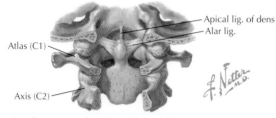

Atlas (C1)

Axis (C2)

Apical lig. of dens
Alar lig.

Cruciate lig. removed to show deepest ligs.: posterior view

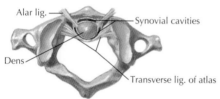

Alar lig.

Dens

Synovial cavities

Transverse lig. of atlas

Median atlanto-axial joint: superior view

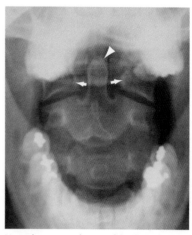

Normal open-mouth view of the dens of C2
(*arrowhead*) and the lateral masses of C1 (*arrows*).

FIGURE 2-6 Craniovertebral Joints and Ligaments. (From *Atlas of human anatomy,* ed 6, Plate 23; radiograph from Major
N: *A practical approach to radiology,* Philadelphia, 2006, Saunders-Elsevier.)

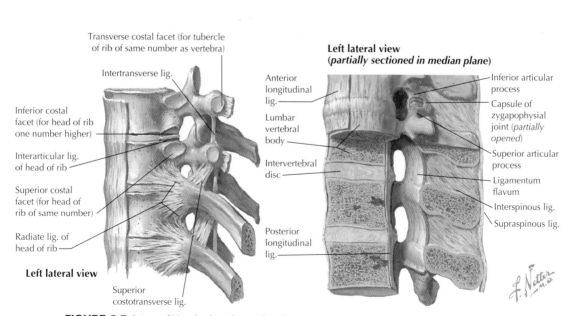

Transverse costal facet (for tubercle
of rib of same number as vertebra)

Intertransverse lig.

Inferior costal
facet (for head of rib
one number higher)

Interarticular lig.
of head of rib

Superior costal
facet (for head of
rib of same number)

Radiate lig. of
head of rib

Left lateral view

Superior
costotransverse lig.

**Left lateral view
(*partially sectioned in median plane*)**

Anterior
longitudinal
lig.

Lumbar
vertebral
body

Intervertebral
disc

Posterior
longitudinal
lig.

Inferior articular
process

Capsule of
zygapophysial
joint (*partially
opened*)

Superior articular
process

Ligamentum
flavum

Interspinous lig.

Supraspinous lig.

FIGURE 2-7 Joints of Vertebral Arches and Bodies. (From *Atlas of human anatomy,* ed 6, Plate 159.)

as a "shock absorber," compressing when load bearing and relaxing when the load is removed. The outer fibrocartilaginous anulus fibrosus, arranged in concentric lamellae, is encircled by a thin ring of collagen and resists compression and shearing forces.

The lumbar are the thickest and the upper thoracic the thinnest intervertebral discs. The anterior and posterior longitudinal ligaments help to stabilize these joints (see Table 2-4).

Clinical Focus 2-4

Osteoporosis

Osteoporosis (porous bone) is the most common bone disease and results from an imbalance in bone resorption and formation, which places bones at a great risk for fracture.

Axial

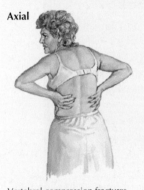

Vertebral compression fractures cause continuous (acute) or intermittent (chronic) back pain from midthoracic to midlumbar region, occasionally to lower lumbar region.

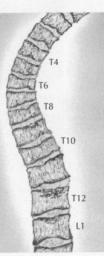

Multiple compression fractures of lower thoracic and upper lumbar vertebrae in patient with severe osteoporosis

T4
T6
T8
T10
T12
L1

Characteristics of Osteoporosis	
Characteristic	**Description**
Etiology	Postmenopausal women, genetics, vitamin D synthesis deficiency, idiopathic
Risk factors	Family history, white female, increasing age, estrogen deficiency, vitamin D deficiency, low calcium intake, smoking, excessive alcohol use, inactive lifestyle
Complications	Vertebral compression fractures, fracture of proximal femur or humerus, ribs, and distal radius (Colles' fracture)

A change in backbone strength over time

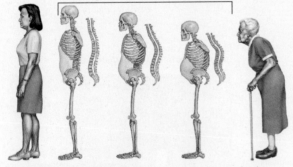

Osteoporosis is the thinning of the bones. Bones become fragile and loss of height is common as the back bones begin to collapse.

Appendicular
Fractures caused by minimal trauma

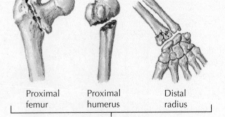

Proximal femur   Proximal humerus   Distal radius

Most common types

Spondylolysis and Spondylolisthesis

Spondylolysis is a congenital defect or an acquired stress fracture of the lamina that presents with no slippage of adjacent articulating vertebrae (most common at L5-S1). Its radiographic appearance suggests a "Scottie dog" (terrier) with a collar (fracture site shown as red collar).

Spondylolisthesis is a bilateral defect (complete dislocation, or luxation) resulting in an anterior displacement of the L5 body and transverse process. The posterior fragment (vertebral laminae and spinous process of L5) remains in proper alignment over the sacrum (S1). This defect has the radiographic appearance of a dog with a broken neck (highlighted in yellow, with the fracture in red). Pressure on spinal nerves often leads to low back and lower limb pain.

Posterior oblique views: Scottie dog profile in yellow and fracture site in red

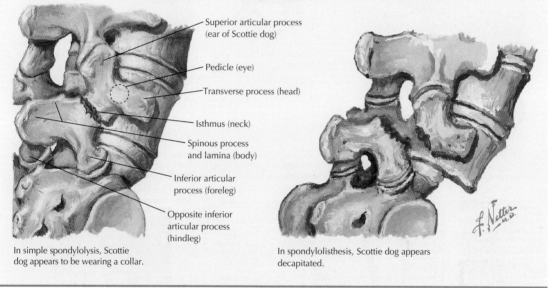

Superior articular process (ear of Scottie dog)

Pedicle (eye)

Transverse process (head)

Isthmus (neck)

Spinous process and lamina (body)

Inferior articular process (foreleg)

Opposite inferior articular process (hindleg)

In simple spondylolysis, Scottie dog appears to be wearing a collar.

In spondylolisthesis, Scottie dog appears decapitated.

Intervertebral Disc Herniation

The intervertebral discs are composed of a central nuclear zone of collagen and hydrated proteoglycans called the **nucleus pulposus**, which is surrounded by concentric lamellae of collagen fibers that compose the **anulus fibrosus**. The nucleus pulposus is hydrated and acts as a "shock absorber," compressing when load bearing and relaxing when the load is removed. Over time, the repeated compression-relaxation cycle of the intervertebral discs can lead to peripheral tears of the anulus fibrosus that allow for the extrusion and herniation of the more gelatinous nucleus pulposus. This often occurs with age, and the nucleus pulposus becomes more dehydrated, thus transferring more of the compression forces to the anulus fibrosus. This added stress may cause thickening of the anulus and tears. Most disc herniations occur in a posterolateral direction because the anulus fibrosus tears often occur at the posterolateral margins of the disc (rim lesions). Moreover, the posterior longitudinal ligament reinforces the anulus such that posterior herniations are much less common; otherwise, the disc would herniate into the vertebral canal and compress the spinal cord or its nerve roots.

Continued

Clinical Focus 2-6

Intervertebral Disc Herniation—cont'd

The most common sites for disc herniation in the cervical region are the C5-C6 and C6-C7 levels, resulting in shoulder and upper limb pain. In the lumbar region the primary sites are the L4-L5 and L5-S1 levels. Lumbar disc herniation is much more common than cervical herniation and results in pain over the sacro-iliac joint, hip, posterior thigh, and leg.

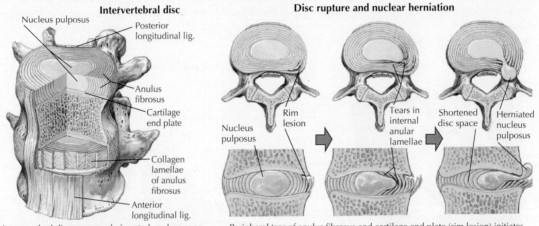

Intervertebral disc

Nucleus pulposus
Posterior longitudinal lig.
Anulus fibrosus
Cartilage end plate
Collagen lamellae of anulus fibrosus
Anterior longitudinal lig.

Intervertebral disc composed of central nuclear zone of collagen and hydrated proteoglycans surrounded by concentric lamellae of collagen fibers

Disc rupture and nuclear herniation

Nucleus pulposus
Rim lesion
Tears in internal anular lamellae
Shortened disc space
Herniated nucleus pulposus

Peripheral tear of anulus fibrosus and cartilage end plate (rim lesion) initiates sequence of events that weaken and tear internal anular lamellae, allowing extrusion and herniation of nucleus pulposus.

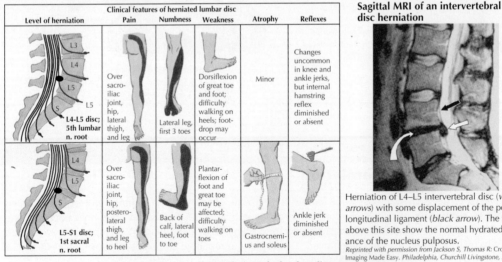

Clinical features of herniated lumbar disc					
Level of herniation	**Pain**	**Numbness**	**Weakness**	**Atrophy**	**Reflexes**
L4-L5 disc; 5th lumbar n. root	Over sacro-iliac joint, hip, lateral thigh, and leg	Lateral leg, first 3 toes	Dorsiflexion of great toe and foot; difficulty walking on heels; foot-drop may occur	Minor	Changes uncommon in knee and ankle jerks, but internal hamstring reflex diminished or absent
L5-S1 disc; 1st sacral n. root	Over sacro-iliac joint, hip, postero-lateral thigh, and leg to heel	Back of calf, lateral heel, foot to toe	Plantar-flexion of foot and great toe may be affected; difficulty walking on toes	Gastrocnemius and soleus	Ankle jerk diminished or absent

Sagittal MRI of an intervertebral disc herniation

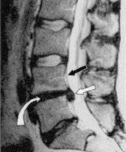

Herniation of L4–L5 intervertebral disc (*white arrows*) with some displacement of the posterior longitudinal ligament (*black arrow*). The two discs above this site show the normal hydrated appearance of the nucleus pulposus.
Reprinted with permission from Jackson S, Thomas R: Cross-Sectional Imaging Made Easy. Philadelphia, Churchill Livingstone, 2004.

Herniation of a lumbar disc

Herniated nucleus pulposus
Nerve root compressed by herniated disc
Disc material removed
Portion of lamina and facet removed

Disc material removed to decompress nerve root

Back Pain Associated with the Zygapophysial (Facet) Joints

Although changes in the vertebral facet joints are not the most common cause of back pain (~15%), such alterations can lead to chronic pain. Although the articular surfaces of the synovial facet joints are not directly innervated, sensory nerve fibers derived from the dorsal rami of spinal nerves do supply the synovial linings of the capsules surrounding the joints. Two examples of painful conditions associated with facet joints are degeneration of the articular cartilage and osteophyte overgrowth of the articular processes.

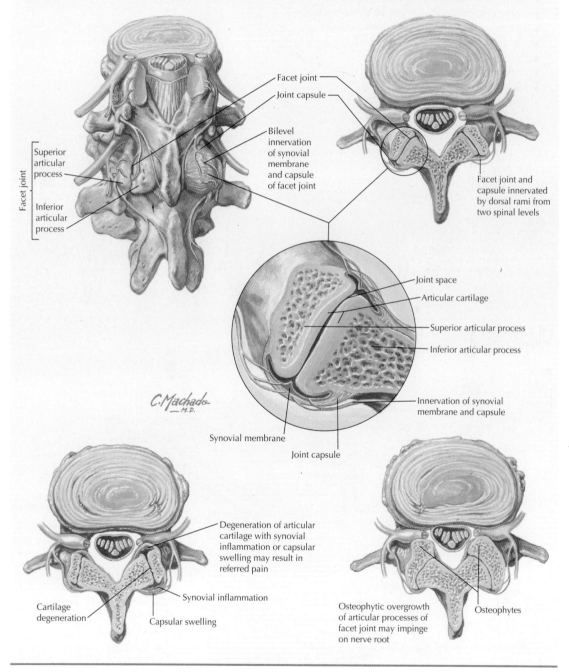

Facet joint

Joint capsule

Bilevel innervation of synovial membrane and capsule of facet joint

Facet joint

Superior articular process

Inferior articular process

Facet joint and capsule innervated by dorsal rami from two spinal levels

Joint space

Articular cartilage

Superior articular process

Inferior articular process

Innervation of synovial membrane and capsule

Synovial membrane

Joint capsule

C. Machado
—M.D.

Degeneration of articular cartilage with synovial inflammation or capsular swelling may result in referred pain

Synovial inflammation

Cartilage degeneration

Capsular swelling

Osteophytic overgrowth of articular processes of facet joint may impinge on nerve root

Osteophytes

Low Back Pain

Low back pain, the most common musculoskeletal disorder, can have various causes. Physical examination, although not always revealing a definite cause, may provide clues to the level of spinal nerve involvement and relative sensitivity to pain. The following causes are identified most often:

- Intervertebral disc rupture and herniation
- Nerve inflammation or compression
- Degenerative changes in vertebral facet joints
- Sacro-iliac joint and ligament involvement
- Metabolic bone disease
- Psychosocial factors
- Abdominal aneurysm
- Metastatic cancer
- Myofascial disorders

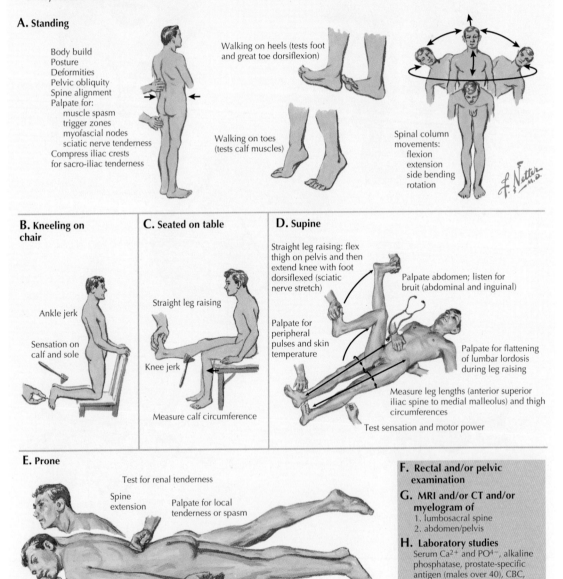

A. Standing

Body build
Posture
Deformities
Pelvic obliquity
Spine alignment
Palpate for:
   muscle spasm
   trigger zones
   myofascial nodes
   sciatic nerve tenderness
Compress iliac crests
for sacro-iliac tenderness

Walking on heels (tests foot and great toe dorsiflexion)

Walking on toes (tests calf muscles)

Spinal column movements:
   flexion
   extension
   side bending
   rotation

B. Kneeling on chair

Ankle jerk

Sensation on calf and sole

C. Seated on table

Straight leg raising

Knee jerk

Measure calf circumference

D. Supine

Straight leg raising: flex thigh on pelvis and then extend knee with foot dorsiflexed (sciatic nerve stretch)

Palpate for peripheral pulses and skin temperature

Palpate abdomen; listen for bruit (abdominal and inguinal)

Palpate for flattening of lumbar lordosis during leg raising

Measure leg lengths (anterior superior iliac spine to medial malleolus) and thigh circumferences

Test sensation and motor power

E. Prone

Test for renal tenderness

Spine extension

Palpate for local tenderness or spasm

F. Rectal and/or pelvic examination

G. MRI and/or CT and/or myelogram of
1. lumbosacral spine
2. abdomen/pelvis

H. Laboratory studies
Serum Ca^{2+} and PO^{4-}, alkaline phosphatase, prostate-specific antigen (males over 40), CBC, ESR, and urinalysis

Movements of the Spine

The essential movements of the spine are flexion, extension, lateral flexion (lateral bending), and rotation (Fig. 2-8). The greatest freedom of movement occurs in the cervical and lumbar spine, with the neck having the greatest range of motion. Flexion is greatest in the cervical region, and extension is greatest in the lumbar region. The thoracic region is relatively stable, as is the sacrum.

Again, the atlanto-occipital joint permits flexion and extension (e.g., nodding in acknowledgment), and the atlanto-axial joint allows side-to-side movements (rotation; e.g., indicating "no"). This is accomplished by a uniaxial synovial joint between the dens of the axis and its articulation with the anterior arch of the atlas. The **dens** functions as a pivot that permits the atlas and attached occipital bone of the skull to rotate on the axis. **Alar ligaments** limit this side-to-side movement so that rotation of the atlanto-axial joint occurs with the skull and atlas rotating as a single unit on the axis (see Fig. 2-6).

Movements of the spine are a function of the following features:

- Size and compressibility of the intervertebral discs
- Tightness of the joint capsules
- Orientation of the articular facets (zygapophysial joints)
- Muscle and ligament function
- Articulations with the thoracic cage
- Limitations imposed by the adjacent tissues and increasing age

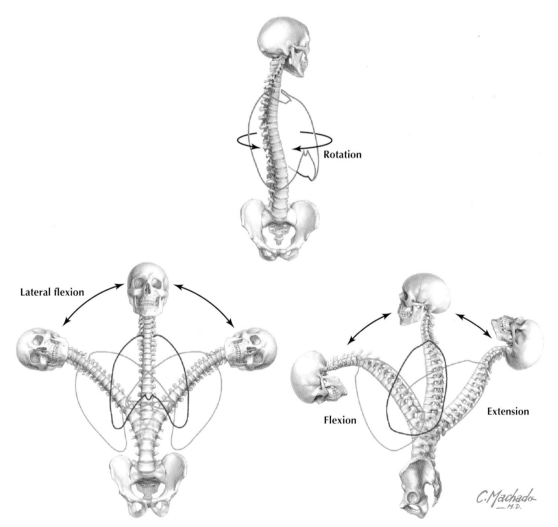

FIGURE 2-8 Movements of the Spine.

Whiplash Injury

"Whiplash" is a nonmedical term for a **cervical hyperextension** injury, which is usually associated with a rear-end vehicular crash. The relaxed neck is thrown backward, or hyperextended, as the vehicle accelerates rapidly forward. Rapid recoil of the neck into extreme flexion occurs next. Properly adjusted headrests can greatly reduce the occurrence of this hyperextension injury, which often results in stretched or torn cervical muscles and, in severe cases, ligament, bone, and nerve damage.

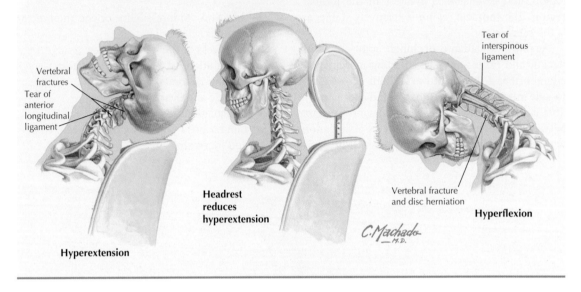

Vertebral fractures

Tear of anterior longitudinal ligament

Hyperextension

Headrest reduces hyperextension

Tear of interspinous ligament

Vertebral fracture and disc herniation

Hyperflexion

C. Machado — M.D.

Blood Supply to the Spine

The spine receives blood from spinal arteries derived from branches of larger arteries that serve each midline region of the body. These major arteries include the following:

- **Vertebral arteries,** arising from the subclavian arteries in the neck
- **Ascending cervical arteries,** from a branch of the subclavian arteries
- **Posterior intercostal arteries,** from the thoracic aorta
- **Lumbar arteries,** from the abdominal aorta
- **Lateral sacral arteries,** from pelvic internal iliac arteries

Spinal arteries arise from these branches and divide into small posterior branches that supply the vertebral arch and small anterior branches that supply the vertebral body (Fig. 2-9). Also, longitudinal branches of **radicular arteries,** which arise from these spinal arteries, course along the inside aspect of the vertebral canal and supply the vertebral column. (Do not confuse these arteries with those that supply the spinal cord, discussed later. In some cases, arteries that do supply the spinal cord also contribute branches that supply the vertebrae.)

Radicular veins receive tributaries from the spinal cord and the internal vertebral veins that course within the vertebral canal; this **internal venous plexus** also anastomoses with a network of **external vertebral veins** (Fig. 2-9). The internal vertebral venous plexus lacks valves, whereas the external vertebral venous plexus has recently been shown to possess some valves, directing blood flow toward the internal venous plexus. The radicular veins then drain blood from the vertebral venous plexus to segmental and intervertebral veins, with the blood ultimately collecting in the segmental branches of the following major venous channels:

- **Superior vena cava:** drains cervical region.
- **Azygos venous system:** drains thoracic region.
- **Inferior vena cava:** drains lumbosacral regions.

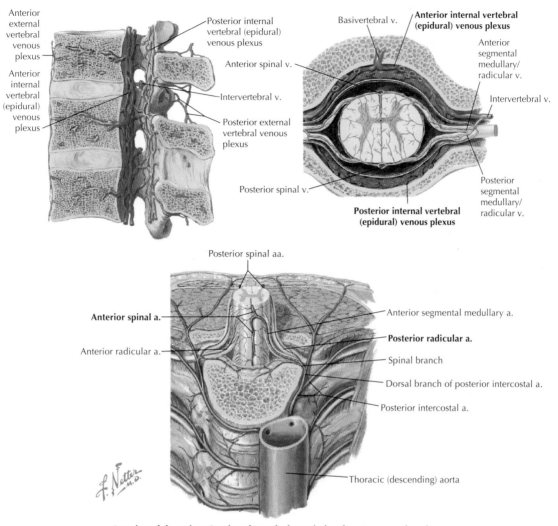

Arteries of the spine: Section through thoracic level: anterosuperior view

FIGURE 2-9 Arteries and Veins of the Spine. (From *Atlas of human anatomy,* ed 6, Plates 168 and 169.)

4. MUSCLES OF THE BACK

Although the spine is the axis of the human body and courses down the body's midline, dividing it into approximately equal right and left halves, it is not midway between the anterior and posterior halves of the body. In fact, most of the body's weight lies anterior to the more posteriorly aligned vertebral column. Consequently, to support the body and spine, most of the muscles associated with the spine attach to its lateral and posterior processes, assisting the spine in maintaining an upright posture that offsets the uneven weight distribution.

The muscles of the back are divided into two major groups, as follows:

Extrinsic back muscles, involved in movements of the upper limb and with respiration.

Intrinsic back muscles, involved in movements of the spine and maintenance of posture.

Extrinsic Back Muscles

The extrinsic muscles of the back are considered "extrinsic" because embryologically they arise from hypaxial myotomes (see Fig. 2-22). The extrinsic back muscles are divided into the following two functional groups (Fig. 2-10 and Table 2-5):

TABLE 2-5 Muscles of the Back

MUSCLE	PROXIMAL ATTACHMENT (ORIGIN)	DISTAL ATTACHMENT (INSERTION)	INNERVATION	MAIN ACTIONS
Extrinsic Back Muscles				
Trapezius	Superior nuchal line, external occipital protuberance, nuchal ligament, and spinous processes of C7-T12	Lateral third of clavicle, acromion, and spine of scapula	Accessory nerve (cranial nerve XI) and C3-C4	Elevates, retracts, and rotates scapula; lower fibers depress scapula
Latissimus dorsi	Spinous processes of T7-L5, sacrum, thoracolumbar fascia, iliac crest, and last three ribs	Humerus (intertubercular groove)	Thoracodorsal nerve (C6-C8)	Extends, adducts, and medially rotates humerus
Levator scapulae	Transverse processes of C1-C4	Superior angle of scapula	C3-C4 and dorsal scapular (C5) nerve	Elevates scapula and tilts glenoid cavity inferiorly
Rhomboid minor and major	*Minor:* nuchal ligament and spinous processes of C7-T1 *Major:* spinous processes of T2-T5	Medial border of scapula	Dorsal scapular nerve (C4-C5)	Retract scapula, rotate it to depress glenoid cavity, and fix scapula to thoracic wall
Serratus posterior superior	Ligamentum nuchae and spinous processes of C7-T3	Superior aspect of ribs 2-5	T1-T4 ventral rami	Elevates ribs
Serratus posterior inferior	Spinous processes of T11-L3	Inferior border ribs 9-12	T9-T12 ventral rami	Depresses ribs
Intrinsic Back Muscles				
Splenius capitis	Nuchal ligament, spinous processes of C7-T4	Mastoid process of temporal bone and lateral third of superior nuchal line	Middle cervical nerves*	Bilaterally: extends head Unilaterally: laterally bends (flexes) and rotates face to same side
Splenius cervicis	Spinous processes of T3-T6	Transverse processes of C1-C3	Lower cervical nerves*	Bilaterally: extends neck Unilaterally: laterally bends (flexes) and rotates neck toward same side
Erector spinae	Posterior sacrum, iliac crest, sacrospinous ligament, supraspinous ligament, and spinous processes of lower lumbar and sacral vertebrae	*Iliocostalis:* angles of lower ribs and cervical transverse processes *Longissimus:* between tubercles and angles of ribs, transverse processes of thoracic and cervical vertebrae, mastoid process *Spinalis:* spinous processes of upper thoracic and midcervical vertebrae	Respective spinal nerves of each region*	Extends and laterally bends vertebral column and head
Semispinalis	Transverse processes of C4-T12	Spinous processes of cervical and thoracic regions	Respective spinal nerves of each region*	Extends head, neck, and thorax and rotates them to opposite side
Multifidi	Sacrum, ilium, and transverse processes of T1-T12 and articular processes of C4-C7	Spinous processes of vertebrae above, spanning two to four segments	Respective spinal nerves of each region*	Stabilizes spine during local movements
Rotatores	Transverse processes of cervical, thoracic, and lumbar regions	Lamina and transverse process or spine above, spanning one or two segments	Respective spinal nerves of each region*	Stabilize, extend, and rotate spine

*Dorsal rami of spinal nerves.

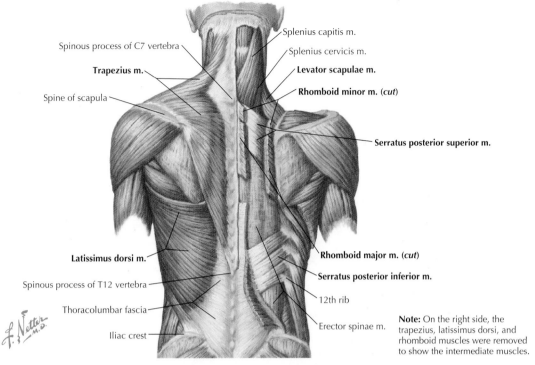

Splenius capitis m.

Splenius cervicis m.

Levator scapulae m.

Rhomboid minor m. (*cut*)

Spinous process of C7 vertebra

Trapezius m.

Spine of scapula

Serratus posterior superior m.

Latissimus dorsi m.

Spinous process of T12 vertebra

Thoracolumbar fascia

Iliac crest

Rhomboid major m. (*cut*)

Serratus posterior inferior m.

12th rib

Erector spinae m.

Note: On the right side, the trapezius, latissimus dorsi, and rhomboid muscles were removed to show the intermediate muscles.

FIGURE 2-10 Extrinsic Muscles of the Back. (From *Atlas of human anatomy*, ed 6, Plate 171.)

- **Superficial muscles,** involved in movements of the upper limb (trapezius, latissimus dorsi, levator scapulae, two rhomboids), attach the pectoral girdle (clavicle, scapula, humerus) to the axial skeleton (skull, ribs, spine).
- **Intermediate muscles,** thin accessory muscles of respiration (serratus posterior superior and inferior) that assist with movements of the rib cage, lie deep to the superficial muscles, and extend from the spine to the ribs.

Intrinsic Back Muscles

The intrinsic back muscles are the "true" muscles of the back because they develop from epaxial myotomes, function in movements of the spine, and help maintain posture. The intrinsic muscles are enclosed within a deep fascial layer that extends in the midline from the medial crest of the sacrum to the nuchal ligament and skull, and that spreads laterally to the transverse processes and angles of the ribs. In the thoracic and lumbar regions, the deep fascia makes up a distinct sheath known as the **thoracolumbar fascia** (Figs. 2-10 and 2-11).

In the lumbar region, this fascial sheath has the following three layers (see also Fig. 4-31):

- **Posterior layer,** extending from the lumbar and sacral spinous processes laterally over the surface of the erector spinae muscles.
- **Middle layer,** extending from the lumbar transverse processes to the iliac crest inferiorly and to the 12th rib superiorly.
- **Anterior layer,** covering the quadratus lumborum muscle of the posterior abdominal wall and extending to the lumbar transverse processes, iliac crest, and superiorly, forming the lateral arcuate ligament for attachment of the abdominal diaphragm.

The intrinsic back muscles also are among the few muscles of the body that are innervated by dorsal rami of a spinal nerve. From superficial to deep, the intrinsic muscles include the following three layers (Fig. 2-11 and Table 2-5):

- **Superficial layer,** including the splenius muscles that occupy the lateral and posterior neck (spinotransversales muscles).
- **Intermediate layer,** including the erector spinae muscles that mainly extend the spine.

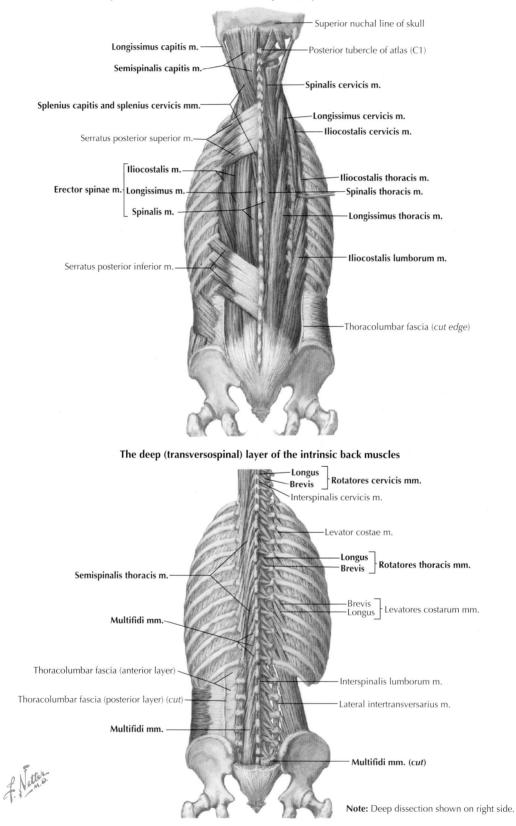

FIGURE 2-11 Intrinsic Muscles of the Back. (From *Atlas of human anatomy*, ed 6, Plates 172 and 173.)

- **Deep layer,** including the transversospinales muscles that fill the spaces between the transverse processes and spinous processes.

The intermediate, or **erector spinae,** layer of muscles is the largest group of the intrinsic back muscles and is important for maintaining posture and extending the spine. These muscles are divided into three major groups, as follows (Fig. 2-11):

- **Iliocostalis**, most laterally located and associated with attachments to the ribs and cervical transverse processes.
- **Longissimus**, intermediate and largest column of the erector spinae muscles.
- **Spinalis**, most medially located and smallest of the erector spinae group, with attachments to the vertebral spinous processes.

These three groups are further subdivided into regional divisions—lumborum, thoracis, cervicis, and capitis—based on their attachments as one proceeds superiorly (Fig. 2-11).

The transversospinales (transversospinal) muscles (deep layer) are often simply called the "paravertebral" muscles because they form a solid mass of muscle tissue interposed and running obliquely between the transverse and spinous processes (Fig. 2-11). The transversospinal muscles comprise the following three groups:

- **Semispinalis group:** thoracis, cervicis, and capitis muscles; the most superficial transversospinal muscles, found in the thoracic and cervical regions superior to the occipital bone.
- **Multifidus group:** found deep to the semispinalis group and in all spinal regions, but most prominent in the lumbar region.
- **Rotatores group:** deepest transversospinal muscles; present in all spinal regions, but most prominent in the thoracic region.

Deep to the transversospinal muscles lies a relatively small set of segmental muscles that assist in elevating the ribs (levatores costarum) and stabilizing adjacent vertebrae while larger muscle groups act on the spine (interspinales, intertransversarii) (Fig. 2-11).

Suboccipital Muscles

In the back of the neck, deep to the trapezius, splenius, and semispinalis muscles, several small muscles that move the head are attached to the skull, the atlas, and the axis (Fig. 2-12 and Table 2-6). These muscles are the **suboccipital muscles,** innervated by the suboccipital nerve (dorsal ramus of C1) and forming a (suboccipital) triangle with the following muscle boundaries:

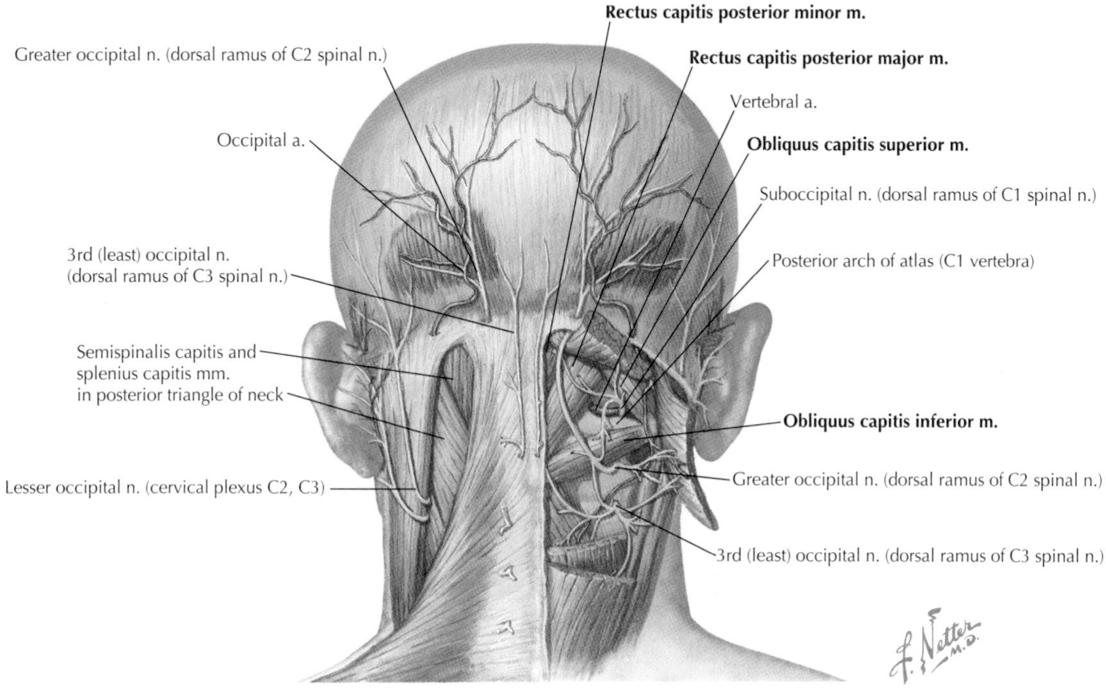

FIGURE 2-12 Suboccipital Triangle and Associated Musculature. (From *Atlas of human anatomy,* ed 6, Plate 175.)

TABLE 2-6 Suboccipital Muscles

MUSCLE	PROXIMAL ATTACHMENT (ORIGIN)	DISTAL ATTACHMENT (INSERTION)	INNERVATION	MAIN ACTIONS
Rectus capitis posterior major	Spine of axis	Lateral inferior nuchal line	Suboccipital nerve (C1)	Extends head and rotates to same side
Rectus capitis posterior minor	Tubercle of posterior arch of atlas	Median inferior nuchal line	Suboccipital nerve (C1)	Extends head
Obliquus capitis superior	Atlas transverse process	Occipital bone	Suboccipital nerve (C1)	Extends head and bends it laterally
Obliquus capitis inferior	Spine of axis	Atlas transverse process	Suboccipital nerve (C1)	Rotates head to same side

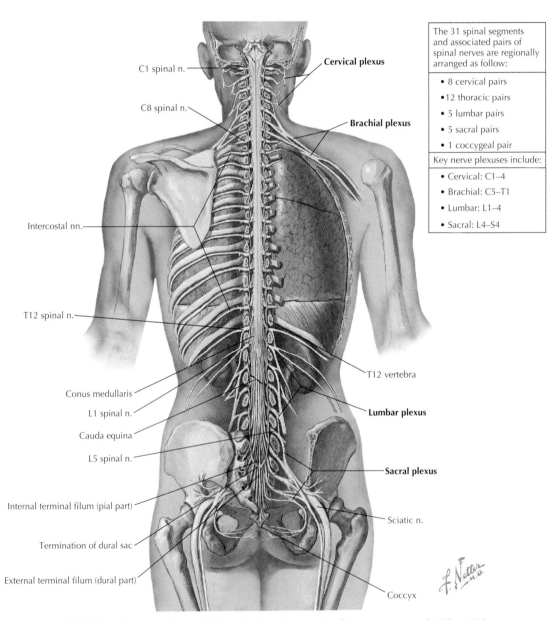

The 31 spinal segments and associated pairs of spinal nerves are regionally arranged as follow:

- 8 cervical pairs
- 12 thoracic pairs
- 5 lumbar pairs
- 5 sacral pairs
- 1 coccygeal pair

Key nerve plexuses include:

- Cervical: C1–4
- Brachial: C5–T1
- Lumbar: L1–4
- Sacral: L4–S4

C1 spinal n.
C8 spinal n.
Intercostal nn.
T12 spinal n.
Conus medullaris
L1 spinal n.
Cauda equina
L5 spinal n.
Internal terminal filum (pial part)
Termination of dural sac
External terminal filum (dural part)

Cervical plexus
Brachial plexus
T12 vertebra
Lumbar plexus
Sacral plexus
Sciatic n.
Coccyx

FIGURE 2-13 Spinal Cord and Nerves In Situ. (From *Atlas of human anatomy*, ed 6, Plate 160.)

- **Rectus capitis posterior major**
- **Obliquus capitis superior** (superior oblique muscle of head)
- **Obliquus capitis inferior** (inferior oblique muscle of head)

Deep within the suboccipital triangle, the **vertebral artery,** a branch of the subclavian artery in the lower anterior neck, passes through the transverse foramen of the atlas and loops medially to enter the foramen magnum of the skull to supply the brainstem. The first three pairs of spinal nerves are also found in this region (Fig. 2-12).

5. SPINAL CORD

The spinal cord is a direct continuation of the medulla oblongata, extending below the foramen magnum at the base of the skull and passing through the vertebral (spinal) canal formed by the articulated vertebrae (Fig. 2-13).

The spinal cord has a slightly larger diameter in the cervical and lumbar regions, primarily because of increased numbers of neurons and axons in these regions for innervation of the many muscles in the upper and lower limbs. The spinal cord ends as a tapered region called the **conus medullaris,** which is situated at about the L1-L2 vertebral level (or L3 in neonate). From this point inferiorly, the nerve rootlets course to their respective levels and form a bundle called the **cauda equina** ("horse's tail"). The spinal cord is anchored inferiorly by the **terminal filum,** which is attached to the coccyx. The terminal filum is a pial extension that picks up a layer of dura mater after passing through the dural sac (L2 vertebral level) before attaching to the coccyx (see Spinal Meninges). Features of the spinal cord include the following:

- The 31 pairs of spinal nerves that comprise 8 cervical, 12 thoracic, 5 lumbar, and 5 sacral pairs and 1 coccygeal pair.
- Each spinal nerve is formed by a dorsal (posterior) and a ventral (anterior) root.
- Motor neurons reside in the spinal cord gray matter (anterior horn).
- Sensory neurons reside in the spinal dorsal root ganglia.
- Ventral rami of spinal nerves often converge to form **plexuses** (mixed networks of nerve axons; cervical, brachial, lumbar, sacral) or segmental thoracic nerves (intercostal nerves and the subcostal nerve).

- Dorsal rami of spinal nerves are small and innervate the intrinsic back muscles and the suboccipital region (epaxial muscles of embryo) and a narrow band of skin above the intrinsic muscles.

Typical Spinal Nerve

The typical scheme for a **somatic** (innervates skin and skeletal muscle) peripheral nerve shows a motor neuron in the spinal cord anterior horn (gray matter) sending a myelinated axon through a **ventral** (anterior) **root** and into a peripheral nerve, which ends at a neuromuscular junction on a skeletal muscle (Fig. 2-14). Likewise, a nerve ending in the skin sends a sensory axon toward the spinal cord in a peripheral nerve. (Sensory axons also arise from the muscle spindles and joints and are similarly conveyed back to the spinal cord.) Thus, each peripheral nerve contains hundreds or thousands of motor and sensory axons. The sensory neuron is a pseudounipolar neuron that resides in a **dorsal root ganglion** (a ganglion in the periphery is a collection of neurons, just as a "nucleus" is in the brain) and sends its central axon into the posterior horn (gray matter) of the spinal cord. At each level of the spinal cord, the gray matter is visible as a butterfly-shaped central collection of neurons, exhibiting a posterior and an anterior horn (Fig. 2-14).

The spinal cord gives rise to 31 pairs of spinal nerves, which then form two major branches (rami), as follows:

- **Dorsal ramus:** a small ramus that courses dorsally to the back and conveys motor and sensory information to and from the skin and the intrinsic back muscles and suboccipital skeletal muscles.
- **Ventral ramus:** a much larger ramus that courses laterally and ventrally and innervates all the remaining skin and skeletal muscles of the neck, limbs, and trunk.

Once nerve fibers (sensory or motor) are beyond, or peripheral to, the spinal cord proper, the fibers then reside in nerves of the peripheral nervous system (PNS). Components of the PNS include the following (see Nervous System, Chapter 1):

- **Somatic nervous system:** sensory and motor fibers to skin, skeletal muscle, and joints (Fig. 2-15, left side).

Segment of the spinal cord showing the dorsal and ventral roots, membranes removed: anterior view (*greatly magnified*)

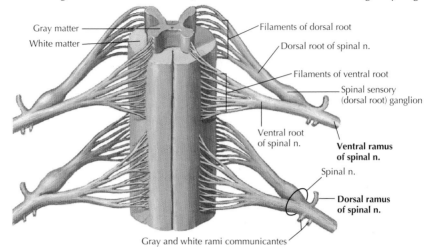

Schematic of a typical peripheral nerve showing the somatic axons (autonomic axons not shown)

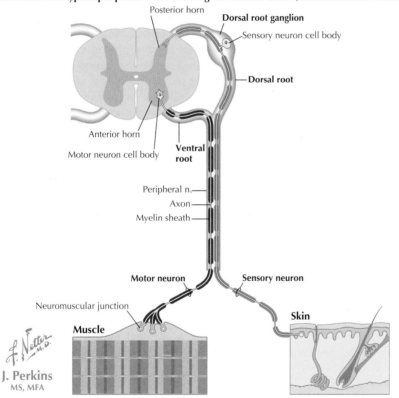

J. Perkins
MS, MFA

FIGURE 2-14 Typical Spinal Nerve.

- **Autonomic nervous system** (ANS): sensory and motor fibers to all smooth muscle (including viscera and vasculature), cardiac muscle (heart), and glands (Fig. 2-15, right side).
- **Enteric nervous system:** plexuses and ganglia of the gastrointestinal tract that regulate bowel secretion, absorption, and

motility (originally, considered part of the ANS); linked to the ANS for optimal regulation (see Fig. 1-26).

Thus, each peripheral nerve arising from the spinal cord contains hundreds or thousands of three types of axons (Fig. 2-15, left and right sides):

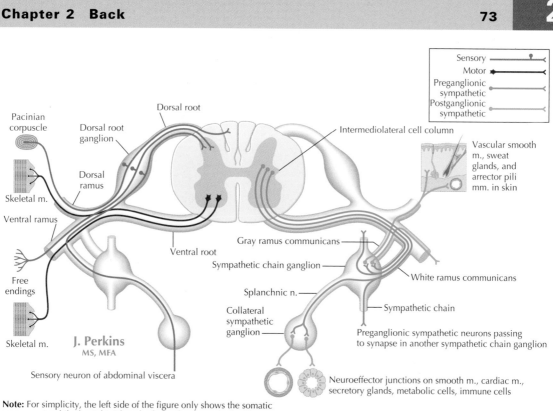

Note: For simplicity, the left side of the figure only shows the somatic components while the right side only shows the sympathetic efferent components.

FIGURE 2-15 Structural Anatomy of a Thoracic Spinal Nerve.

- **Somatic efferent** (motor) axons to skeletal muscle
- **Afferent** (sensory) axons from the skin, skeletal muscle, and joints or viscera
- **Postganglionic sympathetic efferent** axons to smooth muscle (vascular smooth muscle and arrector pili muscles in the skin) and glands (sweat and sebaceous skin glands)

Each of the 31 pairs of spinal nerves exits the spinal cord and passes through an opening in the vertebral column to gain access to the periphery. The C1 nerve pair passes between the skull and the atlas, with subsequent cervical nerve pairs exiting the intervertebral foramen above the vertebra of the same number; C2 nerve exits via the intervertebral foramen superior to the C2 vertebra, and so on, until one reaches the C8 nerve, which then exits the intervertebral foramen above the T1 vertebra. All the remaining thoracic, lumbar, and sacral nerves exit via the intervertebral foramen below the vertebra of the same number (Fig. 2-16).

As it divides into its small dorsal ramus and larger ventral ramus, the spinal nerve also gives off several small recurrent meningeal branches that reenter the intervertebral foramen and innervate the dura mater, intervertebral discs, ligaments, and blood vessels associated with the spinal cord and vertebral column (see Fig. 2-18).

Dermatomes

The region of skin innervated by the somatic sensory nerve axons associated with a single dorsal root ganglion at a single spinal cord level is called a **dermatome.** (Likewise, over the antero-lateral head, the skin is innervated by one of the three divisions of the trigeminal cranial nerve, as discussed later.) The neurons that give rise to these sensory fibers are pseudounipolar neurons that reside in the single dorsal root ganglion associated with the specific spinal cord level. (Note that for each level, we are speaking of a pair of nerves, roots, and ganglia, with 31 pairs of spinal nerves, one pair for each spinal cord level.) The first cervical spinal cord level, C1, does possess sensory fibers, but these provide minimal if any contribution to the skin, so at the top of the head the

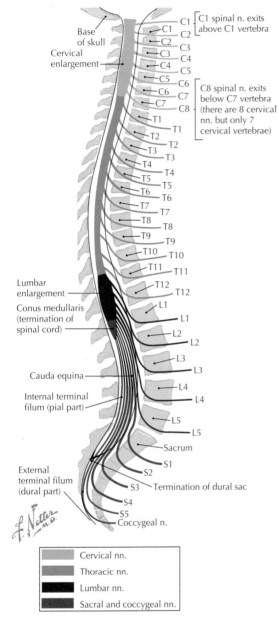

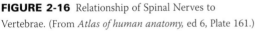

	Cervical nn.
	Thoracic nn.
	Lumbar nn.
	Sacral and coccygeal nn.

FIGURE 2-16 Relationship of Spinal Nerves to Vertebrae. (From *Atlas of human anatomy,* ed 6, Plate 161.)

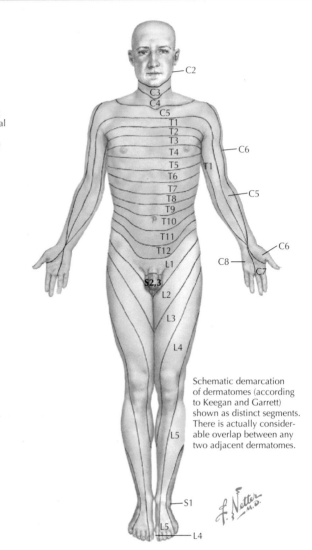

FIGURE 2-17 Distribution of dermatomes. (From *Atlas of human anatomy,* ed 6, Plate 162.)

Schematic demarcation of dermatomes (according to Keegan and Garrett) shown as distinct segments. There is actually considerable overlap between any two adjacent dermatomes.

TABLE 2-7 Key Dermatomes as Related to Body Surface

VERTEBRA(E)	BODY SURFACE
C5	Clavicles
C5-C7	Lateral upper limb
C6	Thumb
C7	Middle finger
C8	Little finger
C8-T1	Medial upper limb
T4	Nipple
T10	Umbilicus (navel)
T12-L1	Inguinal/groin region
L1-L4	Anterior and inner surfaces of lower limbs
L4	Medial side of big toe; knee
L4-S1	Foot
S1-S2	Posterior lower limb
S2-S4	Perineum

dermatome pattern begins with the C2 dermatome (Fig. 2-17 and Table 2-7).

The dermatomes encircle the body in segmental fashion, corresponding to the spinal cord level that receives sensory input from that segment of skin. The sensation conveyed by touching the skin is largely that of pressure and pain. Knowledge of the dermatome pattern is useful in localizing specific spinal cord segments and in assessing the

Herpes Zoster

Herpes zoster, or *shingles,* is the most common infection of the peripheral nervous system. It is an acute neuralgia confined to the dermatome distribution of a specific spinal or cranial sensory nerve root.

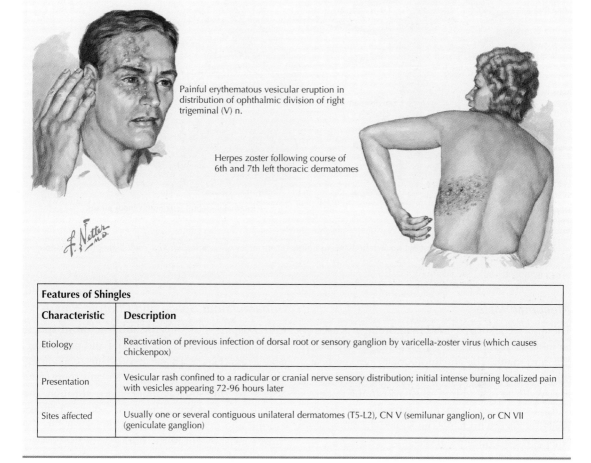

Painful erythematous vesicular eruption in distribution of ophthalmic division of right trigeminal (V) n.

Herpes zoster following course of 6th and 7th left thoracic dermatomes

Features of Shingles	
Characteristic	**Description**
Etiology	Reactivation of previous infection of dorsal root or sensory ganglion by varicella-zoster virus (which causes chickenpox)
Presentation	Vesicular rash confined to a radicular or cranial nerve sensory distribution; initial intense burning localized pain with vesicles appearing 72-96 hours later
Sites affected	Usually one or several contiguous unilateral dermatomes (T5-L2), CN V (semilunar ganglion), or CN VII (geniculate ganglion)

integrity of the spinal cord at that level (intact or "lesioned").

The sensory nerve fibers that innervate a segment of skin and constitute the "dermatome" exhibit some overlap of nerve fibers. Consequently, a segment of skin is innervated primarily by fibers from a single spinal cord level, but there will be some overlap with sensory fibers from the level above and below the primary cord level. For example, dermatome T5 will have some overlap with sensory fibers associated with the T4 and T6 levels. Thus, dermatomes provide a good approximation of cord levels, but variation is common and overlap exists (Table 2-7).

Spinal Meninges

The brain and spinal cord are covered by three membranes called the **meninges** and are bathed in **cerebrospinal fluid** (CSF) (Fig. 2-18). The three meningeal layers are the dura, arachnoid, and pia mater ("mother").

Dura Mater

The dura mater is a thick outer covering that is richly innervated by sensory nerve endings and that extends around the spinal cord down to the level of the S2 vertebra, where the dural sac ends. The **epidural (extradural) space** lies between the vertebral canal walls and the spinal dural sac and contains fat and blood vessels (Fig. 2-18).

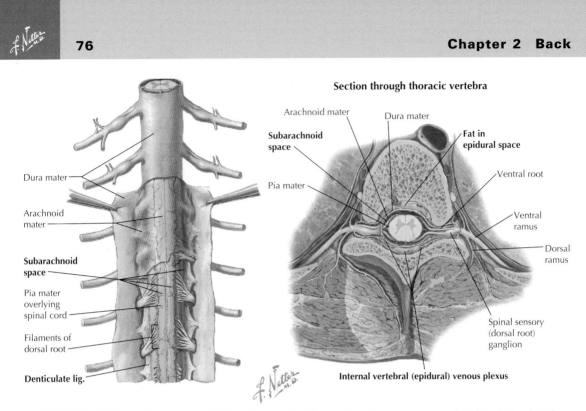

FIGURE 2-18 Spinal Meninges and Relationship to Spine. (From *Atlas of human anatomy*, ed 6, Plates 165 and 166.)

Arachnoid Mater

The fine, weblike arachnoid membrane is avascular and lies directly beneath, but is not attached to, the dura mater. The arachnoid mater also ends at the level of the S2 vertebra. Wispy threads of connective tissue extend from this layer to the underlying pia mater and span the **subarachnoid space,** which is filled with CSF. The subarachnoid space ends at the S2 vertebral level.

Pia Mater

The pia mater is a delicate, transparent inner layer that intimately covers the spinal cord. At the cervical and thoracic levels, extensions of pia form approximately 21 pairs of triangular **denticulate** ("having small teeth") **ligaments** that extend laterally and help to anchor the cord to the dural sac. At the conus medullaris, the pia mater forms the **terminal filum,** a single cord of tissue that pierces the dural sac at the S2 vertebral level, acquires a dural covering, and then attaches to the coccyx to anchor the spinal cord inferiorly.

Subarachnoid Space and Choroid Plexus

Cerebrospinal fluid fills the **subarachnoid space**, which lies between the arachnoid and pia meningeal layers (Figs. 2-18 and 2-19). Thus, CSF circulates through the brain ventricles and then gains access to the subarachnoid space through the lateral and median apertures, where it flows around and over the brain and spinal cord to the most caudal extent of the dural sac at the S2 vertebral level.

Cerebrospinal fluid is secreted by the **choroid plexus**, and most CSF is absorbed primarily by the **arachnoid granulations** (associated with superior sagittal dural venous sinus) and secondarily by small veins on the surface of the pia mater throughout the central nervous system (Fig. 2-19). With about 500 mL produced daily, CSF supports and cushions the spinal cord and brain, fulfills some of the functions normally provided by the lymphatic system, and fills the 150-mL volume of the subarachnoid space.

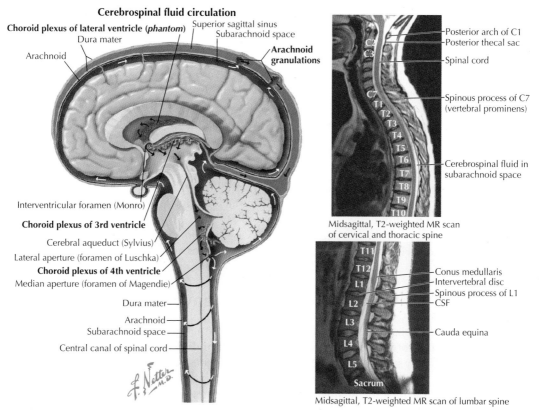

Cerebrospinal fluid circulation

Choroid plexus of lateral ventricle (*phantom*)
Dura mater
Arachnoid
Interventricular foramen (Monro)
Choroid plexus of 3rd ventricle
Cerebral aqueduct (Sylvius)
Lateral aperture (foramen of Luschka)
Choroid plexus of 4th ventricle
Median aperture (foramen of Magendie)
Dura mater
Arachnoid
Subarachnoid space
Central canal of spinal cord

Superior sagittal sinus
Subarachnoid space
Arachnoid granulations

Posterior arch of C1
Posterior thecal sac
Spinal cord
Spinous process of C7 (vertebral prominens)
Cerebrospinal fluid in subarachnoid space

Midsagittal, T2-weighted MR scan of cervical and thoracic spine

Conus medullaris
Intervertebral disc
Spinous process of L1
CSF
Cauda equina

Midsagittal, T2-weighted MR scan of lumbar spine

FIGURE 2-19 Cerebrospinal Fluid Circulation. (From *Atlas of human anatomy,* 6th ed, Plate 110; MR images from Kelley LL, Petersen C: *Sectional anatomy for imaging professionals,* St Louis, 2007, Mosby-Elsevier.)

Clinical Focus 2-11

Lumbar Puncture and Epidural Anesthesia

Cerebrospinal fluid may be sampled and examined clinically by performing a lumbar puncture (spinal tap). A spinal needle is inserted into the subarachnoid space of the lumbar cistern, in the midline between the L3 and L4 or the L4 and L5 vertebral spinal processes. Because the spinal cord ends at approximately the L1 or L2 vertebral level, the needle will not pierce and damage the cord. Anesthetic agents may be directly delivered into the epidural space (above dura mater) to anesthetize the nerve fibers of the cauda equina; this common form of anesthesia is used during childbirth in most Western countries. The epidural anesthetic infiltrates the dural sac to reach the nerve roots and is usually administered at the same levels as the lumbar puncture.

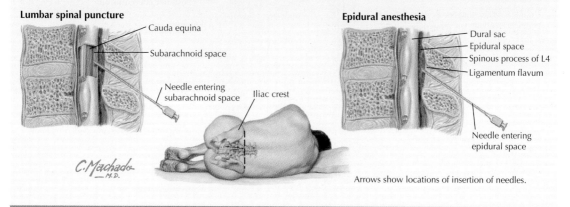

Lumbar spinal puncture
Cauda equina
Subarachnoid space
Needle entering subarachnoid space
Iliac crest

Epidural anesthesia
Dural sac
Epidural space
Spinous process of L4
Ligamentum flavum
Needle entering epidural space

Arrows show locations of insertion of needles.

Blood Supply to Spinal Cord

The spinal cord receives blood from spinal arteries derived from branches of larger arteries that serve each midline region of the body (Fig. 2-20). These major arteries include the following:

- **Vertebral arteries,** arising from the subclavian arteries in the neck
- **Ascending cervical arteries,** from a branch of the subclavian arteries
- **Posterior intercostal arteries,** from the thoracic aorta
- **Lumbar arteries,** from the abdominal aorta
- **Lateral sacral arteries,** from pelvic internal iliac arteries

A single **anterior spinal artery** and two **posterior spinal arteries,** originating intracranially from the vertebral arteries, run longitudinally along the length of the cord and are joined segmentally in each region by segmental arteries (Fig. 2-20). The largest of these segmental branches is the **major segmental artery** (of Adamkiewicz),

found in the lower thoracic or upper lumbar region; it is the major blood supply for the lower two thirds of the spinal cord. The dorsal and ventral roots are supplied by segmental **radicular** (medullary) **arteries.**

Multiple **anterior** and **posterior spinal veins** run the length of the cord and drain into segmental (medullary) radicular veins (see Fig. 2-9). **Radicular veins** receive tributaries from the internal vertebral veins that course within the vertebral canal. Radicular veins then drain into **segmental veins,** with the blood ultimately collecting in the following locations:

- Superior vena cava
- Azygos venous system of the thorax
- Inferior vena cava

6. EMBRYOLOGY

Most of the bones inferior to the skull form by **endochondral** bone formation, that is, from a cartilaginous precursor that becomes ossified. The embryonic development of the musculoskeletal components of the back represents a classic

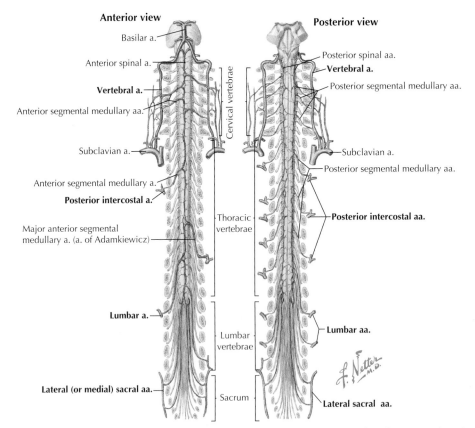

Anterior view

Basilar a.

Anterior spinal a.

Vertebral a.

Anterior segmental medullary aa.

Subclavian a.

Anterior segmental medullary a.

Posterior intercostal a.

Major anterior segmental medullary a. (a. of Adamkiewicz)

Lumbar a.

Lateral (or medial) sacral aa.

Cervical vertebrae

Thoracic vertebrae

Lumbar vertebrae

Sacrum

Posterior view

Posterior spinal aa.

Vertebral a.

Posterior segmental medullary aa.

Subclavian a.

Posterior segmental medullary aa.

Posterior intercostal aa.

Lumbar aa.

Lateral sacral aa.

FIGURE 2-20 Blood Supply to Spinal Cord. (From *Atlas of human anatomy,* ed 6, Plates 167 and 168.)

example of segmentation, with each segment corresponding to the distribution of peripheral nerves. This process begins around the end of the third week of embryonic development (day 19), during the period called gastrulation (see Chapter 1).

Development of Myotomes, Dermatomes, and Sclerotomes

The bones, muscles, and connective tissues of the embryo arise from the following sources:

- Primitive streak mesoderm (somites)
- Lateral plate mesoderm
- Diffuse collections of mesenchyme

As the neural groove invaginates along the posterior midline of the embryonic disc, it is flanked on either side by masses of mesoderm called **somites.** About 42 to 44 pairs of somites develop along this central axis and subsequently develop into the following (Fig. 2-21):

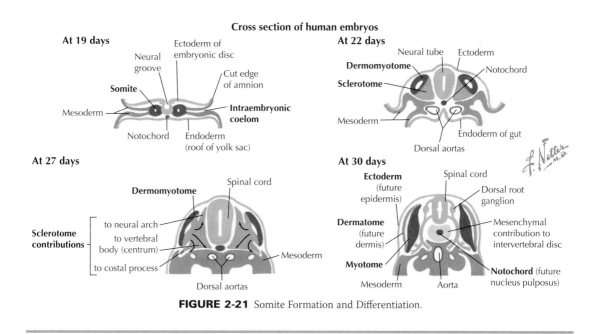

FIGURE 2-21 Somite Formation and Differentiation.

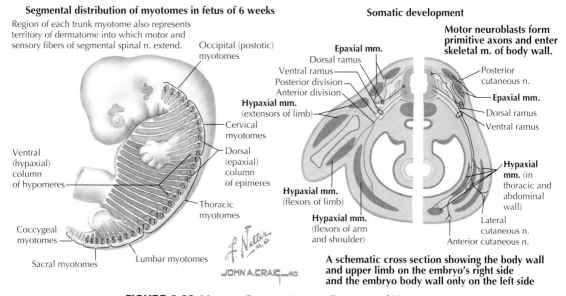

FIGURE 2-22 Myotome Segmentation into Epimeres and Hypomeres.

- **Dermomyotomes:** divide further to form **dermatomes,** which become the dermis of the skin, and **myotomes,** which differentiate into segmental masses of skeletal muscle.
- **Sclerotomes:** medial part of each somite that, along with the notochord, migrates around the neural tube and forms the cartilaginous precursors of the axial skeleton.

As in the somites from which they are derived, the myotomes have a segmental distribution. Each segment is innervated by a pair of nerves originating from the spinal cord segment. A small dorsal portion of the myotome becomes an **epimere** (epaxial) mass of skeletal muscle that will form the true, intrinsic muscles of the back (e.g., erector spinae) and are innervated by a dorsal ramus of the spinal nerve (Fig. 2-22).

A much larger ventral segment becomes the **hypomere** (hypaxial) mass of skeletal muscle, which will form the muscles of the trunk wall and limb muscles, all innervated by a ventral ramus of

the spinal nerve. Adjacent myotome segments often merge so that an individual skeletal muscle derived from those myotomes is innervated by more than one spinal cord segment. For example, the latissimus dorsi muscle is innervated by the thoracodorsal nerve, which is composed of nerves from spinal cord segments C6-C8.

Vertebral Column Development

Each vertebra first appears as a hyaline cartilage model that then ossifies, beginning in a **primary ossification center** (Fig. 2-23). Ossification centers include the following:

- **Body:** forms the vertebral body; important for support of body weight.
- **Costal process:** forms the ribs, or in vertebrae without rib articulation, part of the transverse process; important for movement and muscle attachment.
- **Neural arch:** includes the pedicle and lamina, for protection of the spinal cord,

Fate of body, costal process, and neural arch components of vertebral column, with sites and time of appearance of ossification centers

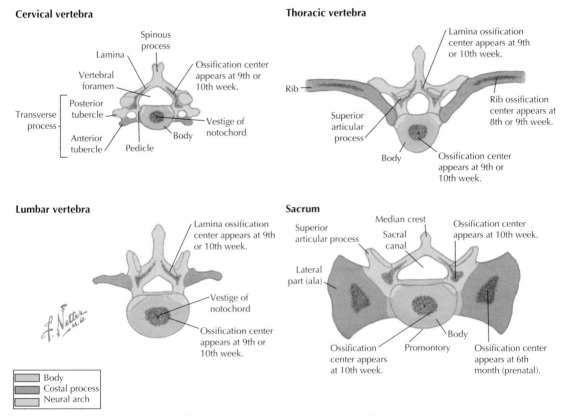

FIGURE 2-23 Ossification of Vertebral Column.

and the spinous process, for movement and muscle attachment.

The body of the vertebra does not develop from a single sclerotome but rather from the fusion of two adjacent sclerotomes (i.e., fusion of caudal half of sclerotome above with cranial half of sclerotome below). The intervertebral foramen thus lies over this fusion and provides the opening for the exiting of a spinal nerve that will innervate the myotome at that particular segment.

The **notochord** initially is in the central portion of each vertebral body but disappears. The notochord persists only as the central portion (nucleus pulposus) of each intervertebral disc, surrounded by concentric lamellae of fibrocartilage.

Neurulation and Development of the Spinal Cord

Neurulation (neural tube formation) begins concurrently with **gastrulation** (formation of trilaminar embryonic disc during third week of development). As the primitive streak recedes caudally, the midline surface ectoderm thickens to form the **neural plate,** which then invaginates to form the **neural groove** (Fig. 2-24, *A*). The **neural crest** forms at the dorsal aspect of the neural groove (Fig. 2-24, *B*) and fuses in the midline as the groove sinks below the surface and pinches off to form the **neural tube** (Fig. 2-24, *C*). The neural tube forms the following:

- Neurons of central nervous system (CNS: brain, spinal cord)
- Supporting cells of CNS
- Somatomotor neurons (innervate skeletal muscle) of PNS
- Presynaptic autonomic neurons of PNS

The **neural crest** gives rise to the following (Fig. 2-24, *D* and *E*):

- Sensory neurons of PNS found in dorsal root ganglia

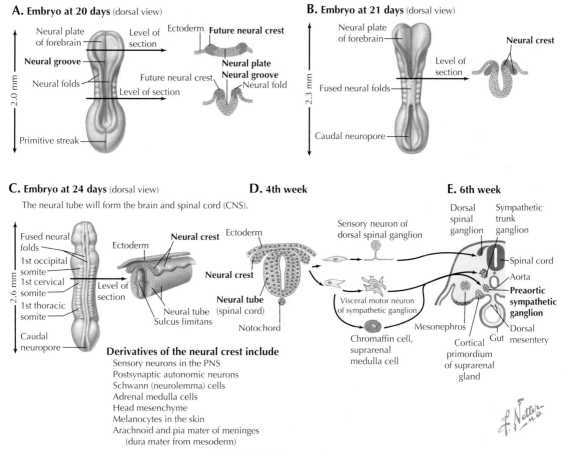

FIGURE 2-24 Neurulation.

- Postsynaptic autonomic neurons
- Schwann cells of PNS
- Adrenal medullary cells
- Head mesenchyme and portions of heart
- Melanocytes in skin
- Arachnoid and pia mater meninges (dura from mesenchyme)

The cells in the walls of the neural tube compose the **neuroepithelium,** which develops into three zones, as follows:

- **Ependymal zone:** inner layer lining central canal of spinal cord (also lines ventricles of brain).
- **Mantle:** intermediate zone that develops into gray matter of spinal cord.

- **Marginal zone:** outer layer that becomes white matter of spinal cord.

Glial cells are found primarily in the mantle and marginal zone. The neural tube is distinguished by a longitudinal groove on each side that forms the **sulcus limitans** and divides the tube into a dorsal **alar plate** and a ventral **basal plate** (Fig. 2-25). The dorsal alar plate forms the sensory derivatives of the spinal cord, and the ventral basal plate gives rise to the somatic and autonomic motor neurons, whose axons will leave the spinal cord and pass into the peripheral tissues. The sensory neurons of the dorsal root ganglia are formed from neural crest cells.

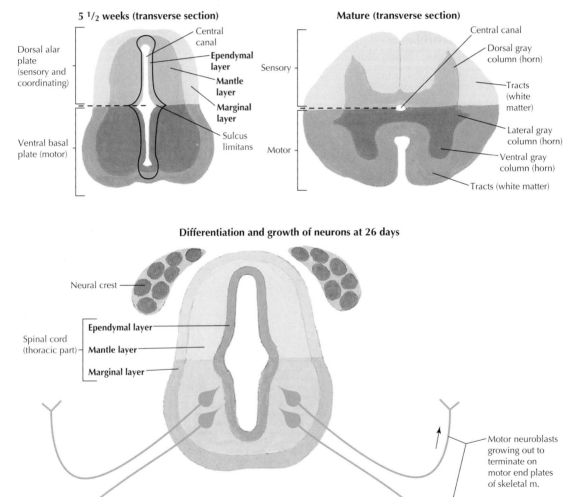

FIGURE 2-25 Alar and Basal Plates of Spinal Cord.

Spina Bifida

Spina bifida, one of several neural tube defects, is linked to low folic acid ingestion during the first trimester of pregnancy. Spina bifida is a congenital defect in which the neural tube remains too close to the surface such that the sclerotome cells do not migrate over the tube and form the neural arch of the vertebra (**spina bifida occulta**). This defect occurs most often at the L5 or S1 vertebral level and may present with neurologic findings. If the meninges and CSF protrude as a cyst (**meningocele**) or if the meninges and the cord itself reside in the cyst (**meningomyelocele**), significant neurologic problems often develop.

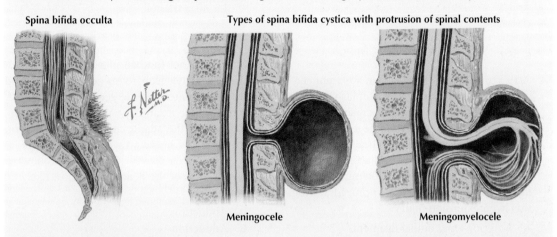

Spina bifida occulta

Types of spina bifida cystica with protrusion of spinal contents

Meningocele

Meningomyelocele

Available Online

2-13 Myofascial Pain

2-14 Acute Spinal Syndromes

Additional figures available online (see inside front cover for details).

Challenge Yourself Questions

1. Besides his other apparent mental deficits, the "hunchback of Notre Dame" also suffered from which of the following conditions?

   A. Halitosis
   B. Kyphosis
   C. Lordosis
   D. Osmosis
   E. Scoliosis

2. You are asked to assist a resident with a lumbar puncture procedure to withdraw a cerebrospinal fluid sample for analysis. Which of the following surface landmarks will help you determine where along the midline of the spine you will insert the spinal needle?

   A. An imaginary line crossing the two iliac crests
   B. An imaginary line crossing the two posterior superior iliac spines
   C. At the level of the 5th lumbar spinous process
   D. At the level of the umbilicus
   E. At the level of the vertebra prominens

3. A 56-year-old man presents with a history of pain for the last 18 months over the right buttock and radiating down the posterior aspect of the thigh and leg. A radiographic examination reveals a herniated disc between the L5 and the S1 vertebral levels. Which of the following nerves is most likely affected by this herniated disc?

   A. L3
   B. L4
   C. L5
   D. S1
   E. S2

4. A 19-year-old man sustained an apparent cervical spine hyperextension ("whiplash") injury after a rear-end roller-coaster crash at a local amusement park. Radiographic examination reveals several cervical vertebral body fractures and the rupture of an adjacent vertebral ligament. Which of the following vertebral ligaments was most likely ruptured during this hyperextension injury?

   A. Anterior longitudinal ligament
   B. Cruciate ligament
   C. Interspinous ligament
   D. Ligamentum flavum
   E. Nuchal ligament

5. A 34-year-old woman presents with a spider bite and a circumscribed area of inflammation on the back of her neck over the T4 dermatome region. Which of the following types of nerve fibers mediate this sensation?

   A. Somatic afferents in T4 ventral root
   B. Somatic afferents in T4 dorsal root
   C. Somatic afferents in T4 ventral ramus
   D. Somatic efferents in T4 ventral root
   E. Somatic efferents in T4 dorsal root
   F. Somatic efferents in T4 ventral ramus

6. A newborn female presents with a congenital neural tube defect likely caused by folic acid deficiency and characterized by failure of the sclerotome to form the neural arch. Which of the following conditions is consistent with this congenital defect?

   A. Osteophyte overgrowth
   B. Osteoporosis
   C. Scoliosis
   D. Spina bifida
   E. Spondylolysis

7. After an automobile crash, a 39-year-old man presents with a headache and midback pain. A radiographic examination reveals trauma to the thoracic spine and bleeding from the anterior and posterior internal vertebral venous plexus. In which of the following regions is this bleeding most likely accumulating?

   A. Central spinal canal
   B. Epidural space
   C. Lumbar triangle
   D. Subarachnoid space
   E. Subdural space

8. A high school football player receives a helmet-to-helmet blow to his head and neck and is brought into the emergency department. A radiographic examination reveals a mild dislocation of the atlanto-axial joint. When you examine his neck, you notice his range of motion is decreased. Which of following movements of the head would most likely be affected?

   A. Abduction
   B. Adduction
   C. Extension
   D. Flexion
   E. Rotation

9. A patient is admitted to the emergency department with a sharp penetrating wound in the upper back region just lateral to the thoracic spine. Based on a quick examination, the physician concludes that several of the dorsal root ganglia are clearly damaged. Which of the following neural elements are most likely compromised by this injury?

   A. Postganglionic efferents
   B. Somatic afferents only
   C. Somatic afferents and efferents
   D. Somatic and visceral afferents
   E. Somatic efferents only

10. A congenital defect that involves the neural crest cells would potentially involve the normal development of which of the following structures?

   A. Anterior spinal artery
   B. Choroid plexus
   C. Dura mater
   D. Intrinsic back muscles
   E. Schwann cells

For each of the following conditions (11-20), select the muscle (A-K) most likely responsible.

A. Erector spinae
B. Latissimus dorsi
C. Levator scapulae
D. Obliquus capitis inferior
E. Rectus capitis posterior major
F. Rhomboid major
G. Rotatores
H. Semispinalis
I. Serratus posterior superior
J. Splenius capitis
K. Trapezius

_____ 11. A work-related injury results in a weakness against resistance in elevation of the scapula and atrophy of one of the lateral neck muscles. The physician suspects damage to a cranial nerve.

_____ 12. An injury results in significant weakness in extension and lateral rotation along the entire length of the spine.

_____ 13. After an automobile crash, a patient presents with radiating pain around the shoulder blades and weakness in elevating the ribs on deep breathing.

_____ 14. An injury to the back results in a weakened ability to extend and medially rotate the upper limb.

_____ 15. Sharp trauma to the back of the neck damages the suboccipital nerve, resulting in a weakened ability to extend and rotate the head to the same side against resistance.

_____ 16. Malformation to the craniocervical portion of the embryonic epaxial (epimere) muscle group that attaches to the ligamentum nuchae results in a weakened ability to extend the neck bilaterally.

_____ 17. Trauma to the lateral neck results in a lesion to the dorsal scapular nerve and a weakened ability to shrug the shoulders.

_____ 18. The loss of innervation to this pair of hypaxial (hypomere) muscles results in a bilateral weakened ability to retract the scapulae but does not affect the ability to elevate the scapulae.

_____ 19. During spinal surgery, these small intrinsic back muscles must be retracted from the lamina and transverse processes of one or two vertebral segments.

_____ 20. During surgery in the neck, the vertebral artery is observed passing just deep to this muscle prior to the artery entering the foramen magnum.

Answers to Challenge Yourself Questions

1. **B.** Kyphosis, or "humpback (hunchback)," is one of several accentuated spinal curvatures. It is commonly observed in the thoracic spine. Halitosis refers to bad breath, and lordosis to the lumbar curvature, either the normal curvature or an accentuated lordosis similar to that observed in women during the third trimester of pregnancy. Osmosis is the passage of a solvent through a semipermeable membrane based on solute concentration, and scoliosis is an abnormal lateral curvature of the spine.

2. **A.** An imaginary line connecting the two iliac crests demarcates the space between the L3 and L4 spinous processes with patients on their side and the spine flexed. Lumbar punctures are usually performed between the L3-L4 or L4-L5 levels to avoid injury to the spinal cord proper, which usually ends as the conus medullaris at the L1-L2 vertebral levels. Below the L2 vertebral level, the nerve roots comprise the cauda equina, suspended in the CSF-filled subarachnoid space.

3. **D.** The nucleus pulposus of the intervertebral discs usually herniates in a posterolateral direction, where it can impinge on the nerve roots passing through the intervertebral foramen. A disc herniating at the L4-L5 level usually impinges on the L5 roots, and herniation at the L5-S1 level involves the S1 roots.

4. **A.** Hyperextension-hyperflexion (whiplash) of the cervical spine can occur when the relaxed neck is thrown backward (hyperextension), tearing the anterior longitudinal ligament. Hyperflexion is usually limited when one's chin hits the sternum. Properly adjusted headrests, if available, can limit the hyperextension.

5. **B.** Sensation from the skin is mediated by somatic afferents (fibers in dorsal root), and the cell bodies of these sensory neurons (pseudounipolar) associated with the T4 dermatome reside in the T4 dorsal root ganglion.

6. **D.** Sclerotome-derived mesoderm normally contributes to the formation of the neural arch (pedicle, lamina, and spinous process), and a folic acid deficiency in the first trimester of pregnancy may contribute to this congenital malformation (spina bifida occulta).

7. B. The internal vertebral venous plexus (Batson's plexus) resides in the epidural fat surrounding the meningeal-encased spinal cord. The epidural space lies between the bony vertebral spinal canal and the dura mater.

8. E. The atlanto-axial joint (atlas and axis) functions in the axial rotational movements of the head. The cranium and atlas move as a unit and rotate side to side on the uniaxial synovial pivot joint between the axis (C2) and atlas (C1).

9. D. The dorsal root ganglia between T1-L2 contain sensory neurons for both somatic and visceral (autonomic) afferent fibers, so both of these modalities would be compromised. Efferent (motor) fibers are not associated with the dorsal root ganglia.

10. E. Of the options, only Schwann cells are derived from the neural crest. While the arachnoid and pia mater are derived from neural crest cells (neither of these choices are options), the dura mater is from mesoderm.

11. K. The only muscle of this group innervated by a cranial nerve is the trapezius, by the accessory nerve (CN XI). The other neck muscle innervated by CN XI is the sternocleidomastoid muscle in the lateral neck.

12. A. The major extensors along the entire length of the spine, also involved in lateral rotation or bending when unilaterally contracted, are the erector spinae group of muscles (spinalis, longissimus, and iliocostalis).

13. I. The only muscles in the list that are associated with the shoulder blades (scapula), attach to the ribs, and elevate them during inspiration are the serratus posterior superior group. These muscles are considered respiratory muscles because they assist in respiratory movements of the ribs.

14. B. The latissimus dorsi extends and medially rotates the upper limb at the shoulder and is the only muscle in this list with these combined actions on the upper limb.

15. E. The suboccipital nerve (dorsal ramus of C1) innervates the suboccipital muscles in the posterior neck, and the rectus capitis posterior major is the only one in the list that extends and rotates the head to the same side.

16. J. The splenius capitis is the only epaxial (intrinsic back muscles innervated by dorsal rami of the spinal nerves) in this list that has significant attachment to the ligamentum nuchae (origin) and exclusively extends the neck when it contracts bilaterally.

17. C. The levator scapulae is innervated by the dorsal scapular nerve (C5) and assists the superior portion of the trapezius in shrugging the shoulders.

18. F. Hypaxial muscles are innervated by the ventral rami of spinal nerves, and the rhomboid major is a hypaxial muscle that retracts the scapulae.

19. G. The rotatores muscles are part of the transversospinales group of muscles that largely fill the spaces between the transverse processes and the spinal processes. Specifically, the rotatores extend between the lamina and transverse processes and stabilize, extend, and rotate the spine.

20. E. The vertebral arteries ascend in the neck by passing through the transverse foramina of C6 to C1, then loop medially and superiorly to the posterior arch of the atlas (C1), pass deep (anterior) to the rectus capitis posterior major muscle, and enter the foramen magnum to supply the posterior portion of the brainstem and brain, and the cerebellum by forming the basilar artery and its branches.

Thorax

1. INTRODUCTION

The thorax lies between the neck and abdomen, encasing the great vessels, heart, and lungs, and provides a conduit for structures passing between the head and neck superiorly and the abdomen, pelvis, and lower limbs inferiorly. Functionally, the thorax and its encased visceral structures are involved in the following:

- **Protection:** the thoracic cage and its muscles protect the vital structures in the thorax.
- **Support:** the thoracic cage provides muscular support for the upper limb.
- **Conduit:** the thorax provides for a superior and an inferior thoracic aperture and a central mediastinum.
- **Segmentation:** the thorax provides an excellent example of segmentation, a hallmark of the vertebrate body plan.
- **Breathing:** movements of the diaphragm and intercostal muscles are essential for expanding the thoracic cavity to facilitate the entry of air into the lungs in the process of breathing.
- **Pumping blood:** the thorax contains the heart, which pumps blood through the pulmonary and systemic circulations.

The sternum, ribs (12 pairs), and thoracic vertebrae (12) encircle the thoracic contents and provide a stable thoracic cage that both protects the visceral structures of the thorax and offers assistance with breathing. Because of the lower extent of the rib cage, the thorax also offers protection for some of the abdominal viscera, including the liver and gallbladder on the right side, the stomach and spleen on the left side, and the adrenal (suprarenal) glands and upper poles of the kidneys on both sides.

The **superior thoracic aperture** (the anatomical *thoracic inlet*) conveys large vessels, important nerves, the thoracic lymphatic duct, the trachea, and the esophagus between the neck and thorax. Clinicians often refer to "thoracic outlet syndrome," which describes symptoms associated with compression of the brachial plexus as it passes over the first rib (specifically, the T1 ventral ramus). Technically, this is a misnomer because these nerves are not exiting the superior thoracic aperture (thoracic inlet). The **inferior thoracic aperture** (the anatomical *thoracic outlet*) conveys the inferior vena cava (IVC), aorta, esophagus, nerves, and thoracic lymphatic duct between the thorax and the abdominal cavity. Additionally, the thorax contains two pleural cavities laterally and a central "middle space" called the **mediastinum,** which is divided as follows (Fig. 3-1):

- **Superior mediastinum:** a midline compartment that lies above an imaginary horizontal plane that passes through the manubrium of the sternum (sternal angle of Louis) and the intervertebral disc between the T4 and T5 vertebrae
- **Inferior mediastinum:** the midline compartment below this same horizontal plane, which is further subdivided into an anterior, middle (contains the heart), and posterior mediastinum

2. SURFACE ANATOMY

Key Landmarks

Key surface landmarks for thoracic structures include the following (Fig. 3-2):

- **Jugular (suprasternal) notch:** a notch marking the level of the second thoracic vertebra, the top of the manubrium, and the

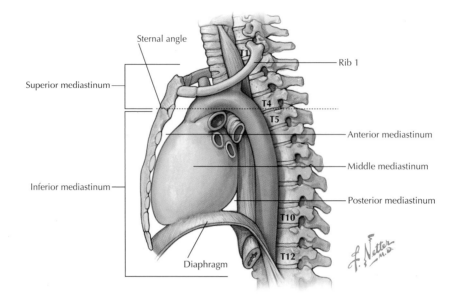

FIGURE 3-1 Subdivisions of the Mediastinum. (From *Atlas of human anatomy*, ed 6, Plate 230.)

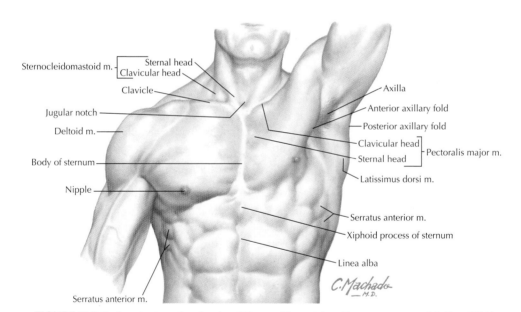

FIGURE 3-2 Surface Anatomy Landmarks of Thorax. (From *Atlas of human anatomy*, ed 6, Plate 178.)

midpoint between the articulation of the two clavicles. The trachea is palpable in the suprasternal notch.

- **Sternal angle (of Louis):** marks the articulation between the manubrium and body of the sternum, the dividing line between the superior and the inferior mediastinum, and the site of articulation of the second ribs (useful for counting ribs and intercostal spaces).

- **Nipple:** marks the T4 dermatome and approximate level of the dome of the diaphragm on the right side.

- **Xiphoid process:** marks the inferior extent of the sternum and the anterior attachment point of the diaphragm.

Planes of Reference

In addition to the sternal angle of Louis, physicians often use other imaginary planes of reference to assist in locating underlying visceral structures of clinical importance. Important vertical planes of reference include the following (Fig. 3-3):

- Midclavicular line
- Anterior axillary line: inferolateral margin of the pectoralis major muscle; demarcates the anterior axillary fold.
- Midaxillary line
- Posterior axillary line: margin of the latissimus dorsi and teres major muscles; demarcates the posterior axillary fold.
- Scapular line: intersects the inferior angles of the scapula.
- Midvertebral line: also called the "posterior median" line.

3. THORACIC WALL

Thoracic Cage

The thoracic cage, which is part of the axial skeleton, includes the thoracic vertebrae, the midline sternum, the 12 pairs of ribs (each with a **head, neck, tubercle,** and **body;** floating ribs 11 and 12 are short and do not have a neck or tubercle), and the costal cartilages (Fig. 3-4). This bony framework provides the scaffolding for attachment of the chest wall muscles and the pectoral girdle, which includes the clavicle and scapula and forms the attachment of the upper limb to the thoracic cage at the shoulder joint (Table 3-1).

Rib fractures can be a painful injury (we must continue to breathe) but are less common in

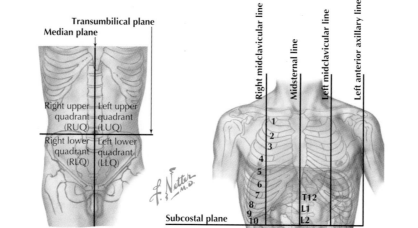

FIGURE 3-3 Planes of Reference for Visceral Structures. (From *Atlas of human anatomy,* ed 6, Plate 244.)

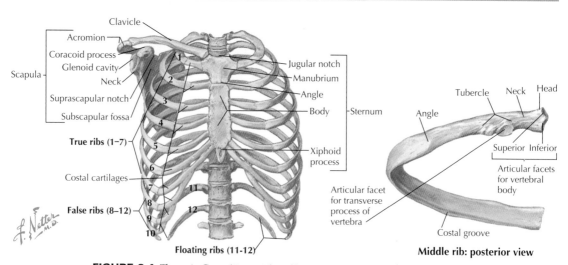

FIGURE 3-4 Thoracic Cage. (From *Atlas of human anatomy,* ed 6, Plates 183 and 184.)

children because their thoracic wall is still fairly elastic. The weakest part of the rib is the angle.

Joints of Thoracic Cage

Joints of the thoracic cage include articulations between the ribs and the sternum and thoracic vertebrae and between the sternum and the clavicle and are summarized in Figure 3-5 and Table 3-2.

Muscles of Anterior Thoracic Wall

The musculature of the anterior thoracic wall include several muscles that attach to the thoracic cage but that actually are muscles that act on the upper limb (Fig. 3-6). These muscles are as follows (for a review, see Chapter 7):

- Pectoralis major
- Pectoralis minor
- Serratus anterior

The *true* anterior thoracic wall muscles fill the intercostal spaces or support the ribs, act on the ribs (elevate or depress the ribs), and keep the intercostal spaces rigid, thereby preventing them

from bulging out during expiration and being drawn in during inspiration (Fig. 3-6 and Table 3-3). Note that the external intercostal muscles are replaced by the anterior intercostal membrane at the costochondral junction anteriorly, and that the internal intercostal muscles extend posteriorly to the angle and then are replaced by the posterior intercostal membrane. The innermost intercostal muscles lie deep to the internal intercostals and extend from the midclavicular line to about the angles of the ribs posteriorly.

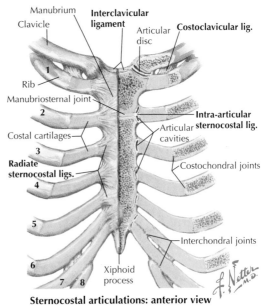

Sternocostal articulations: anterior view

Note: On left side of the rib cage, the sternum and proximal ribs have been shaved down and the ligaments removed to show the bone marrow and articular cavities.

FIGURE 3-5 Joints of Thoracic Cage. (From *Atlas of human anatomy*, ed 6, Plate 184.)

TABLE 3-1 Features of the Thoracic Cage	
STRUCTURE	**CHARACTERISTICS**
Sternum	Long, flat bone composed of the manubrium, body, and xiphoid process
True ribs	Ribs 1-7: articulate with the sternum directly
False ribs	Ribs 8-12: articulate to costal cartilages of the ribs above
Floating ribs	Ribs 11 and 12: articulate with vertebrae only

TABLE 3-2 Joints of the Thoracic Cage		
LIGAMENT	**ATTACHMENT**	**COMMENT**
Sternoclavicular (Saddle-Type Synovial) Joint with an Articular Disc		
Capsule	Clavicle and manubrium	Allows elevation, depression, protraction, retraction, circumduction
Sternoclavicular	Clavicle and manubrium	Consists of anterior and posterior ligaments
Interclavicular	Between both clavicles	Connects two sternoclavicular joints
Costoclavicular	Clavicle to first rib	Anchors clavicle to first rib
Sternocostal (Primary Cartilaginous [Synchondroses]) Joints		
First sternocostal	First rib to manubrium	Allows no movement at this joint
Radiate sternocostal	Ribs 2-7 with sternum	Permit some gliding or sliding movement at these synovial plane joints
Costochondral (Primary Cartilaginous) Joints		
Cartilage	Costal cartilage to rib	Allow no movement at these joints
Interchondral (Synovial Plane) Joints		
Interchondral	Between costal cartilages	Allow some gliding movement

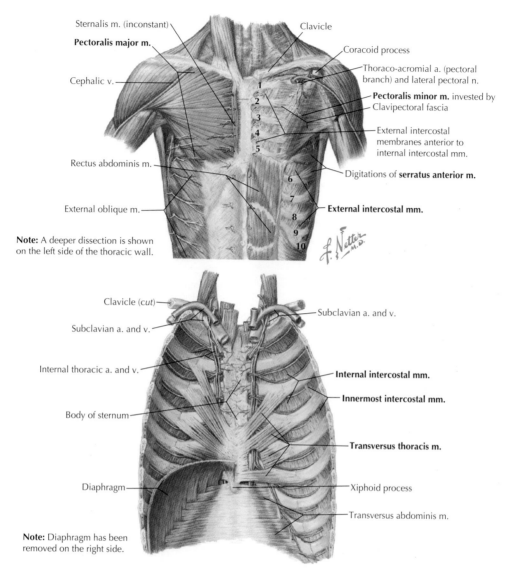

Sternalis m. (inconstant)

Pectoralis major m.

Cephalic v.

Rectus abdominis m.

External oblique m.

Note: A deeper dissection is shown on the left side of the thoracic wall.

Clavicle

Coracoid process

Thoraco-acromial a. (pectoral branch) and lateral pectoral n.

Pectoralis minor m. invested by Clavipectoral fascia

External intercostal membranes anterior to internal intercostal mm.

Digitations of **serratus anterior m.**

External intercostal mm.

Clavicle (*cut*)

Subclavian a. and v.

Internal thoracic a. and v.

Body of sternum

Diaphragm

Note: Diaphragm has been removed on the right side.

Subclavian a. and v.

Internal intercostal mm.

Innermost intercostal mm.

Transversus thoracis m.

Xiphoid process

Transversus abdominis m.

FIGURE 3-6 Muscles of Anterior Thoracic Wall. (From *Atlas of human anatomy,* ed 6, Plates 185 and 187.)

TABLE 3-3 Muscles of the Anterior Thoracic Wall

MUSCLE	SUPERIOR ATTACHMENT (ORIGIN)	INFERIOR ATTACHMENT (INSERTION)	INNERVATION	MAIN ACTIONS
External intercostal	Inferior border of rib above	Superior border of rib below	Intercostal nerves	Elevate ribs, supports intercostal space
Internal intercostal	Inferior border of rib above	Superior border of rib below	Intercostal nerves	Elevate ribs (upper four and five); others depress ribs
Innermost intercostal	Inferior border of rib above	Superior border of rib below	Intercostal nerves	Acts with internal intercostals
Transversus thoracis	Posterior surface of lower sternum	Internal surface of costal cartilages 2-6	Intercostal nerves	Depress ribs
Subcostal	Internal surface of lower rib near their angles	Superior borders of second or third ribs below	Intercostal nerves	Depress ribs
Levator costarum	Transverse processes of C7 and T1-T11	Subjacent ribs between tubercle and angle	Dorsal primary rami of C8-T11	Depress ribs and costal cartilages

Clinical Focus 3-1

Thoracic Cage Injuries

Thoracic cage injuries usually result from trauma and often involve rib fractures (ribs 1 and 2 and 11 and 12 are more protected and often escape being fractured), crush injuries with rib fractures, and penetrating chest wounds such as gunshot and stab wounds. The pain caused by rib fractures can be intense because of the expansion and contraction of the rib cage during respiration, sometimes requiring palliation by anesthetizing the intercostal nerve (nerve block).

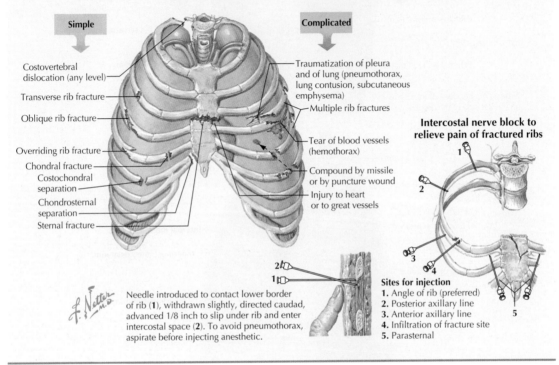

Simple

Costovertebral dislocation (any level)

Transverse rib fracture

Oblique rib fracture

Overriding rib fracture

Chondral fracture
Costochondral separation

Chondrosternal separation

Sternal fracture

Complicated

Traumatization of pleura and of lung (pneumothorax, lung contusion, subcutaneous emphysema)

Multiple rib fractures

Tear of blood vessels (hemothorax)

Compound by missile or by puncture wound

Injury to heart or to great vessels

Intercostal nerve block to relieve pain of fractured ribs

Needle introduced to contact lower border of rib (**1**), withdrawn slightly, directed caudad, advanced 1/8 inch to slip under rib and enter intercostal space (**2**). To avoid pneumothorax, aspirate before injecting anesthetic.

Sites for injection
1. Angle of rib (preferred)
2. Posterior axillary line
3. Anterior axillary line
4. Infiltration of fracture site
5. Parasternal

Intercostal Vessels and Nerves

The **intercostal neurovascular bundles** (vein, artery, and nerve) lie inferior to each rib, running in the costal groove deep to the internal intercostal muscles (Fig. 3-7 and Table 3-4). The veins largely correspond to the arteries and drain into the azygos system of veins or the internal thoracic veins. The intercostal arteries form an anastomotic loop between the internal thoracic artery (branches of anterior intercostal arteries arise here) and the thoracic aorta posteriorly. Posterior intercostal arteries arise from the aorta, except for the first two, which arise from the supreme intercostal artery, a branch of the costocervical trunk of the subclavian artery.

The **intercostal nerves** are the ventral rami of the first 11 thoracic spinal nerves. The 12th thoracic nerve gives rise to the subcostal nerve, which courses inferior to the 12th rib. The nerves give rise to lateral and anterior cutaneous branches

TABLE 3-4 Arteries of the Internal Thoracic Wall	
ARTERY	**COURSE**
Internal thoracic	Arises from subclavian and terminates by dividing into superior epigastric and musculophrenic arteries.
Intercostals	First two posterior branches derived from superior intercostal branch of costocervical trunk and lower nine from thoracic aorta; these anastomose with anterior branches derived from internal thoracic artery (1st-6th spaces) or its musculophrenic branch (7th-9th spaces); the lowest two spaces only have posterior branches.
Subcostal	From aorta, courses inferior to the 12th rib.
Pericardiacophrenic	From internal thoracic and accompanies phrenic nerve.

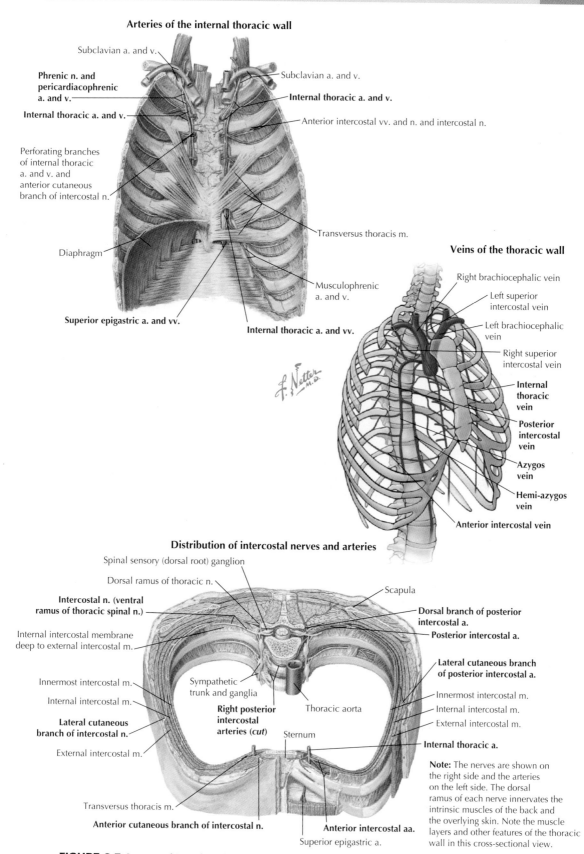

Arteries of the internal thoracic wall

Subclavian a. and v.

Phrenic n. and pericardiacophrenic a. and v.

Internal thoracic a. and v.

Subclavian a. and v.

Internal thoracic a. and v.

Anterior intercostal vv. and n. and intercostal n.

Perforating branches of internal thoracic a. and v. and anterior cutaneous branch of intercostal n.

Transversus thoracis m.

Diaphragm

Veins of the thoracic wall

Right brachiocephalic vein

Left superior intercostal vein

Left brachiocephalic vein

Right superior intercostal vein

Musculophrenic a. and v.

Superior epigastric a. and vv.

Internal thoracic a. and vv.

Internal thoracic vein

Posterior intercostal vein

Azygos vein

Hemi-azygos vein

Anterior intercostal vein

Distribution of intercostal nerves and arteries

Spinal sensory (dorsal root) ganglion

Dorsal ramus of thoracic n.

Intercostal n. (ventral ramus of thoracic spinal n.)

Internal intercostal membrane deep to external intercostal m.

Innermost intercostal m.

Internal intercostal m.

Lateral cutaneous branch of intercostal n.

External intercostal m.

Sympathetic trunk and ganglia

Right posterior intercostal arteries (cut)

Transversus thoracis m.

Anterior cutaneous branch of intercostal n.

Scapula

Dorsal branch of posterior intercostal a.

Posterior intercostal a.

Lateral cutaneous branch of posterior intercostal a.

Innermost intercostal m.

Internal intercostal m.

External intercostal m.

Internal thoracic a.

Thoracic aorta

Sternum

Anterior intercostal aa.

Superior epigastric a.

Note: The nerves are shown on the right side and the arteries on the left side. The dorsal ramus of each nerve innervates the intrinsic muscles of the back and the overlying skin. Note the muscle layers and other features of the thoracic wall in this cross-sectional view.

FIGURE 3-7 Intercostal Vessels and Nerves. (From *Atlas of human anatomy*, ed 6, Plates 187, 188, and 189.)

and branches innervating the intercostal muscles (Fig. 3-7).

Female Breast

The female breast extends from approximately the second to the sixth ribs and from the sternum medially to the midaxillary line laterally. Mammary tissue is composed of compound tubuloacinar glands organized into about 15 to 20 lobes, which are supported and separated from each other by fibrous connective tissue septae (the **suspensory**

ligaments of Cooper) and fat. Each lobe is divided in lobules of secretory acini and their ducts. Features of the breast include the following (Fig. 3-8):

- **Breast:** fatty tissue containing glands that produce milk; lies in the superficial fascia above the **retromammary space,** which lies above the deep pectoral fascia enveloping the pectoralis major muscle.
- **Areola:** circular pigmented skin surrounding the nipple; it contains modified

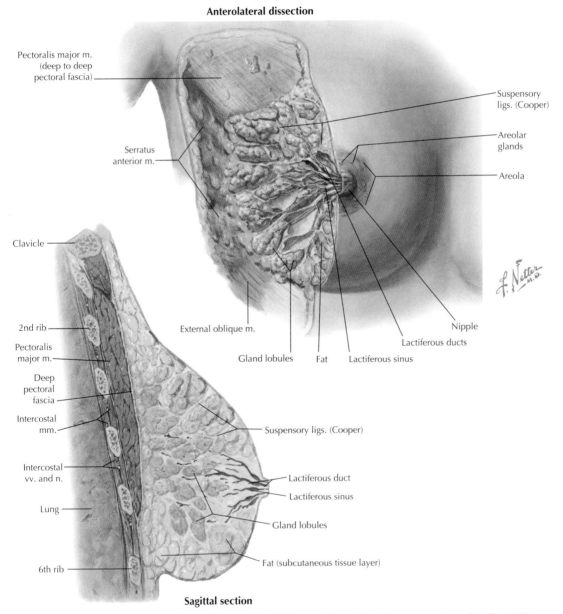

Anterolateral dissection

Pectoralis major m. (deep to deep pectoral fascia)

Serratus anterior m.

Suspensory ligs. (Cooper)

Areolar glands

Areola

Clavicle

2nd rib

Pectoralis major m.

Deep pectoral fascia

Intercostal mm.

Intercostal vv. and n.

Lung

6th rib

External oblique m.

Gland lobules

Fat

Lactiferous sinus

Nipple

Lactiferous ducts

Suspensory ligs. (Cooper)

Lactiferous duct

Lactiferous sinus

Gland lobules

Fat (subcutaneous tissue layer)

Sagittal section

FIGURE 3-8 Anterolateral and Sagittal Views of Female Breast. (From *Atlas of human anatomy,* ed 6, Plate 179.)

sebaceous and sweat glands (glands of Montgomery) that lubricate the nipple and keep it supple.

- **Nipple:** site of opening for the lactiferous ducts; usually lies at about the level of the fourth intercostal space.
- **Axillary tail** (of Spence): extension of mammary tissue superolaterally toward the axilla.
- **Lymphatic system:** lymph is drained from breast tissues; about 75% of lymphatic drainage is to the axillary lymph nodes (Fig. 3-9; see also Fig. 7-11), and the remainder drains to infraclavicular, pectoral, or parasternal nodes.

The primary **arterial supply** to the breast includes the following:

- Anterior intercostal branches of the internal thoracic (mammary) arteries (from the subclavian artery)
- Lateral mammary branches of the lateral thoracic artery (a branch of the axillary artery)
- Thoraco-acromial artery (branch of the axillary artery)

The venous drainage (Fig. 3-9) largely parallels the arterial supply, finally draining into the internal thoracic, axillary, and adjacent intercostal veins.

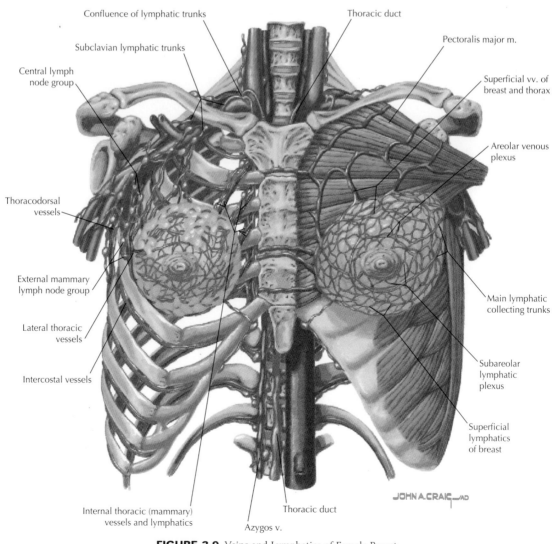

Confluence of lymphatic trunks

Thoracic duct

Subclavian lymphatic trunks

Pectoralis major m.

Central lymph node group

Superficial vv. of breast and thorax

Areolar venous plexus

Thoracodorsal vessels

External mammary lymph node group

Main lymphatic collecting trunks

Lateral thoracic vessels

Subareolar lymphatic plexus

Intercostal vessels

Superficial lymphatics of breast

JOHN A. CRAIG—AD

Internal thoracic (mammary) vessels and lymphatics

Thoracic duct

Azygos v.

FIGURE 3-9 Veins and Lymphatics of Female Breast.

Clinical Focus 3-2

Fibrocystic Breast Disease

Fibrocystic change (disease) is a general term covering a large group of benign conditions occurring in about 80% of women that are often related to cyclic changes in maturation and involution of glandular tissue. **Fibroadenoma,** the second most common tumor of the breast after carcinoma, is a benign neoplasm of glandular epithelium and is usually accompanied by a significant increase in connective tissue stroma. Both conditions present as palpable masses and warrant follow-up evaluation.

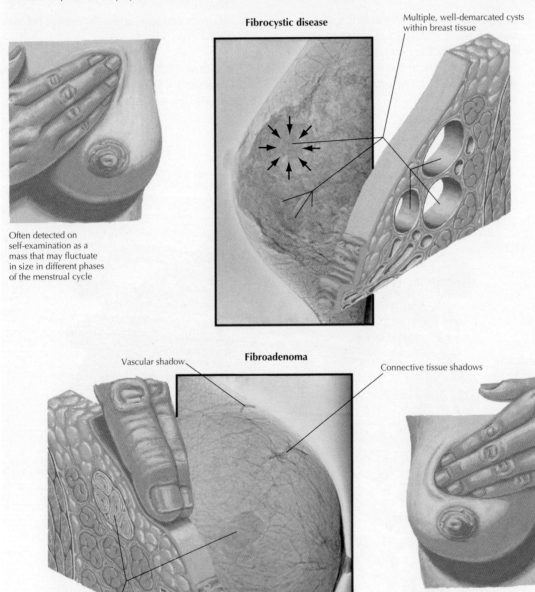

Fibrocystic disease

Multiple, well-demarcated cysts within breast tissue

Often detected on self-examination as a mass that may fluctuate in size in different phases of the menstrual cycle

Fibroadenoma

Vascular shadow

Connective tissue shadows

Fibroadenoma

Usually palpated as a solitary, smooth, firm, well-demarcated nodule

JOHN A.CRAIG__AD

Breast Cancer

Breast cancer is the most common malignancy in women; approximately two thirds of all cases occur in postmenopausal women. Invasive carcinoma may involve the suspensory ligaments, causing retraction of the ligaments and dimpling of the overlying skin. Additionally, invasion and obstruction of the subcutaneous lymphatics can result in dilation and skin edema, creating an "orange peel" appearance (peau d'orange). About 50% of cancers develop in the upper outer quadrant (quadrant closest to the axilla, which includes the axillary tail). Distant sites of metastasis include the following:

- Lungs and pleura
- Liver
- Bones
- Brain

Nipple retraction

Carcinomatous involvement of mammary ducts may cause duct shortening and retraction or inversion of nipple.

Retraction of nipple

Carcinoma involving mammary ducts

Retraction of nipple

Skin edema

Carcinoma

Subcutaneous lymphatics

Skin edema with peau d'orange appearance

Lymph accumulation

Skin gland orifices

Involvement and obstruction of subcutaneous lymphatic by tumor result in lymphatic dilatation and lymph accumulation in the skin. Resultant edema creates "orange peel" appearance due to prominence of skin gland orifices.

JOHN A. CRAIG—AD

Skin dimpling

Dimpling of skin over a carcinoma is caused by involvement and retraction of suspensory (Cooper's) ligaments.

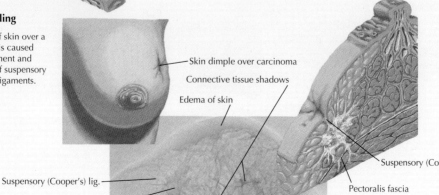

Skin dimple over carcinoma

Connective tissue shadows

Edema of skin

Suspensory (Cooper's) lig.

Pectoralis fascia

Suspensory (Cooper's) lig.

Carcinoma

Partial Mastectomy

Several clinical options are available to treat breast cancer, including systemic approaches (chemotherapy, hormonal therapy, immunotherapy) and "local" approaches (radiation therapy, surgery). In a partial mastectomy, also called "lumpectomy" or "quadrantectomy," the surgeon performs a breast-conserving surgery that removes the portion of the breast that harbors the tumor along with a halo of normal surrounding breast tissue. Because of the possibility of lymphatic spread, especially to the **axillary nodes,** an incision also may be made for a sentinel node biopsy to examine the first axillary node, which is likely to be invaded by metastatic cancer cells from the breast.

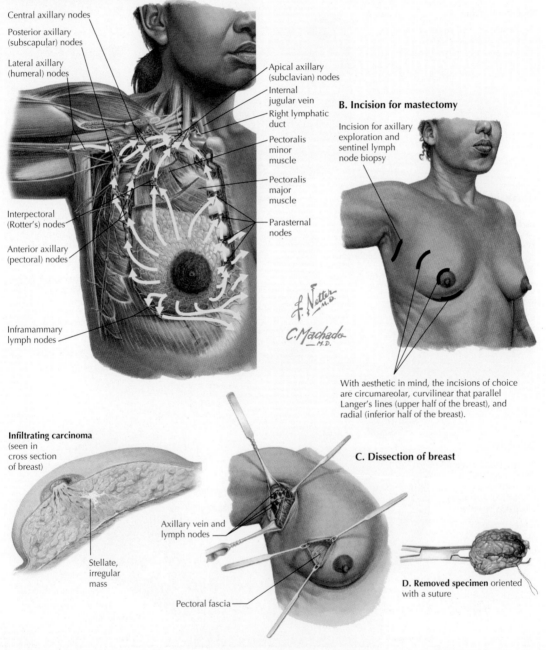

A. Breast nodes and carcinoma

Central axillary nodes

Posterior axillary (subscapular) nodes

Lateral axillary (humeral) nodes

Apical axillary (subclavian) nodes

Internal jugular vein

Right lymphatic duct

Pectoralis minor muscle

Pectoralis major muscle

Interpectoral (Rotter's) nodes

Anterior axillary (pectoral) nodes

Parasternal nodes

Inframammary lymph nodes

B. Incision for mastectomy

Incision for axillary exploration and sentinel lymph node biopsy

With aesthetic in mind, the incisions of choice are circumareolar, curvilinear that parallel Langer's lines (upper half of the breast), and radial (inferior half of the breast).

Infiltrating carcinoma (seen in cross section of breast)

Stellate, irregular mass

C. Dissection of breast

Axillary vein and lymph nodes

Pectoral fascia

D. Removed specimen oriented with a suture

Modified Radical Mastectomy

In addition to breast-conserving surgery, several more invasive mastectomy approaches may be indicated, depending on a variety of factors, as follows:

- **Total (simple) mastectomy:** the whole breast is removed, with or without some axillary lymph nodes if indicated, down to the retromammary space.
- **Modified radical mastectomy** (illustrated here): the whole breast is removed along with most of the axillary and pectoral lymph nodes, axillary fat, and the investing fascia over the chest wall muscles. Care is taken to preserve the pectoralis, serratus anterior, and latissimus dorsi muscles and the long thoracic and thoracodorsal nerves to the latter two, respectively. Damage to the long thoracic nerve results in "winging" of the scapula, and damage to the thoracodorsal nerve weakens extension at the shoulder.
- **Radical mastectomy:** the whole breast is removed along with the axillary lymph nodes, fat, and chest wall muscles (pectoralis major and minor); use of the radical surgical approach is much less common now.

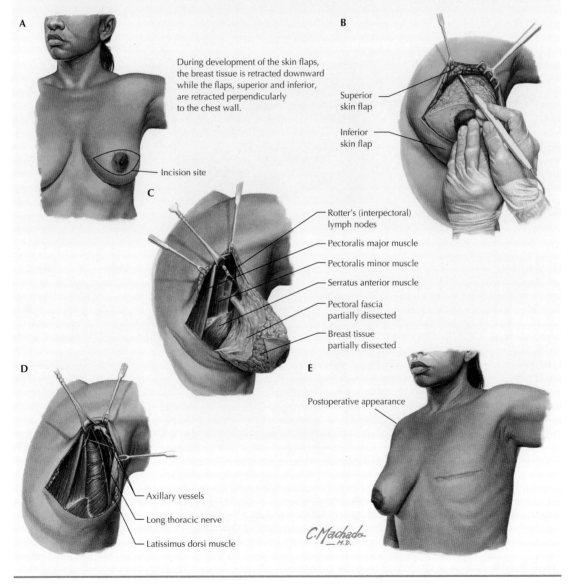

A

During development of the skin flaps, the breast tissue is retracted downward while the flaps, superior and inferior, are retracted perpendicularly to the chest wall.

Incision site

B

Superior skin flap

Inferior skin flap

C

Rotter's (interpectoral) lymph nodes

Pectoralis major muscle

Pectoralis minor muscle

Serratus anterior muscle

Pectoral fascia partially dissected

Breast tissue partially dissected

D

Axillary vessels

Long thoracic nerve

Latissimus dorsi muscle

E

Postoperative appearance

C. Machado
—M.D.

4. PLEURA AND LUNGS

Pleural Spaces (Cavities)

The thorax is divided into the following three compartments:

- Right pleural space
- Left pleural space
- Mediastinum: a "middle space" lying between the pleural spaces

The lungs lie within the **pleural cavity** (right and left) (Fig. 3-10). This "potential space" is between the investing **visceral pleura,** which closely envelops each lung, and the **parietal pleura,** which reflects off each lung and lines the inner aspect of the thoracic wall, the superior surface of the diaphragm, and the sides of the pericardial sac (Table 3-5). Normally, the pleural cavity contains a small amount of serous fluid, which lubricates the surfaces and reduces friction

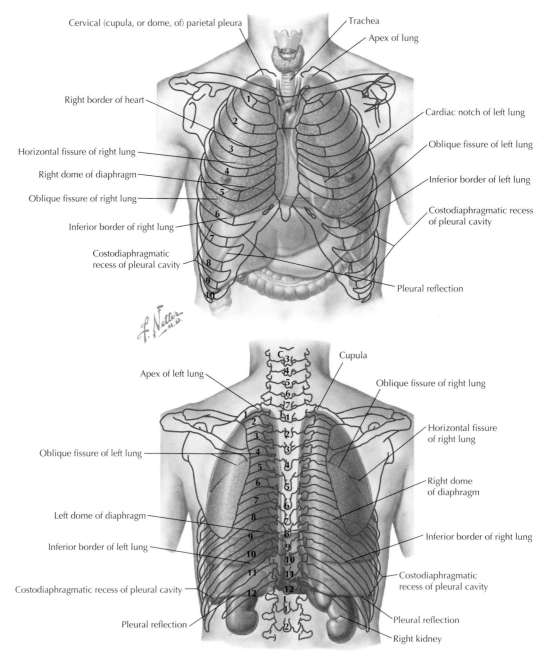

FIGURE 3-10 Anterior and Posterior Topography of the Pleura and Lungs. (From *Atlas of human anatomy,* ed 6, Plates 193 and 194.)

TABLE 3-5 Pleural Features and Recesses

STRUCTURE	DEFINITION
Cupula	Dome of cervical parietal pleura extending above the first rib
Parietal pleura	Membrane that in descriptive terms includes costal, mediastinal, diaphragmatic, and cervical (cupula) pleura
Pleural reflections	Points at which parietal pleurae reflect off one surface and extend onto another (e.g., costal to diaphragmatic)
Pleural recesses	Reflection points at which lung does not fully extend into the pleural space (e.g., costodiaphragmatic, costomediastinal)

during respiration. The parietal pleura is richly innervated with afferent fibers that course in the somatic intercostal nerves and, over the surface of the diaphragm, the phrenic nerve (C3-C5); the visceral pleura has few, if any, pain fibers.

Clinically, it is important for physicians to be able to "visualize" the extent of the lungs and pleural cavities topographically on the surface of their patients (Fig. 3-10). The lungs lie adjacent to the parietal pleura inferiorly to the sixth costal cartilage. (Note the presence of the cardiac notch on the left side.) Beyond this point, the lungs do not occupy the full extent of the pleural cavity during quiet respiration. These points are important to know if one needs access to the pleural cavity without injuring the lungs (Table 3-6), such as to drain inflammatory exudate **(pleural effusion),** hemorrhage into the cavity **(hemothorax),** or air **(pneumothorax).** In quiet respiration, the lung margins reside two ribs above the extent of the pleural cavity at the midclavicular, midaxillary, and midscapular lines.

The Lungs

The paired lungs are invested in the visceral pleura and are attached to mediastinal structures (trachea

TABLE 3-6 Surface Landmarks of the Pleura and Lungs

LANDMARK	MARGIN OF LUNG	MARGIN OF PLEURA
Midclavicular line	6th rib	8th rib
Midaxillary line	8th rib	10th rib
Midscapular line	10th rib	12th rib

and heart) at their hilum. Each lung possesses the following surfaces:

- **Apex:** superior part of the upper lobe that extends into the root of the neck (above the clavicles).
- **Hilum:** area located on the medial aspect through which structures enter and leave the lung.
- **Costal:** anterior, lateral, and posterior aspects of the lung in contact with the costal elements of the internal thoracic cage.
- **Diaphragmatic:** inferior part of the lung in contact with the underlying diaphragm.

The right lung has three lobes and is slightly larger than the left lung, which has two lobes. Both lungs are composed of spongy and elastic tissue, which readily expands and contracts to conform to the internal contours of the thoracic cage (Fig. 3-11 and Table 3-7).

The lung's parenchyma is supplied by several small **bronchial arteries** that arise from the proximal portion of the descending thoracic aorta. Usually, one small right bronchial artery and a pair of left bronchial arteries (superior and inferior) can be found on the posterior aspect of the main bronchi. Although much of this blood returns to the heart via the pulmonary veins, some also collects into small **bronchial veins** that drain into the azygos system of veins (see Fig. 3-25).

The lymphatic drainage of both lungs is to **pulmonary** (intrapulmonary) and **bronchopulmonary** (hilar) nodes (i.e., from distal sites to the proximal hilum). Lymph then drains into **tracheobronchial** nodes at the tracheal bifurcation and into right and left **paratracheal** nodes (Fig. 3-12).

As visceral structures, the lungs are innervated by the autonomic nervous system. **Sympathetic bronchodilator** fibers, which relax smooth muscle, arise from upper thoracic spinal cord segments. **Parasympathetic bronchoconstrictor** fibers, which contract smooth muscle and increase mucus secretion, arise from the vagus nerve.

Respiration

During *quiet inspiration* the contraction of the diaphragm alone accounts for most of the decrease in intrapleural pressure, allowing air to expand the lungs. Active inspiration occurs when the diaphragm and intercostal muscles together increase the diameter of the thoracic wall, decreasing

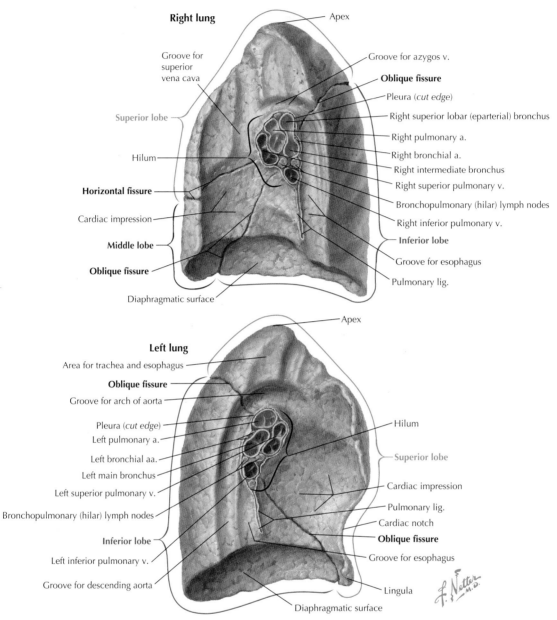

FIGURE 3-11 Features of Medial Aspect of the Lungs. (From *Atlas of human anatomy,* ed 6, Plate 196.)

TABLE 3-7 External Features of the Lungs

STRUCTURE	CHARACTERISTICS	STRUCTURE	CHARACTERISTICS
Lobes	Three lobes (superior, middle, inferior) in right lung; two in left lung	Lingula	Tongue-shaped feature of left lung
		Cardiac notch	Indentation for the heart, in left lung
Horizontal fissure	Only on right lung, extends along line of fourth rib	Pulmonary ligament	Double layer of parietal pleura hanging from the hilum that marks reflection of visceral pleura to parietal pleura
Oblique fissure	On both lungs, extends from T2 vertebra to sixth costal cartilage		
Impressions	Made by adjacent structures, in fixed lungs	Bronchopulmonary segment	10 functional segments in each lung supplied by a segmental bronchus and a segmental artery from the pulmonary artery
Hilum	Points at which structures (bronchus, vessels, nerves, lymphatics) enter or leave lungs		

Chest Drainage Tubes

A chest tube provides a way to evacuate air or fluids (blood, pus) from the pleural cavity, thus reapposing the parietal and visceral pleura and enhancing the patient's ability to breathe normally. Following administration of a local anesthetic, the tube is inserted close to the upper border of a rib to avoid the neurovascular bundle, which runs in the costal groove at the inferior margin of each rib.

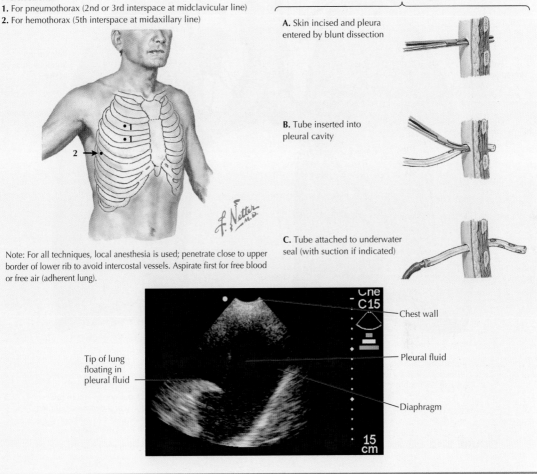

Preferred sites
1. For pneumothorax (2nd or 3rd interspace at midclavicular line)
2. For hemothorax (5th interspace at midaxillary line)

Hemostat technique

A. Skin incised and pleura entered by blunt dissection

B. Tube inserted into pleural cavity

C. Tube attached to underwater seal (with suction if indicated)

Note: For all techniques, local anesthesia is used; penetrate close to upper border of lower rib to avoid intercostal vessels. Aspirate first for free blood or free air (adherent lung).

Chest wall

Pleural fluid

Tip of lung floating in pleural fluid

Diaphragm

Cne C15

15 cm

---

intrapleural pressure even more. Although the first rib is stationary, ribs 2 to 6 tend to increase the anteroposterior diameter of the chest wall, and the lower ribs mainly increase the transverse diameter. Accessory muscles of inspiration that attach to the thoracic cage may also assist in very deep inspiration.

During *quiet expiration* the elastic recoil of the lungs and thoracic cage expel the air. In forced expiration the abdominal muscles contract and, by compressing the abdominal viscera superiorly,

raise the intraabdominal pressure and force the diaphragm upward. Having the "wind knocked out of you" shows how forceful this maneuver can be.

Trachea and Bronchi

The **trachea** is a single midline airway that extends from the cricoid cartilage to its bifurcation at the sternal angle of Louis. It lies anterior to the esophagus and is rigidly supported by 16 to 20 **C**-shaped cartilaginous rings (Fig. 3-13 and Table 3-8). The

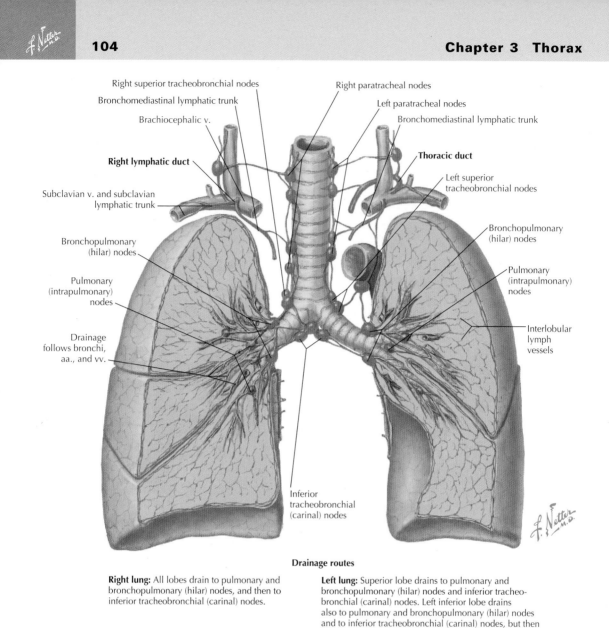

Right superior tracheobronchial nodes

Bronchomediastinal lymphatic trunk

Brachiocephalic v.

Right lymphatic duct

Subclavian v. and subclavian
lymphatic trunk

Bronchopulmonary
(hilar) nodes

Pulmonary
(intrapulmonary)
nodes

Drainage
follows bronchi,
aa., and vv.

Right paratracheal nodes

Left paratracheal nodes

Bronchomediastinal lymphatic trunk

Thoracic duct

Left superior
tracheobronchial nodes

Bronchopulmonary
(hilar) nodes

Pulmonary
(intrapulmonary)
nodes

Interlobular
lymph
vessels

Inferior
tracheobronchial
(carinal) nodes

Drainage routes

Right lung: All lobes drain to pulmonary and bronchopulmonary (hilar) nodes, and then to inferior tracheobronchial (carinal) nodes.

Left lung: Superior lobe drains to pulmonary and bronchopulmonary (hilar) nodes and inferior tracheo-bronchial (carinal) nodes. Left inferior lobe drains also to pulmonary and bronchopulmonary (hilar) nodes and to inferior tracheobronchial (carinal) nodes, but then mostly to right superior tracheobronchial nodes, where it follows same route as lymph from right lung.

FIGURE 3-12 Lymphatic Drainage Routes of the Lungs. (From *Atlas of human anatomy*, ed 6, Plate 205.)

trachea may be displaced if adjacent structures become enlarged (usually the thyroid gland or aortic arch).

The trachea bifurcates inferiorly into a **right main bronchus** and a **left main bronchus,** which enter the hilum of the right lung and the left lung, respectively, and immediately divide into **lobar (secondary) bronchi** (Fig. 3-13). The right main bronchus often gives rise to the superior lobar (eparterial) bronchus just before entering the hilum of the right lung. Each lobar bronchus then divides again into **tertiary bronchi** supplying the 10 bronchopulmonary segments of each lung (sometimes the left lung may have 8 to 10

segments) (Fig. 3-13 and Tables 3-7 and 3-8). The **bronchopulmonary segments** are lung segments that are supplied by a tertiary bronchus and a segmental artery of the pulmonary artery that passes to each lung. The bronchi and respiratory airways continue to divide into smaller and smaller passageways until they terminate in alveolar sacs (about 23 divisional generations from the right and left main bronchi). Gas exchange occurs only in these most distal respiratory regions.

The right main bronchus is shorter, more vertical, and wider than the left main bronchus. Therefore, aspirated objects often pass more easily into the right main bronchus and right lung.

Pulmonary Embolism

The lungs naturally filter **venous clots** larger than circulating blood cells and can usually accommodate small clots because of their fibrinolytic ("clot buster") mechanisms. However, pulmonary embolism (PE) is the cause of death in 10% to 15% of hospitalized patients. **Thromboemboli** originate from deep leg veins in approximately 95% of cases. Major causes are called *Virchow's triad* and include the following:

- Venous stasis (e.g., caused by extended bed rest)
- Trauma (e.g., fracture, tissue injury)
- Coagulation disorders (inherited or acquired)

Other contributors to PE include postoperative and postpartum immobility and some hormone medications that increase the risk of blood clots. About 60% to 80% of PEs are "silent" because they are small; larger emboli may obstruct medium-sized vessels and lead to infarction or even obstruction of a vessel as large as the pulmonary trunk (saddle embolism). PE without infarction is common and presents as tachypnea, anxiety, dyspnea, and vague substernal pressure. Saddle embolus, on the other hand, is an emergency that can precipitate acute cor pulmonale (right-sided heart failure) and circulatory collapse.

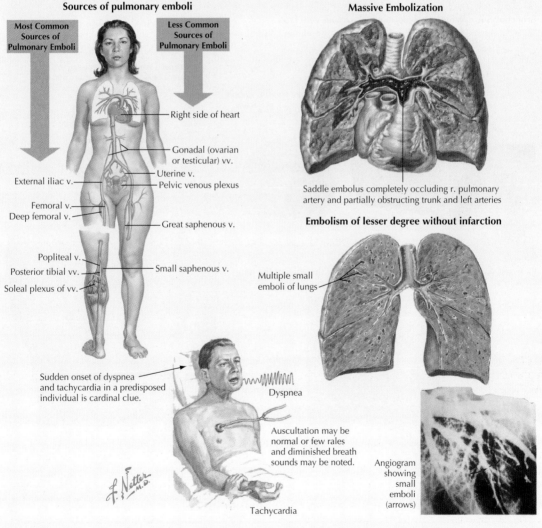

Sources of pulmonary emboli

Most Common Sources of Pulmonary Emboli

Less Common Sources of Pulmonary Emboli

Right side of heart

Gonadal (ovarian or testicular) vv.

Uterine v.

External iliac v.

Pelvic venous plexus

Femoral v.

Deep femoral v.

Great saphenous v.

Popliteal v.

Posterior tibial vv.

Small saphenous v.

Soleal plexus of vv.

Massive Embolization

Saddle embolus completely occluding r. pulmonary artery and partially obstructing trunk and left arteries

Embolism of lesser degree without infarction

Multiple small emboli of lungs

Sudden onset of dyspnea and tachycardia in a predisposed individual is cardinal clue.

Dyspnea

Auscultation may be normal or few rales and diminished breath sounds may be noted.

Angiogram showing small emboli (arrows)

Tachycardia

Clinical Focus 3-8

Lung Cancer

Lung cancer is the leading cause of cancer-related death. It arises either from alveolar lining cells of the lung parenchyma or from the epithelium of the tracheobronchial tree. Although there are a number of types, **squamous cell (bronchiogenic) carcinoma** and **adenocarcinoma** (from intrapulmonary bronchi) are the most common types. Bronchiogenic carcinoma may impinge on adjacent anatomical structures. For example, in **Pancoast syndrome** the tumor may spread to involve the sympathetic trunk and compromise the sympathetic tone to the head. This may lead to **Horner's syndrome,** characterized by the following symptoms on the affected side:

- **Miosis:** constricted pupil
- **Ptosis:** minor drooping of the upper eyelid
- **Anhidrosis:** lack of sweating
- **Flushing:** subcutaneous vasodilation

Additionally, the neurovascular components passing into the upper limb (trunks of the brachial plexus and subclavian artery) may be affected, resulting in paresthesia in the neck, head, shoulder, and limb, with 90% affecting areas of ulnar nerve distribution (C8-T1).

Bronchogenic carcinoma: epidermoid (squamous cell) type

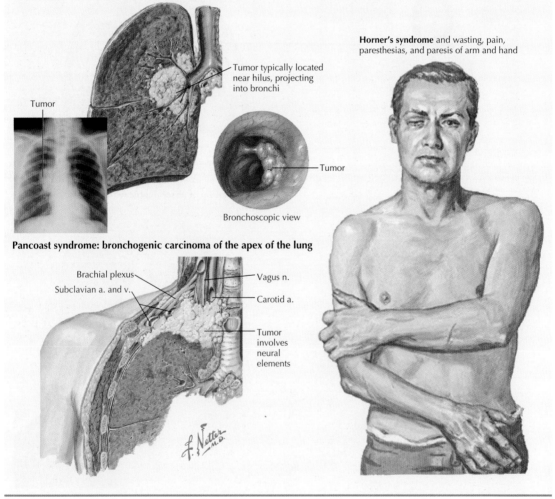

Tumor

Tumor typically located near hilus, projecting into bronchi

Tumor

Bronchoscopic view

Horner's syndrome and wasting, pain, paresthesias, and paresis of arm and hand

Pancoast syndrome: bronchogenic carcinoma of the apex of the lung

Brachial plexus

Subclavian a. and v.

Vagus n.

Carotid a.

Tumor involves neural elements

Clinical Focus 3-9

Chronic Obstructive Pulmonary Disease

Chronic obstructive pulmonary disease (COPD) is a broad classification of obstructive lung diseases, the most familiar being **chronic bronchitis, asthma,** and **emphysema.** Emphysema is characterized by permanent enlargement of air spaces at and distal to the respiratory bronchioles, with destruction of the bronchiole walls by inflammation. As a result, lung compliance increases because the elastic recoil of the lung decreases, causing collapse of the airways during expiration. This increases the work of expiration as patients try to force air from their diseased lungs. This can lead to a "barrel-chested" appearance caused by hypertrophy of the intercostal muscles. Smoking is a major risk factor for COPD.

Gross specimen. Involvement tends to be most marked in upper part of lung.

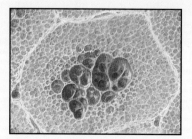

Magnified section. Distended, intercommunicating, saclike spaces in central area of acini.

Clinical Focus 3-10

Idiopathic Pulmonary Fibrosis

Idiopathic pulmonary fibrosis is a chronic restrictive lung disease. Chronic restrictive lung diseases account for approximately 15% of noninfectious lung diseases and include a diverse group of disorders with reduced compliance that cause chronic inflammation, fibrosis, and the need for more pressure to inflate the stiffened lungs. This is a poorly understood **interstitial fibrotic disorder,** perhaps caused by an injurious environmental or occupational agent, which leads to hypoxemia and cyanosis. Men are affected more often than women, and most patients are diagnosed between ages 30 and 50.

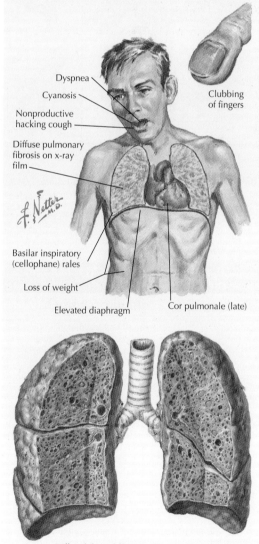

Dyspnea

Cyanosis

Nonproductive hacking cough

Diffuse pulmonary fibrosis on x-ray film

Clubbing of fingers

Basilar inspiratory (cellophane) rales

Loss of weight

Elevated diaphragm

Cor pulmonale (late)

Diffuse bilateral fibrosis of lungs with multiple small cysts giving honeycomb appearance

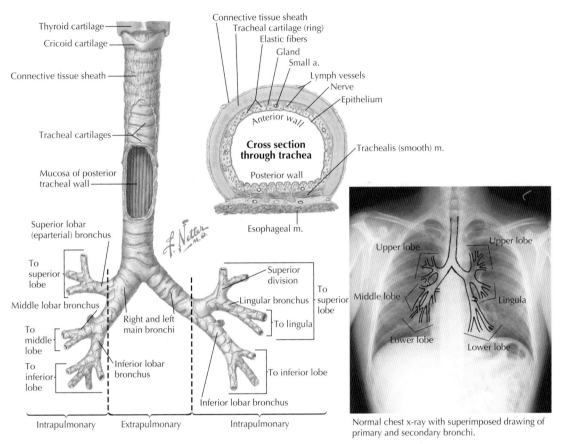

Normal chest x-ray with superimposed drawing of primary and secondary bronchi.

FIGURE 3-13 Trachea and Bronchi. (From *Atlas of human anatomy*, ed 6, Plate 199; chest radiograph from Major NM: *A practical approach to radiology*, Philadelphia, 2006, Saunders.)

TABLE 3-8 Features of the Trachea and Bronchi

STRUCTURE	CHARACTERISTICS
Trachea	Approximately 5 inches (10 cm) long and 1 inch in diameter; courses inferiorly anterior to esophagus and posterior to aortic arch
Cartilaginous rings	Are 16-20 C-shaped rings
Bronchus	Divides into right and left main (primary) bronchi at level of sternal angle of Louis
Right bronchus	Shorter, wider, and more vertical than left bronchus; aspirated foreign objects more likely to pass into right bronchus
Carina	Internal, keel-like cartilage at bifurcation of trachea
Secondary bronchi	Supply lobes of each lung (three on right, two on left)
Tertiary bronchi	Supply bronchopulmonary segments (10 for each lung)

5. PERICARDIUM AND HEART

The Pericardium

The pericardium and heart lie within the **middle mediastinum.** The heart is enclosed within a fibroserous pericardial pouch that extends and blends into the adventitia of the great vessels that enter or leave the heart. The pericardium has a **fibrous outer layer** that is lined internally by a serous layer, the **parietal serous layer,** which then reflects onto the heart and becomes the **visceral serous layer,** which is the outer covering of the heart itself, also known as the **epicardium** (Fig. 3-14 and Table 3-9). These two serous layers form a potential space known as the **pericardial sac (cavity).**

The Heart

The heart is essentially two muscular pumps in series. The two atria contract in unison, followed

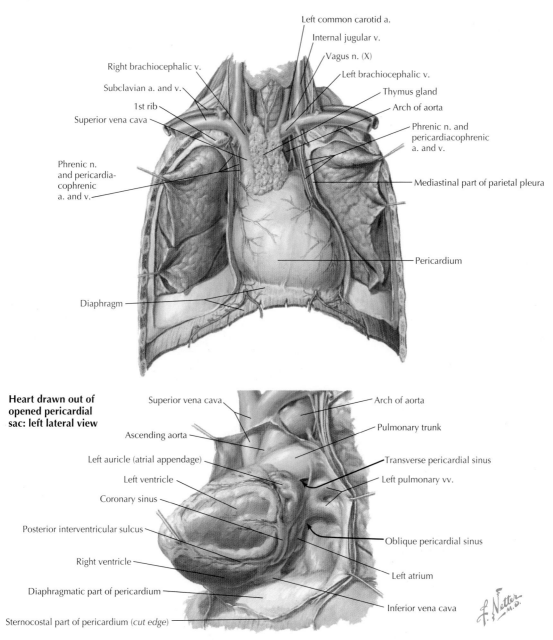

FIGURE 3-14 Pericardium and Pericardial Sac. (From *Atlas of human anatomy,* ed 6, Plates 208 and 212.)

TABLE 3-9 Features of the Pericardium			
STRUCTURE	**DEFINITION**	**STRUCTURE**	**DEFINITION**
Fibrous pericardium	Tough, outer layer that reflects onto great vessels	Transverse sinus	Space posterior to aorta and pulmonary trunk; can clamp vessels with fingers in this sinus and above
Serous pericardium	Layer that lines inner aspect of fibrous pericardium (parietal layer); reflects onto heart as epicardium (visceral layer)		
		Oblique sinus	Pericardial space posterior to heart
Innervation	Phrenic nerve (C3-C5) for conveying pain; vasomotor innervation via sympathetics		

Clinical Focus 3-11

Cardiac Tamponade

Cardiac tamponade can result from fluid accumulation or bleeding into the pericardial sac. Bleeding may be caused by a ruptured aortic aneurysm, a ruptured myocardial infarct, or a penetrating injury that compromises the beating heart and decreases venous return and cardiac output. The fluid can be removed by a **pericardial tap** (i.e., withdrawn by a needle and syringe).

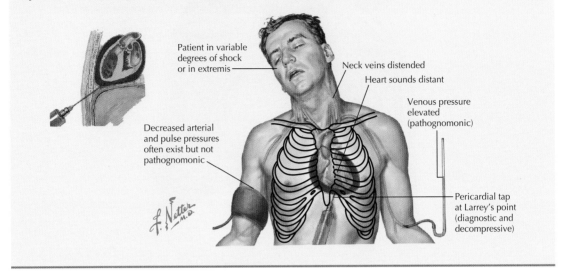

Patient in variable degrees of shock or in extremis

Decreased arterial and pulse pressures often exist but not pathognomonic

Neck veins distended

Heart sounds distant

Venous pressure elevated (pathognomonic)

Pericardial tap at Larrey's point (diagnostic and decompressive)

---

by contraction of the two ventricles. The right side of the heart receives the blood from the systemic circulation and pumps it into the pulmonary circulation of the lungs. The left side of the heart receives the blood from the pulmonary circulation and pumps it into the systemic circulation, thus perfusing the organs and tissues of the entire body, including the heart itself. In situ, the heart is oriented in the middle mediastinum and has the following descriptive relationships (Fig. 3-15):

- **Anterior (sternocostal):** the right atrium, right ventricle, and part of the left ventricle
- **Posterior (base):** the left atrium
- **Inferior (diaphragmatic):** some of the right ventricle and most of the left ventricle
- **Acute angle:** the sharp right ventricular margin of the heart
- **Obtuse angle:** the more rounded left margin of the heart
- **Apex:** the inferolateral part of the left ventricle at the fourth to fifth intercostal space

The **atrioventricular groove** (coronary sulcus) separates the two atria from the ventricles and marks the locations of the right coronary artery and the circumflex branch of the left coronary artery. The **anterior** and **posterior interventricular grooves** mark the locations of the left anterior descending (anterior interventricular) branch of the left coronary artery and the posterior descending (posterior interventricular) artery, respectively.

Coronary Arteries and Cardiac Veins

The right and left coronary arteries arise immediately superior to the right and left cusps, respectively, of the aortic semilunar valve (Fig. 3-16). The **right coronary artery** passes between the pulmonary trunk and right atrium in the right atrioventricular groove and passes around the acute angle of the heart. The **left coronary artery** passes behind the pulmonary trunk, reaches the left atrioventricular groove and divides into the anterior interventricular and circumflex branches. During ventricular diastole, blood enters the coronary arteries to supply the myocardium of each chamber. About 5% of the cardiac output goes to the heart itself.

The corresponding **great cardiac vein, middle cardiac vein,** and **small cardiac vein** parallel the left anterior descending (LAD) branch of the left coronary artery, the posterior descending artery

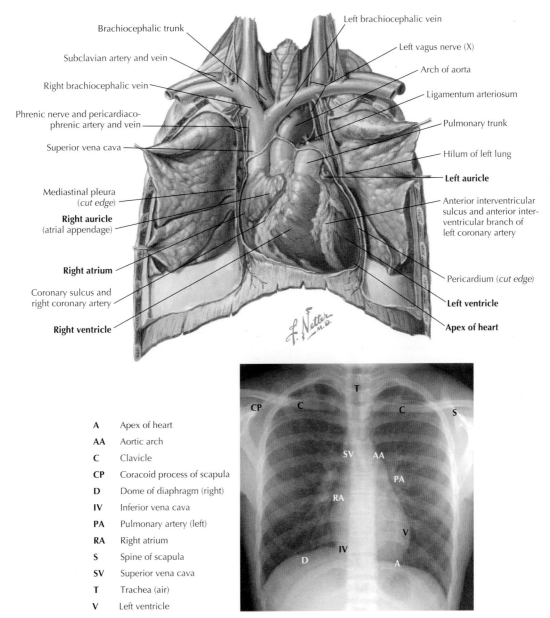

FIGURE 3-15 Anterior In Situ Exposure of the Heart. (From *Atlas of human anatomy,* ed 6, Plate 209.)

The labels in the figure include:

Brachiocephalic trunk
Subclavian artery and vein
Right brachiocephalic vein
Phrenic nerve and pericardiaco-phrenic artery and vein
Superior vena cava
Mediastinal pleura (*cut edge*)
Right auricle (atrial appendage)
Right atrium
Coronary sulcus and right coronary artery
Right ventricle

Left brachiocephalic vein
Left vagus nerve (X)
Arch of aorta
Ligamentum arteriosum
Pulmonary trunk
Hilum of left lung
Left auricle
Anterior interventricular sulcus and anterior interventricular branch of left coronary artery
Pericardium (*cut edge*)
Left ventricle
Apex of heart

A	Apex of heart
AA	Aortic arch
C	Clavicle
CP	Coracoid process of scapula
D	Dome of diaphragm (right)
IV	Inferior vena cava
PA	Pulmonary artery (left)
RA	Right atrium
S	Spine of scapula
SV	Superior vena cava
T	Trachea (air)
V	Left ventricle

TABLE 3-10 Coronary Arteries and Cardiac Veins

VESSEL	COURSE	VESSEL	COURSE
Right coronary artery	Consists of major branches: sinu-atrial (SA) nodal, right marginal, posterior interventricular (posterior descending), atrioventricular (AV) nodal	Middle cardiac vein	Parallels posterior descending artery (PDA), and drains into coronary sinus
Left coronary artery	Consists of major branches: circumflex, anterior interventricular (left anterior descending [LAD]), left marginal	Small cardiac vein	Parallels right marginal artery and drains into coronary sinus
		Anterior cardiac veins	Several small veins that drain directly into right atrium
Great cardiac vein	Parallels LAD artery and drains into coronary sinus	Smallest cardiac veins	Drain through the cardiac wall directly into all four heart chambers

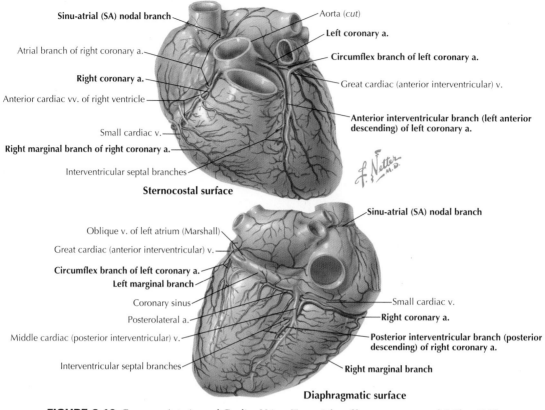

Sinu-atrial (SA) nodal branch

Atrial branch of right coronary a.

Right coronary a.

Anterior cardiac vv. of right ventricle

Small cardiac v.

Right marginal branch of right coronary a.

Interventricular septal branches

Aorta (*cut*)

Left coronary a.

Circumflex branch of left coronary a.

Great cardiac (anterior interventricular) v.

Anterior interventricular branch (left anterior descending) of left coronary a.

Sternocostal surface

Oblique v. of left atrium (Marshall)

Great cardiac (anterior interventricular) v.

Circumflex branch of left coronary a.

Left marginal branch

Coronary sinus

Posterolateral a.

Middle cardiac (posterior interventricular) v.

Interventricular septal branches

Sinu-atrial (SA) nodal branch

Small cardiac v.

Right coronary a.

Posterior interventricular branch (posterior descending) of right coronary a.

Right marginal branch

Diaphragmatic surface

FIGURE 3-16 Coronary Arteries and Cardiac Veins. (From *Atlas of human anatomy*, ed 6, Plate 215.)

(PDA) of the right coronary artery, and the marginal branch of the right coronary artery, respectively. Each of these cardiac veins then empties into the **coronary sinus** on the posterior aspect of the atrioventricular groove (Table 3-10). The coronary sinus empties into the right atrium. Additionally, numerous **small cardiac veins** (thebesian veins) empty venous blood into all four chambers of the heart.

Clinical Focus 3-12

Dominant Coronary Circulation

About 70% of individuals have a "right dominant" coronary circulation. This means that the right coronary artery gives rise to the PDA and the posterolateral artery, as shown in **Figure 3-16.** When these two arteries arise from the left coronary artery's circumflex branch, the heart is considered "left dominant." If both the right and the left coronary arteries contribute to these two branches, the circulation is considered "balanced."

Chambers of the Heart

The human heart has four chambers, each with unique internal features related to their function (Fig. 3-17 and Table 3-11). The right side of the heart is composed of the **right atrium** and **right ventricle.** These chambers receive blood from the systemic circulation and pump it to the pulmonary circulation for gas exchange.

The **left atrium** and **left ventricle** receive blood from the pulmonary circulation and pump it to the systemic circulation (Fig. 3-18 and Table 3-12).

In both ventricles the **papillary muscles** and their **chordae tendineae** provide a structural mechanism that prevents the **atrioventricular valves** (**tricuspid** and **mitral**) from everting (prolapsing) during ventricular systole. The papillary muscles (actually part of the ventricular muscle) contract as the ventricles contract and pull the valve leaflets into alignment. This prevents them from prolapsing into the atrial chamber above as the pressure in the ventricle increases. During ventricular diastole, the muscle relaxes and the

Opened right atrium: right lateral view

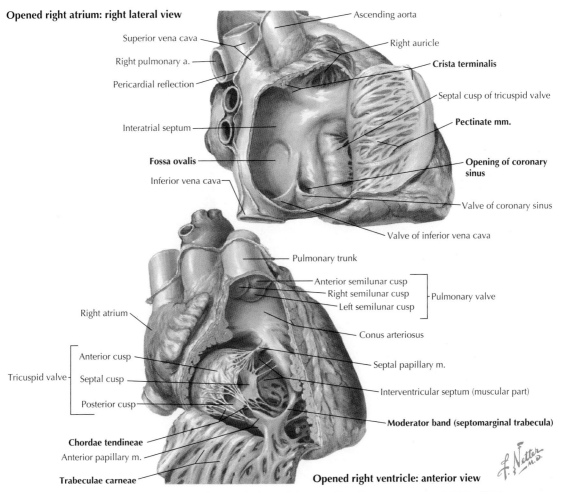

Ascending aorta

Superior vena cava

Right auricle

Right pulmonary a.

Crista terminalis

Pericardial reflection

Septal cusp of tricuspid valve

Interatrial septum

Pectinate mm.

Fossa ovalis

Opening of coronary sinus

Inferior vena cava

Valve of coronary sinus

Valve of inferior vena cava

Pulmonary trunk

Anterior semilunar cusp
Right semilunar cusp — Pulmonary valve
Left semilunar cusp

Right atrium

Conus arteriosus

Anterior cusp

Septal papillary m.

Tricuspid valve — Septal cusp

Interventricular septum (muscular part)

Posterior cusp

Moderator band (septomarginal trabecula)

Chordae tendineae

Anterior papillary m.

Trabeculae carneae

Opened right ventricle: anterior view

FIGURE 3-17 Right Atrium and Ventricle Opened. (From *Atlas of human anatomy*, ed 6, Plate 217.)

TABLE 3-11 General Features of Right Atrium and Right Ventricle

STRUCTURE	DEFINITION	STRUCTURE	DEFINITION
Right Atrium		Papillary muscles	Anterior, posterior, and septal projections of myocardium extending into ventricular cavity; prevent valve leaflet prolapse
Auricle	Pouchlike appendage of atrium; embryonic heart tube derivative		
Pectinate muscles	Ridges of myocardium inside auricle		
Crista terminalis	Ridge that runs from inferior vena cava (IVC) to superior vena cava (SVC) openings; its superior extent marks site of SA node	Chordae tendineae	Fibrous cords that connect papillary muscles to valve leaflets
		Moderator band	Muscular band that conveys AV bundle from septum to base of ventricle at site of anterior papillary muscle
Fossa ovalis	Depression in interatrial septum; former site of foramen ovale		
Atrial openings	One each for SVC, IVC, and coronary sinus (venous return from cardiac veins)	Ventricular openings	One to pulmonary trunk through pulmonary valve; one to receive blood from right atrium through tricuspid valve
Right Ventricle			
Trabeculae carneae	Irregular ridges of ventricular myocardium		

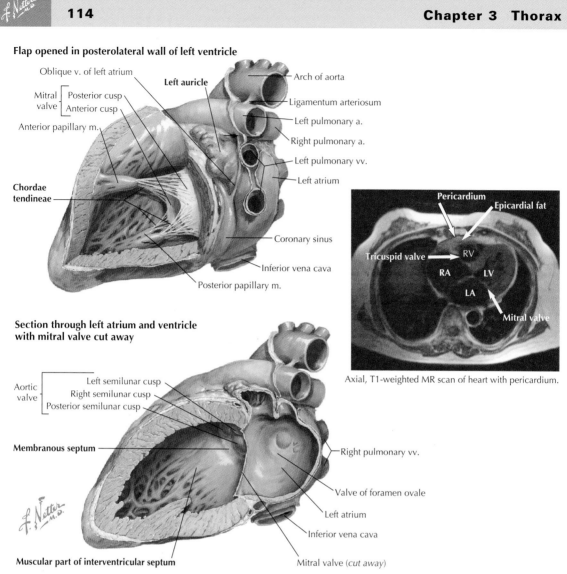

Flap opened in posterolateral wall of left ventricle

Oblique v. of left atrium

Mitral ⎡ Posterior cusp
valve ⎣ Anterior cusp

Left auricle

Arch of aorta

Ligamentum arteriosum

Left pulmonary a.

Right pulmonary a.

Left pulmonary vv.

Left atrium

Anterior papillary m.

**Chordae
tendineae**

Coronary sinus

Inferior vena cava

Posterior papillary m.

Pericardium   **Epicardial fat**

Tricuspid valve   RV

RA   LV

LA

Mitral valve

Axial, T1-weighted MR scan of heart with pericardium.

**Section through left atrium and ventricle
with mitral valve cut away**

Aortic ⎡ Left semilunar cusp
valve ⎢ Right semilunar cusp
       ⎣ Posterior semilunar cusp

Membranous septum

Right pulmonary vv.

Valve of foramen ovale

Left atrium

Inferior vena cava

Muscular part of interventricular septum

Mitral valve (cut away)

FIGURE 3-18 Left Atrium and Ventricle Opened. (From *Atlas of human anatomy,* ed 6, Plate 218; MR image from Kelley LL, Petersen C: *Sectional anatomy for imaging professionals,* St Louis, 2007, Mosby.)

TABLE 3-12 General Features of Left Atrium and Left Ventricle

STRUCTURE	DEFINITION	STRUCTURE	DEFINITION
Left Atrium		Chordae tendineae	Fibrous cords that connect papillary muscles to valve leaflets
Auricle	Small appendage representing primitive embryonic atrium whose wall has pectinate muscle	Ventricular wall	Wall much thicker than that of right ventricle
Atrial wall	Wall slightly thicker than thin-walled right atrium	Membranous septum	Very thin superior portion of IVS and site of most ventricular septal defects (VSDs)
Atrial openings	Usually four openings for four pulmonary veins	Ventricular openings	One to aorta through aortic valve; one to receive blood from left atrium through mitral valve
Left Ventricle			
Papillary muscles	Anterior and posterior muscles, larger than those of right ventricle		

Clinical Focus 3-13

Angina Pectoris (the Referred Pain of Myocardial Ischemia)

Angina pectoris is usually described as pressure, discomfort, or a feeling of choking or breathlessness in the left chest or substernal region that radiates to the left shoulder and arm, as well as the neck, jaw and teeth, abdomen, and back. The pain also may radiate to the right arm. This radiating pattern is an example of **referred pain,** in which visceral afferents from the heart enter the upper thoracic spinal cord along with somatic afferents, both converging in the spinal cord's dorsal horn. The higher brain center's interpretation of this visceral pain may initially be confused with somatic sensations from the same spinal cord levels.

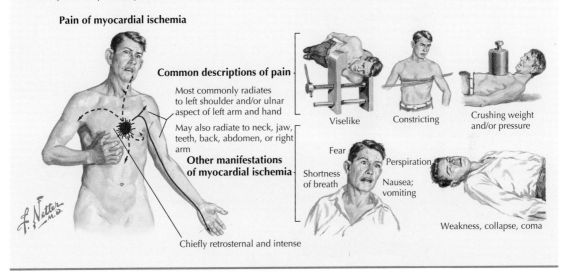

Pain of myocardial ischemia

Common descriptions of pain
- Most commonly radiates to left shoulder and/or ulnar aspect of left arm and hand
- May also radiate to neck, jaw, teeth, back, abdomen, or right arm

Viselike   Constricting   Crushing weight and/or pressure

Other manifestations of myocardial ischemia
- Fear
- Shortness of breath
- Perspiration
- Nausea; vomiting
- Weakness, collapse, coma

Chiefly retrosternal and intense

Clinical Focus 3-14

Coronary Bypass

A **coronary artery bypass graft** (CABG), also called "the cabbage procedure," offers a surgical approach for revascularization. Veins or arteries from elsewhere in the patient's body are grafted to the coronary arteries to improve blood supply. In a *saphenous vein graft* a portion of the great saphenous vein is harvested from the patient's lower limb. Alternatives include internal thoracic artery and radial artery grafts.

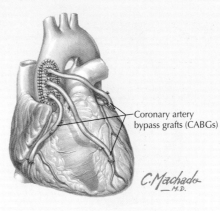

If indicated the physician may prefer to use coronary angioplasty to widen the partially occluded artery, which may include using a stent to keep the artery open.

Coronary artery bypass grafts (CABGs)

Coronary Angiogenesis

Angiogenesis occurs by the budding of new blood vessels. Hypoxia and inflammation are the two major stimuli for new vessel growth. Revascularization of the myocardium after an ischemic episode, bypass surgery, or percutaneous coronary intervention is vital for establishing new vessels **(angiogenesis)** and for creating **anastomoses** (interconnections) with existing vessels.

Angiogenesis occurs by the budding of new blood vessels. Hypoxia and inflammation are the two major stimuli for new vessel growth.

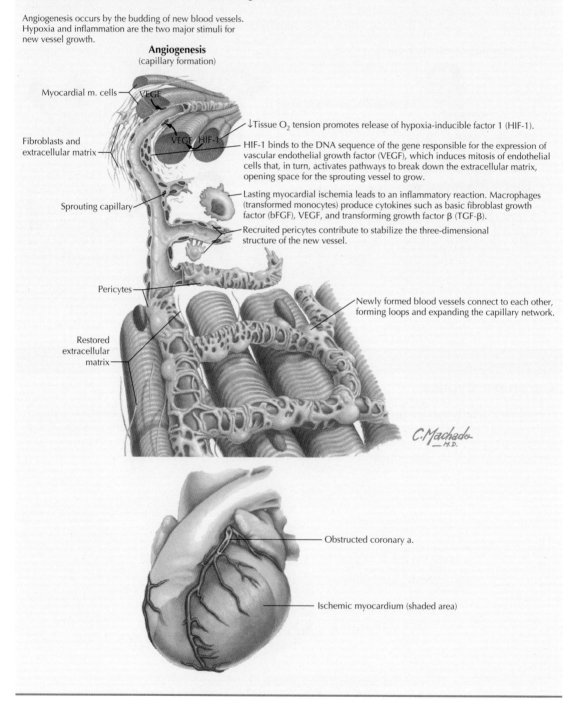

Angiogenesis
(capillary formation)

Myocardial m. cells — VEGF

Fibroblasts and extracellular matrix

VEGF HIF-1

Sprouting capillary

Pericytes

Restored extracellular matrix

↓Tissue O_2 tension promotes release of hypoxia-inducible factor 1 (HIF-1).

HIF-1 binds to the DNA sequence of the gene responsible for the expression of vascular endothelial growth factor (VEGF), which induces mitosis of endothelial cells that, in turn, activates pathways to break down the extracellular matrix, opening space for the sprouting vessel to grow.

Lasting myocardial ischemia leads to an inflammatory reaction. Macrophages (transformed monocytes) produce cytokines such as basic fibroblast growth factor (bFGF), VEGF, and transforming growth factor β (TGF-β).

Recruited pericytes contribute to stabilize the three-dimensional structure of the new vessel.

Newly formed blood vessels connect to each other, forming loops and expanding the capillary network.

Obstructed coronary a.

Ischemic myocardium (shaded area)

tricuspid and mitral valves open normally to facilitate blood flow into the ventricles.

Cardiac Skeleton and Cardiac Valves

The heart has four valves that, along with the myocardium, are attached to fibrous rings of dense collagen that make up the **fibrous skeleton of the heart** (Fig. 3-19 and Table 3-13). In addition to providing attachment points for the valves, the cardiac skeleton separates the atrial myocardium from the ventricular myocardium (which originate from the fibrous skeleton) and electrically isolates the atria from the ventricles. Only the atrioventricular bundle (of His) conveys electrical impulses between the atria and the ventricles. The following sounds result from valve closure:

- **First heart sound (S_1):** results from the closing of the mitral and tricuspid valves.
- **Second heart sound (S_2):** results from the closing of the aortic and pulmonary valves.

Conduction System of the Heart

The heart's conduction system is formed by specialized cardiac muscle cells that form nodes and by unidirectional conduction pathways that initiate and coordinate excitation and contraction of the myocardium (Fig 3-20). The system includes the following four elements:

- **Sinu-atrial (SA) node:** the "pacemaker" of the heart, where initiation of action potential occurs; located at the superior end of the crista terminalis near the superior vena cava (SVC) opening.
- **Atrioventricular (AV) node:** the area of the heart that receives impulses from the SA node and conveys them to the common **atrioventricular bundle (of His);** located between the opening of the coronary sinus and the origin of the septal cusp of the tricuspid valve.
- **Common atrioventricular bundle and bundle branches:** a collection of specialized heart muscle cells; AV bundle divides into right and left bundle branches,

TABLE 3-13 Features of the Heart Valves

VALVE	CHARACTERISTIC
Tricuspid	(Right AV) Between right atrium and right ventricle; has three cusps
Pulmonary	(Semilunar) Between right ventricle and pulmonary trunk; has three semilunar cusps (leaflets)
Mitral	(Bicuspid) Between left atrium and left ventricle; has two cusps
Aortic	(Semilunar) Between left ventricle and aorta; has three semilunar cusps

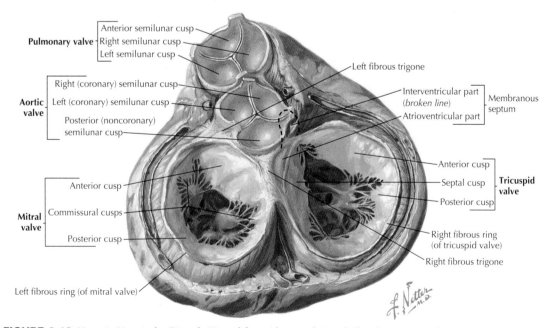

FIGURE 3-19 Heart in Ventricular Diastole Viewed from Above with Atrial Chambers Removed. (From *Atlas of human anatomy*, ed 6, Plate 219.)

Clinical Focus 3-16

Myocardial Infarction

Myocardial infarction (MI) is a major cause of death. Coronary artery **atherosclerosis** and **thrombosis,** the major causes of MI, precipitate local ischemia and necrosis of a defined myocardial area. Necrosis usually occurs approximately 20 to 30 minutes after coronary artery occlusion. Usually, MI begins in the subendocardium because this region is the most poorly perfused part of the ventricular wall.

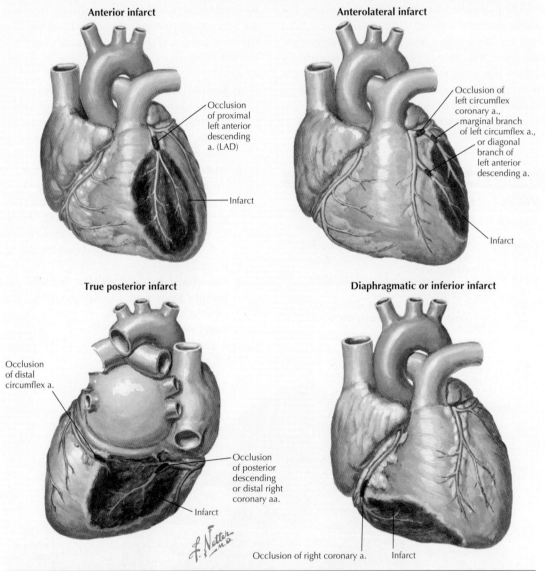

Anterior infarct

Occlusion of proximal left anterior descending a. (LAD)

Infarct

Anterolateral infarct

Occlusion of left circumflex coronary a., marginal branch of left circumflex a., or diagonal branch of left anterior descending a.

Infarct

True posterior infarct

Occlusion of distal circumflex a.

Occlusion of posterior descending or distal right coronary aa.

Infarct

Diaphragmatic or inferior infarct

Occlusion of right coronary a.

Infarct

Artery and Area Affected by MI	
Artery occluded	**Frequency and affected area**
LAD	40–50%; affects anterior and apical left ventricle and anterior two thirds of interventricular septum (IVS)
Right coronary	30–40%; affects posterior wall of left ventricle, posterior one third of IVS (if right-dominant coronary circulation)
Left circumflex	15–20%; affects lateral wall of left ventricle (can also affect posterior wall if left dominant coronary circulation)

Cardiac Auscultation

Auscultation of the heart requires not only an understanding of normal and abnormal heart sounds but also knowledge of the optimal location to detect the sounds. Sounds are best heard by auscultating the area where **turbulent blood flow radiates** (i.e., distal to the valve through which the blood has just passed).

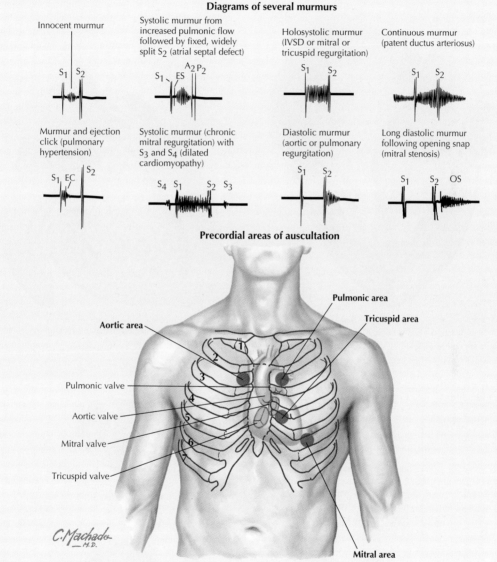

Diagrams of several murmurs

Innocent murmur

Systolic murmur from increased pulmonic flow followed by fixed, widely split S_2 (atrial septal defect)

Holosystolic murmur (IVSD or mitral or tricuspid regurgitation)

Continuous murmur (patent ductus arteriosus)

S_1 S_2

A_2 P_2 S_1 ES

S_1 S_2

S_1 S_2

Murmur and ejection click (pulmonary hypertension)

Systolic murmur (chronic mitral regurgitation) with S_3 and S_4 (dilated cardiomyopathy)

Diastolic murmur (aortic or pulmonary regurgitation)

Long diastolic murmur following opening snap (mitral stenosis)

S_1 EC S_2

S_4 S_1 S_2 S_3

S_1 S_2

S_1 S_2 OS

Precordial areas of auscultation

Pulmonic area

Tricuspid area

Aortic area

Pulmonic valve

Aortic valve

Mitral valve

Tricuspid valve

1
2
3
4
5
6
7

C. Machado
—M.D.

Mitral area

Features of Various Heart Sounds	
Area	Comment
Aortic	Upper right sternal border; aortic stenosis
Pulmonary	Upper left sternal border to below left clavicle; second heart sound, pulmonary valve murmurs, VSD murmur, continuous murmur of patent ductus arteriosus (PDA)
Tricuspid	Left fourth intercostal space; tricuspid and aortic regurgitation
Mitral	Left fifth intercostal space, apex; first heart sound, murmurs of mitral or aortic valves, third and fourth heart sounds

Valvular Heart Disease

Although each valve may be involved in disease, the mitral and aortic valves are most frequently involved. Major problems include **stenosis** (narrowing) or **insufficiency** (compromised valve function, often leading to regurgitation).

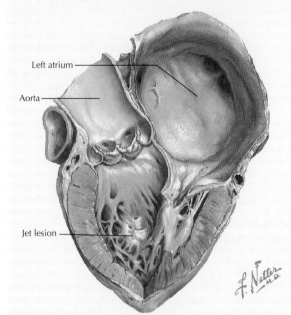

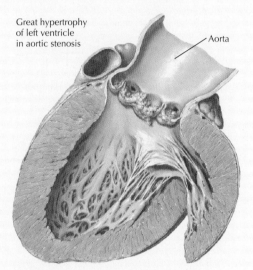

Thickened stenotic mitral valve: anterior cusp has typical convexity; enlarged left atrium; "jet lesion" on left ventricular wall

Elongation of left ventricle with tension on chordae tendineae, which may prevent full closure of mitral valve

Condition	Comment
Aortic stenosis	Leads to left ventricular overload and hypertrophy; caused by rheumatic heart disease (RHD), calcific stenosis, congenital bicuspid valve (1–2%)
Aortic regurgitation (insufficiency)	Caused by congenitally malformed leaflets, RHD, IE, ankylosing spondylitis, Marfan's syndrome, aortic root dilation
Mitral stenosis	Leads to left atrial dilation; usually caused by RHD
Mitral regurgitation (insufficiency)	Caused by abnormalities of valve leaflets, rupture of papillary muscle or chordae tendineae, papillary muscle fibrosis, IE, left ventricular enlargement

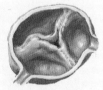

Stenosis and insufficiency (fusion of all commissures)

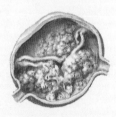

Calcific stenosis

IE, infective endocarditis (infection of cardiac valves)

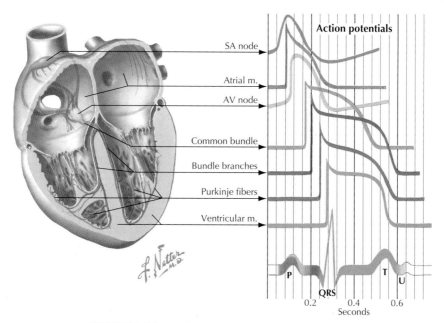

FIGURE 3-20 Conduction System and Electrocardiogram.

which course down the interventricular septum.

- **Subendocardial (Purkinje) system**: the ramification of bundle branches in the ventricles of the heart's conduction system; distributes into a subendocardial network of conduction cells that supply the ventricular walls and papillary muscles.

Autonomic Innervation of the Heart

Parasympathetic fibers from the vagus nerve (CN X) course as preganglionic nerves that synapse on postganglionic neurons in the cardiac plexus or within the heart wall itself (Fig. 3-21). Parasympathetic stimulation:

- Decreases heart rate.
- Decreases the force of contraction.
- Vasodilates coronary resistance vessels (although most vagal effects are restricted directly to the SA node region).

Sympathetic fibers arise from the upper thoracic cord levels (intermediolateral cell column of T1-T4/T5) and enter the sympathetic trunk (Fig. 3-21). These preganglionic fibers synapse in the upper cervical and thoracic sympathetic chain ganglia, and then postganglionic fibers pass to the cardiac plexus. Sympathetic stimulation:

- Increases the heart rate.
- Increases the force of contraction.
- Minimally vasoconstricts the coronary resistance vessels (via alpha adrenoceptors).

Vasoconstriction, however, *is masked by a powerful metabolic coronary vasodilation* (mediated by adenosine release from myocytes), which is important because coronary arteries must dilate to supply blood to the heart as it increases its workload.

A bilateral thoracic sympathetic chain of ganglia **(sympathetic trunk)** passes through the posterior mediastinum across the neck of the upper thoracic ribs and, as it proceeds inferiorly, aligns itself along the lateral bodies of the lower thoracic vertebrae (see also Fig. 4-29). Each of the 11 or 12 ganglia (number varies) is connected to the ventral ramus of the spinal nerve by a white ramus communicans (conveys preganglionic sympathetic fibers from the spinal gray matter to the ganglion) and a gray ramus communicans (conveys postganglionic sympathetic fibers back into the spinal nerve and its ventral and dorsal rami) (see Chapter 1). Additionally, the upper thoracic sympathetic trunk conveys small thoracic cardiac branches (postganglionic sympathetic fibers from the upper thoracic ganglia, T1-T4 or T5) to the cardiac plexus, where they mix with preganglionic

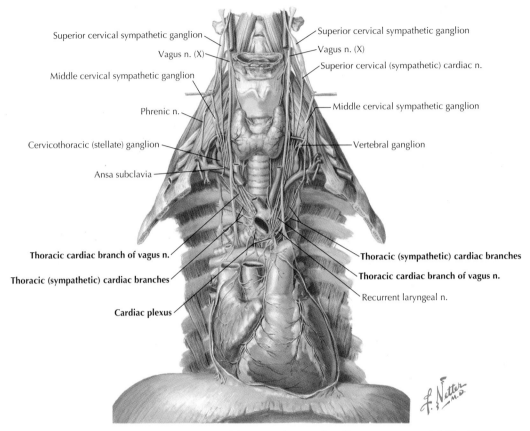

FIGURE 3-21 Autonomic Innervation of the Heart. (From *Atlas of human anatomy*, ed 6, Plate 223.)

Clinical Focus 3-19

Cardiac Pacemakers

Cardiac pacemakers consist of a pulse generator and one or two endocardial leads with an electrode (passive or active fixation lead). The lead is threaded through the subclavian vein, brachiocephalic vein, superior vena cava, and right atrium and is either embedded there or threaded in the trabeculae carneae of the right ventricular wall. Depending on the device and its programming, the lead may sense as well as pace the cardiac chamber in which it is embedded. In pacing, the electrode impulses generated by the pulse generator depolarize the myocardium and initiate contractions at a prescribed rate.

Implantable cardiac pacemaker (dual-chamber cardiac pacing)

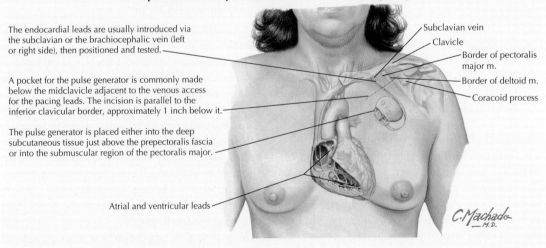

The endocardial leads are usually introduced via the subclavian or the brachiocephalic vein (left or right side), then positioned and tested.

A pocket for the pulse generator is commonly made below the midclavicle adjacent to the venous access for the pacing leads. The incision is parallel to the inferior clavicular border, approximately 1 inch below it.

The pulse generator is placed either into the deep subcutaneous tissue just above the prepectoralis fascia or into the submuscular region of the pectoralis major.

Atrial and ventricular leads

Subclavian vein
Clavicle
Border of pectoralis major m.
Border of deltoid m.
Coracoid process

Clinical Focus 3-20

Cardiac Defibrillators

An implantable cardioverter defibrillator is used for survivors of **sudden cardiac death,** patients with **sustained ventricular tachycardia** (a dysrhythmia originating from a ventricular focus with a heart rate typically greater than 120 beats/min), those at high risk for developing ventricular arrhythmias (ischemic dilated cardiomyopathy), and other indications. In addition to sensing arrhythmias and providing defibrillation to stop them, the device can function as a pacemaker for postdefibrillation bradycardia or atrioventricular dissociation.

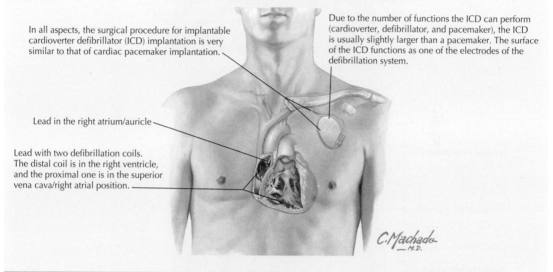

Implantable cardiac defibrillator (dual-chamber leads)

In all aspects, the surgical procedure for implantable cardioverter defibrillator (ICD) implantation is very similar to that of cardiac pacemaker implantation.

Due to the number of functions the ICD can perform (cardioverter, defibrillator, and pacemaker), the ICD is usually slightly larger than a pacemaker. The surface of the ICD functions as one of the electrodes of the defibrillation system.

Lead in the right atrium/auricle

Lead with two defibrillation coils. The distal coil is in the right ventricle, and the proximal one is in the superior vena cava/right atrial position.

parasympathetic fibers from the vagus nerve (Fig. 3-21). Three other pairs of thoracic splanchnic nerves arise from the lower seven thoracic ganglia and send their preganglionic sympathetic fibers inferiorly to abdominal ganglia. The thoracic splanchnic nerves (ganglia levels can vary) (see Chapter 4) include the following:

- **Greater splanchnic nerve:** usually arises from T5-T9 sympathetic ganglia.
- **Lesser splanchnic nerve:** usually arises from T10-T11 sympathetic ganglia.
- **Least splanchnic nerve:** usually arises from T12 sympathetic ganglia.

Visceral afferents for pain are conveyed back to the upper thoracic spinal cord, usually levels T1-T4 or T5, via the sympathetic fiber pathways (see Clinical Focus 3-13). Visceral afferents mediating cardiopulmonary reflexes (stretch receptors, baroreflexes, and chemoreflexes) are conveyed back to the brainstem via the vagus nerve.

6. MEDIASTINUM

The mediastinum ("middle space") is the middle region of the thoracic cavity and is divided into a superior and an inferior mediastinum by an imaginary horizontal line extending from the sternal angle of Louis to the intervertebral disc between T4 and T5 (Fig. 3-22; see also Fig. 3-1). The superior mediastinum lies behind the manubrium of the sternum, anterior to the first four thoracic vertebrae, and contains the following:

- Thymus gland (largely involuted and replaced by fat in older adults)
- Brachiocephalic veins
- Superior vena cava
- Aortic arch and its three arterial branches

Superior mediastinum and lungs

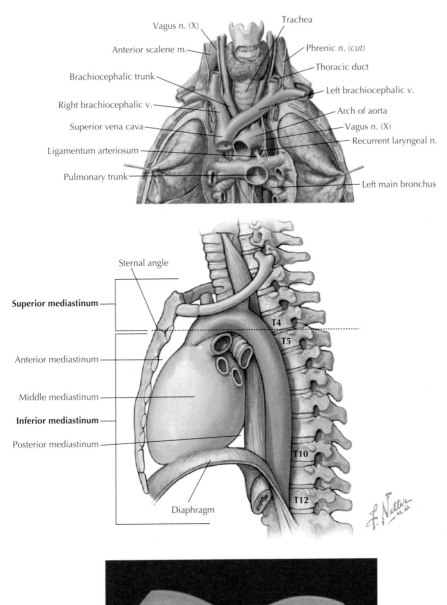

Vagus n. (X)
Trachea
Anterior scalene m.
Phrenic n. (*cut*)
Brachiocephalic trunk
Thoracic duct
Right brachiocephalic v.
Left brachiocephalic v.
Superior vena cava
Arch of aorta
Ligamentum arteriosum
Vagus n. (X)
Pulmonary trunk
Recurrent laryngeal n.
Left main bronchus

Sternal angle

Superior mediastinum

T4

T5

Anterior mediastinum

Middle mediastinum

Inferior mediastinum

Posterior mediastinum

T10

T12

Diaphragm

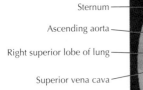

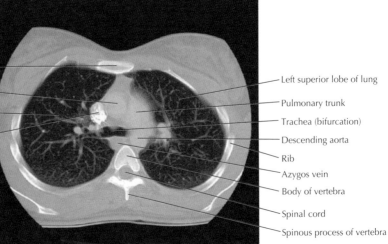

Sternum
Ascending aorta
Right superior lobe of lung
Superior vena cava

Left superior lobe of lung
Pulmonary trunk
Trachea (bifurcation)
Descending aorta
Rib
Azygos vein
Body of vertebra
Spinal cord
Spinous process of vertebra

FIGURE 3-22 Mediastinum. (From *Atlas of human anatomy*, ed 6, Plates 203 and 230.)

- Trachea
- Esophagus
- Phrenic and vagus nerves
- Thoracic duct and lymphatics

The inferior mediastinum is further subdivided as follows (Fig. 3-23):

- **Anterior mediastinum:** the region posterior to the body of the sternum and anterior to the pericardium (substernal region); contains a variable amount of fat.
- **Middle mediastinum:** the region containing the pericardium and heart.
- **Posterior mediastinum:** the region posterior to the heart and anterior to the bodies of the T5-T12 vertebrae; contains the esophagus and its nerve plexus, thoracic aorta, azygos system of veins, sympathetic trunks and thoracic splanchnic nerves, lymphatics, and thoracic duct.

Esophagus and Thoracic Aorta

The **esophagus** extends from the pharynx (throat) to the stomach and enters the thorax posterior to the trachea. As it descends, the esophagus gradually slopes to the left of the median plane, lying anterior to the thoracic aorta (Fig. 3-24), and pierces the diaphragm at the T10 vertebral level. The esophagus is about 10 cm (4 inches) long and has four points along its course where foreign

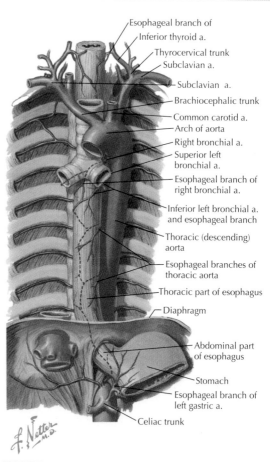

Esophageal branch of
Inferior thyroid a.
Thyrocervical trunk
Subclavian a.
Subclavian a.
Brachiocephalic trunk
Common carotid a.
Arch of aorta
Right bronchial a.
Superior left bronchial a.
Esophageal branch of right bronchial a.
Inferior left bronchial a. and esophageal branch
Thoracic (descending) aorta
Esophageal branches of thoracic aorta
Thoracic part of esophagus
Diaphragm
Abdominal part of esophagus
Stomach
Esophageal branch of left gastric a.
Celiac trunk

FIGURE 3-24 Esophagus and Thoracic Aorta. (From *Atlas of human anatomy*, ed 6, Plate 233.)

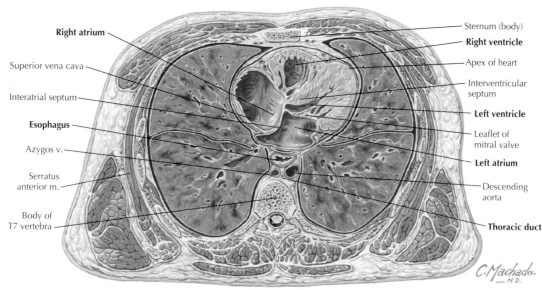

Transverse section: level of T7, 3rd interchondral space

Right atrium
Superior vena cava
Interatrial septum
Esophagus
Azygos v.
Serratus anterior m.
Body of T7 vertebra

Sternum (body)
Right ventricle
Apex of heart
Interventricular septum
Left ventricle
Leaflet of mitral valve
Left atrium
Descending aorta
Thoracic duct

FIGURE 3-23 Inferior Mediastinum. (From *Atlas of human anatomy*, ed 6, Plate 241.)

bodies may become lodged: (1) at its most proximal site at the level of the C6 vertebra (level of the cricoid cartilage), (2) at the point where it is crossed by the aortic arch, (3) at the point where it is crossed by the left main bronchus, and (4) distally at the point where it passes through the diaphragm at the level of the T10 vertebra. The esophagus receives its blood supply from the inferior thyroid artery, esophageal branches of the thoracic aorta, and branches of the left gastric artery (a branch of the celiac trunk in the abdomen).

The **thoracic aorta** descends alongside and slightly to the left of the esophagus and gives rise to the following arteries before piercing the diaphragm at the T12 vertebral level:

- **Pericardial arteries:** small arteries that branch from the thoracic aorta and supply the posterior pericardium; variable in number.
- **Bronchial arteries:** arteries that supply blood to the lungs; usually one artery to the right and two to the left, but variable in number.

- **Esophageal arteries:** arteries that supply the esophagus; variable in number.
- **Mediastinal arteries:** small branches that supply the lymph nodes, nerves, and connective tissue of the posterior mediastinum.
- **Posterior intercostal arteries:** paired arteries that supply blood to the lower nine intercostal spaces.
- **Superior phrenic arteries:** small arteries to the superior surface of the diaphragm; anastomose with the musculophrenic and pericardiacophrenic arteries (which arise from the internal thoracic artery).
- **Subcostal arteries:** paired arteries that lie below the inferior margin of the last rib; anastomose with superior epigastric, lower intercostal, and lumbar arteries.

Azygos System of Veins

The azygos venous system drains the posterior thorax and forms an important venous conduit between the inferior and the superior vena cava (IVC and SVC) (Fig. 3-25). This system represents the deep venous drainage characteristic of veins

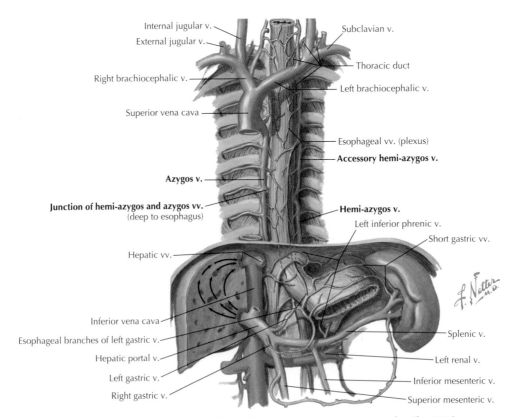

FIGURE 3-25 Azygos System of Veins. (From *Atlas of human anatomy*, ed 6, Plate 234.)

throughout the body. Its branches, although variable, largely drain the same regions supplied by the thoracic aorta's branches described earlier. The key veins include the **azygos vein,** with its right ascending lumbar, subcostal, and intercostal tributaries (sometimes the azygos vein also arises from the IVC before the ascending lumbar and subcostal tributaries join it), the **hemi-azygos vein,** and the **accessory hemi-azygos vein.** (If present, it usually begins at the fourth intercostal space.) A small left superior intercostal vein (a tributary of the left brachiocephalic vein) may also connect with the hemi-azygos vein. Ultimately, most of the thoracic venous drainage passes into the azygos vein, which ascends right of the midline to empty into the SVC.

Clinical Focus 3-21

Mediastinal Masses

Some of the more common mediastinal masses and their signs and symptoms are noted here.

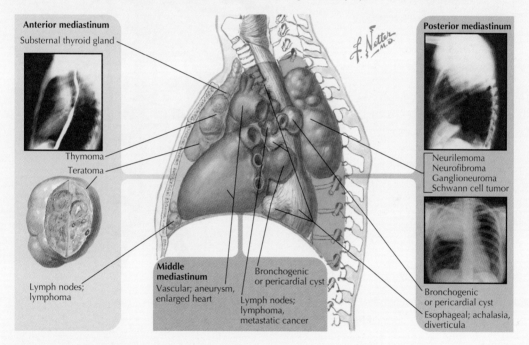

Anterior mediastinum
Substernal thyroid gland

Thymoma
Teratoma

Lymph nodes; lymphoma

Middle mediastinum
Vascular; aneurysm, enlarged heart

Bronchogenic or pericardial cyst

Lymph nodes; lymphoma, metastatic cancer

Posterior mediastinum

Neurilemoma
Neurofibroma
Ganglioneuroma
Schwann cell tumor

Bronchogenic or pericardial cyst
Esophageal; achalasia, diverticula

Types of Mediastinal Masses	
Type of mass	**Comment**
Anterior Mediastinum (retrosternal pain, cough, dyspnea, SVC syndrome, choking sensation)	
Thymoma	Thymus tumors (<50% malignant), often associated with myasthenia gravis
Thyroid mass	Mass that may cause enlarged gland to extend inferiorly and displace trachea
Teratoma	Benign and malignant tumors of totipotent cells, often containing all three germ cell types (ectoderm, mesoderm, and endoderm)
Lymphoma	Hodgkin's, non-Hodgkin's, and primary mediastinal B-cell tumors
Middle Mediastinum (signs and symptoms similar to those of anterior masses)	
Lymph nodes	Enlarged nodes resulting from infections or malignancy
Aortic aneurysm	Aneurysm that is atherosclerotic in origin, may rupture, and can be in any part of the mediastinum
Vascular dilatation	Enlarged pulmonary trunk or cardiomegaly
Cysts	Bronchogenic (at tracheal bifurcation) cysts, pericardial cysts
Posterior Mediastinum (pain, neurologic symptoms, or swallowing difficulty)	
Neurogenic tumors	Tumors of peripheral nerves or sheath cells (e.g., schwannomas)
Esophageal lesions	Diverticula and tumors

1. **Heart (Left Ventricle)***

2. **Ascending Aorta**

3. **Aortic Arch**

4. **Descending Aorta**

5. **Thoracic Aorta**

   Bronchial arteries (branches)

   Esophageal arteries

   Pericardial arteries

   Mediastinal arteries

   Superior phrenic arteries

   Posterior intercostal arteries (lower 9 spaces)

      Dorsal branch

         Medial cutaneous branch

         Lateral cutaneous branch

         Spinal branches

            Postcentral branch

            Prelaminar branch

            Posterior radicular artery

            Anterior radicular artery

            Segmental medullary artery

   Posterior intercostal arteries

      Collateral branch

      Lateral cutaneous branch

      Lateral mammary branches

   Subcostal artery (inferior to rib 12)

      Dorsal branch

      Spinal branch

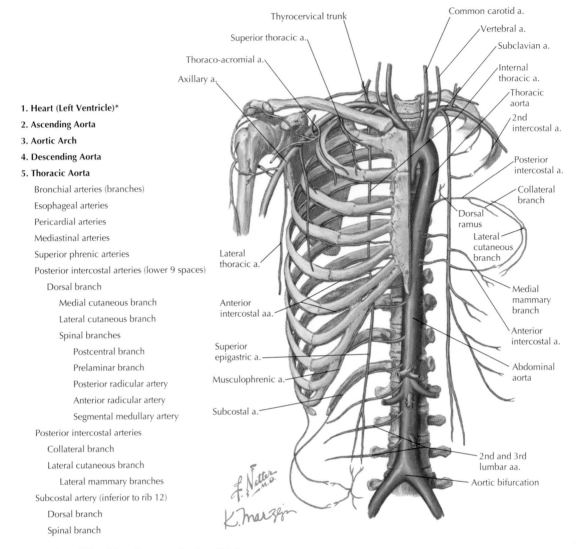

*Direction of blood flow from proximal to distal

FIGURE 3-26 Arteries of the Thoracic Aorta.

Arteriovenous Overview

Arteries of the Thoracic Aorta (Fig. 3-26)

The **heart (1)** gives rise to the **ascending aorta (2)**, which receives blood from the left ventricle. The right and left coronary arteries immediately arise from the aorta and supply the heart itself. The **aortic arch (3)** connects the ascending aorta and the **descending aorta (4)** and is found in the superior mediastinum. The descending aorta then continues inferiorly as the **thoracic aorta (5)**. The thoracic aorta gives rise to branches to the lungs, esophagus, pericardium, mediastinum, diaphragm, and posterior intercostal branches to the thoracic wall. The posterior intercostal arteries course along the inferior aspect of each rib (in the costal groove) and supply spinal branches (to thoracic vertebrae and thoracic spinal cord), lateral branches, and branches to the mammary glands. The intercostals anastomose with the anterior intercostal branches from the internal thoracic artery, a branch of the subclavian artery (see Fig. 8-64). The thoracic aorta lies to the left of the thoracic vertebral bodies as it descends in the thorax, so the left intercostals are shorter than the right intercostal arteries. As it approaches the diaphragm, the aorta then shifts closer to the midline of the lower thoracic vertebrae. The lower portion of the esophagus passes anterior to the lower portion of the thoracic aorta **(5)** on its way to the diaphragm and stomach. The thoracic aorta pierces the diaphragm at the level of the T12

Posterior internal vertebral venous plexus*

Post. and ant. spinal veins

Veins of spinal cord

Basivertebral veins

Anterior internal vertebral venous plexus

Ant. and post. external vertebral venous plexus

Posterior intercostal veins (left 4–8th)

Bronchial veins (left)

1. Accessory Hemi-azygos Vein

Ascending lumbar vein (left)

Posterior intercostal veins (left 8–12th)

Esophageal veins

Mediastinal veins

Superior phrenic veins (left)

2. Hemi-azygos Vein

Ascending lumbar vein (right)

Posterior intercostal veins (right 5–11th)

Esophageal veins

Mediastinal veins

Pericardial veins

Bronchial veins (right)

Right superior intercostal vein

3. Azygos Vein

4. Superior Vena Cava

5. Heart (Right Atrium)

*Distal (vertebral and intercostal veins)
to Heart (right atrium)

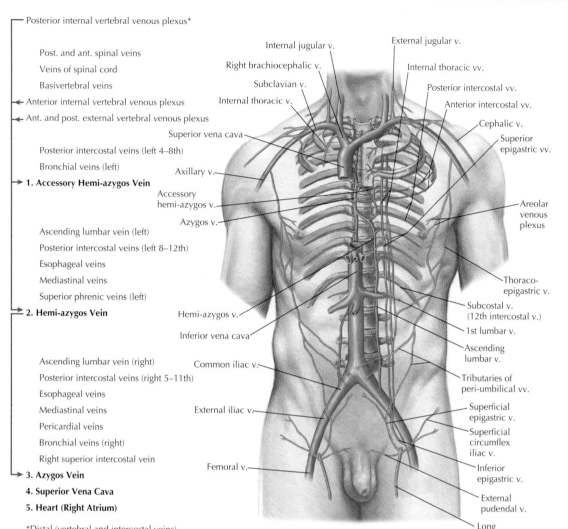

Internal jugular v.
Right brachiocephalic v.
Subclavian v.
Internal thoracic v.
Superior vena cava
Axillary v.
Accessory hemi-azygos v.
Azygos v.
Hemi-azygos v.
Inferior vena cava
Common iliac v.
External iliac v.
Femoral v.

External jugular v.
Internal thoracic vv.
Posterior intercostal vv.
Anterior intercostal vv.
Cephalic v.
Superior epigastric vv.
Areolar venous plexus
Thoraco-epigastric v.
Subcostal v. (12th intercostal v.)
1st lumbar v.
Ascending lumbar v.
Tributaries of peri-umbilical vv.
Superficial epigastric v.
Superficial circumflex iliac v.
Inferior epigastric v.
External pudendal v.
Long saphenous v.

FIGURE 3-27 Veins of the Thorax.

vertebra and passes through the aortic hiatus to enter the abdominal cavity. The aortic arch gives off very small branches to the aortic body chemoreceptors (not listed in the outline; function similar to the carotid body chemoreceptors).

Veins of the Thorax (Fig. 3-27)

The venous drainage begins with the **vertebral venous plexus** draining the vertebral column and spinal cord. This plexus includes both an internal and an external vertebral venous plexus. While most of these veins are valveless, recent evidence suggests that some valves do exist in variable numbers in some of these veins. The **posterior intercostal veins** parallel the posterior intercostal arteries as the veins course in the costal groove at

the inferior margin of each rib. The intercostal veins drain largely into **hemi-azygos veins (2)** and **azygos veins (3)** in the posterior mediastinum. An **ascending lumbar vein** from the upper abdominal cavity collects venous blood segmentally and often from the left renal vein; it is an important connection between these abdominal caval veins and the azygos system in the thorax. A number of mediastinal veins exist in the posterior mediastinum and drain the diaphragm, pericardium, esophagus, and main bronchi. These veins ultimately drain into the **accessory hemi-azygos veins (1)** and hemia-zygos veins just to the left of the thoracic vertebral bodies or into the azygos vein just to the right of the vertebral bodies. About midway in the thorax, the hemi-azygos vein crosses the midline and drains into the **azygos vein,** although the hemi-azygos usually maintains its connection with the accessory hemi-azygos vein as well. Veins tend to connect with one another where possible, and many connections are small, variable, and not readily recognizable. The azygos vein delivers venous blood to the **superior vena cava (4)** just before the SVC enters the **right atrium of the heart (5).** The accessory hemi-azygos vein also often has connections with the left brachiocephalic vein, providing another venous pathway back to the right side of the heart. Flow in the azygos system of veins is pressure dependent and, being essentially valveless veins, the flow can go in either direction. As with other regional veins, the number of veins of the azygos system can be variable.

Mediastinal Lymphatics

The thoracic lymphatic duct begins in the abdomen at the **cisterna chyli** (found between the abdominal aorta and the right crus of the diaphragm), ascends through the posterior mediastinum posterior to the esophagus, crosses to the left of the median plane at approximately the T5-T6 vertebral level, and empties into the venous system at the junction of the left internal jugular and left subclavian veins (Fig. 3-28).

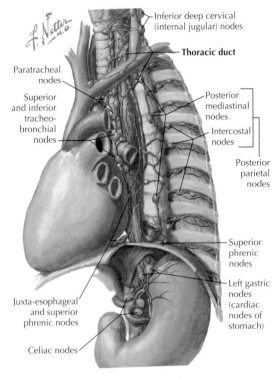

Inferior deep cervical (internal jugular) nodes

Thoracic duct

Paratracheal nodes

Superior and inferior tracheo-bronchial nodes

Posterior mediastinal nodes

Intercostal nodes

Posterior parietal nodes

Superior phrenic nodes

Left gastric nodes (cardiac nodes of stomach)

Juxta-esophageal and superior phrenic nodes

Celiac nodes

FIGURE 3-28 Mediastinal Lymphatics. (From *Atlas of human anatomy,* ed 6, Plate 235.)

7. EMBRYOLOGY

Respiratory System

The airway and lungs begin developing during the fourth week of gestation. Key features of this development include the following (Fig. 3-29):

- Formation of the **laryngotracheal diverticulum** from the ventral foregut, just inferior to the last pair of pharyngeal pouches
- Division of the laryngotracheal diverticulum into the **left and right lung (bronchial) buds,** each with a primary bronchus
- Division of the lung buds to form the definitive lobes of the lungs (three lobes in the right lung, two lobes in the left lung)
- Formation of segmental bronchi and 10 bronchopulmonary segments in each lung (by weeks 6 to 7)

The airway passages are lined by epithelium derived from the **endoderm of the foregut,** while mesoderm forms the stroma of each lung. By 6 months of gestation, the alveoli are mature enough for gas exchange, but the production of **surfactant,** which reduces surface tension and helps prevent alveolar collapse, may not be sufficient to support respiration. A premature infant's ability to keep its airways open often is the limiting factor if the premature birth occurs before adequate surfactant cells (type II pneumocytes) are present.

Early Embryonic Vasculature

Toward the end of the third week of development, the embryo establishes a primitive vascular system to meet its growing needs for oxygen and nutrients (Fig. 3-30). Blood leaving the embryonic heart enters a series of paired arteries called the **aortic arches,** which are associated with the pharyngeal arches. The blood then flows from these arches into the single midline **aorta** (formed by the fusion of two dorsal aortae), coursing along the length of the embryo. Some of the blood enters the **vitelline arteries** to supply the future bowel (still the yolk sac at this stage), and some passes to the placenta via a pair of **umbilical arteries,** where gases, nutrients, and metabolic wastes are exchanged.

Blood returning from the placenta is oxygenated and carries nutrients back to the heart

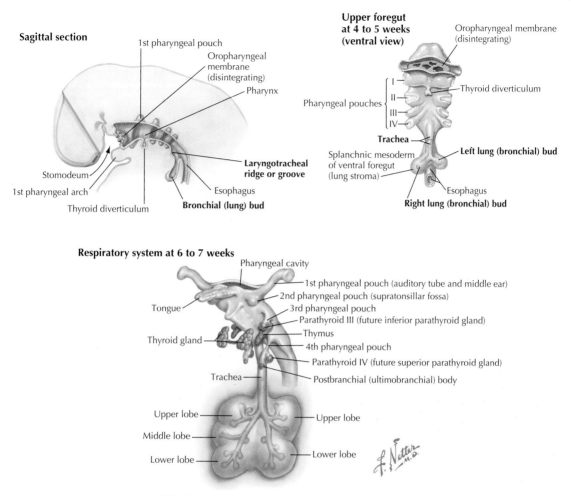

FIGURE 3-29 Embryology of the Respiratory System.

through the single **umbilical vein.** Blood also returns to the heart through the following veins:

- **Vitelline veins:** drain blood from yolk sac; will become the **portal system** draining the gastrointestinal tract through the liver.
- **Cardinal veins:** form SVC and IVC (and azygos system of veins) and their tributaries; will become the **caval system** of venous return.

Aortic Arches

Blood pumped from the primitive embryonic heart passes into **aortic arches** that are associated with the pharyngeal arches (Fig. 3-31). The right and left dorsal aortas caudal to the pharyngeal arches fuse to form the single midline aorta, while the aortic arches give rise to the arteries summarized in Table 3-14.

Development of Embryonic Heart Tube and Heart Chambers

The primitive heart begins its development as a single unfolded tube, much like an artery develops (Fig. 3-32). The **heart tube** receives blood from the embryonic body, which passes through its heart tube segments in the following sequence:

- **Sinus venosus:** receives all the venous return from the embryonic body and placenta to the heart tube.
- **Atrium:** receives blood from the sinus venosus and passes it to the ventricle.
- **Ventricle:** receives atrial blood and passes it to the bulbus cordis.
- **Bulbus cordis:** receives ventricular blood and passes it to the truncus arteriosus.
- **Truncus arteriosus:** receives blood and passes it to the aortic arch system for distribution to the body.

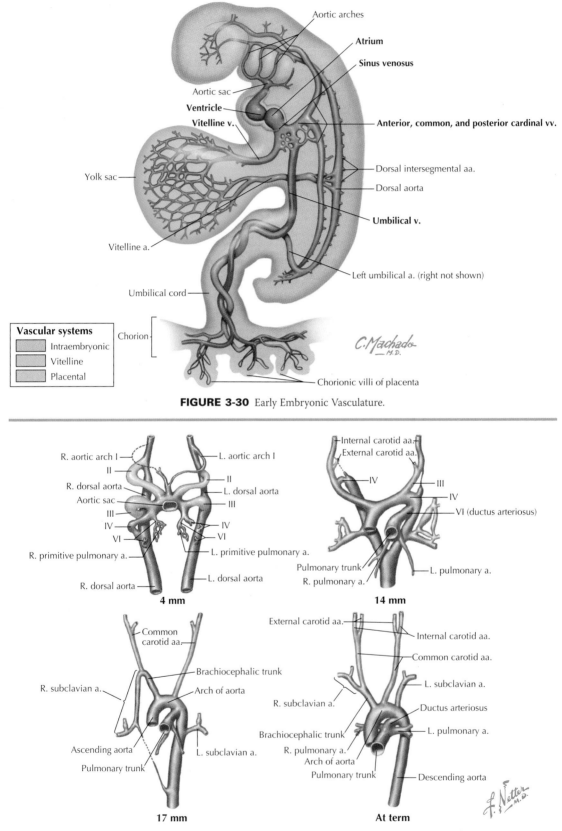

FIGURE 3-30 Early Embryonic Vasculature.

FIGURE 3-31 Sequential Development of Aortic Arch Derivatives (color-coded).

TABLE 3-14 Aortic Arch Derivatives

ARCH	DERIVATIVE
1	Largely disappears (part of maxillary artery in head)
2	Largely disappears
3	Common and internal carotid arteries
4	Right subclavian artery and aortic arch (on left side)
5	Disappears
6	Ductus arteriosus and proximal part of pulmonary arteries

This primitive heart tube soon begins to fold on itself in an "S-bend." The ventricle folds downward and to the right, and the atrium and sinus venosus fold upward and to the left, thus forming the definitive positions of the heart's future chambers (atria and ventricles) (Fig. 3-32 and Table 3-15).

The four chambers of the heart (two atria and two ventricles) are formed by the internal septation of the single atrium and ventricle of the primitive heart tube. Because most of the blood does not perfuse the lungs in utero (the lungs are filled with amniotic fluid and are partially collapsed), blood in the right atrium passes directly to the left atrium via a small opening in the interatrial septum called the **foramen ovale.** The **interatrial septum** is formed by the fusion of a septum primum and a septum secundum (develops on the right atrial side of the septum primum) (Fig. 3-33). This fusion occurs after birth when the left atrial pressure exceeds that of the right atrium (blood now passes into the lungs and returns to the left atrium, raising the pressure on the left side) and pushes the two septae together, thus forming the **fossa ovalis** of the postnatal heart. The **ventricular septum** forms from the superior growth of the muscular interventricular septum from the base of the heart toward the downward growth of a thin membranous septum from the

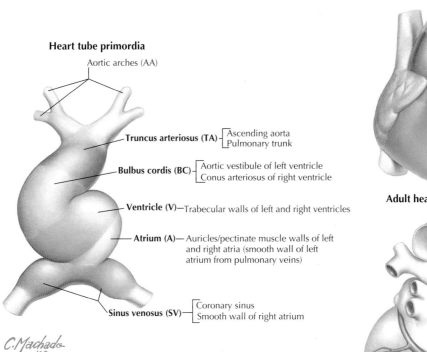

Heart tube derivatives

Heart tube primordia

Aortic arches (AA)

Truncus arteriosus (TA)—⎡Ascending aorta
　　　　　　　　　　　⎣Pulmonary trunk

Bulbus cordis (BC)—⎡Aortic vestibule of left ventricle
　　　　　　　　　　⎣Conus arteriosus of right ventricle

Ventricle (V)—Trabecular walls of left and right ventricles

Atrium (A)—Auricles/pectinate muscle walls of left and right atria (smooth wall of left atrium from pulmonary veins)

Sinus venosus (SV)—⎡Coronary sinus
　　　　　　　　　　⎣Smooth wall of right atrium

C. Machado
　—M.D.

Adult heart, anterior view

Adult heart, posterior view

FIGURE 3-32 Primitive Heart Tube Formation.

TABLE 3-15 Adult Heart Derivatives of Embryonic Heart Tube

STRUCTURE	DERIVATIVES
Truncus arteriosus	Aorta
	Pulmonary trunk
Bulbus cordis	Smooth part of right ventricle (conus arteriosus)
	Smooth part of left ventricle (aortic vestibule)
Primitive ventricle	Trabeculated part of right ventricle
	Trabeculated part of left ventricle
Primitive atrium	Pectinate wall of right atrium
	Pectinate wall of left atrium
Sinus venosus	Smooth part of right atrium (sinus venarum)*
	Coronary sinus
	Oblique vein of left atrium

From Dudek R: *High-yield embryology: a collaborative project of medical students and faculty*, Philadelphia, 2006, Lippincott Williams & Wilkins.

*The smooth part of the left atrium is formed by incorporation of parts of the pulmonary veins into the atrial wall. The junction of the pectinated and smooth parts of the right atrium is called the *crista terminalis*.

endocardial cushion (Fig. 3-34). Simultaneously, the **bulbus cordis** and **truncus arteriosus** form the outflow tracts of the ventricles, pulmonary trunk, and aorta.

Fetal Circulation

The pattern of fetal circulation is one of gas exchange and nutrient/metabolic waste exchange across the placenta with the maternal blood (but not the exchange of blood cells), and distribution of oxygen and nutrient-rich blood to the tissues of the fetus (Fig. 3-35). Various shunts allow fetal blood to bypass the liver (not needed for metabolic processing in utero) and lungs (not needed for gas exchange in utero) so that the blood may gain direct access to the left side of the heart and be pumped into the fetal arterial system. At or shortly after birth, these shunts close, resulting in the normal pattern of pulmonary and systemic circulation.

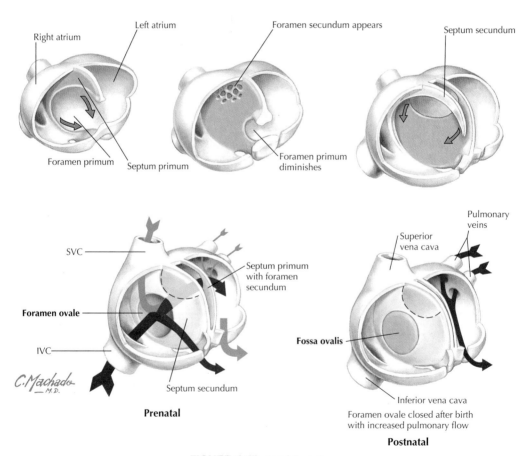

FIGURE 3-33 Atrial Septation.

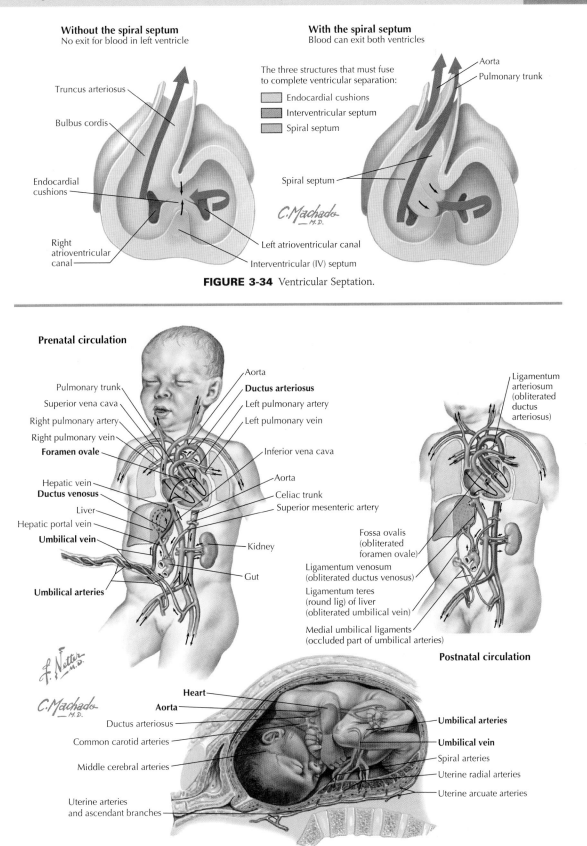

Without the spiral septum
No exit for blood in left ventricle

With the spiral septum
Blood can exit both ventricles

Truncus arteriosus

Bulbus cordis

Aorta
Pulmonary trunk

The three structures that must fuse
to complete ventricular separation:

Endocardial cushions
Interventricular septum
Spiral septum

Endocardial
cushions

Spiral septum

Right
atrioventricular
canal

Left atrioventricular canal

Interventricular (IV) septum

C. Machado
_M.D._

FIGURE 3-34 Ventricular Septation.

Prenatal circulation

Pulmonary trunk
Superior vena cava
Right pulmonary artery
Right pulmonary vein
Foramen ovale

Hepatic vein
Ductus venosus
Liver
Hepatic portal vein
Umbilical vein

Umbilical arteries

Aorta
Ductus arteriosus
Left pulmonary artery
Left pulmonary vein

Inferior vena cava

Aorta
Celiac trunk
Superior mesenteric artery

Kidney

Gut

Ligamentum
arteriosum
(obliterated
ductus
arteriosus)

Fossa ovalis
(obliterated
foramen ovale)
Ligamentum venosum
(obliterated ductus venosus)
Ligamentum teres
(round lig) of liver
(obliterated umbilical vein)
Medial umbilical ligaments
(occluded part of umbilical arteries)

Postnatal circulation

f. Netter
_M.D._

C. Machado
_M.D._

Heart
Aorta
Ductus arteriosus
Common carotid arteries
Middle cerebral arteries

Uterine arteries
and ascendant branches

Umbilical arteries
Umbilical vein
Spiral arteries
Uterine radial arteries
Uterine arcuate arteries

FIGURE 3-35 Fetal Circulation Pattern and Changes at Birth. (From *Atlas of human anatomy,* ed 6, Plate 226.)

Ventricular Septal Defect

Ventricular septal defect (VSD) is the most common congenital heart defect, representing about 30% of all heart defects. Approximately 80% of cases are **perimembranous** (occur where the muscular septum and membranous septum of the endocardial cushion should fuse). This results in a left-to-right shunt, which may precipitate congestive heart failure. The repair illustrated in the figure is through the right atrial approach.

Transatrial repair of ventricular septal defect

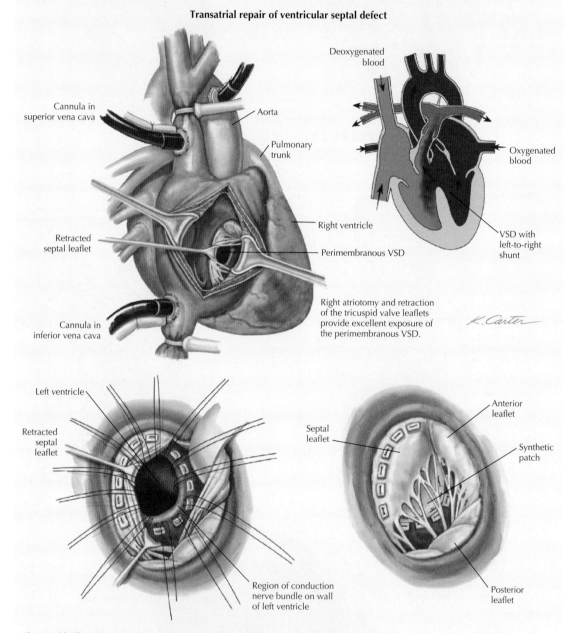

Right atriotomy and retraction of the tricuspid valve leaflets provide excellent exposure of the perimembranous VSD.

The septal leaflet of the tricuspid valve may need to be bisected to permit placement of pledgetted sutures at its junction with the VSD. Superficial sutures are placed along the inferior border of the VSD to prevent injury to the conduction system.

The VSD is closed with a synthetic patch and pledgetted sutures. The septal leaflet, if detached, is then repaired with a running suture.

Clinical Focus 3-23

Atrial Septal Defect

Atrial septal defects make up approximately 10% to 15% of congenital cardiac anomalies. Repair of these defects (other than fossa ovalis defects) can be achieved surgically by using a relatively new transcatheter approach through the IVC and into the atria, where a septal occluder is deployed and secured. By threading it through the IVC, the catheter is positioned to pass directly into the defect, which mimics the direction of flow of the fetal blood passing from the IVC through the foramen ovale and into the left atrium.

The Amplatzer Septal Occluder is deployed from its delivery sheath forming two discs, one for either side of the septum, and a central waist available in varying diameters to seat on the rims of the atrial septal defect.

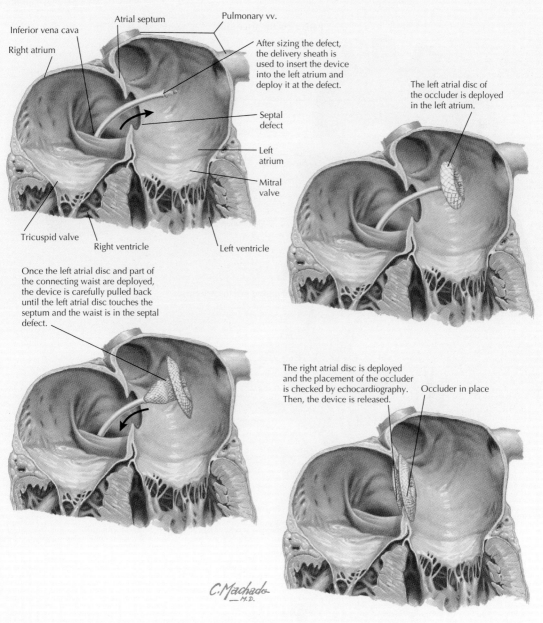

Atrial septum

Pulmonary vv.

Inferior vena cava

Right atrium

After sizing the defect, the delivery sheath is used to insert the device into the left atrium and deploy it at the defect.

The left atrial disc of the occluder is deployed in the left atrium.

Septal defect

Left atrium

Mitral valve

Tricuspid valve

Right ventricle

Left ventricle

Once the left atrial disc and part of the connecting waist are deployed, the device is carefully pulled back until the left atrial disc touches the septum and the waist is in the septal defect.

The right atrial disc is deployed and the placement of the occluder is checked by echocardiography. Then, the device is released.

Occluder in place

C. Machado
—M.D.

Patent Ductus Arteriosus

Patent ductus arteriosus (PDA) is failure of the ductus arteriosus to close shortly after birth. This results in a shunt of blood from the **aorta into the pulmonary trunk,** which may lead to congestive heart failure. PDA accounts for approximately 10% of congenital heart defects and can be treated medically (or surgically if necessary). Surgical treatment is by direct ligation or a less invasive, catheter-based device that is threaded through the vasculature and positioned to occlude the PDA. Often, children with a PDA may be fine until they become more active and then experience trouble breathing when exercising and demonstrate a failure to thrive. A continuous murmur usually is evident over the left sternal border to just below the clavicle (see Clinical Focus 3-17).

Patent ductus arteriosus

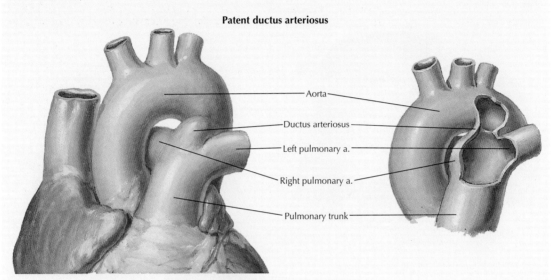

Aorta

Ductus arteriosus

Left pulmonary a.

Right pulmonary a.

Pulmonary trunk

Pathophysiology of patent ductus arteriosus

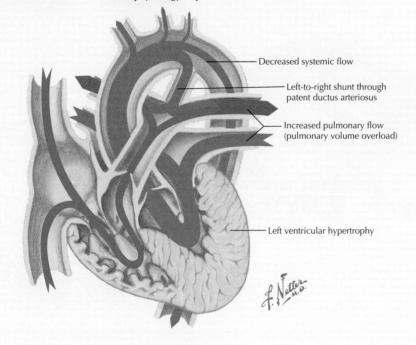

Decreased systemic flow

Left-to-right shunt through patent ductus arteriosus

Increased pulmonary flow (pulmonary volume overload)

Left ventricular hypertrophy

Repair of Tetralogy of Fallot

Tetralogy of Fallot usually results from a maldevelopment of the spiral septum that normally divides the truncus arteriosus into the pulmonary trunk and aorta. This defect involves the following:

- Pulmonary stenosis or narrowing of the right ventricular outflow tract
- Overriding (transposed) aorta
- Right ventricular hypertrophy
- Ventricular septal defect (VSD)

Surgical repair is done on cardiopulmonary bypass to close the VSD and provide unobstructed flow into the pulmonary trunk. The stenotic pulmonary outflow tract is widened by inserting a patch into the wall (pericardial), thus increasing the volume of the subpulmonic stenosis and/or the pulmonary artery stenosis.

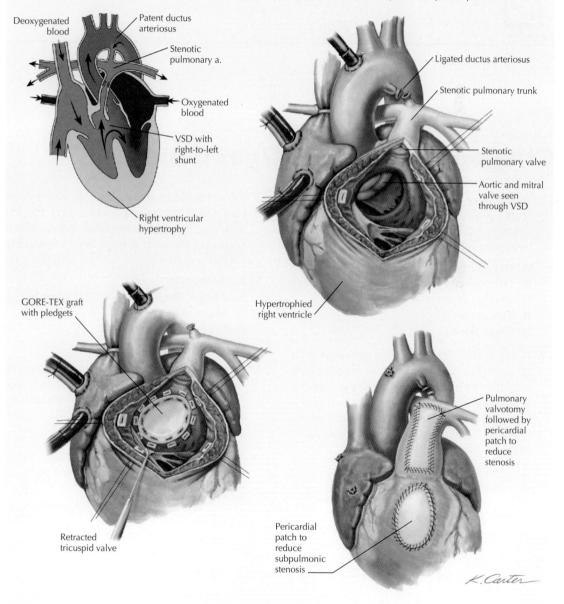

K. Carter

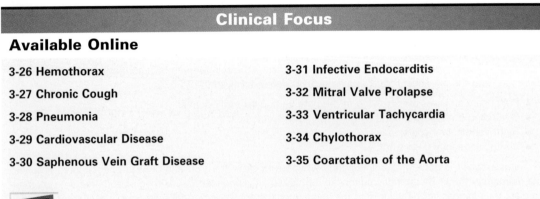

Clinical Focus

Available Online

3-26 Hemothorax

3-27 Chronic Cough

3-28 Pneumonia

3-29 Cardiovascular Disease

3-30 Saphenous Vein Graft Disease

3-31 Infective Endocarditis

3-32 Mitral Valve Prolapse

3-33 Ventricular Tachycardia

3-34 Chylothorax

3-35 Coarctation of the Aorta

Additional figures available online (see inside front cover for details).

Challenge Yourself Questions

1. During open-heart surgery, the pericardial sac is cut open by a longitudinal incision. If a horizontal incision is used, which of the following structures might be transected?

   A. Azygos vein
   B. Inferior vena cava
   C. Internal thoracic artery
   D. Phrenic nerves
   E. Vagus nerves

2. A small, thin, 4-year-old boy presents with an audible continuous murmur that is heard near the left proximal clavicle and is present throughout the cardiac cycle. The murmur is louder in systole than diastole. Which of the following conditions is most likely the cause of this murmur?

   A. Atrial septal defect
   B. Mitral stenosis
   C. Patent ductus arteriosus
   D. Right ventricular hypertrophy
   E. Ventricular septal defect

3. A 61-year-old man presents with severe chest pain and a rhythmic pulsation over the left midclavicular, fifth intercostal space. Which portion of the heart is most likely responsible for this pulsation?

   A. Aortic arch
   B. Apex of the heart
   C. Mitral valve
   D Pulmonary valve
   E. Right atrium

4. After a boating accident, a young child needs an emergency tracheotomy because of injuries to his upper body. Which of the following structures is most at risk for injury during this procedure?

   A. Left brachiocephalic vein
   B. Phrenic nerve
   C. Thoracic duct
   D. Thymus gland
   E. Vagus nerve

Multiple-choice and short-answer review questions available online; see inside front cover for details.

5. A coronary artery angiogram for a patient about to undergo coronary bypass surgery shows significant blockage of a vessel that supplies the right and left bundle branches of the heart's conduction system. Which of the following arteries is most likely involved?

   A. Anterior interventricular
   B. Circumflex
   C. Posterior interventricular
   D. Right marginal
   E. Sinu-atrial nodal branch

6. An infant presents with left-to-right shunting of blood and evidence of pulmonary hypertension. Which of the following conditions is most likely responsible for this condition?

   A. Atrial septal defect
   B. Mitral stenosis
   C. Patent ductus arteriosus
   D. Patent ductus venosus
   E. Ventricular septal defect

7. An elderly woman presents with valvular stenosis and a particularly loud first heart sound (S₁). Which of the following heart valves are responsible for S₁?

   A. Aortic and mitral
   B. Mitral and tricuspid
   C. Tricuspid and pulmonary
   D. Pulmonary and aortic
   E. Aortic and tricuspid

8. Endoscopic examination of a 52-year-old man with a history of smoking reveals a malignancy in the right main bronchus. Which of the following lymph structures will most likely be infiltrated first by cancerous cells emanating from this malignancy?

   A. Bronchomediastinal trunk
   B. Bronchopulmonary (hilar) nodes
   C. Inferior tracheobronchial (carinal) nodes
   D. Pulmonary (intrapulmonary) nodes
   E. Right paratracheal nodes

9. Auscultation of the lungs of a 31-year-old woman reveal crackles heard on the back along the right medial border of the scapula, just above the inferior scapular angle, during late inspiration. Which of the following lobes are most likely involved in this pathology?

   A. Lower lobe of the right lung
   B. Lower lobes of both lungs
   C. Middle lobe of the right lung
   D. Upper lobe of the right lung
   E. Upper lobes of both lungs

10. A penetrating injury in the lower left neck just superior to the medial third of the clavicle results in the collapse of the left lung. Which of the following respiratory structures was most likely injured, resulting in this pneumothorax?

   A. Costal pleura
   B. Cupula
   C. Left main bronchus
   D. Left posterior lobe
   E. Mediastinal parietal pleura

For each condition described below (11-16), select the cardiac feature from the list (A-O) that is most likely responsible.

   (A) Aortic valve
   (B) Chordae tendineae
   (C) Conus arteriosus
   (D) Crista terminalis
   (E) Fossa ovalis
   (F) Membranous ventricular septum
   (G) Mitral valve
   (H) Moderator band
   (I) Opening of coronary sinus
   (J) Papillary muscles
   (K) Pectinate muscle
   (L) Pulmonary valve
   (M) Sinu-atrial node
   (N) Trabeculae carneae
   (O) Tricuspid valve

____ 11. During strenuous exercise, this feature of the right ventricle ensures coordinated contraction of the anterior papillary muscle.

____ 12. An implantable cardiac defibrillator can function as a pacemaker should this structure be unable to initiate the normal cardiac rhythm.

____ 13. Most atrial septal defects occur at this site.

____ 14. Some of the venous blood returning to the right atrium gains access through this feature.

____ 15. Radiographic contrast imaging of the heart highlights this roughened internal feature of each ventricular wall.

____ 16. This feature is the postnatal manifestation of the primitive embryonic atrial cardiac muscle.

17. A 67-year-old man experiences chest pain indicative of angina pectoris and myocardial ischemia. The visceral sensory neurons mediating this pain would most likely be found in which of the following locations?

   A. Dorsal root ganglion of T1-T2
   B. Intermediolateral gray matter of the upper thorax spinal cord
   C. Medial brachial cutaneous nerve
   D. Sympathetic chain ganglia
   E. Vagal sensory ganglion

18. Cardiomyopathy results in the enlargement of the left atrium. Which of the following structures is most likely to be compressed by this expansion?

   A. Azygos vein
   B. Esophagus
   C. Left pulmonary artery
   D. Superior vena cava
   E. Sympathetic trunk

19. A woman is diagnosed with metastatic breast cancer with lymph node involvement. Most of the lymphatic drainage of the breast passes to which of the following lymph nodes?

   A. Abdominal
   B. Axillary
   C. Infraclavicular
   D. Parasternal
   E. Pulmonary

20. The sternal angle (of Louis) is an important clinical surface landmark on the anterior chest wall, dividing the thorax into the superior and inferior mediastinum. Which of the following features also is found at the level of the sternal angle?

   A. Articulation of first rib
   B. Azygos vein
   C. Descending aorta
   D. Sinu-atrial node
   E. Tracheal bifurcation

Chapter 3: Thorax

1. **D.** The phrenic nerves course from superior to inferior along the lateral sides of the pericardium, anterior to the root structures entering or leaving the lungs. A longitudinal incision would run parallel to these nerves while a horizontal incision might potentially run across the nerves, unless the surgeon is very careful.

2. **C.** This continuous murmur is caused by the sound of blood rushing through a patent ductus arteriosus from the aorta into the pulmonary trunk (higher to lower pressure vessel). This is best heard over the left proximal clavicular area. Normally, the ductus narrows and closes shortly after birth to form the ligamentum arteriosum.

3. **B.** The apex (lower left ventricle) of the heart lies in the left midclavicular line at the fifth intercostal space. Its forceful contraction as it pumps blood into the aorta and systemic circulation is easily heard over this area.

4. **A.** The left brachiocephalic vein passes across the trachea and is very near the sixth cervical vertebra; moreover, in a young child it can lie above the level of the manubrium of the sternum. A tracheotomy is made below the cricoid cartilage and thyroid gland and just superior to this vein at about the level of the C6 vertebra.

5. **A.** The major blood supply to the interventricular septum and the right and left bundle branches is by the LAD (left anterior descending or anterior interventricular) coronary artery. The posterior interventricular branch supplies the remainder of the interventricular septum.

6. **E.** Ventricular septal defects (VSDs) are the most common congenital heart defect and the shunting of blood from the left to right ventricle results in right ventricular hypertrophy and pulmonary hypertension.

7. **B.** The first heart sound is made by the closing of the two atrioventricular valves (tricuspid and mitral). The stenosis (narrowing) most likely involves the mitral valve.

8. **C.** The "carinal" nodes are located at the inferior aspect of the tracheal bifurcation and would be the first nodes involved as lymph moves from the hilar nodes to the carinal nodes.

9. **A.** At this position on the right side of the back, the lower lobe of the right lung would be the location of the crackles. The oblique fissure dividing the right lung into superior and inferior lobes begins posteriorly at the level of T2, well above this level.

10. B. The cupula is the dome of cervical pleura surrounding the apex of the lung and it extends above the medial portion of the clavicle and the first rib.

11. H. The moderator band (septomarginal trabecula) extends from the lower interventricular septum to the base of the anterior papillary muscle in the right ventricle. It conveys the right AV bundle to this distal papillary muscle and probably assists in its coordinated contraction.

12. M. The "pacemaker" of the heart is the sinuatrial or SA node. It initiates the action potential that will pass through the atria and down into the ventricles.

13. E. Most atrial septal defects (ASDs) occur at the site of the foramen ovale in the fetal heart (fossa ovalis). If the foramen ovale (foramen secundum) remains open after birth, blood can pass from the left into the right atrium.

14. I. Venous blood returning from the coronary circulation returns to the right atrium via the coronary sinus.

15. N. The roughened appearance of the muscular bundles of the ventricular walls is called the trabeculae carneae (fleshy woody beams).

16. K. The roughened muscular walls of the atria (pectinate muscle) represent the "true" embryonic atrium while the smooth portion of each atrium is derived from the embryonic sinus venosus.

17. A. Sensory nerve cell bodies conveying somatic or visceral pain are found in the dorsal root ganglia (DRG). Those sensory pain fibers (visceral pain) from myocardial ischemia are conveyed to the upper portion of the sympathetic component of the ANS and reside in the T1-T2 DRG.

18. B. The esophagus lies directly posterior to the left atrium and may be compressed by enlargement of this heart chamber.

19. B. About three quarters of all the lymph from the breast passes to the axillary lymph nodes. Lymph can also pass laterally, inferiorly, and superiorly, but most passes to the axilla.

20. E. The sternal angle is a good landmark for determining the level of the tracheal bifurcation, the location of the aortic arch, and the articulation of the second ribs with the sternum.

Abdomen

1. INTRODUCTION
2. SURFACE ANATOMY
3. ANTEROLATERAL ABDOMINAL
   WALL

4. INGUINAL REGION
5. ABDOMINAL VISCERA
6. POSTERIOR ABDOMINAL
   WALL AND VISCERA

7. EMBRYOLOGY
CHALLENGE YOURSELF
   QUESTIONS

1. INTRODUCTION

The abdomen is the region between the thorax superiorly and the pelvis inferiorly. The abdomen is composed of the following:

- Layers of skeletal muscle that line the abdominal walls and assist in respiration and, by increasing intraabdominal pressure, facilitate micturition (urination), defecation (bowel movement), and childbirth.
- The abdominal cavity, a peritoneal lined cavity that is continuous with the pelvic cavity inferiorly and contains the abdominal viscera (organs).
- Visceral structures that lie within the abdominal peritoneal cavity (intraperitoneal) and include the gastrointestinal (GI) tract and its associated organs, the spleen, and the urinary system (kidneys and ureters), which is located retroperitoneally behind and outside the cavity but anterior to the posterior abdominal wall muscles.

In your study of the abdomen, first focus on the abdominal wall and note the continuation of the three muscle layers of the thorax (intercostal muscles) as they blend into the abdominal flank musculature.

Next, note the disposition of the abdominal organs. For example, you should know the region or quadrant of the abdominal cavity in which the organs reside; whether an organ is suspended in a mesentery or lies retroperitoneally (refer to embryology of abdominal viscera, i.e., foregut, midgut, or hindgut derivatives); the blood supply and autonomic innervation pattern to the organs; and features of the organs that will allow you to readily identify which organ or part of an organ you are viewing (particularly important in laparoscopic surgery). Also, you should understand the

dual venous drainage of the abdomen by the caval and hepatic portal systems and the key anastomoses between these two systems that facilitate venous return to the heart.

Lastly, study the posterior abdominal wall musculature, and identify the components and distribution of the lumbar plexus of somatic nerves.

2. SURFACE ANATOMY

Key Landmarks

Key surface anatomy features of the anterolateral abdominal wall include the following (Fig. 4-1):

- **Rectus sheath:** a fascial sheath containing the rectus abdominis muscle, which runs from the pubic symphysis and crests to the xiphoid process and fifth to seventh costal cartilages.
- **Linea alba:** literally the "white line"; a relatively avascular midline subcutaneous band of fibrous tissue where the fascial aponeuroses of the rectus sheath from each side interdigitate in the midline.
- **Semilunar line:** the lateral border of the rectus abdominis muscle in the rectus sheath.
- **Tendinous intersections:** transverse skin grooves that demarcate transverse fibrous attachment points of the rectus sheath to the underlying rectus abdominis muscle.
- **Umbilicus:** the site that marks the T10 dermatome, lying at the level of the intervertebral disc between L3 and L4; the former attachment site of the umbilical cord.
- **Iliac crest:** the rim of the ilium, which lies at about the level of the L4 vertebra.
- **Inguinal ligament:** a ligament composed of the aponeurotic fibers of the external abdominal oblique muscle, which lies deep to a skin crease that marks the division

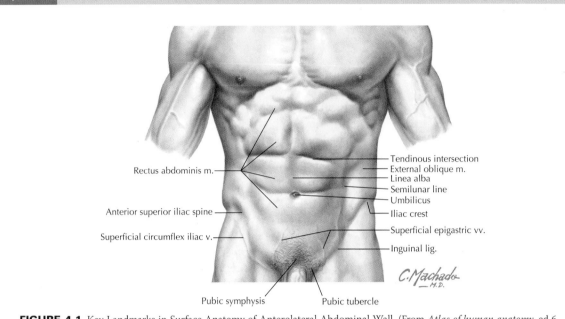

FIGURE 4-1 Key Landmarks in Surface Anatomy of Anterolateral Abdominal Wall. (From *Atlas of human anatomy,* ed 6, Plate 242.)

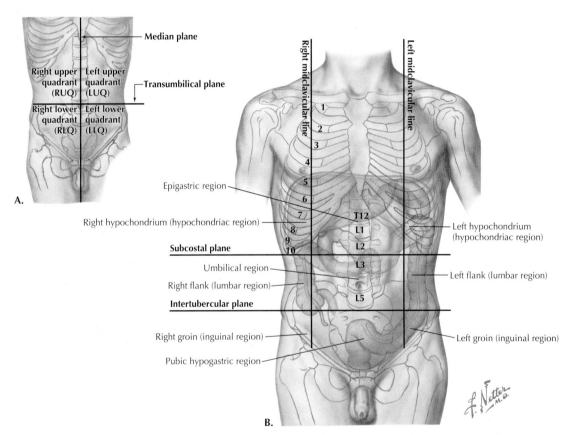

FIGURE 4-2 Four-Quadrant (A) and Nine-Region (B) Abdominal Planes. (From *Atlas of human anatomy,* ed 6, Plate 244.)

TABLE 4-1 Clinical Planes of Reference for Abdomen

PLANE OF REFERENCE	DEFINITION
Median	Vertical plane from xiphoid process to pubic symphysis
Transumbilical	Horizontal plane across umbilicus; these planes divide the abdomen into quadrants.
Subcostal	Horizontal plane across inferior margin of 10th costal cartilage
Intertubercular	Horizontal plane across tubercles of ilium and body of L5 vertebra
Midclavicular	Two vertical planes through midpoint of clavicles; these planes divide the abdomen into nine regions.

between the lower abdominal wall and thigh of the lower limb.

Surface Topography

Clinically, the abdominal wall is divided descriptively into quadrants or regions so that both the underlying visceral structures and the pain or pathology associated with these structures can be localized and topographically described. Common clinical descriptions use either **quadrants** or the **nine descriptive regions,** demarcated by two vertical midclavicular lines and two horizontal lines: the subcostal and intertubercular planes (Fig. 4-2 and Table 4-1).

3. ANTEROLATERAL ABDOMINAL WALL

Layers

The layers of the abdominal wall include the following:

- **Skin:** epidermis and dermis
- **Superficial fascia** (subcutaneous tissue): a single, fatty connective tissue layer below the level of the umbilicus that divides into a more superficial fatty layer (Camper's fascia) and a deeper membranous layer (Scarpa's fascia; see Fig. 4-11).
- **Investing fascia:** tissue that covers the muscle layers.
- **Abdominal muscles:** three flat layers, similar to the thoracic wall musculature, except in the anterior midregion where the

vertically oriented rectus abdominis muscle lies in the rectus sheath.

- **Endoabdominal fascia:** tissue that is unremarkable except for a thicker portion called the **transversalis fascia,** which usually lines the inner aspect of the transversus abdominis muscle; it is continuous with fascia on the underside of the diaphragm, fascia of the posterior abdominal muscles, and fascia of the pelvic muscles.
- **Extraperitoneal (fascia) fat:** connective tissue that is variable in thickness and contains a variable amount of fat.
- **Peritoneum:** thin serous membrane that lines the inner aspect of the abdominal wall **(parietal peritoneum)** and occasionally reflects off the walls as a mesentery to invest partially or completely various visceral structures **(visceral peritoneum).**

Muscles

The muscles of the anterolateral abdominal wall include three flat layers that are continuations of the three layers in the thoracic wall (Fig. 4-3). These include two abdominal oblique muscles and the transversus abdominis muscle (Table 4-2). In the midregion a vertically oriented pair of rectus abdominis muscles lies within the rectus sheath and extends from the pubic symphysis and crest to the xiphoid process and costal cartilages 5 to 7 superiorly. The small pyramidalis muscle (Fig. 4-3, *B*) is inconsistent and clinically insignificant.

Rectus Sheath

The rectus sheath encloses the vertically running rectus abdominis muscle (and inconsistent pyramidalis), the superior and inferior epigastric vessels, the lymphatics, and the ventral rami of T7-L1 nerves, which enter the sheath along its lateral margins (Fig. 4-3, *C*). The superior three quarters of the rectus abdominis is completely enveloped within the rectus sheath, and the inferior one quarter is supported posteriorly only by the transversalis fascia, extraperitoneal fat, and peritoneum; the site of this transition is called the *arcuate line* (Fig. 4-4 and Table 4-3).

Innervation and Blood Supply

The segmental innervation of the anterolateral abdominal skin and muscles is by **ventral rami of T7-L1.** The blood supply includes the following arteries (Figs. 4-3, *C,* and 4-5):

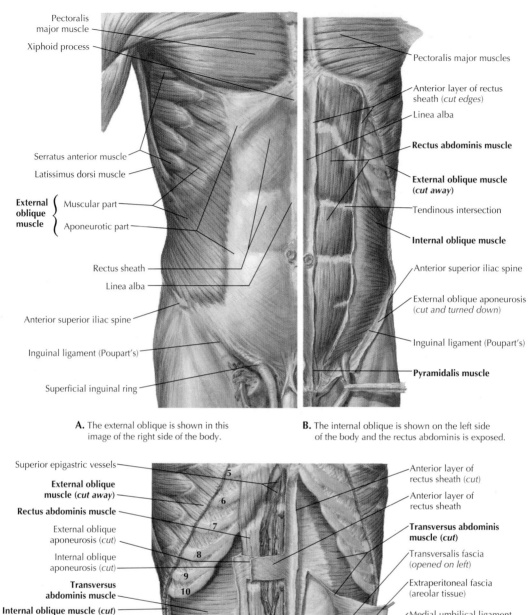

Pectoralis major muscle

Xiphoid process

Serratus anterior muscle

Latissimus dorsi muscle

External oblique muscle { Muscular part

Aponeurotic part

Rectus sheath

Linea alba

Anterior superior iliac spine

Inguinal ligament (Poupart's)

Superficial inguinal ring

Pectoralis major muscles

Anterior layer of rectus sheath (*cut edges*)

Linea alba

Rectus abdominis muscle

External oblique muscle (*cut away*)

Tendinous intersection

Internal oblique muscle

Anterior superior iliac spine

External oblique aponeurosis (*cut and turned down*)

Inguinal ligament (Poupart's)

Pyramidalis muscle

A. The external oblique is shown in this image of the right side of the body.

B. The internal oblique is shown on the left side of the body and the rectus abdominis is exposed.

Superior epigastric vessels

External oblique muscle (*cut away*)

Rectus abdominis muscle

External oblique aponeurosis (*cut*)

Internal oblique aponeurosis (*cut*)

Transversus abdominis muscle

Internal oblique muscle (*cut*)

Posterior layer of rectus sheath

Arcuate line

Inferior epigastric vessels

Anterior superior iliac spine

Inguinal ligament (Poupart's)

5
6
7
8
9
10

Anterior layer of rectus sheath (*cut*)

Anterior layer of rectus sheath

Transversus abdominis muscle (*cut*)

Transversalis fascia (*opened on left*)

Extraperitoneal fascia (areolar tissue)

Medial umbilical ligament (occluded part of umbilical artery)

Inferior epigastric artery and vein (*cut*)

Inguinal ligament (Poupart's)

C. The transversus abdominis muscle is shown on the right side of the body and is partially reflected on the left side to reveal the underlying transversalis fascia.

FIGURE 4-3 Muscles of Anterolateral Abdominal Wall. (From *Atlas of human anatomy,* ed 6, Plates 245 to 247.)

TABLE 4-2 Principal Muscles of Anterolateral Abdominal Wall

MUSCLE	PROXIMAL ATTACHMENT (ORIGIN)	DISTAL ATTACHMENT (INSERTION)	INNERVATION	MAIN ACTIONS
External oblique	External surfaces of 5th to 12th ribs	Linea alba, pubic tubercle, and anterior half of iliac crest	Inferior six thoracic nerves and subcostal nerve	Compresses and supports abdominal viscera; flexes and rotates trunk
Internal oblique	Thoracolumbar fascia, anterior two thirds of iliac crest, and lateral half of inguinal ligament	Inferior borders of 10th to 12th ribs, linea alba, and pubis via conjoint tendon	Ventral rami of inferior six thoracic nerves and 1st lumbar nerve	Compresses and supports abdominal viscera; flexes and rotates trunk
Transversus abdominis	Internal surfaces of costal cartilages 7-12, thoracolumbar fascia, iliac crest, and lateral third of inguinal ligament	Linea alba with aponeurosis of internal oblique, pubic crest, and pecten pubis via conjoint tendon	Ventral rami of inferior six thoracic nerves and 1st lumbar nerve	Compresses and supports abdominal viscera
Rectus abdominis	Pubic symphysis and pubic crest	Xiphoid process and costal cartilages 5-7	Ventral rami of inferior six thoracic nerves	Compresses abdominal viscera and flexes trunk

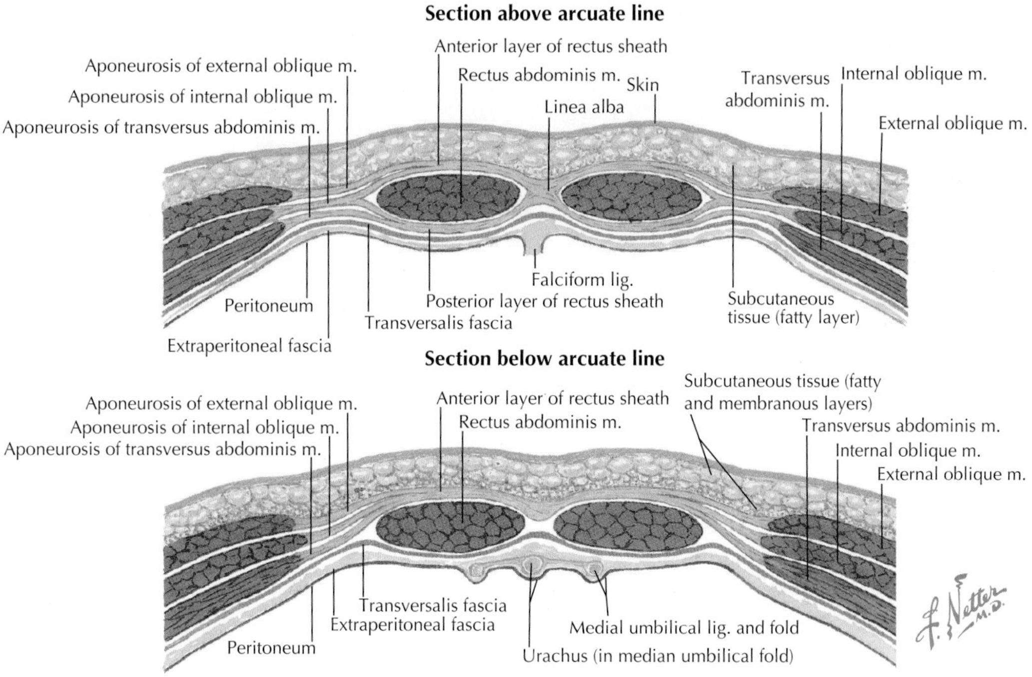

Section above arcuate line

Aponeurosis of external oblique m.
Aponeurosis of internal oblique m.
Aponeurosis of transversus abdominis m.
Anterior layer of rectus sheath
Rectus abdominis m. Skin
Linea alba
Transversus abdominis m. Internal oblique m.
External oblique m.
Peritoneum
Extraperitoneal fascia
Falciform lig.
Posterior layer of rectus sheath
Transversalis fascia
Subcutaneous tissue (fatty layer)

Section below arcuate line

Aponeurosis of external oblique m.
Aponeurosis of internal oblique m.
Aponeurosis of transversus abdominis m.
Anterior layer of rectus sheath
Rectus abdominis m.
Subcutaneous tissue (fatty and membranous layers)
Transversus abdominis m.
Internal oblique m.
External oblique m.
Transversalis fascia
Extraperitoneal fascia
Peritoneum
Medial umbilical lig. and fold
Urachus (in median umbilical fold)

FIGURE 4-4 Features of Rectus Sheath. (*Atlas of human anatomy,* ed 6, Plate 248.)

TABLE 4-3 Aponeuroses and Layers Forming Rectus Sheath*

LAYER	COMMENT	LAYER	COMMENT
Anterior lamina above arcuate line	Formed by fused aponeuroses of external and internal abdominal oblique muscles	Below arcuate line	All three muscle aponeuroses fuse to form anterior lamina, with rectus abdominis in contact only with transversalis fascia posteriorly
Posterior lamina above arcuate line	Formed by fused aponeuroses of internal abdominal oblique and transversus abdominis muscles		

*See Figure 4-4.

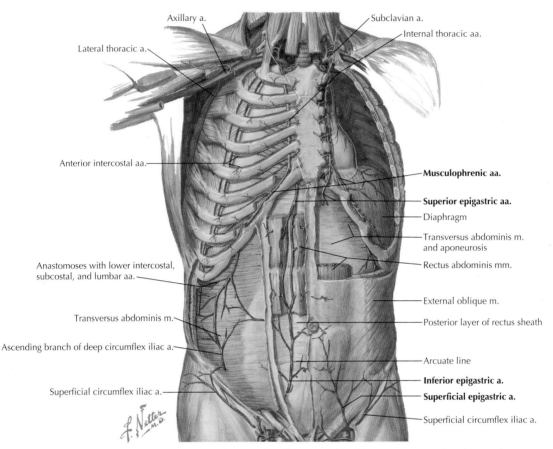

FIGURE 4-5 Arteries of Anterolateral Abdominal Wall. (From *Atlas of human anatomy,* ed 6, Plate 251.)

- **Musculophrenic:** a terminal branch of the internal thoracic artery that courses along the costal margin.
- **Superior epigastric:** arises from the terminal end of the internal thoracic artery and anastomoses with the inferior epigastric artery at the level of the umbilicus.
- **Inferior epigastric:** arises from the external iliac artery and anastomoses with the superior epigastric artery.
- **Superficial circumflex iliac:** arises from the femoral artery and anastomoses with the deep circumflex iliac artery.
- **Superficial epigastric:** arises from the femoral artery and courses toward the umbilicus.
- **External pudendal:** arises from the femoral artery and courses toward the pubis.

Superficial and deeper veins accompany these arteries, but, as elsewhere in the body, they form extensive anastomoses with each other to facili-tate venous return to the heart (Fig. 4-6 and Table 4-4).

Lymphatic drainage of the abdominal wall parallels the venous drainage, with the lymph ultimately coursing to the following lymph node collections:

- **Axillary nodes:** superficial drainage above the umbilicus
- **Superficial inguinal nodes:** superficial drainage below the umbilicus
- **Parasternal nodes:** deep drainage along the internal thoracic vessels
- **Lumbar nodes:** deep drainage internally to the nodes along the abdominal aorta
- **External iliac nodes:** deep drainage along the external iliac vessels

4. INGUINAL REGION

The inguinal region, or groin, is the transition zone between the lower abdomen and the upper

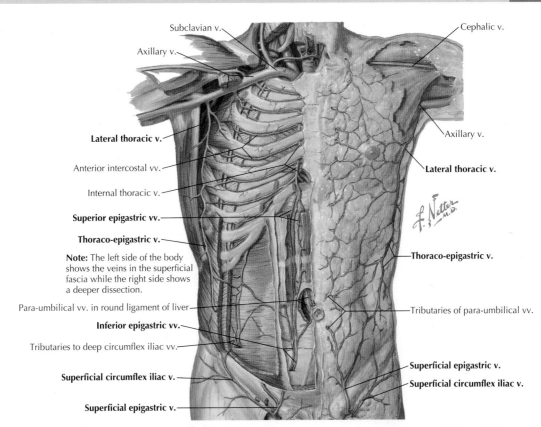

FIGURE 4-6 Veins of Anterolateral Abdominal Wall. (From *Atlas of human anatomy*, ed 6, Plate 252.)

TABLE 4-4 Principal Veins of Anterolateral Abdominal Wall

VEIN	COURSE
Superficial epigastric	Drains into femoral vein
Superficial circumflex iliac	Drains into femoral vein and parallels inguinal ligament
Inferior epigastric	Drains into external iliac vein
Superior epigastric	Drains into internal thoracic vein
Thoraco-epigastric	Anastomoses between superficial epigastric and lateral thoracic
Lateral thoracic	Drains into axillary vein

thigh. This region, especially in males, is characterized by a weakened area of the lower abdominal wall that renders this region particularly susceptible to inguinal hernias. Although occurring in either gender, inguinal hernias are much more common in males because of the descent of the testes into the scrotum, which occurs along this boundary region.

The inguinal region is demarcated by the **inguinal ligament,** the inferior border of the external abdominal oblique aponeurosis, which is folded under on itself and attaches to the anterior superior iliac spine and extends inferomedially to attach to the pubic tubercle (see Figs. 4-1 and 4-3, *B*). Medially, the inguinal ligament flares into the crescent-shaped **lacunar ligament** that attaches to the pecten pubis of the pubic bone (Fig. 4-7). Fibers from the lacunar ligament also course internally along the pelvic brim as the **pectineal ligament** (see Clinical Focus 4-2). A thickened inferior margin of the transversalis fascia, called the **iliopubic tract,** runs parallel to the inguinal ligament but deep to it and reinforces the medial portion of the inguinal canal.

Inguinal Canal

The gonads in both genders initially develop retroperitoneally from a mass of intermediate mesoderm called the *urogenital ridge*. As the gonads begin to descend toward the pelvis, a peritoneal pouch called the **processus vaginalis** extends through the various layers of the anterior abdominal wall and acquires a covering from each layer, except for the transversus abdominis muscle because the pouch passes beneath this muscle layer. The processus vaginalis and its coverings form the fetal **inguinal canal,** a tunnel or

Clinical Focus 4-1

Abdominal Wall Hernias

Abdominal wall hernias often are called **ventral hernias** to distinguish them from inguinal hernias. However, all are technically abdominal wall hernias. Other than inguinal hernias, which are discussed separately, the most common types of abdominal hernias include:

- **Umbilical hernia:** usually seen up to age 3 years and after 40.
- **Linea alba hernia:** often seen in the epigastric region and more common in males; rarely contains visceral structures (e.g., bowel).
- **Linea semilunaris (spigelian) hernia:** usually occurs in midlife and develops slowly.
- **Incisional hernia:** occurs at the site of a previous laparotomy scar.

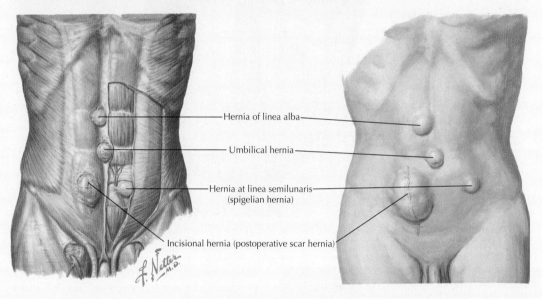

Hernia of linea alba

Umbilical hernia

Hernia at linea semilunaris (spigelian hernia)

Incisional hernia (postoperative scar hernia)

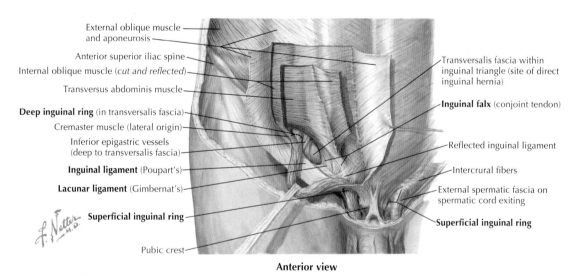

External oblique muscle and aponeurosis

Anterior superior iliac spine

Internal oblique muscle (*cut and reflected*)

Transversus abdominis muscle

Deep inguinal ring (in transversalis fascia)

Cremaster muscle (lateral origin)

Inferior epigastric vessels (deep to transversalis fascia)

Inguinal ligament (Poupart's)

Lacunar ligament (Gimbernat's)

Superficial inguinal ring

Pubic crest

Transversalis fascia within inguinal triangle (site of direct inguinal hernia)

Inguinal falx (conjoint tendon)

Reflected inguinal ligament

Intercrural fibers

External spermatic fascia on spermatic cord exiting

Superficial inguinal ring

Anterior view

FIGURE 4-7 Adult Inguinal Canal and Retracted Spermatic Cord. (From *Atlas of human anatomy*, ed 6, Plate 255.)

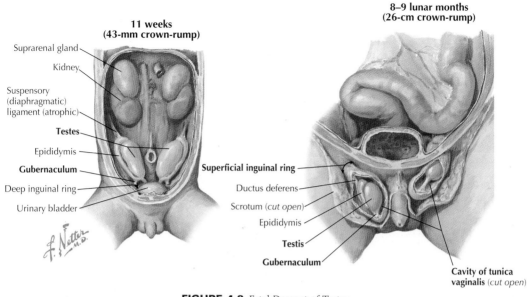

FIGURE 4-8 Fetal Descent of Testes.

passageway through the anterior abdominal wall. In females the ovaries are attached to the **gubernaculum,** the other end of which terminates in the labioscrotal swellings (which will form the labia majora in females or the scrotum in males). The ovaries descend into the pelvis, where they remain, tethered between the lateral pelvic wall and the uterus medially (by the ovarian ligament, a derivative of the gubernaculum). The gubernaculum then reflects off the uterus as the **round ligament of the uterus,** passes through the inguinal canal, and ends as a fibrofatty mass in the future labia majora.

In males the testes descend into the pelvis but then continue their descent through the inguinal canal (formed by the processus vaginalis) and into the scrotum, which is the male homologue of the female labia majora (Fig. 4-8). This descent through the inguinal canal occurs around the 26th week of development, usually over several days. The **gubernaculum** terminates in the scrotum and anchors the testis to the floor of the scrotum. A small pouch of the processus vaginalis called the **tunica vaginalis** persists and partially envelops the testis. In both genders the processus vaginalis then normally seals itself and is obliterated. Sometimes this fusion does not occur or is incomplete, especially in males, probably caused by descent of the testes through the inguinal canal. Consequently, a weakness may persist in the abdominal wall that can lead to inguinal hernias.

As the testes descend, they bring their accompanying spermatic cord along with them and, as these structures pass through the inguinal canal, they too become ensheathed within the layers of the anterior abdominal wall (Fig. 4-9). The spermatic cord enters the inguinal canal at the **deep inguinal ring** (an outpouching in the transversalis fascia lateral to the inferior epigastric vessels) and exits the 4-cm-long canal via the **superficial inguinal ring** (superior to the pubic tubercle) before passing into the scrotum, where it suspends the testis. In females the only structure in the inguinal canal is the fibrofatty remnant of the round ligament of the uterus, which terminates in the labia majora. The contents in the spermatic cord include the following (Fig. 4-9):

- Ductus (vas) deferens
- Testicular artery, artery of the ductus deferens, and cremasteric artery
- Pampiniform plexus of veins (testicular veins)
- Autonomic nerve fibers (sympathetic efferents and visceral afferents) coursing on the arteries and ductus deferens
- Genital branch of the genitofemoral nerve (innervates cremaster muscle)
- Lymphatics

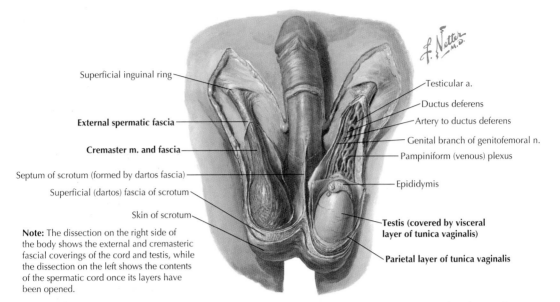

Superficial inguinal ring

External spermatic fascia

Cremaster m. and fascia

Septum of scrotum (formed by dartos fascia)

Superficial (dartos) fascia of scrotum

Skin of scrotum

Note: The dissection on the right side of
the body shows the external and cremasteric
fascial coverings of the cord and testis, while
the dissection on the left shows the contents
of the spermatic cord once its layers have
been opened.

Testicular a.

Ductus deferens

Artery to ductus deferens

Genital branch of genitofemoral n.

Pampiniform (venous) plexus

Epididymis

**Testis (covered by visceral
layer of tunica vaginalis)**

Parietal layer of tunica vaginalis

FIGURE 4-9 Layers of Spermatic Cord and Contents. (From *Atlas of human anatomy*, ed 6, Plate 365.)

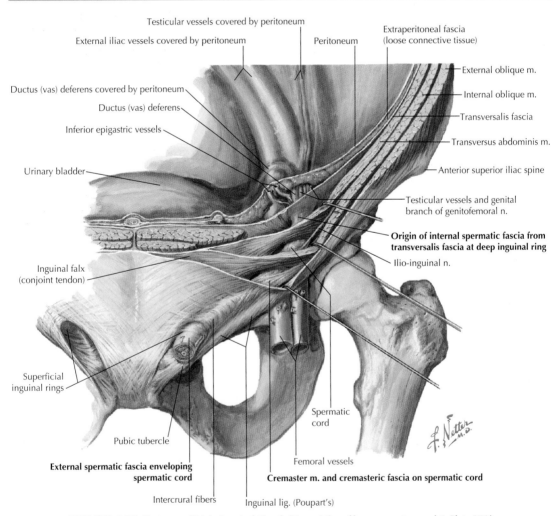

Testicular vessels covered by peritoneum

External iliac vessels covered by peritoneum

Peritoneum

Extraperitoneal fascia
(loose connective tissue)

Ductus (vas) deferens covered by peritoneum

Ductus (vas) deferens

Inferior epigastric vessels

Urinary bladder

External oblique m.

Internal oblique m.

Transversalis fascia

Transversus abdominis m.

Anterior superior iliac spine

Testicular vessels and genital
branch of genitofemoral n.

**Origin of internal spermatic fascia from
transversalis fascia at deep inguinal ring**

Ilio-inguinal n.

Inguinal falx
(conjoint tendon)

Superficial
inguinal rings

Pubic tubercle

**External spermatic fascia enveloping
spermatic cord**

Intercrural fibers

Inguinal lig. (Poupart's)

Spermatic
cord

Femoral vessels

Cremaster m. and cremasteric fascia on spermatic cord

FIGURE 4-10 Features of Male Inguinal Canal. (From *Atlas of human anatomy*, ed 6, Plate 256.)

Layers of the spermatic cord include the following (see Fig. 4-9):

- **External spermatic fascia:** derived from the external abdominal oblique aponeurosis
- **Cremasteric (middle spermatic) fascia:** derived from the internal abdominal oblique muscle
- **Internal spermatic fascia:** derived from the transversalis fascia

The features of the inguinal canal include its anatomical boundaries, as shown in Figure 4-10 and summarized in Table 4-5. Note that the **deep inguinal ring** begins internally as an outpouching of the transversalis fascia lateral to the inferior epigastric vessels, and that the **superficial inguinal ring** is the opening in the aponeurosis of the external abdominal oblique muscle. Aponeurotic fibers at the superficial ring envelop the emerging spermatic cord medially **(medial crus),** over its top **(intercrural fibers),** and laterally **(lateral crus)** (Fig. 4-10).

5. ABDOMINAL VISCERA

Peritoneal Cavity

The abdominal viscera are contained within a serous membrane–lined recess called the **abdominopelvic cavity** (sometimes just "abdominal" or "peritoneal" cavity) or lie in a retroperitoneal position adjacent to this cavity, often with only their anterior surface covered by peritoneum (e.g., the kidneys and ureters). The abdominopelvic cavity extends from the abdominal diaphragm inferiorly to the floor of the pelvis (Fig. 4-11).

The walls of the abdominopelvic cavity are lined by **parietal peritoneum,** which can reflect off the abdominal walls in a double layer called a **mesentery,** which embraces and suspends a visceral structure. As the mesentery wraps around the viscera, it becomes **visceral peritoneum.** Viscera suspended by a mesentery are considered intraperitoneal, whereas viscera covered on only one side by peritoneum are considered retroperitoneal.

The parietal peritoneum lines the inner aspect of the abdominal wall and thus is innervated by somatic afferent fibers of the ventral rami of the spinal nerves innervating the abdominal musculature. Inflammation or trauma to the parietal peritoneum therefore presents as well-localized pain. The visceral peritoneum, on the other hand, is

TABLE 4-5 Features and Boundaries of Inguinal Canal

FEATURE	COMMENT
Superficial ring	Medial opening in external abdominal oblique aponeurosis
Deep ring	Evagination of transversalis fascia lateral to inferior epigastric vessels, forming internal layer of spermatic fascia
Inguinal canal	Tunnel extending from deep to superficial ring, paralleling inguinal ligament; transmits spermatic cord in males or round ligament of uterus in females)
Anterior wall	Aponeuroses of external and internal abdominal oblique muscles
Posterior wall	Transversalis fascia; medially includes conjoint tendon
Roof	Arching muscle fibers of internal abdominal oblique and transversus abdominis muscles
Floor	Medial half of inguinal ligament, and medially by lacunar ligament, an expanded extension of the ligament
Inguinal ligament	Ligament extending between anterior superior iliac spine and pubic tubercle; folded inferior border of external abdominal oblique aponeurosis

innervated by visceral afferent fibers carried in the sympathetic and parasympathetic nerves. Pain associated with visceral peritoneum thus is more poorly localized, giving rise to *referred pain* (see Table 4-12).

Anatomists refer to the peritoneal cavity as a "potential space" because it normally contains only a small amount of serous fluid that lubricates its surface. If excessive fluid collects in this space because of edema **(ascites)** or hemorrhage, it becomes a "real space." Many clinicians, however, view the cavity only as a real space because it does contain serous fluid, although they qualify this distinction further when ascites or hemorrhage occurs.

The abdominopelvic cavity is further subdivided into the following (Figs. 4-11 and 4-12):

- **Greater sac:** most of the abdominopelvic cavity
- **Lesser sac:** also called the **omental bursa;** an irregular part of the peritoneal cavity that forms a cul-de-sac space posterior to the stomach and anterior to the retroperitoneal pancreas; it communicates with the greater sac via the **epiploic foramen** (of Winslow).

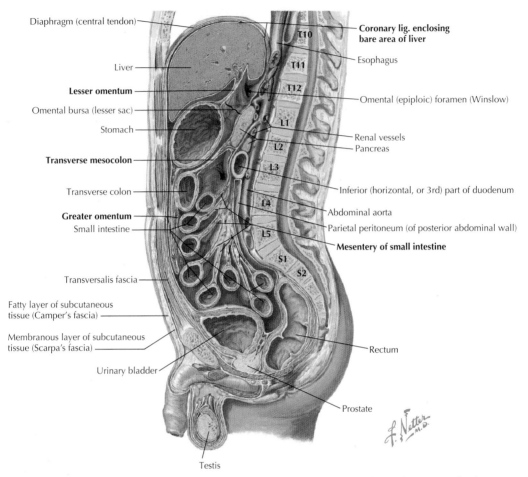

FIGURE 4-11 Sagittal Section of Peritoneal Cavity. Observe the parietal peritoneum lining the cavity walls, the mesenteries suspending various portions of the viscera, and the lesser and greater sacs. (From *Atlas of human anatomy*, ed 6, Plate 321.)

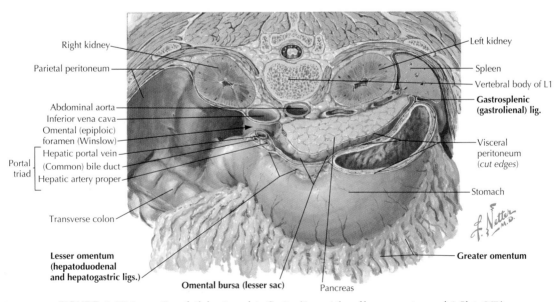

FIGURE 4-12 Lesser Sac of Abdominopelvic Cavity. (From *Atlas of human anatomy*, ed 6, Plate 267.)

Inguinal Hernias

The protrusion of peritoneal contents (mesentery, fat, and/or a portion of bowel) through the abdominal wall in the groin region is termed an *inguinal hernia*. Inguinal hernias are distinguished by their relationship to the inferior epigastric vessels. There are two types of inguinal hernia:

- **Indirect (congenital) hernia:** represents 75% of inguinal hernias; occurs lateral to the inferior epigastric vessels, passes through the deep inguinal ring and inguinal canal as a protrusion along the spermatic cord, and lies within the internal spermatic fascia.
- **Direct (acquired) hernia:** occurs medial to the inferior epigastric vessels, passes directly through the posterior wall of the inguinal canal, and is separate from the spermatic cord and its coverings derived from the abdominal wall.

Many indirect inguinal hernias arise from incomplete closure or weakness of the processus vaginalis. The herniated peritoneal contents may extend into the scrotum (or labia majora, but much less common in females) if the processus vaginalis is patent along its entire course.

Direct inguinal hernias pass through the **inguinal (Hesselbach's) triangle**, demarcated internally by the inferior epigastric vessels laterally, the rectus abdominis muscle medially, and the inguinal ligament inferiorly. Often, direct hernias are more limited in the extent to which they can protrude through the inferomedial abdominal wall. They occur not because of a patent processus vaginalis but because of an "acquired" weakness in the lower abdominal wall. Direct inguinal hernias can exit at the superficial ring and acquire a layer of external spermatic fascia, with the rare potential to herniate into the scrotum.

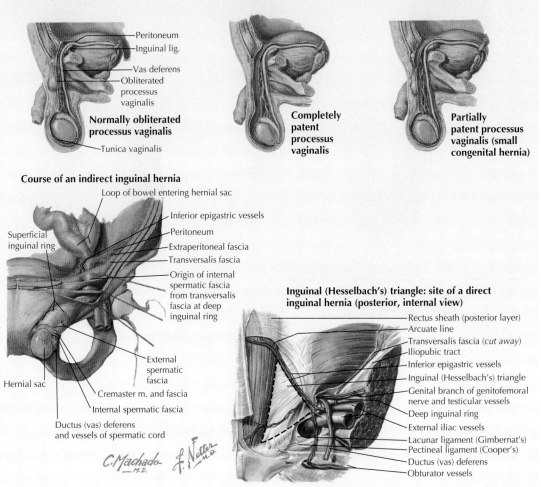

Peritoneum
Inguinal lig.

Vas deferens
Obliterated processus vaginalis

Normally obliterated processus vaginalis

Tunica vaginalis

Completely patent processus vaginalis

Partially patent processus vaginalis (small congenital hernia)

Course of an indirect inguinal hernia

Loop of bowel entering hernial sac

Inferior epigastric vessels

Superficial inguinal ring

Peritoneum
Extraperitoneal fascia
Transversalis fascia
Origin of internal spermatic fascia from transversalis fascia at deep inguinal ring

Inguinal (Hesselbach's) triangle: site of a direct inguinal hernia (posterior, internal view)

External spermatic fascia

Hernial sac

Cremaster m. and fascia
Internal spermatic fascia

Ductus (vas) deferens and vessels of spermatic cord

Rectus sheath (posterior layer)
Arcuate line
Transversalis fascia (*cut away*)
Iliopubic tract
Inferior epigastric vessels
Inguinal (Hesselbach's) triangle
Genital branch of genitofemoral nerve and testicular vessels
Deep inguinal ring
External iliac vessels
Lacunar ligament (Gimbernat's)
Pectineal ligament (Cooper's)
Ductus (vas) deferens
Obturator vessels

C. Machado
F. Netter
M.D.

Clinical Focus 4-3

Hydrocele and Varicocele

The most common cause of scrotal enlargement is **hydrocele,** an excessive accumulation of serous fluid within the tunica vaginalis (usually a potential space). This small sac of peritoneum is originally from the processus vaginalis that covers about two thirds of the testis. An infection in the testis or epididymis, trauma, or a tumor may lead to a hydrocele, or it may be idiopathic.

   Varicocele is an abnormal dilation and tortuosity of the pampiniform venous plexus within the spermatic cord. Almost all varicoceles are on the left side, perhaps because the left testicular vein drains into the left renal vein rather than the larger inferior vena cava, as the right testicular vein does. A varicocele is evident at physical examination when a patient stands, but it often resolves when the patient is recumbent.

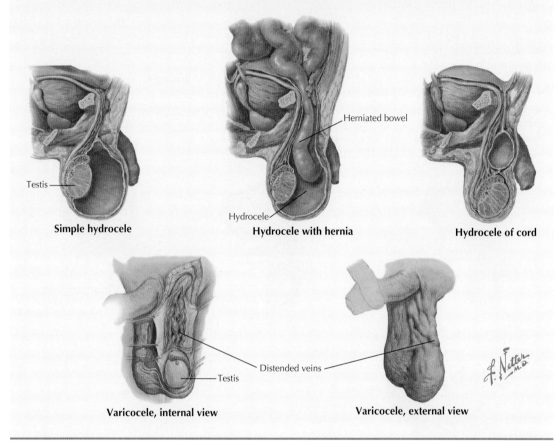

Testis

Simple hydrocele

Herniated bowel

Hydrocele

Hydrocele with hernia

Hydrocele of cord

Distended veins

Testis

Varicocele, internal view

Varicocele, external view

   In addition to the mesenteries that suspend the bowel, the peritoneal cavity contains a variety of double-layered folds of peritoneum, including the **omenta** (attached to the stomach) and **peritoneal ligaments.** These are not "ligaments" in the traditional sense but rather short, distinct mesenteries that connect structures (for which they are named) together or to the abdominal wall (Table 4-6). Some of these structures are shown in Figures 4-11 and 4-12, and we will encounter the others later in the chapter as we describe the abdominal contents.

Abdominal Organs

Abdominal Esophagus and Stomach

The distal end of the esophagus passes through the right crus of the abdominal diaphragm at about the level of the T10 vertebra and terminates in the cardiac portion of the stomach (Fig. 4-13).

   The stomach is a dilated, saclike portion of the GI tract that exhibits significant variation in size and configuration, terminating at the thick, smooth muscle sphincter (**pyloric sphincter**) by joining the first portion of the duodenum. The

TABLE 4-6 Mesenteries, Omenta, and Peritoneal Ligaments

FEATURE	DESCRIPTION	FEATURE	DESCRIPTION
Greater omentum	Double layer of peritoneum comprised of the gastrocolic, gastrosplenic, gastrophrenic and splenorenal ligaments, and upper anterior part of transverse mesocolon; also includes an apron of mesentery folding upon itself and draped over the bowels	Gastrophrenic ligament	Portion of greater omentum that extends from fundus to diaphragm
		Phrenocolic ligament	Extends from left colic flexure to diaphragm
		Hepatorenal ligament	Connects liver to right kidney
Lesser omentum	Double layer of peritoneum extending from lesser curvature of stomach and proximal duodenum to inferior surface of liver	Hepatogastric ligament	Portion of lesser omentum that extends from liver to lesser curvature of stomach
		Hepatoduodenal ligament	Portion of lesser omentum that extends from liver to 1st part of duodenum
Mesenteries	Double fold of peritoneum suspending parts of bowel and conveying vessels, lymphatics, and nerves of bowel (meso-appendix, transverse mesocolon, sigmoid mesocolon)	Falciform ligament	Extends from liver to anterior abdominal wall
		Ligamentum teres hepatis	Obliterated left umbilical vein in free margin of falciform ligament
		Coronary ligaments	Reflections of peritoneum from superior aspect of liver to diaphragm
Peritoneal ligaments	Double layer of peritoneum attaching viscera to walls or to other viscera	Ligamentum venosum	Fibrous remnant of obliterated ductus venosus
Gastrocolic ligament	Portion of greater omentum that extends from greater curvature of stomach to transverse colon	Suspensory ligament of ovary	Extends from lateral pelvic wall to ovary
Gastrosplenic ligament	Left part of greater omentum that extends from hilum of spleen to greater curvature of stomach	Ovarian ligament	Connects ovary to uterus (part of gubernaculum)
Splenorenal ligament	Connects spleen and left kidney	Round ligament of uterus	Extends from uterus to deep inguinal ring (part of gubernaculum)

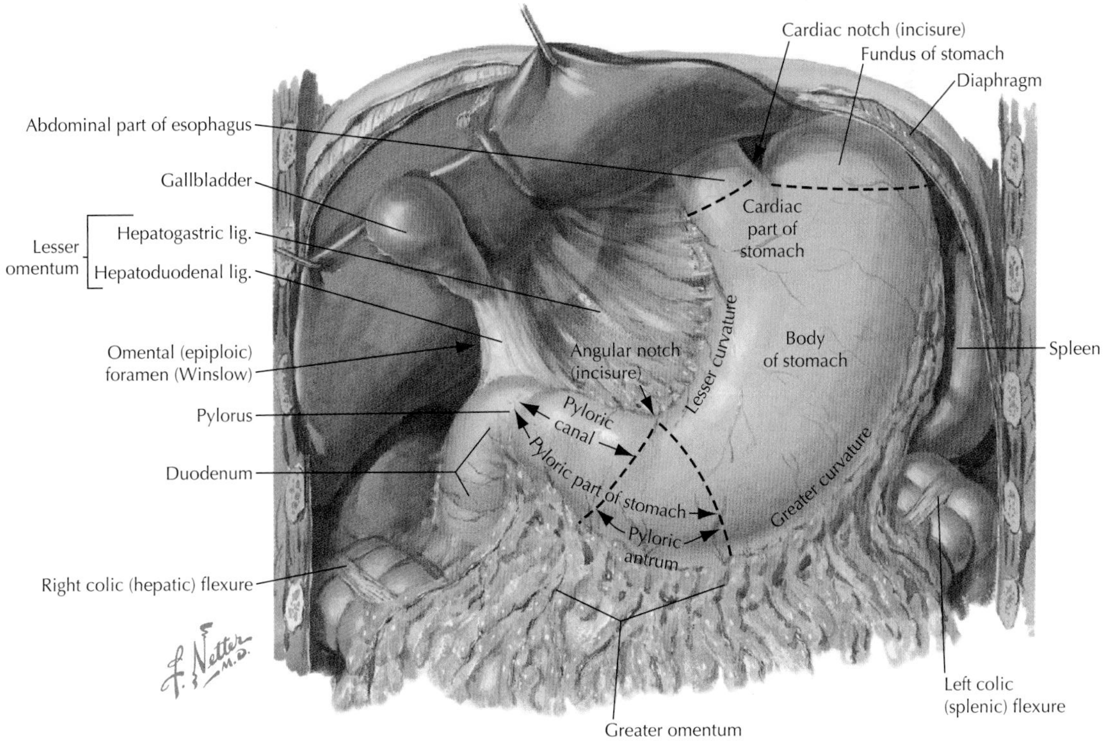

FIGURE 4-13 Abdominal Esophagus and Regions of the Stomach. (From *Atlas of human anatomy*, ed 6, Plate 269.)

stomach is tethered superiorly by the **lesser omentum** (gastrohepatic ligament portion; Table 4-6) extending from its lesser curvature and is attached along its greater curvature to the **greater omentum** and the **gastrosplenic ligament** (see Figs. 4-12 and 4-13). Generally, the J-shaped stomach is divided into the following regions (Fig. 4-13 and Table 4-7):

- **Cardiac region**
- **Fundus**
- **Body**
- **Pyloric region (antrum and canal)**

The interior of the unstretched stomach is lined with prominent longitudinal mucosal gastric folds called **rugae,** which become more evident as they approach the pyloric region. As an embryonic foregut derivative, the stomach's blood supply comes from the **celiac trunk** and its major branches (see Embryology).

Small Intestine

The small intestine measures about 6 meters in length (somewhat shorter in the fixed cadaver) and is divided into the following three parts:

- **Duodenum:** about 25 cm long and largely retroperitoneal
- **Jejunum:** about 2.5 meters long and suspended by a mesentery
- **Ileum:** about 3.5 meters long and suspended by a mesentery

The **duodenum** is the first portion of the small intestine and descriptively is divided into four parts (Table 4-8). Most of the C-shaped duodenum is retroperitoneal and ends at the duodenojejunal flexure, where it is tethered by a musculoperitoneal fold called the **suspensory ligament of the duodenum** (ligament of Treitz) (Fig. 4-14).

The **jejunum** and **ileum** are both suspended in an elaborate mesentery. The jejunum is recognizable from the ileum because the jejunum (Fig. 4-15):

- Occupies the left upper quadrant of the abdomen.
- Is larger in diameter than the ileum.
- Has thicker walls.
- Has mesentery with less fat.
- Has arterial branches with fewer arcades and longer vasa recta.
- Internally has mucosal folds that are higher and more numerous, which increases the surface area for absorption.

The small intestine ends at the **ileocecal junction,** where a sphincter called the **ileocecal valve** controls the passage of ileal contents into the cecum (Fig. 4-16). The valve is actually two internal mucosal folds that cover a thickened smooth muscle sphincter.

The small intestine is a derivative of the embryonic midgut and receives its arterial supply from the **superior mesenteric artery** and its branches. An exception to this generalization is the first part of the duodenum, and sometimes the second part, which receives arterial blood from the gastroduodenal branch (from the common hepatic artery of the celiac trunk). This overlap reflects the embryonic transition from the foregut and midgut derivatives (stomach to first portions of duodenum).

TABLE 4-7 Descriptive Features of the Stomach

FEATURE	DESCRIPTION
Lesser curvature	Right border of stomach; lesser omentum attaches here and extends to liver
Greater curvature	Convex border with greater omentum suspended from its margin
Cardiac part	Area of stomach that communicates with esophagus superiorly
Fundus	Superior part just under left dome of diaphragm
Body	Main part between fundus and pyloric antrum
Pyloric part	Portion divided into proximal antrum and distal canal
Pylorus	Site of pyloric sphincter muscle; joins 1st part of duodenum

TABLE 4-8 Features of the Duodenum

PART OF DUODENUM	DESCRIPTION
Superior	First part; attachment site for hepatoduodenal ligament of lesser omentum; technically not retroperitoneal for the first 1 or 2 inches (2.5-5 cm)
Descending	Second part; site where bile and pancreatic ducts empty
Inferior	Third part; crosses inferior vena cava and aorta and is crossed anteriorly by mesenteric vessels
Ascending	Fourth part; tethered by suspensory ligament at duodenojejunal flexure

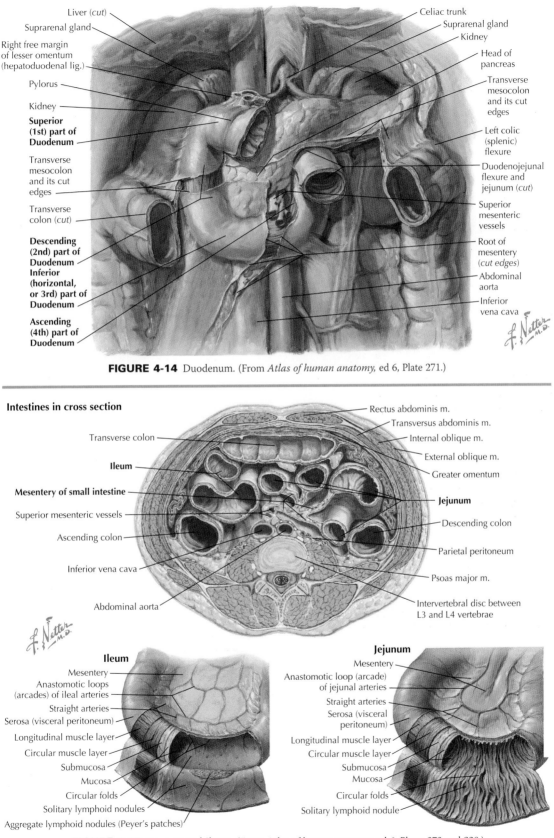

Liver (*cut*)
Suprarenal gland
Right free margin of lesser omentum (hepatoduodenal lig.)
Pylorus
Kidney
Superior (1st) part of Duodenum
Transverse mesocolon and its cut edges
Transverse colon (*cut*)
Descending (2nd) part of Duodenum
Inferior (horizontal, or 3rd) part of Duodenum
Ascending (4th) part of Duodenum

Celiac trunk
Suprarenal gland
Kidney
Head of pancreas
Transverse mesocolon and its cut edges
Left colic (splenic) flexure
Duodenojejunal flexure and jejunum (*cut*)
Superior mesenteric vessels
Root of mesentery (*cut edges*)
Abdominal aorta
Inferior vena cava

FIGURE 4-14 Duodenum. (From *Atlas of human anatomy*, ed 6, Plate 271.)

Intestines in cross section

Transverse colon
Ileum
Mesentery of small intestine
Superior mesenteric vessels
Ascending colon
Inferior vena cava
Abdominal aorta

Rectus abdominis m.
Transversus abdominis m.
Internal oblique m.
External oblique m.
Greater omentum
Jejunum
Descending colon
Parietal peritoneum
Psoas major m.
Intervertebral disc between L3 and L4 vertebrae

Ileum
Mesentery
Anastomotic loops (arcades) of ileal arteries
Straight arteries
Serosa (visceral peritoneum)
Longitudinal muscle layer
Circular muscle layer
Submucosa
Mucosa
Circular folds
Solitary lymphoid nodules
Aggregate lymphoid nodules (Peyer's patches)

Jejunum
Mesentery
Anastomotic loop (arcade) of jejunal arteries
Straight arteries
Serosa (visceral peritoneum)
Longitudinal muscle layer
Circular muscle layer
Submucosa
Mucosa
Circular folds
Solitary lymphoid nodule

FIGURE 4-15 Jejunum and Ileum. (From *Atlas of human anatomy*, ed 6, Plates 272 and 328.)

Large Intestine

The large intestine is about 1.5 meters long, extending from the cecum to the anal canal, and includes the following segments (Figs. 4-16 and 4-17):

- **Cecum:** a pouch that is connected to the ascending colon and the ileum; it extends below the ileocecal junction, although it is not suspended by a mesentery.
- **Appendix:** a narrow tube of variable length (usually 7-10 cm) that contains numerous

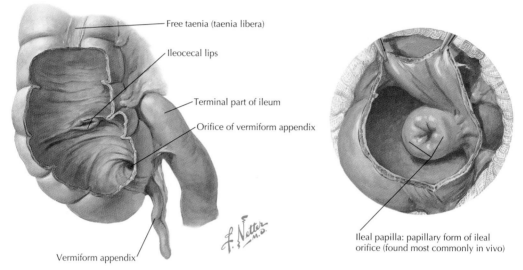

Free taenia (taenia libera)

Ileocecal lips

Terminal part of ileum

Orifice of vermiform appendix

Vermiform appendix

Ileal papilla: papillary form of ileal orifice (found most commonly in vivo)

FIGURE 4-16 Ileocecal Junction and Valve. (From *Atlas of human anatomy*, ed 6, Plate 274.)

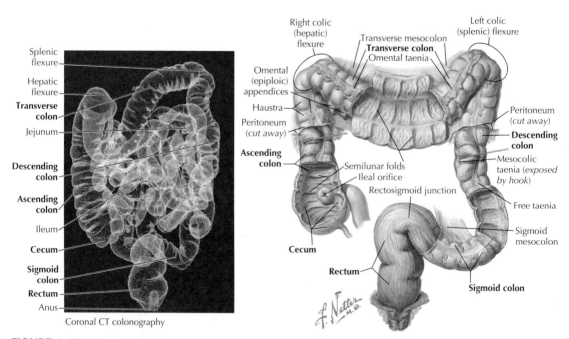

Splenic flexure
Hepatic flexure
Transverse colon
Jejunum
Descending colon
Ascending colon
Ileum
Cecum
Sigmoid colon
Rectum
Anus
Coronal CT colonography

Right colic (hepatic) flexure
Transverse mesocolon
Transverse colon
Omental taenia
Left colic (splenic) flexure

Omental (epiploic) appendices
Haustra
Peritoneum (cut away)
Ascending colon
Semilunar folds
Ileal orifice
Rectosigmoid junction
Cecum
Rectum

Peritoneum (cut away)
Descending colon
Mesocolic taenia (exposed by hook)
Free taenia
Sigmoid mesocolon
Sigmoid colon

FIGURE 4-17 Features and Large Intestine Musculature. (From *Atlas of human anatomy*, ed 6, Plate 276; CT image from Kelley LL, Petersen C: *Sectional anatomy for imaging professionals*, Philadelphia, Mosby, 2007.)

lymphoid nodules and is suspended by mesentery called the **meso-appendix.**

- **Ascending colon:** is retroperitoneal and ascends on the right flank to reach the liver, where it bends into the **right colic (hepatic) flexure.**
- **Transverse colon:** is suspended by a mesentery, the **transverse mesocolon,** and runs transversely from the right hypochondrium to the left, where it bends to form the **left colic (splenic) flexure.**
- **Descending colon:** is retroperitoneal and descends along the left flank to join the sigmoid colon in the left groin region.
- **Sigmoid colon:** is suspended by a mesentery, the **sigmoid mesocolon,** and forms a variable loop of bowel that runs medially to join the midline rectum in the pelvis.
- **Rectum and anal canal:** are retroperitoneal and extend from the middle sacrum to the anus (see Chapter 5).

Lateral to the ascending and the descending colon lie the right and the left paracolic gutters, respectively. These depressions provide conduits for abdominal fluids to pass from region to region, largely dependent on gravity. Functionally the colon (ascending colon through the sigmoid part) absorbs water and important ions from the feces.

It then compacts the feces for delivery to the rectum. Features of the large intestine include the following (Fig. 4-17):

- **Taeniae coli:** three longitudinal bands of smooth muscle that are visible on the cecum and colon's surface and assist in peristalsis.
- **Haustra:** sacculations of the colon created by the contracting taeniae coli.
- **Omental appendices:** small fat accumulations that are covered by visceral peritoneum and hang from the colon.
- **Greater luminal diameter:** the large intestine has a larger luminal diameter than the small intestine.

The arterial supply to the cecum, ascending colon, appendix, and most of the transverse colon is provided by branches of the **superior mesenteric artery;** these portions of the large intestine are derived from the embryonic midgut. The embryonic hindgut gives rise to the distal transverse colon, descending colon, sigmoid colon, rectum, and anal canal. These are supplied by branches of the **inferior mesenteric artery** and, in the case of the distal rectum and anal canal, rectal branches from the internal iliac and internal pudendal arteries (see pages 197-200).

Clinical Focus 4-4

Acute Appendicitis

Appendicitis is a fairly common inflammation of the appendix, often caused by bacterial infection. Initially the patient feels diffuse pain in the periumbilical region. However, as the appendix becomes more inflamed and irritates the parietal peritoneum, the pain becomes well localized to the right lower quadrant (circumscribed tenderness to palpation). Surgical resection is the treatment of choice to prevent life-threatening complications such as abscess and peritonitis.

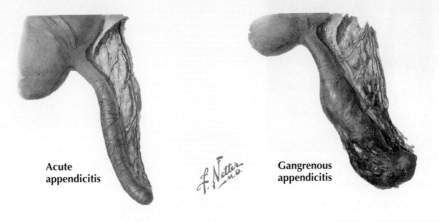

Acute appendicitis

Gangrenous appendicitis

Clinical Focus 4-5

Gastroesophageal Reflux Disease (GERD)

The terminal end of the esophagus possesses a **lower esophageal sphincter** (specialized smooth muscle that is physiologically different from the smooth muscle lining the lower esophagus). It prevents the reflux of gastric contents into the lower esophagus. However, it can become compromised, usually by a loss of muscle tone or a sliding hiatal hernia, leading to GERD and inflammation of the esophageal lining. GERD often presents with upper abdominal pain, dyspepsia, gas, heartburn, dysphagia, bronchospasm, or asthma.

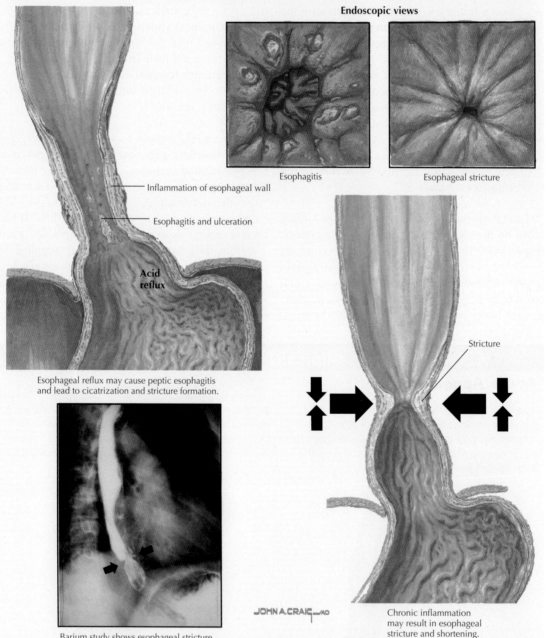

Endoscopic views

Esophagitis

Esophageal stricture

Inflammation of esophageal wall

Esophagitis and ulceration

Acid reflux

Stricture

Esophageal reflux may cause peptic esophagitis and lead to cicatrization and stricture formation.

JOHN A. CRAIG—AD

Chronic inflammation may result in esophageal stricture and shortening.

Barium study shows esophageal stricture.

Clinical Focus 4-6

Hiatal Hernia

Herniation of the diaphragm that involves the stomach is referred to as a hiatal hernia. A widening of the space between the muscular right crus forming the esophageal hiatus allows protrusion of part of the stomach superiorly into the posterior mediastinum of the thorax. The two anatomical types are as follows:

- Sliding, rolling, or axial hernia (95% of hiatal hernias): appears as a bell-shaped protrusion
- Para-esophageal, or nonaxial hernia: usually involves the gastric fundus

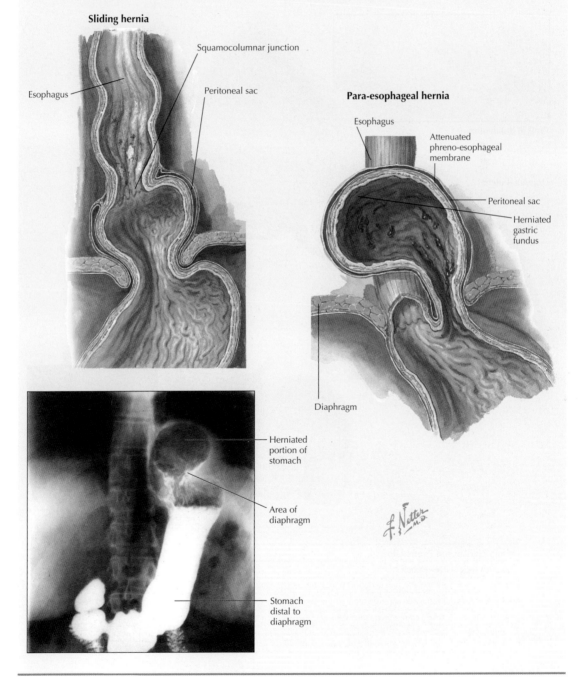

Sliding hernia

Squamocolumnar junction

Esophagus

Peritoneal sac

Para-esophageal hernia

Esophagus

Attenuated phreno-esophageal membrane

Peritoneal sac

Herniated gastric fundus

Diaphragm

Herniated portion of stomach

Area of diaphragm

Stomach distal to diaphragm

Peptic Ulcer Disease

Peptic ulcers are GI lesions that extend through the muscularis mucosae and are remitting, relapsing lesions. (*Erosions*, on the other hand, affect only the superficial epithelium.) Acute lesions are small and shallow, whereas chronic ulcers may erode into the muscularis externa or perforate the serosa. Although they may occur in the stomach, most occur in the first part of the duodenum, which is referred to by clinicians as the *duodenal cap.*

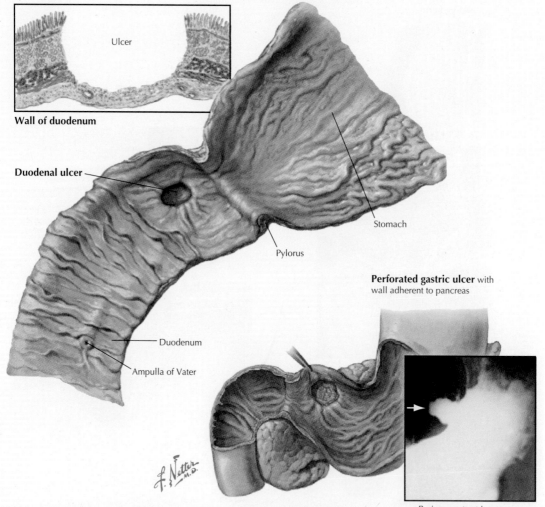

Ulcer

Wall of duodenum

Duodenal ulcer

Stomach

Pylorus

Perforated gastric ulcer with wall adherent to pancreas

Duodenum

Ampulla of Vater

Barium contrast image of perforated ulcer

Characteristics of Peptic Ulcers	
Characteristic	**Description**
Site	98% in first part of duodenum or stomach, in ratio of approximately 4:1
Prevalence	Worldwide approximately 5%; in United States approximately 2% in males and 1.5% in females
Age	Young adults, increasing with age
Aggravating factors	Mucosal exposure to gastric acid and pepsin; *H. pylori* infection (almost 80% of duodenal ulcers and 70% of gastric ulcers); use of nonsteroidal antiinflammatory drugs, aspirin, or alcohol; smoking

Clinical Focus 4-8

Bariatric Surgery

In some cases of morbid obesity, bariatric surgery may offer a viable alternative to failed dieting. The following three approaches may be considered:

- **Gastric stapling** (vertical banded gastroplasty) involves creating a small stomach pouch in conjunction with stomach stapling and banding; this approach is performed less frequently in preference to other options.
- **Gastric bypass** (Roux-en-Y) spares a small region of the fundus and attaches it to the proximal jejunum; the main portion of the stomach is stapled off, and the duodenum is reattached to a more distal section of jejunum, allowing for the mixture of digestive juices from the liver and pancreas.
- **Adjustable gastric banding** restricts the size of the proximal stomach, limiting the amount of food that can enter; the band can be tightened or relaxed via a subcutaneous access port if circumstances warrant.

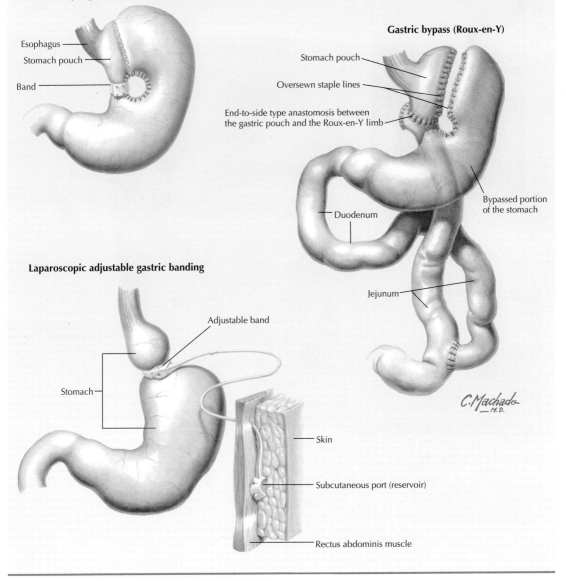

Gastric stapling (vertical banded gastroplasty)

Esophagus

Stomach pouch

Band

Gastric bypass (Roux-en-Y)

Stomach pouch

Oversewn staple lines

End-to-side type anastomosis between the gastric pouch and the Roux-en-Y limb

Duodenum

Bypassed portion of the stomach

Laparoscopic adjustable gastric banding

Adjustable band

Jejunum

Stomach

C. Machado
—M.D.

Skin

Subcutaneous port (reservoir)

Rectus abdominis muscle

Clinical Focus 4-9

Crohn Disease

Crohn disease is an idiopathic inflammatory bowel disease that can affect any segment of the GI tract but usually involves the small intestine (terminal ileum) and colon. Young adults of northern European ancestry are more often affected. Transmural edema, follicular lymphocytic infiltrates, epithelioid cell granulomas, and fistulation characterize Crohn disease. Signs and symptoms include the following:

- Diffuse abdominal pain (para-umbilical and right lower quadrant)
- Diarrhea
- Fever
- Dyspareunia (pain during sexual intercourse)
- Urinary tract infection (UTI)
- Malabsorption

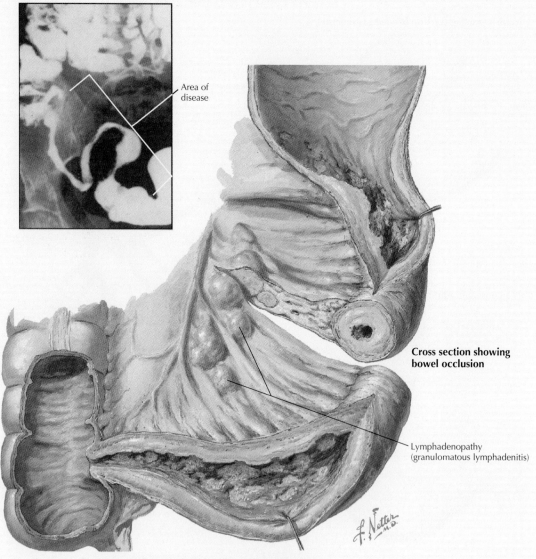

Area of disease

Cross section showing bowel occlusion

Lymphadenopathy (granulomatous lymphadenitis)

Regional enteritis confined to terminal ileum

Ulcerative Colitis

As with Crohn disease, ulcerative colitis is an idiopathic inflammatory bowel disease that begins in the rectum and extends proximally. Usually the inflammation is limited to the mucosal and submucosal layers of the bowel.

Intestinal complications

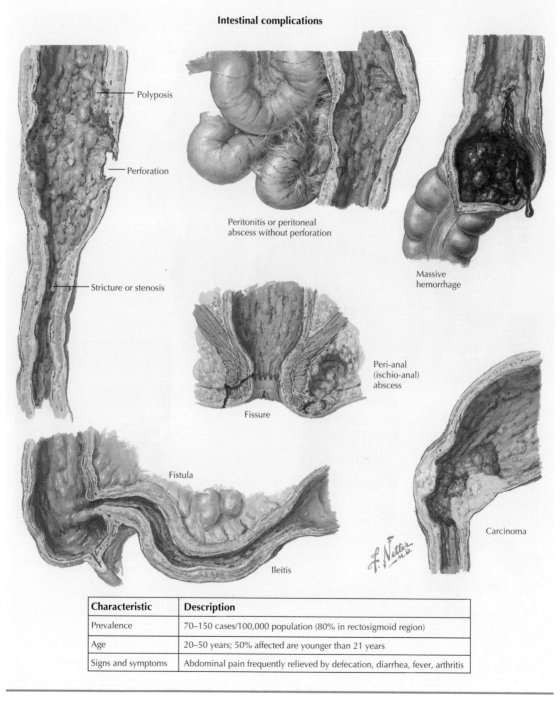

Polyposis

Perforation

Stricture or stenosis

Peritonitis or peritoneal abscess without perforation

Massive hemorrhage

Peri-anal (ischio-anal) abscess

Fissure

Fistula

Ileitis

Carcinoma

Characteristic	Description
Prevalence	70–150 cases/100,000 population (80% in rectosigmoid region)
Age	20–50 years; 50% affected are younger than 21 years
Signs and symptoms	Abdominal pain frequently relieved by defecation, diarrhea, fever, arthritis

Clinical Focus 4-11

Diverticulosis

Diverticulosis is a herniation of colonic mucosa and submucosa through the muscular wall, with a diverticular expansion in the adventitia of the bowel visible on its external surface. Common sites of development occur where neurovascular bundles penetrate the muscular wall of the bowel.

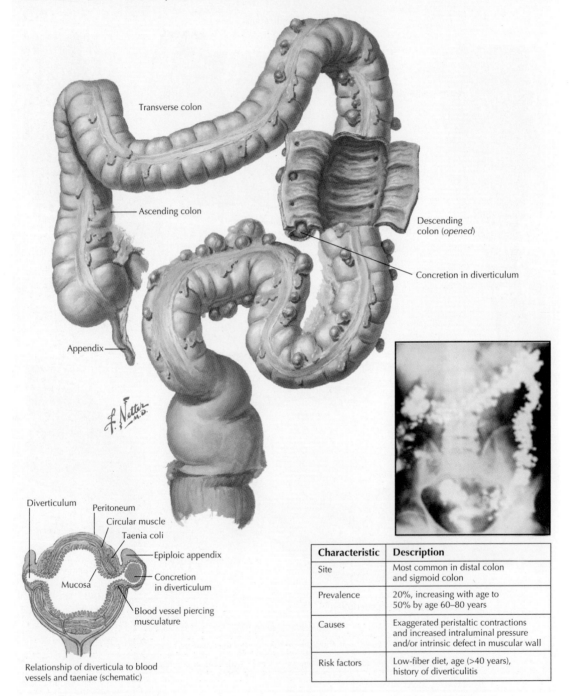

Transverse colon

Ascending colon

Descending colon (*opened*)

Concretion in diverticulum

Appendix

Diverticulum

Peritoneum

Circular muscle

Taenia coli

Epiploic appendix

Mucosa

Concretion in diverticulum

Blood vessel piercing musculature

Relationship of diverticula to blood vessels and taeniae (schematic)

Characteristic	Description
Site	Most common in distal colon and sigmoid colon
Prevalence	20%, increasing with age to 50% by age 60–80 years
Causes	Exaggerated peristaltic contractions and increased intraluminal pressure and/or intrinsic defect in muscular wall
Risk factors	Low-fiber diet, age (>40 years), history of diverticulitis

Clinical Focus 4-12

Colorectal Cancer

Colorectal cancer is second only to lung cancer in site-specific mortality and accounts for almost 15% of cancer-related deaths in the United States. The cancer appears as polypoid and ulcerating, and spreads by infiltration through the colonic wall, by regional lymph nodes, and to the liver through portal venous tributaries.

Relative regional incidence of carcinoma of large bowel

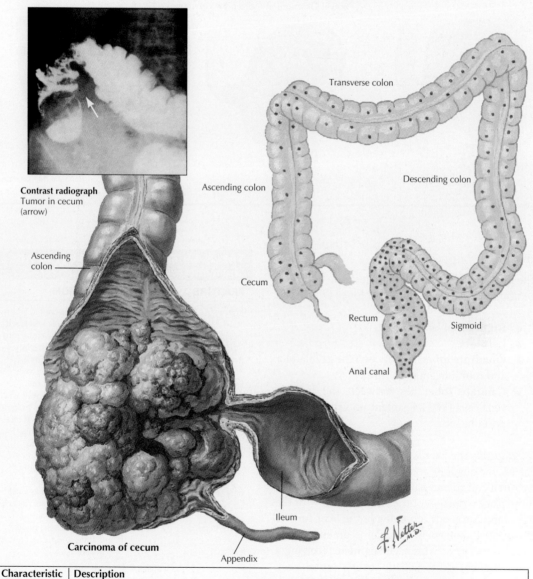

Contrast radiograph
Tumor in cecum
(arrow)

Ascending
colon

Cecum

Carcinoma of cecum

Appendix

Ileum

Transverse colon

Ascending colon

Descending colon

Cecum

Rectum

Sigmoid

Anal canal

Characteristic	Description
Site	98% adenocarcinomas: 25% in cecum-ascending colon, 25% in sigmoid colon, 25% in rectum, 25% elsewhere
Prevalence	Highest in United States, Canada, Australia, New Zealand, Denmark, Sweden; males affected 20% more than females
Age	Peak incidence at 60–70 years
Risk factors	Heredity, high-fat diet, increasing age, inflammatory bowel disease, polyps

Clinical Focus 4-13

Volvulus

Volvulus is the twisting of a bowel loop that may cause bowel obstruction and constriction of its vascular supply, which may lead to infarction. Volvulus affects the small intestine more often than the large, and the sigmoid colon is the most common site in the large intestine; the mesenteric mobility of these portions of the bowel account for this higher occurrence at these sites. Volvulus is associated with dietary habits, perhaps a bulky vegetable diet that results in an increased fecal load.

Bowel Obstruction Caused by Volvulus

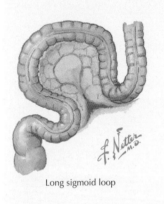

Long sigmoid loop   Contraction of base of mesosigmoid   Torsion, obstruction, strangulation, distention

Liver

The liver is the largest solid organ in the body and *anatomically* is divided into four lobes (Fig. 4-18):

- **Right lobe:** largest lobe
- **Left lobe**
- **Quadrate lobe:** lies between the gallbladder and round ligament of liver.
- **Caudate lobe:** lies between the inferior vena cava (IVC), ligamentum venosum, and porta hepatis.

Surgically the liver is divided into right and left halves. The quadrate and caudate anatomical lobes are often considered part of the left half, although some place a portion of the caudate lobe with the right lobe. Surgeons often divide the liver further into eight independent vascular segments based on its vasculature, with each segment receiving a major branch of the hepatic artery, portal vein, hepatic vein (drains the liver's blood into the IVC), and biliary drainage. The external demarcation of the two liver halves runs in an imaginary sagittal plane passing through the gallbladder and IVC (Table 4-9).

The liver is important as it receives the venous drainage from the GI tract, its accessory organs, and the spleen via the **portal vein** (see

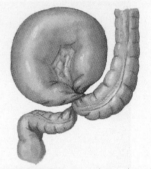

TABLE 4-9 Features of the Liver and Its Ligaments

FEATURE	DESCRIPTION
Lobes	Divisions, in functional terms, into right and left lobes, with anatomical subdivisions into quadrate and caudate lobes
Round ligament	Ligament that contains obliterated umbilical vein
Falciform ligament	Peritoneal reflection off anterior abdominal wall with round ligament in its margin
Ligamentum venosum	Ligamentous remnant of fetal ductus venosus, allowing fetal blood from placenta to bypass liver
Coronary ligaments	Reflections of peritoneum from liver to diaphragm
Bare area	Area of liver pressed against diaphragm that lacks visceral peritoneum
Porta hepatis	Site at which vessels, ducts, lymphatics, and nerves enter or leave liver

Fig. 4-25). The liver serves the following important functions:

- Storage of energy sources (glycogen, fat, protein, and vitamins)
- Production of cellular fuels (glucose, fatty acids, and keto acids)

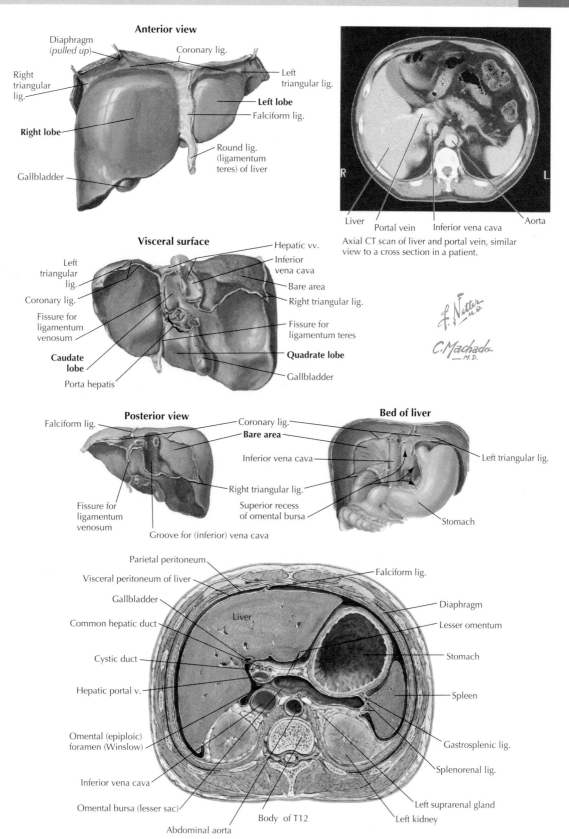

Anterior view

Diaphragm (*pulled up*)
Coronary lig.
Right triangular lig.
Left triangular lig.
Left lobe
Falciform lig.
Right lobe
Round lig. (ligamentum teres) of liver
Gallbladder

Liver   Portal vein   Inferior vena cava   Aorta

Axial CT scan of liver and portal vein, similar view to a cross section in a patient.

Visceral surface

Hepatic vv.
Inferior vena cava
Left triangular lig.
Bare area
Coronary lig.
Right triangular lig.
Fissure for ligamentum venosum
Fissure for ligamentum teres
Caudate lobe
Quadrate lobe
Porta hepatis
Gallbladder

Posterior view

Falciform lig.
Coronary lig.
Bare area
Inferior vena cava
Right triangular lig.
Fissure for ligamentum venosum
Superior recess of omental bursa
Groove for (inferior) vena cava

Bed of liver

Left triangular lig.
Stomach

Parietal peritoneum
Falciform lig.
Visceral peritoneum of liver
Gallbladder
Diaphragm
Liver
Common hepatic duct
Lesser omentum
Stomach
Cystic duct
Hepatic portal v.
Spleen
Omental (epiploic) foramen (Winslow)
Gastrosplenic lig.
Splenorenal lig.
Inferior vena cava
Left suprarenal gland
Omental bursa (lesser sac)
Left kidney
Body of T12
Abdominal aorta

FIGURE 4-18 Various Views of the Liver and Bed of the Liver. (From *Atlas of human anatomy,* ed 6, Plate 277; CT image from Kelley LL, Petersen C: *Sectional anatomy for imaging professionals,* Philadelphia, Mosby, 2007.)

- Production of plasma proteins and clotting factors
- Metabolism of toxins and drugs
- Modification of many hormones
- Production of bile acids
- Excretion of substances (bilirubin)
- Storage of iron and many vitamins
- Phagocytosis of foreign materials that enter the portal circulation from the bowel

The liver is a derivative of the foregut and receives its arterial supply from branches of the **celiac trunk.** Its right and left hepatic arteries arise from the **hepatic artery proper,** a branch of the common hepatic from the celiac trunk. The hepatic artery proper lies in the **hepatoduodenal ligament** with the **common bile duct** and **portal vein** (Figs. 4-18 and 4-19).

Gallbladder

The gallbladder is composed of a **fundus, body, and neck.** Its function is to receive, store, and concentrate bile. Bile secreted by the hepatocytes of the liver passes through the extrahepatic duct system (Fig. 4-19) as follows:

- Collects in the **right** and **left hepatic ducts** after draining the right and left liver lobes.
- Enters the **common hepatic duct.**
- Enters the **cystic duct** and is stored and concentrated in the gallbladder.
- On stimulation, largely by vagal efferents and cholecystokinin (CCK), leaves the gallbladder and enters the cystic duct.
- Passes inferiorly down the **common bile duct.**
- Enters the **hepatopancreatic ampulla** (of Vater).
- Empties into the second part of the duodenum (major duodenal papilla).

The liver produces about 900 mL of bile per day. Between meals, most of the bile is stored in the gallbladder, which has a capacity of 30 to 50 mL and where the bile is also concentrated.

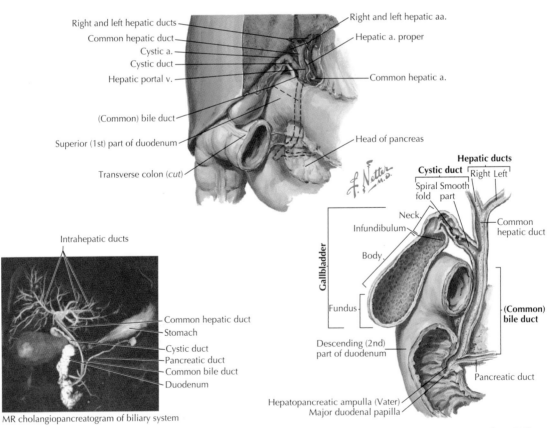

FIGURE 4-19 Gallbladder and Extrahepatic Ducts. (From *Atlas of human anatomy,* ed 6, Plate 280; MR image from Kelley LL, Petersen C: *Sectional anatomy for imaging professionals,* Philadelphia, Mosby, 2007.)

Intussusception

Intussusception is the invagination, or telescoping, of one bowel segment into a contiguous distal segment. In children the cause may be linked to excessive peristalsis. In adults an intraluminal mass such as a tumor may become trapped during a peristaltic wave and pull its attachment site forward into the more distal segment. Intestinal obstruction and infarction may occur.

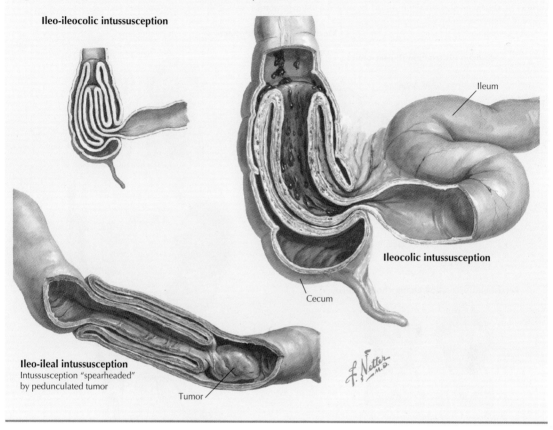

Ileo-ileocolic intussusception

Ileum

Ileocolic intussusception

Cecum

Ileo-ileal intussusception
Intussusception "spearheaded"
by pedunculated tumor

Tumor

Consequently, bile that reaches the duodenum is a mixture of the more dilute bile directly flowing from the liver and the concentrated bile from the gallbladder.

As a derivative of the embryonic foregut, the gallbladder is supplied by the **cystic artery,** usually a branch of the right hepatic artery, a branch of the hepatic artery proper (**celiac trunk distribution,** typical of foregut derivatives). The cystic artery lies in a triangle formed by the liver, cystic duct, and common hepatic duct, clinically referred to as **Calot's triangle** (Figs. 4-19 and 4-23). Variations in the biliary system (ducts and vessels) are common, and surgeons must proceed with caution in this area.

Pancreas

The pancreas is an exocrine and endocrine organ that lies posterior to the stomach in the floor of the lesser sac. It is a retroperitoneal organ, except for the distal tail, which is in contact with the spleen (Fig. 4-20). The anatomical parts of the pancreas include the following:

- **Head:** nestled within the C-shaped curve of the duodenum, with its **uncinate process** lying posterior to the superior mesenteric vessels.
- **Neck:** lies anterior to the mesenteric vessels, deep to the pylorus of the stomach.

Clinical Focus 4-15

Gallstones (Cholelithiasis)

Cholelithiasis results from stone formation in the gallbladder and extrahepatic ducts. Acute pain (biliary colic) can be referred to several sites. Common sites include the back just below the right scapula (T6-T9 dermatomes) or even the right shoulder region, if an inflamed gallbladder **(cholecystitis)** irritates the diaphragm. Obstruction of bile flow **(bile stasis)** can lead to numerous complications and **jaundice,** a yellow discoloration of the skin and sclera caused by bilirubin accumulation in the blood plasma.

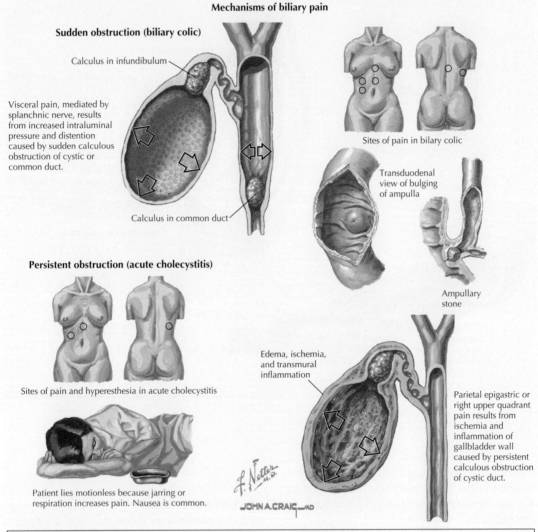

Mechanisms of biliary pain

Sudden obstruction (biliary colic)

Calculus in infundibulum

Visceral pain, mediated by splanchnic nerve, results from increased intraluminal pressure and distention caused by sudden calculous obstruction of cystic or common duct.

Calculus in common duct

Sites of pain in biliary colic

Transduodenal view of bulging of ampulla

Ampullary stone

Persistent obstruction (acute cholecystitis)

Sites of pain and hyperesthesia in acute cholecystitis

Edema, ischemia, and transmural inflammation

Parietal epigastric or right upper quadrant pain results from ischemia and inflammation of gallbladder wall caused by persistent calculous obstruction of cystic duct.

Patient lies motionless because jarring or respiration increases pain. Nausea is common.

Features of Cholelithiasis	
Characteristic	**Description**
Prevalence	10–20% of adults in developed countries
Types	Cholesterol stones: 80% (crystalline cholesterol monohydrate) Pigment stones: 20% (bilirubin calcium salts)
Risk factors	Increased age, obesity, female, rapid weight loss, estrogenic factors, gallbladder stasis
Complications	Gallbladder inflammation (cholecystitis), obstructive cholestasis or pancreatitis, empyema

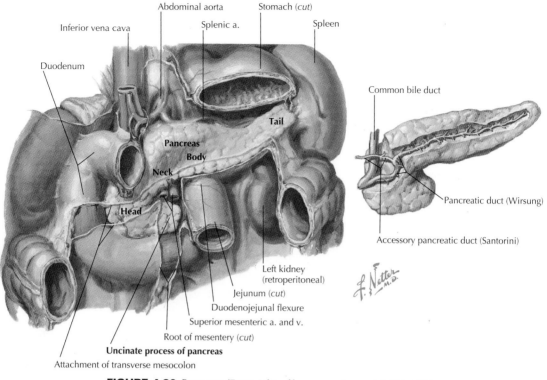

Abdominal aorta   Stomach (*cut*)
Inferior vena cava   Splenic a.   Spleen
Duodenum   Common bile duct
Tail
Pancreas
Body
Neck   Pancreatic duct (Wirsung)
Head
Accessory pancreatic duct (Santorini)
Left kidney (retroperitoneal)
Jejunum (*cut*)
Duodenojejunal flexure
Superior mesenteric a. and v.
Root of mesentery (*cut*)
Uncinate process of pancreas
Attachment of transverse mesocolon

FIGURE 4-20 Pancreas. (From *Atlas of human anatomy*, ed 6, Plate 281.)

- **Body:** extends above the duodenojejunal flexure and across the superior part of the left kidney.
- **Tail:** terminates at the hilum of the spleen in the splenorenal ligament.

The acinar cells of the exocrine pancreas secrete a number of enzymes necessary for digestion of proteins, starches, and fats. The pancreatic ductal cells secrete fluid with a high bicarbonate content that serves to neutralize the acid entering the duodenum from the stomach. Pancreatic secretion is under neural (vagus nerve) and hormonal (secretin and CCK) control, and the exocrine secretions empty primarily into the **main pancreatic duct,** which joins the common bile duct at the hepatopancreatic ampulla (of Vater). A smaller **accessory pancreatic duct** also empties into the second part of the duodenum above the major duodenal papilla (Fig. 4-20).

The endocrine pancreas is represented by clusters of islet cells (of Langerhans), a heterogeneous population of cells responsible for the elaboration and secretion primarily of insulin, glucagon, somatostatin, and several lesser hormones.

The pancreas is a derivative of the embryonic foregut but receives its arterial supply primarily from the **celiac trunk** (splenic artery and gastroduodenal branch from the common hepatic branch of the celiac artery), but also from branches of the **superior mesenteric artery** (inferior pancreaticoduodenal branches; see Fig. 4-23).

Spleen

The spleen is slightly larger than a clenched fist and weighs about 180 to 250 grams. It lies in the left upper quadrant of the abdomen and is tucked posterolateral to the stomach under the protection of the lower-left rib cage and diaphragm (Figs. 4-20 and 4-21). Simplistically, the spleen is a large lymph node, becoming larger during infections, although it is also involved in the following very important functions:

- Lymphocyte proliferation (B and T cells)
- Immune surveillance and response
- Blood filtration
- Destruction of old or damaged red blood cells (RBCs)
- Destruction of damaged platelets

Clinical Focus 4-16

Pancreatic Cancer

Carcinoma of the pancreas is the fifth leading cause of cancer death in the United States. Pancreatic carcinomas, which are mostly adenocarcinomas, arise from the exocrine part of the organ (cells of the duct system); 60% of cancers are found in the pancreatic head and often cause **obstructive jaundice.** Islet tumors of the endocrine pancreas are less common. Because of the anatomical position of the pancreas, adjacent sites may be directly involved (duodenum, stomach, liver, colon, spleen), and pancreatic metastases via the lymphatic network are common and extensive.

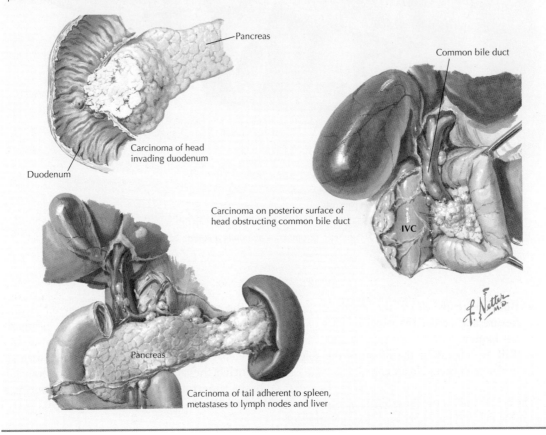

Pancreas

Common bile duct

Carcinoma of head invading duodenum

Duodenum

Carcinoma on posterior surface of head obstructing common bile duct

IVC

Pancreas

Carcinoma of tail adherent to spleen, metastases to lymph nodes and liver

- Recycling iron and globin
- Providing a reservoir for blood
- Providing a source of RBCs in early fetal life

The spleen is tethered between the stomach by the **gastrosplenic ligament** and the left kidney by the **splenorenal ligament.** Vessels, nerves, and lymphatics enter or leave the spleen at the hilum (Fig. 4-21). The arterial supply is via the splenic artery from the celiac trunk. Although supplied by the **celiac trunk,** the spleen is not a foregut embryonic derivative. The spleen is derived from mesoderm, unlike the ductal and epithelial linings

of the abdominal GI tract and its accessory organs (liver, gallbladder, pancreas).

Arterial Supply

The arterial supply and the innervation pattern of the abdominal viscera are directly reflected in the embryology of the GI tract, which is discussed later at the end of the chapter. The abdominal GI tract is derived from the following three embryonic gut regions:

- **Foregut**: gives rise to the abdominal esophagus, stomach, proximal half of the duodenum, liver, gallbladder, and pancreas

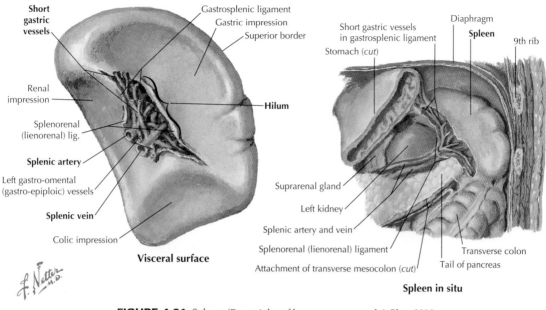

Short gastric vessels

Gastrosplenic ligament

Gastric impression

Superior border

Renal impression

Splenorenal (lienorenal) lig.

Splenic artery

Left gastro-omental (gastro-epiploic) vessels

Splenic vein

Colic impression

Hilum

Visceral surface

Short gastric vessels in gastrosplenic ligament

Stomach (*cut*)

Diaphragm

Spleen

9th rib

Suprarenal gland

Left kidney

Splenic artery and vein

Splenorenal (lienorenal) ligament

Attachment of transverse mesocolon (*cut*)

Transverse colon

Tail of pancreas

Spleen in situ

FIGURE 4-21   Spleen. (From *Atlas of human anatomy*, ed 6, Plate 282.)

Rupture of the Spleen

Trauma to the left upper quadrant can lead to splenic rupture. The adventitial capsule of the spleen is very thin, making traumatic rupture a medical emergency, as the spleen receives a rich vascular supply and can bleed profusely.

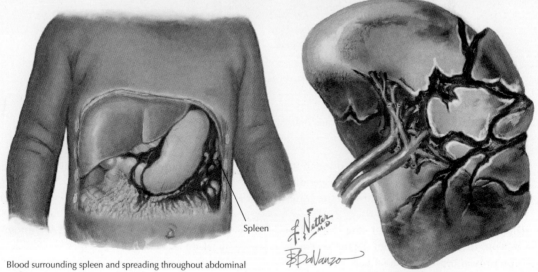

Spleen

Blood surrounding spleen and spreading throughout abdominal cavity

Multiple lacerations in spleen

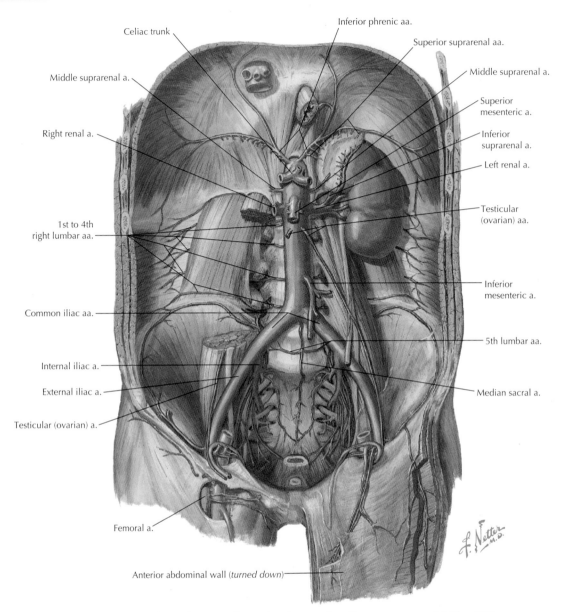

FIGURE 4-22 Abdominal Aorta and Branches. (From *Atlas of human anatomy,* ed 6, Plate 259.)

- **Midgut**: distal half of the duodenum, jejunum, ileum, cecum, appendix, ascending colon, and proximal two-thirds of the transverse colon
- **Hindgut**: distal third of the transverse colon, descending colon, sigmoid colon, rectum, and proximal anal canal

The following three large arteries arise from the anterior aspect of the **abdominal aorta;** each artery supplies the derivatives of the three embryonic gut regions (Fig. 4-22):

- **Celiac trunk** (artery): foregut derivatives and the spleen
- **Superior mesenteric artery (SMA):** midgut derivatives
- **Inferior mesenteric artery (IMA):** hindgut derivatives

The **celiac trunk** arises from the aorta immediately inferior to the diaphragm and divides into the following three main branches (Fig. 4-23):

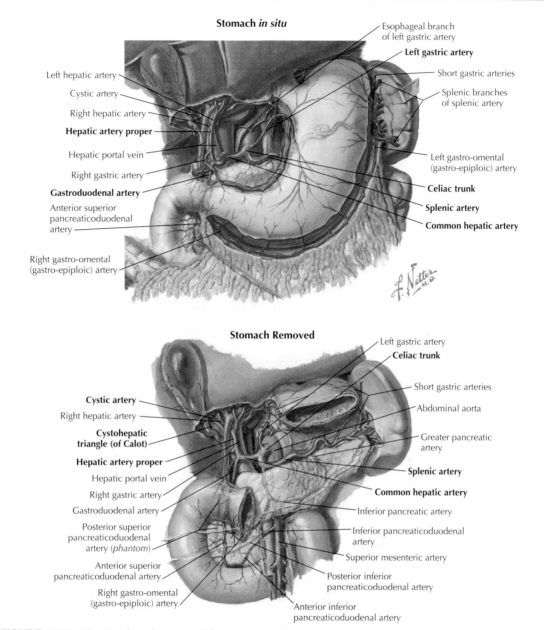

FIGURE 4-23 Celiac Trunk, with Major and Secondary Branches. (From *Atlas of human anatomy*, ed 6, Plates 283 and 284.)

- **Common hepatic artery:** supplies the liver, gallbladder, stomach, duodenum, and pancreas (head and neck).
- **Left gastric artery:** the smallest branch; supplies the stomach and esophagus.
- **Splenic artery:** the largest branch; takes a tortuous course along the superior margin of the pancreas and supplies the spleen, stomach, and pancreas (neck, body, tail).

The **SMA** arises from the aorta about one finger's breadth inferior to the celiac trunk. It then passes posterior to the neck of the pancreas and anterior to the distal duodenum. Its major branches include the following (Fig. 4-24):

- **Inferior pancreaticoduodenal artery:** supplies the head of the pancreas and duodenum

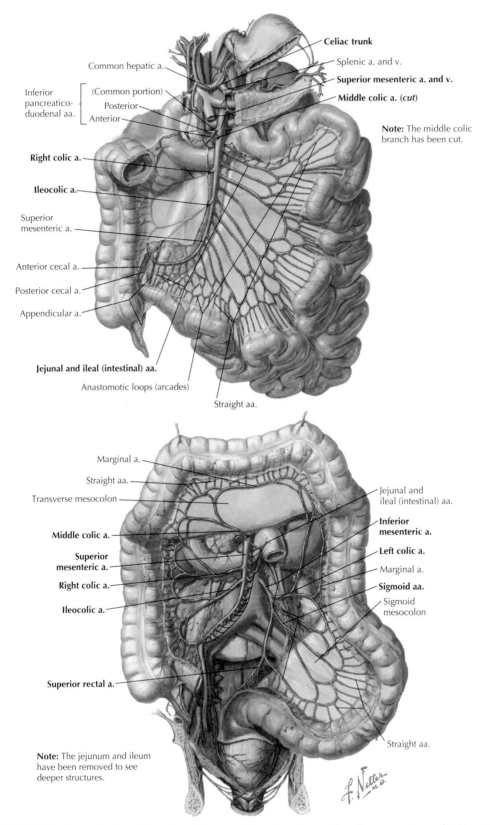

Celiac trunk

Common hepatic a.

Splenic a. and v.

Superior mesenteric a. and v.

Inferior pancreatico-duodenal aa.

(Common portion)

Posterior

Anterior

Middle colic a. (*cut*)

Note: The middle colic branch has been cut.

Right colic a.

Ileocolic a.

Superior mesenteric a.

Anterior cecal a.

Posterior cecal a.

Appendicular a.

Jejunal and ileal (intestinal) aa.

Anastomotic loops (arcades)

Straight aa.

Marginal a.

Straight aa.

Transverse mesocolon

Jejunal and ileal (intestinal) aa.

Inferior mesenteric a.

Middle colic a.

Superior mesenteric a.

Left colic a.

Marginal a.

Right colic a.

Sigmoid aa.

Ileocolic a.

Sigmoid mesocolon

Superior rectal a.

Note: The jejunum and ileum have been removed to see deeper structures.

Straight aa.

FIGURE 4-24 Superior and Inferior Mesenteric Arteries and Branches. (From *Atlas of human anatomy,* ed 6, Plates 287 and 288.)

- **Jejunal and ileal branches:** give rise to 15 to 18 intestinal branches; they run in the mesentery tethering the jejunum and ileum
- **Middle colic artery:** runs in the transverse mesocolon; supplies the transverse colon
- **Right colic artery:** courses retroperitoneally to the right side; supplies the ascending colon; is variable in location
- **Ileocolic artery:** passes to the right iliac fossa and supplies the ileum, cecum, appendix, and proximal ascending colon; terminal branch of the SMA

The **IMA** arises from the anterior aorta at about the level of the L3 vertebra (the aorta divides anterior to L4), angles to the left, and gives rise to the following branches (Fig. 4-24):

- **Left colic artery:** courses to the left and ascends retroperitoneally; supplies the distal transverse colon (by an ascending branch that enters the transverse mesocolon) and the descending colon

- **Sigmoid arteries:** a variable number of arteries (two to four) that enter the sigmoid mesocolon; supply the sigmoid colon
- **Superior rectal artery:** a small terminal branch; supplies the distal sigmoid colon and proximal rectum

Along the extent of the abdominal GI tract, the branches of each of these arteries anastomose with each other, providing alternative routes of arterial supply. For example, the **marginal artery** (of Drummond) (Fig. 4-24) is a large, usually continuous branch that interconnects the right, middle, and left colic branches supplying the large intestine.

Venous Drainage

The **hepatic portal system** drains the abdominal GI tract, pancreas, gallbladder, and spleen and ultimately drains into the liver and its sinusoids (Fig. 4-25). By definition, a *portal system* implies that arterial blood flows into a capillary system (in this case the bowel and its accessory organs), then

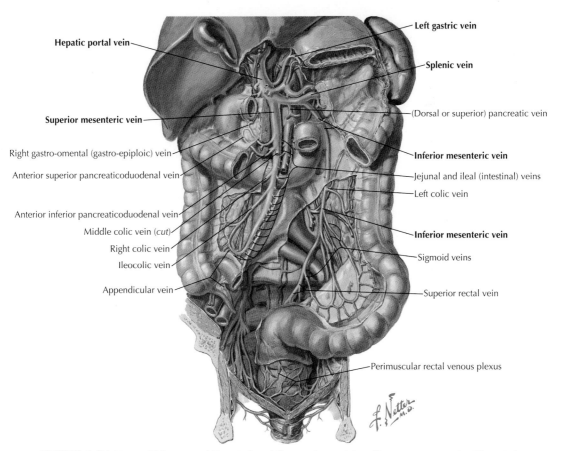

FIGURE 4-25 Venous Tributaries of Hepatic Portal System. (From *Atlas of human anatomy,* ed 6, Plate 291.)

into larger veins (portal tributaries), and then again into another capillary (or sinusoids) system (liver), before ultimately being collected into larger veins (hepatic veins, IVC) that return the blood to the heart.

The **portal vein** ascends from behind the pancreas (superior neck) and courses superiorly in the **hepatoduodenal ligament** (which also contains the common bile duct and hepatic artery proper) to the hilum of the liver; it is formed by the following veins (Figs. 4-25 and 4-26):

- **Superior mesenteric vein (SMV):** large vein that lies to the right of the SMA and drains portions of the foregut and all of the midgut derivatives.
- **Splenic vein:** large vein that lies inferior to the splenic artery, parallels its course, and drains the spleen, pancreas, foregut, and,

usually, hindgut derivatives (via the inferior mesenteric vein).

The **inferior mesenteric vein (IMV),** while usually draining into the splenic vein (see Fig. 4-25), also may drain into the junction of the SMV and splenic vein or drain directly into the SMV.

Typical of most veins in the body, the portal system has numerous anastomoses with other veins, specifically in this case with the tributaries of the caval system (IVC and azygos system of veins; Fig. 4-26). These anastomoses allow for the rerouting of venous return to the heart (these veins do not possess valves) should a major vein become occluded. The most important portosystemic anastomoses are around the lower esophagus (veins can enlarge and form varices), around the rectum and anal canal (present as hemorrhoids), and in the para-umbilical region (present as a caput medusae).

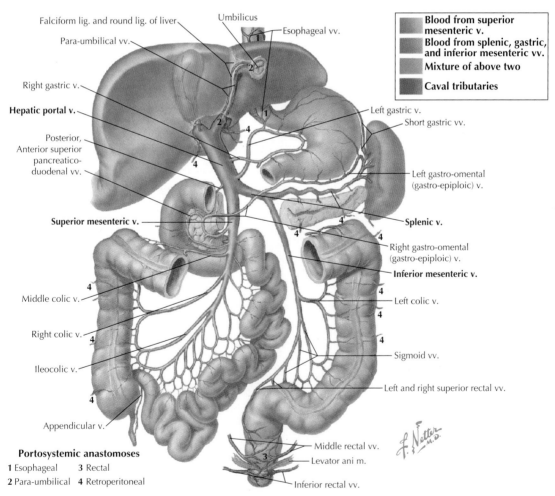

FIGURE 4-26 Hepatic Portal System and Important Portacaval Anastomoses. (From *Atlas of human anatomy,* ed 6, Plate 292.)

Cirrhosis of the Liver

Cirrhosis is a largely irreversible disease characterized by diffuse fibrosis, parenchymal nodular regeneration, and disturbed hepatic architecture. Progressive fibrosis disrupts the portal blood flow, leading to portal hypertension. Major causes of cirrhosis include the following:

- Alcoholic liver disease (60% to 70%)
- Viral hepatitis (10%)
- Biliary diseases (5% to 10%)
- Genetic hemochromatosis (5%)
- Cryptogenic cirrhosis (10% to 15%)

Portal hypertension can lead to **esophageal** and **rectal varices** (tortuous enlargement of the esophageal and rectal veins) as the portal venous blood is shunted into the caval system using portosystemic anastomoses (see Fig. 4-26). Additionally, the engorgement of the superficial venous channels in the subcutaneous tissues of the abdominal wall (see Fig. 4-6, via the para-umbilical portosystemic route) can appear as a **caput medusae** (tortuous subcutaneous varices that resemble the snakes of Medusa's head).

Changes resulting from cirrhosis and portal hypertension

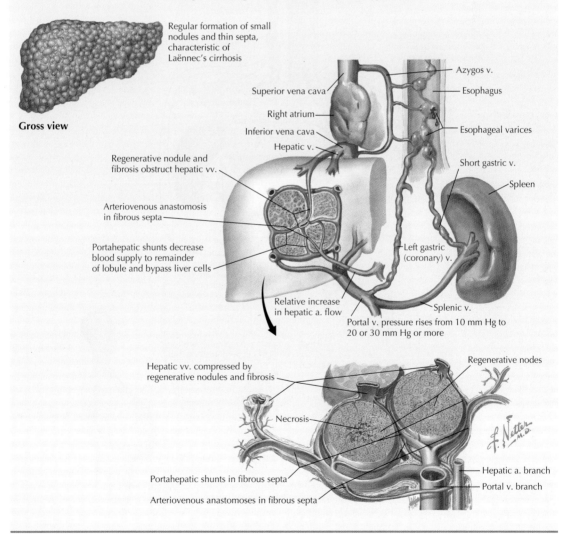

Regular formation of small nodules and thin septa, characteristic of Laënnec's cirrhosis

Gross view

Superior vena cava

Right atrium

Inferior vena cava

Hepatic v.

Regenerative nodule and fibrosis obstruct hepatic vv.

Arteriovenous anastomosis in fibrous septa

Portahepatic shunts decrease blood supply to remainder of lobule and bypass liver cells

Relative increase in hepatic a. flow

Azygos v.

Esophagus

Esophageal varices

Short gastric v.

Spleen

Left gastric (coronary) v.

Splenic v.

Portal v. pressure rises from 10 mm Hg to 20 or 30 mm Hg or more

Hepatic vv. compressed by regenerative nodules and fibrosis

Necrosis

Regenerative nodes

Portahepatic shunts in fibrous septa

Arteriovenous anastomoses in fibrous septa

Hepatic a. branch

Portal v. branch

Clinical Focus 4-19

Portal Hypertension

If the portal vein becomes occluded or its blood cannot pass through the hepatic sinusoids, a significant increase in portal venous pressure will ensue, resulting in portal hypertension. Normal portal venous pressure is 3 to 6 mm Hg but can exceed 12 mm Hg (portal hypertension), resulting in dilated, tortuous veins (varices) and variceal rupture. Three major mechanisms are defined as follows:

- **Prehepatic:** obstructed blood flow to the liver
- **Posthepatic:** obstructed blood flow from the liver to the heart
- **Intrahepatic:** cirrhosis or another liver disease, affecting hepatic sinusoidal blood flow

Clinical consequences of portal hypertension include the following:

- Ascites, usually detectable when 500 mL of fluid accumulates in the abdomen
- Formation of portosystemic shunts via anastomotic channels (see Fig. 4-26)
- Congestive splenomegaly (becomes engorged with venous blood backing up from the splenic vein)
- Hepatic encephalopathy (neurologic problems caused by inadequate removal of toxins in the blood by the diseased liver)

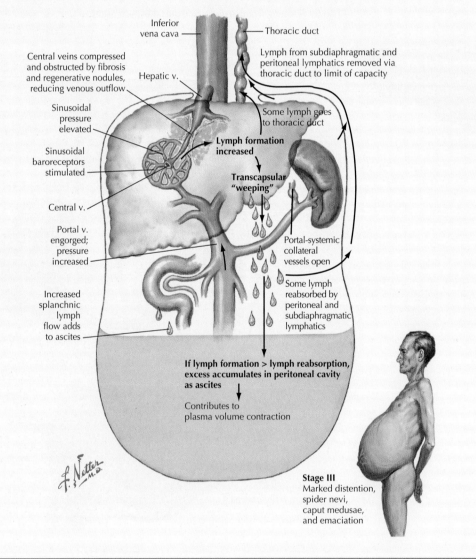

Inferior vena cava

Thoracic duct

Central veins compressed and obstructed by fibrosis and regenerative nodules, reducing venous outflow

Hepatic v.

Lymph from subdiaphragmatic and peritoneal lymphatics removed via thoracic duct to limit of capacity

Sinusoidal pressure elevated

Some lymph goes to thoracic duct

Lymph formation increased

Sinusoidal baroreceptors stimulated

Transcapsular "weeping"

Central v.

Portal v. engorged; pressure increased

Portal-systemic collateral vessels open

Increased splanchnic lymph flow adds to ascites

Some lymph reabsorbed by peritoneal and subdiaphragmatic lymphatics

If lymph formation > lymph reabsorption, excess accumulates in peritoneal cavity as ascites

Contributes to plasma volume contraction

Stage III
Marked distention, spider nevi, caput medusae, and emaciation

Lymphatics

Lymphatic drainage from the stomach, portions of the duodenum, liver, gallbladder, pancreas, and spleen is largely from regional nodes associated with those organs to a central collection of lymph nodes around the celiac trunk (Fig. 4-27). Lymphatic drainage from the midgut derivatives is largely to superior mesenteric nodes adjacent to the superior mesenteric artery, and hindgut derivatives (from the distal transverse colon to the distal rectum) drain to inferior mesenteric nodes adjacent to the artery of the same name (Fig. 4-28). These nodal collections often are referred to as the **pre-aortic** and **para-aortic nodes** and ultimately drain to the **cisterna chyli** (dilated proximal end of the thoracic duct), which is located adjacent to the celiac trunk.

Innervation

The abdominal viscera are innervated by the autonomic nervous system (ANS), and the pattern of innervation closely parallels the arterial supply to the various embryonic gut regions (see Table 4-14). Additionally, the enteric nervous system provides an "intrinsic" network of ganglia with connections to the ANS, which helps coordinate peristalsis and secretion (see Chapter 1). The enteric ganglia and nerve plexuses include the **myenteric plexus** and **submucosal plexus** within the layers of the bowel wall.

The sympathetic innervation of the viscera is derived from the following nerves (Figs. 4-29 and 4-30):

- **Thoracic splanchnic nerves:** greater (T5-T9), lesser (T10-T11), and least (T12) splanchnic nerves (the nerve branches from the thoracic ganglia from which these splanchnic nerves arise often is variable) that convey preganglionic axons to the prevertebral ganglia to innervate the foregut and midgut derivatives.
- **Lumbar splanchnic nerves:** usually several lumbar splanchnic nerves (L1-L2 or L3) that

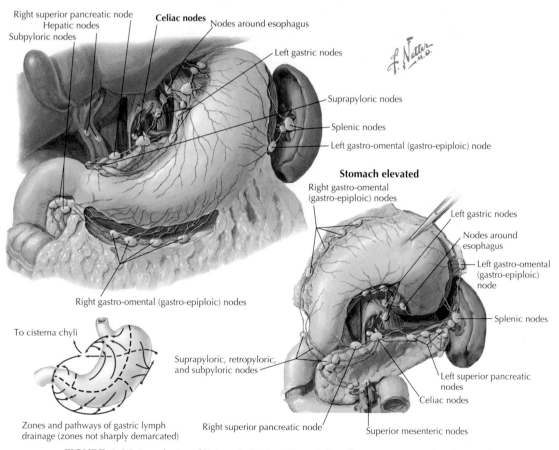

FIGURE 4-27 Lymphatics of Epigastric Region. (From *Atlas of human anatomy*, ed 6, Plate 293.)

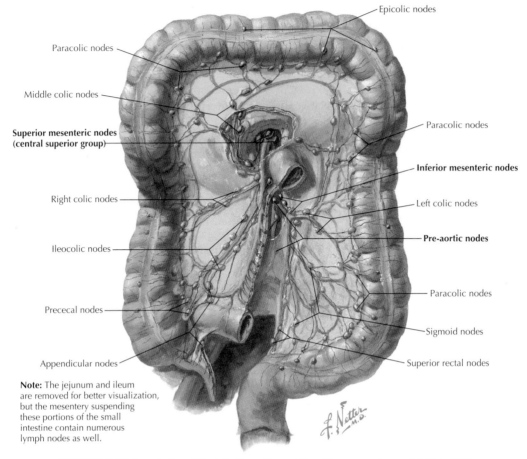

Epicolic nodes

Paracolic nodes

Middle colic nodes

Superior mesenteric nodes
(central superior group)

Paracolic nodes

Inferior mesenteric nodes

Right colic nodes

Left colic nodes

Pre-aortic nodes

Ileocolic nodes

Paracolic nodes

Prececal nodes

Sigmoid nodes

Appendicular nodes

Superior rectal nodes

Note: The jejunum and ileum
are removed for better visualization,
but the mesentery suspending
these portions of the small
intestine contain numerous
lymph nodes as well.

FIGURE 4-28 Lymphatics of the Intestines. (From *Atlas of human anatomy,* ed 6, Plate 296.)

convey preganglionic axons to the prevertebral ganglia and plexus to innervate the hindgut derivatives.

Postganglionic sympathetic axons arise from the postganglionic neurons in the prevertebral ganglia (celiac, superior mesenteric, and inferior mesenteric ganglia) and plexus and travel with the blood vessels to their target viscera. Generally, sympathetic stimulation leads to the following:

- Vasoconstriction to shunt blood to other parts of the body, thus inhibiting digestion
- Reduced bowel motility
- Reduced bowel secretion

The **parasympathetic innervation** of the viscera is derived from the following nerves (see Table 4-14 and Figs. 4-29 and 4-30):

- **Vagus nerves:** anterior and posterior vagal trunks enter the abdomen on the esophagus

and send preganglionic axons directly to postganglionic neurons in the walls of the viscera derived from the foregut and midgut (distal esophagus to the proximal two thirds of the transverse colon).

- **Pelvic splanchnic nerves:** preganglionic axons from S2-S4 travel via these splanchnic nerves to the prevertebral plexus (inferior hypogastric plexus) and distribute to the postganglionic neurons of the hindgut derivatives. (Note: pelvic splanchnic nerves are *not* part of the sympathetic trunk; only sympathetic neurons and axons reside in the sympathetic trunk and chain ganglia.)

Many postganglionic parasympathetic neurons are in the **myenteric** and **submucosal ganglia** and plexuses that compose the enteric nervous system (see Chapter 1). Generally, parasympathetic stimulation leads to the following:

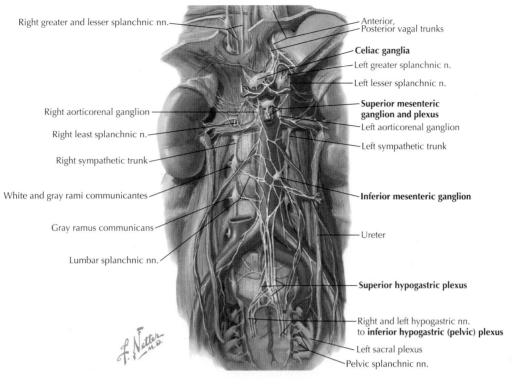

Right greater and lesser splanchnic nn.

Anterior,
Posterior vagal trunks

Celiac ganglia

Left greater splanchnic n.

Left lesser splanchnic n.

Right aorticorenal ganglion

Superior mesenteric ganglion and plexus

Right least splanchnic n.

Left aorticorenal ganglion

Right sympathetic trunk

Left sympathetic trunk

White and gray rami communicantes

Inferior mesenteric ganglion

Gray ramus communicans

Ureter

Lumbar splanchnic nn.

Superior hypogastric plexus

Right and left hypogastric nn.
to **inferior hypogastric (pelvic) plexus**

Left sacral plexus

Pelvic splanchnic nn.

FIGURE 4-29 Abdominal Autonomic Nerves. (From *Atlas of human anatomy*, ed 6, Plate 297.)

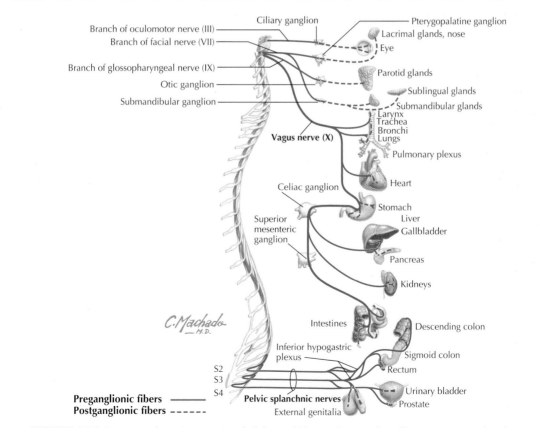

Ciliary ganglion

Pterygopalatine ganglion

Branch of oculomotor nerve (III)

Lacrimal glands, nose

Branch of facial nerve (VII)

Eye

Branch of glossopharyngeal nerve (IX)

Parotid glands

Otic ganglion

Sublingual glands

Submandibular ganglion

Submandibular glands

Larynx
Trachea
Bronchi
Lungs

Vagus nerve (X)

Pulmonary plexus

Heart

Celiac ganglion

Stomach
Liver
Gallbladder

Superior mesenteric ganglion

Pancreas

Kidneys

Intestines

Descending colon

Inferior hypogastric plexus

Sigmoid colon

Rectum

S2
S3
S4

Urinary bladder
Prostate

Preganglionic fibers ———
Postganglionic fibers - - - - -

Pelvic splanchnic nerves

External genitalia

FIGURE 4-30 Parasympathetic Innervation of Abdominal Viscera. (From *Atlas of human anatomy*, ed 6, Plate 164.)

- Increased bowel motility
- Increased secretion
- Increased blood flow

Visceral afferent fibers travel with the ANS components and can be summarized as follows:

- **Pain afferents:** include the pain of distention, inflammation, and ischemia, which is conveyed to the central nervous system (CNS) largely by the sympathetic components to the spinal dorsal root ganglia associated with the T5-L2 spinal cord levels.
- **Reflex afferents:** include information from chemoreceptors, osmoreceptors, and mechanoreceptors, which are conveyed to autonomic centers in the medulla oblongata via the vagus nerves.

Gastrointestinal function is a coordinated effort not only by the "hard-wired" components of the ANS and enteric nervous system, as described earlier, but also by the immune and endocrine systems. In fact, many view the GI tract as the largest endocrine organ in the body, secreting and responding to dozens of GI hormones and other neuroimmune substances.

6. POSTERIOR ABDOMINAL WALL AND VISCERA

Posterior Abdominal Wall

The posterior abdominal wall and its visceral structures lie deep to the parietal peritoneum (retroperitoneal) lining the posterior abdominal cavity. This region contains skeletal structures, muscles, major vascular channels, adrenal glands, the upper urinary system, nerves, and lymphatics.

Fascia and Muscles

Deep to the parietal peritoneum, the muscles of the posterior abdominal wall are enveloped in a layer of investing fascia called the **endoabdominal fascia,** which is continuous laterally with the transversalis fascia of the transversus abdominis muscle. For identification, the fascia is named according to the structures it covers and includes the following layers (Figs. 4-31 and 4-32):

- **Psoas fascia:** covers the psoas major muscle and is thickened superiorly, forming the medial arcuate ligament.
- **Thoracolumbar fascia:** anterior layer covers the quadratus lumborum muscle and is thickened superiorly, forming the lateral arcuate ligament; middle and posterior layers envelop the erector spinae muscles of the back.

The muscles of the posterior abdominal wall have attachments to the lower rib cage, the T12-L5 vertebrae, and bones of the pelvic girdle (Table 4-10 and Fig. 4-32). Note that the **diaphragm** has a central tendinous portion and is attached to the lumbar vertebrae by a right crus and a left crus (leg), which are joined centrally by the median arcuate ligament that passes over the emerging

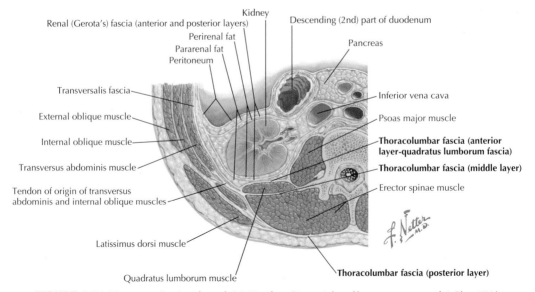

FIGURE 4-31 Transverse Section through L2 Vertebra. (From *Atlas of human anatomy*, ed 6, Plate 176.)

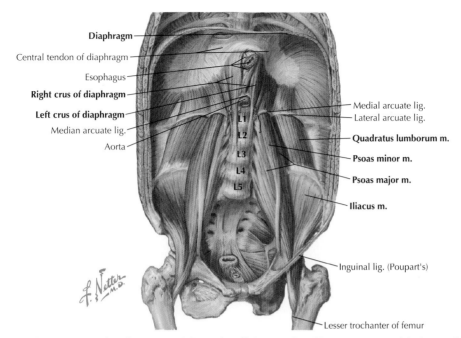

FIGURE 4-32 Muscles of Posterior Abdominal Wall. (From *Atlas of human anatomy*, ed 6, Plate 258.)

TABLE 4-10 Muscles of Posterior Abdominal Wall

MUSCLE	SUPERIOR ATTACHMENT (ORIGIN)	INFERIOR ATTACHMENT (INSERTION)	INNERVATION	ACTIONS
Psoas major	Transverse processes of lumbar vertebrae; sides of bodies of T12-L5 vertebrae, and intervening intervertebral discs	Lesser trochanter of femur	Lumbar plexus via ventral branches of L2-L4 nerves	Acting superiorly with iliacus, flexes hip; acting inferiorly, flexes vertebral column laterally; used to balance trunk in sitting position; acting inferiorly with iliacus, flexes trunk
Iliacus	Superior two thirds of iliac fossa, ala of sacrum, and anterior sacro-iliac ligaments	Lesser trochanter of femur and shaft inferior to it and to psoas major tendon	Femoral nerve (L2-L4)	Flexes hip and stabilizes hip joint; acts with psoas major
Quadratus lumborum	Medial half of inferior border of 12th rib and tips of lumbar transverse processes	Iliolumbar ligament and internal lip of iliac crest	Ventral branches of T12 and L1-L4 nerves	Extends and laterally flexes vertebral column; fixes 12th rib during inspiration
Diaphragm	Thoracic outlet: xiphoid, lower six costal cartilages, L1-L3 vertebrae	Converges into central tendon	Phrenic nerve (C3-C5)	Draws central tendon down and forward during inspiration

abdominal aorta. The **inferior vena cava** passes through the diaphragm at the T8 vertebral level to enter the right atrium of the heart. The right phrenic nerve may accompany the IVC as it passes through the diaphragm, which it innervates. The **esophagus** passes through the diaphragm at the T10 vertebral level, along with the anterior and posterior vagal trunks and left gastric vessels. The **aorta** passes through the diaphragm at the T12

vertebral level and is accompanied by the thoracic duct and often the azygos vein as they course superiorly.

Kidneys and Adrenal (Suprarenal) Glands

The kidneys and adrenal glands are retroperitoneal organs that receive a rich arterial supply

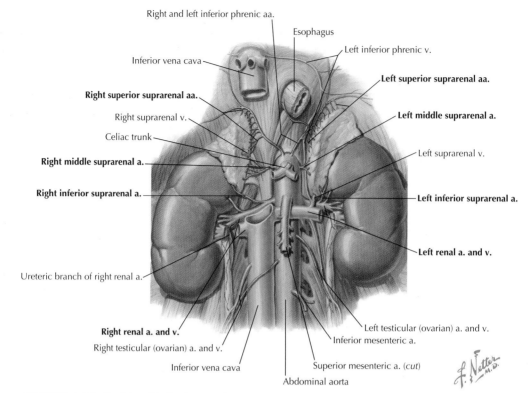

FIGURE 4-33 Blood Supply of Kidneys and Adrenal Glands. (From *Atlas of human anatomy*, ed 6, Plate 310.)

(Fig. 4-33). The right kidney usually lies somewhat lower than the left kidney because of the presence of the liver.

Each **kidney** is enclosed in the following layers of fascia and fat (Figs. 4-31 and 4-34):

- **Renal capsule:** covers each kidney; a thick fibroconnective tissue capsule.
- **Perirenal (perinephric) fat:** directly surrounds the kidney (and adrenal glands) and cushions it.
- **Renal fascia:** surrounds the kidney (and adrenal glands) and perirenal fat; superiorly it is continuous with the fascia covering the diaphragm; inferiorly it may blend with the transversalis fascia; medially the anterior layer blends with the vessels in the renal hilum and the connective tissue of the aorta and IVC.
- **Pararenal (paranephric) fat:** an outer layer of fat that is variable in thickness and is continuous with the extraperitoneal (retroperitoneal) fat.

The kidneys are related posteriorly to the diaphragm and muscles of the posterior abdominal wall, as well as the 11th and 12th (floating) ribs.

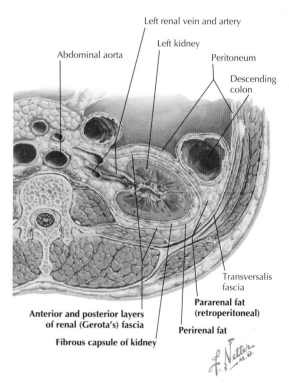

FIGURE 4-34 Renal Fascia and Fat. (From *Atlas of human anatomy*, ed 6, Plate 315.)

They move with respiration, and anteriorly are in relation to the abdominal viscera and mesenteries shown in Figure 4-14. For the right kidney, this includes the liver, second part of the duodenum, and ascending colon. For the left kidney, this includes the stomach, pancreas, spleen, and descending colon. Each kidney also is "capped" by the adrenal (suprarenal) glands. Variability in these relationships is common because of the size of the kidneys and adjacent viscera, disposition of mobile portions of the bowel, and extent of the mesenteries.

Structurally, each kidney has the following gross features (Fig. 4-35):

- **Renal capsule:** a fibroconnective tissue capsule that surrounds the renal cortex.
- **Renal cortex:** outer layer that surrounds the renal medulla and contains nephrons (units of filtration) and renal tubules.

- **Renal medulla:** inner layer (usually appears darker) that contains renal tubules and collecting ducts that convey the filtrate to minor calices; the renal cortex extends as renal columns between the medulla, demarcating the distinctive **renal pyramids** whose apex **(renal papilla)** terminates with a minor calyx.
- **Minor calyx:** structure that receives urine from the collecting ducts of the renal pyramids.
- **Major calyx:** site at which several minor calices drain.
- **Renal pelvis:** point at which several major calices unite; conveys urine to the proximal **ureter.**
- **Hilum:** medial aspect of each kidney, where the renal pelvis emerges from the kidney and where vessels, nerves, and lymphatics enter or leave the kidney.

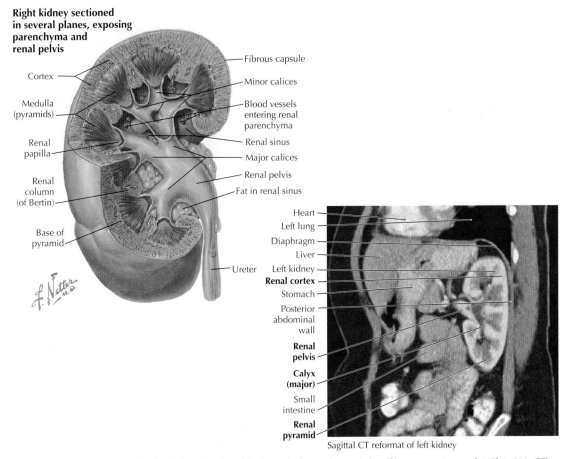

FIGURE 4-35. Features of Right Kidney Sectioned in Several Planes. (From *Atlas of human anatomy*, ed 6, Plate 311; CT image from Kelley LL, Petersen C: *Sectional anatomy for imaging professionals*, Philadelphia, Mosby, 2007.)

Renal Stones (Calculi)

Renal stones may form in the kidney and remain there or more often pass down the ureters to the bladder. When they traverse the ureter, the stones cause significant pain (renal colic) that typically distributes on the side of the insult radiating from "loin to groin." The ureters narrow at three points along their course to the bladder. This is a common location for renal stones to become lodged and cause pain. This pain distribution reflects the pathway of visceral pain afferents (pain is from distention of the ureter) that course to the spinal cord levels T11-L1 via the sympathetic splanchnic nerves. Complications of renal stones include obstruction to the flow of urine, infection, and destruction of the renal parenchyma.

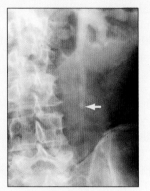

Midureteral obstruction

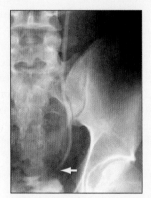

Distal ureteral obstruction

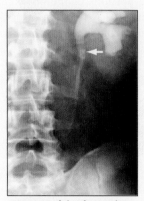

Ureteropelvic obstruction

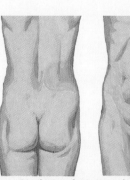

Distribution of pain in renal colic

JOHN A.CRAIG—AD

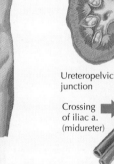

Ureteropelvic
junction

Crossing
of iliac a.
(midureter)

Uretero-
vesical
junction

Common sites of obstruction

Features of Urinary Tract Calculi	
Characteristic	**Description**
Type	75% calcium oxalate (phosphate), 15% magnesium ammonium phosphate, 10% uric acid or cystine
Prevalence	Approximately 12% in the United States, highest in Southeast; 2-3 times more common in men than in women; uncommon in African-Americans and Asians
Risk factors	Concentrated urine, heredity, diet, associated diseases (sarcoidosis, inflammatory bowel disease, cancer)

Clinical Focus 4-21

Obstructive Uropathy

Obstruction to the normal flow of urine, which may occur anywhere from the level of the renal nephrons to the urethral opening, can precipitate pathologic changes that with infection can lead to serious uropathies. This composite figure shows a number of obstructive possibilities and highlights important aspects of the adjacent anatomy one sees along the extent of the urinary tract.

Possible obstructive entities along the urinary tract

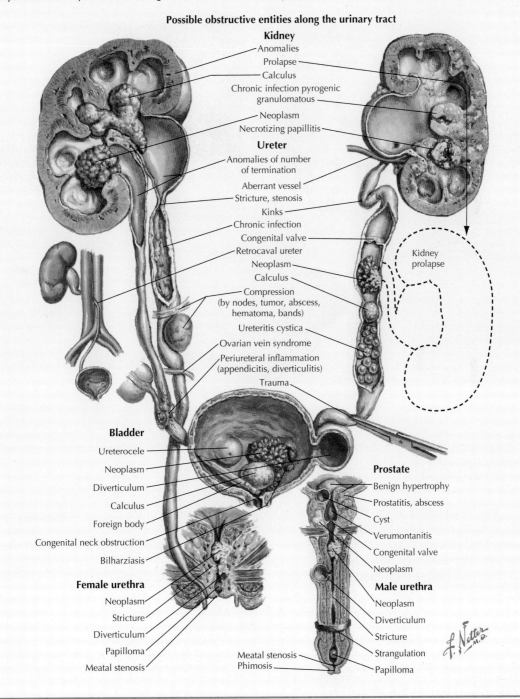

Kidney
Anomalies
Prolapse
Calculus
Chronic infection pyrogenic granulomatous
Neoplasm
Necrotizing papillitis

Ureter
Anomalies of number of termination
Aberrant vessel
Stricture, stenosis
Kinks
Chronic infection
Congenital valve
Retrocaval ureter
Neoplasm
Calculus
Compression (by nodes, tumor, abscess, hematoma, bands)
Ureteritis cystica
Ovarian vein syndrome
Periureteral inflammation (appendicitis, diverticulitis)
Trauma

Kidney prolapse

Bladder
Ureterocele
Neoplasm
Diverticulum
Calculus
Foreign body
Congenital neck obstruction
Bilharziasis

Prostate
Benign hypertrophy
Prostatitis, abscess
Cyst
Verumontanitis
Congenital valve
Neoplasm

Female urethra
Neoplasm
Stricture
Diverticulum
Papilloma
Meatal stenosis

Male urethra
Neoplasm
Diverticulum
Stricture
Strangulation
Papilloma

Meatal stenosis
Phimosis

Clinical Focus 4-22

Malignant Tumors of the Kidney

Of the malignant kidney tumors, 80% to 90% are adenocarcinomas that arise from the tubular epithelium. They account for about 2% of all adult cancers, often occur after age 50, and occur twice as often in men as in women. **Wilms tumor** is the third most common solid tumor in children younger than 10 years and is associated with congenital malformations related to chromosome 11.

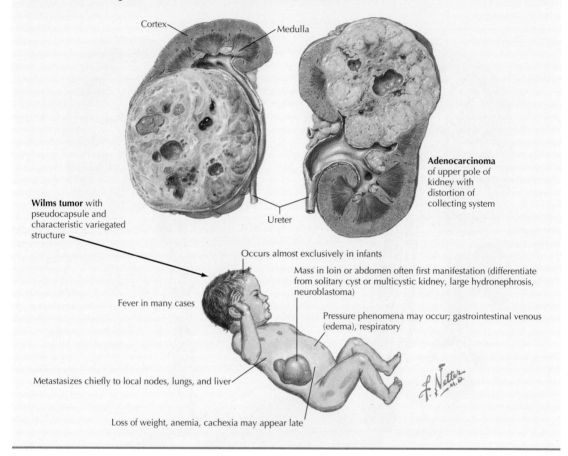

Cortex

Medulla

Adenocarcinoma of upper pole of kidney with distortion of collecting system

Wilms tumor with pseudocapsule and characteristic variegated structure

Ureter

Occurs almost exclusively in infants

Mass in loin or abdomen often first manifestation (differentiate from solitary cyst or multicystic kidney, large hydronephrosis, neuroblastoma)

Fever in many cases

Pressure phenomena may occur; gastrointestinal venous (edema), respiratory

Metastasizes chiefly to local nodes, lungs, and liver

Loss of weight, anemia, cachexia may appear late

The ureters are about 25 cm (10 inches) long, extend from the renal pelvis to the urinary bladder, are composed of a thick layer of smooth muscle, and lie in a retroperitoneal position.

The **right adrenal (suprarenal) gland** often is pyramidal in shape, whereas the left gland is semilunar (see Fig. 4-33). Each adrenal gland "caps" the superior pole of the kidney and is surrounded by perirenal fat and renal fascia. The right adrenal gland is close to the IVC and liver, whereas the stomach, pancreas, and even the spleen can lie anterior to the left adrenal gland.

As endocrine organs, the adrenal glands have a rich vascular supply from superior suprarenal arteries (branches of the inferior phrenic arteries), middle suprarenal arteries directly from the aorta, and inferior suprarenal arteries from the renal arteries (see Fig. 4-36). The kidneys and adrenal glands are innervated by the ANS. Sympathetic nerves arise from the T12-L2 spinal levels and synapse in the superior mesenteric ganglia and superior hypogastric plexuses and send postganglionic fibers to the kidney. Preganglionic fibers from lower thoracic levels travel directly to the adrenal medulla and synapse on the cells of the adrenal medulla (neuroendocrine cells that are the postganglionic part of the sympathetic system). Parasympathetic nerves to the kidneys and adrenal gland travel with the vagus nerves and synapse on postganglionic neurons within the kidney and adrenal cortex (see Figs. 4-29 and 4-30).

Abdominal Vessels

The **abdominal aorta** extends from the aortic hiatus (T12) to the lower level of L4, where it divides into the right and left common iliac arteries (Fig. 4-36). The abdominal aorta gives rise to the following three groups of arteries (Table 4-11):

- **Unpaired visceral arteries** to the GI tract, spleen, pancreas, gallbladder, and liver
- **Paired visceral arteries** to the kidneys, adrenal glands, and gonads
- **Parietal arteries** to musculoskeletal structures

The **inferior vena cava** drains abdominal structures other than the GI tract and the spleen, which are drained by the hepatic portal system (Fig. 4-37). The IVC begins by the union of the two common iliac veins just to the right and slightly inferior of the midline distal abdominal aorta and ascends to pierce the diaphragm at the level of the T8 vertebral level, where it empties into the right atrium. Most of the IVC tributaries parallel the arterial branches of the aorta, but two or three

TABLE 4-11 Branches of Abdominal Aorta

ARTERIAL BRANCH	STRUCTURES SUPPLIED
Unpaired Visceral	
Celiac trunk	Embryonic foregut derivatives and spleen
SMA	Embryonic midgut derivatives
IMA	Embryonic hindgut derivatives
Paired Visceral	
Middle suprarenals	Adrenal (suprarenal) glands
Renals	Kidneys
Gonadal	Ovarian or testicular branches to gonad
Parietal Branches	
Inferior phrenics	Paired arteries to diaphragm
Lumbars	Usually four pairs to posterior abdominal wall and spine
Median sacral	Unpaired artery to sacrum (caudal artery)

SMA, Superior mesenteric artery; *IMA*, inferior mesenteric artery.

hepatic veins also enter the IVC just inferior to the diaphragm. It is important to note that the ascending lumbar veins connect adjacent lumbar veins and drain superiorly into the **azygos venous system** (see Chapter 3). This venous anastomosis is important if the IVC should become obstructed.

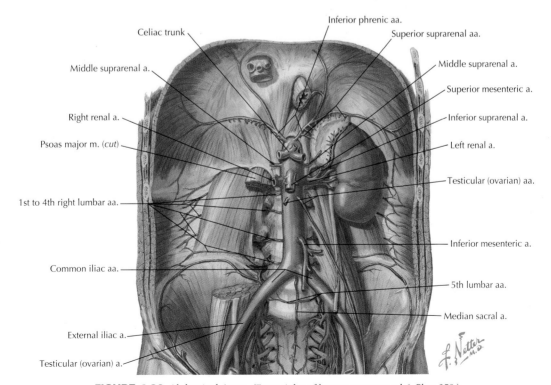

FIGURE 4-36 Abdominal Aorta. (From *Atlas of human anatomy*, ed 6, Plate 259.)

Surgical Management of Abdominal Aortic Aneurysm

Aneurysms (bulges in the arterial wall) usually involve the large arteries. The multifactorial etiology includes family history, hypertension, breakdown of collagen and elastin within the vessel wall (which leads to inflammation and weakening of the arterial wall), and atherosclerosis. The abdominal aorta (infrarenal segment) and iliac arteries are most often involved, but the thoracic aorta and the femoral and popliteal arteries can also have aneurysms. Symptoms include abdominal and back pain, nausea, and early satiety, but up to 75% of patients may be asymptomatic. If surgical repair is warranted, an open procedure may be done using durable synthetic grafts (illustrated) or by an endovascular repair, in which a new synthetic lining is inserted using hooks or stents to hold the lining in place.

Indications for surgery include aneurysm diameter twice
normal aorta, rapid enlargement, or symptomatic aneurysm.

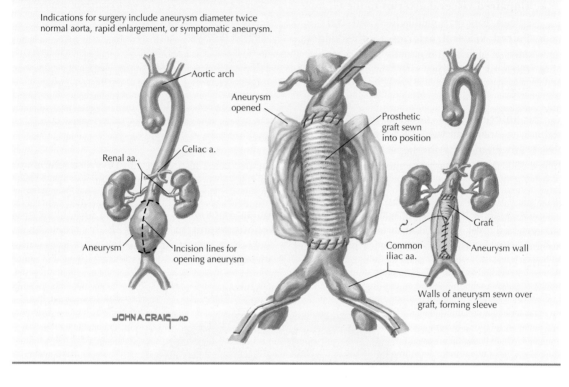

JOHN A. CRAIG—AD

Arteries of the Abdominal Aorta

The **abdominal aorta (1)** is a continuation of the thoracic aorta beginning at about the level of the T12 vertebra, where the aorta passes through the aortic hiatus of the diaphragm. It gives off three sets of **parietal arteries** that supply the diaphragm **(inferior phrenic artery [2])**, usually four pairs of **lumbar arteries (3)**, and an unpaired **median sacral artery (4)**, our equivalent of the "caudal artery" (for the tail) in most other mammals. These arteries arise from the posterolateral aspect of the aorta (Fig. 4-38).

The **abdominal aorta (1)** also gives rise to three **unpaired visceral arteries** that arise from the anterior aspect of the aorta. The **celiac trunk**

(5) supplies the embryonic foregut derivatives of the gastrointestinal tract and its accessory organs, the gallbladder, liver, and pancreas. It also supplies the spleen, an organ of the immune system. The **superior mesenteric artery (6)** supplies the embryonic midgut derivatives (distal duodenum, small intestine, cecum, appendix, ascending colon, and proximal two thirds of the transverse colon) and also portions of the pancreas. The **inferior mesenteric artery (7)** supplies the embryonic hindgut derivatives (distal transverse colon, descending colon, sigmoid colon, and proximal rectum).

The **abdominal aorta (1)** finally gives rise to three **paired visceral arteries** that supply the

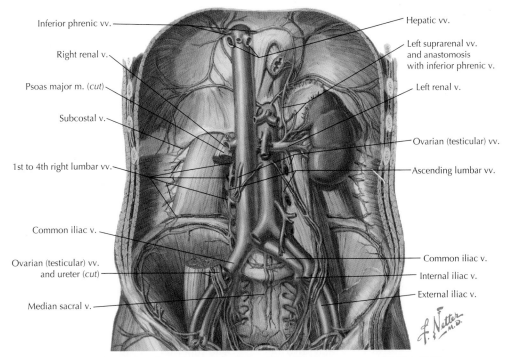

Inferior phrenic vv.

Right renal v.

Psoas major m. (cut)

Subcostal v.

1st to 4th right lumbar vv.

Common iliac v.

Ovarian (testicular) vv. and ureter (cut)

Median sacral v.

Hepatic vv.

Left suprarenal vv. and anastomosis with inferior phrenic v.

Left renal v.

Ovarian (testicular) vv.

Ascending lumbar vv.

Common iliac v.

Internal iliac v.

External iliac v.

FIGURE 4-37 Inferior Vena Cava. (From *Atlas of human anatomy,* ed 6, Plate 260.)

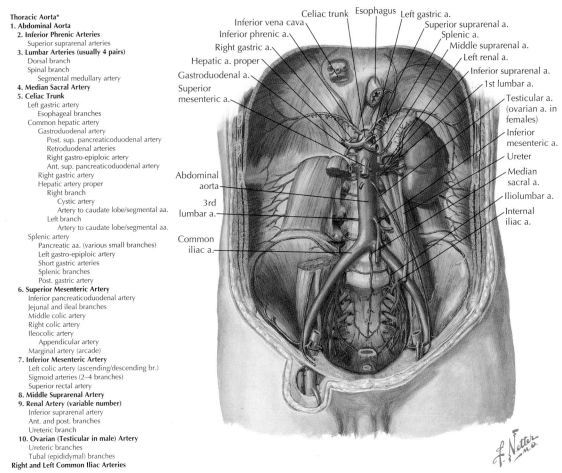

Thoracic Aorta*
1. **Abdominal Aorta**
   2. **Inferior Phrenic Arteries**
      Superior suprarenal arteries
   3. **Lumbar Arteries (usually 4 pairs)**
      Dorsal branch
      Spinal branch
         Segmental medullary artery
   4. **Median Sacral Artery**
   5. **Celiac Trunk**
      Left gastric artery
         Esophageal branches
      Common hepatic artery
         Gastroduodenal artery
            Post. sup. pancreaticoduodenal artery
            Retroduodenal arteries
            Right gastro-epiploic artery
            Ant. sup. pancreaticoduodenal artery
         Right gastric artery
         Hepatic artery proper
            Right branch
               Cystic artery
               Artery to caudate lobe/segmental aa.
            Left branch
               Artery to caudate lobe/segmental aa.
      Splenic artery
         Pancreatic aa. (various small branches)
         Left gastro-epiploic artery
         Short gastric arteries
         Splenic branches
         Post. gastric artery
   6. **Superior Mesenteric Artery**
      Inferior pancreaticoduodenal artery
      Jejunal and ileal branches
      Middle colic artery
      Right colic artery
      Ileocolic artery
         Appendicular artery
      Marginal artery (arcade)
   7. **Inferior Mesenteric Artery**
      Left colic artery (ascending/descending br.)
      Sigmoid arteries (2–4 branches)
      Superior rectal artery
   8. **Middle Suprarenal Artery**
   9. **Renal Artery (variable number)**
      Inferior suprarenal artery
      Ant. and post. branches
      Ureteric branch
   10. **Ovarian (Testicular in male) Artery**
      Ureteric branches
      Tubal (epididymal) branches
Right and Left Common Iliac Arteries

*Proximal (thoracic aorta) to Distal (aortic bifurcation)

Celiac trunk   Esophagus   Left gastric a.
Inferior vena cava   Superior suprarenal a.
Inferior phrenic a.   Splenic a.
Right gastric a.   Middle suprarenal a.
Hepatic a. proper   Left renal a.
Gastroduodenal a.   Inferior suprarenal a.
Superior mesenteric a.   1st lumbar a.
                                Testicular a. (ovarian a. in females)
                                Inferior mesenteric a.
                                Ureter
Abdominal aorta   Median sacral a.
3rd lumbar a.   Iliolumbar a.
Common iliac a.   Internal iliac a.

FIGURE 4-38 Arteries of the Abdominal Aorta.

suprarenal (adrenal) glands via the paired **middle suprarenal artery (8),** the kidneys via the paired **renal artery (9),** and the gonads via the paired **ovarian/testicular artery (10).** The paired visceral branches arise from the lateral aspect of the **abdominal aorta (1).** The aorta then divides into the right and left **common iliac arteries.**

A rich blood supply is common around the stomach, duodenum, and pancreas. The suprarenal glands also receive a rich vascular supply (superior, middle, and inferior suprarenal arteries). The small bowel has a collateral circulation via its arcades and the colon via its marginal artery, although the pattern and supply by these arteries is variable.

In the outline of the arteries (Fig. 4-38), major vessels often dissected in anatomy courses include the first-order arteries (in bold and numbered) and their second-order major branches. In more detailed dissection courses some or all of the third- and/or fourth-order arteries may also be dissected.

Veins of the Abdomen (Caval System)

As elsewhere in the body, the veins of the abdomen possess a deep and superficial group. The deep veins drain essentially the areas supplied by the "parietal and paired visceral" branches of the abdominal aorta (Fig. 4-39). (Note that the "unpaired visceral" branches of the abdominal aorta supplying the GI tract, its accessory organs, and the spleen are drained by the hepatic portal system of veins.)

Beginning at the level of the pelvic brim, the **common iliac vein (1)** is formed by the internal and external iliac veins. The two **common iliac veins (1)** join to form the **inferior vena cava (2),** which receives venous drainage from the gonads, kidneys, posterior abdominal wall (lumbar veins), liver, and diaphragm. The IVC then drains into the **right atrium of the heart (3).**

The superficial set of veins drain the anterolateral abdominal wall, the superficial inguinal

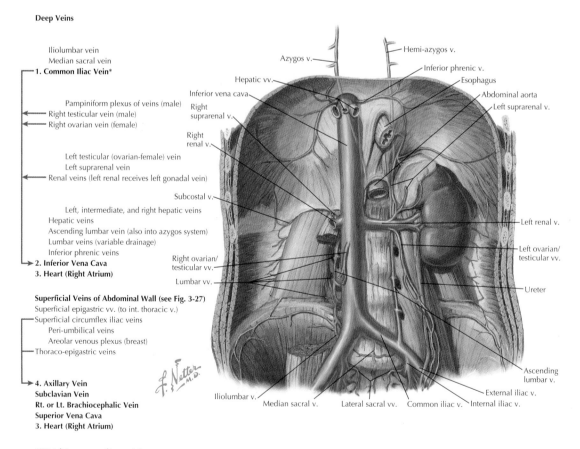

Deep Veins

Iliolumbar vein
Median sacral vein
1. Common Iliac Vein*

Pampiniform plexus of veins (male)
Right testicular vein (male)
Right ovarian vein (female)

Left testicular (ovarian-female) vein
Left suprarenal vein
Renal veins (left renal receives left gonadal vein)

Left, intermediate, and right hepatic veins
Hepatic veins
Ascending lumbar vein (also into azygos system)
Lumbar veins (variable drainage)
Inferior phrenic veins
2. Inferior Vena Cava
3. Heart (Right Atrium)

Superficial Veins of Abdominal Wall (see Fig. 3-27)
Superficial epigastric vv. (to int. thoracic v.)
Superficial circumflex iliac veins
Peri-umbilical veins
Areolar venous plexus (breast)
Thoraco-epigastric veins

4. Axillary Vein
Subclavian Vein
Rt. or Lt. Brachiocephalic Vein
Superior Vena Cava
3. Heart (Right Atrium)

*Distal (common iliac vein)
to Heart (right atrium)

Azygos v.
Hepatic vv.
Inferior vena cava
Right suprarenal v.
Right renal v.
Subcostal v.
Right ovarian/testicular vv.
Lumbar vv.

Hemi-azygos v.
Inferior phrenic v.
Esophagus
Abdominal aorta
Left suprarenal v.
Left renal v.
Left ovarian/testicular vv.
Ureter
Ascending lumbar v.
External iliac v.
Internal iliac v.

Iliolumbar v.
Median sacral v.
Lateral sacral vv.
Common iliac v.

FIGURE 4-39 Veins of the Abdomen.

region, rectus sheath, and lateral thoracic wall. Most of its connections ultimately drain into the **axillary vein (4)** and then into the **subclavian vein**, **brachiocephalic veins**, which form the **superior vena cava**, and then into the **heart (3).** The inferior epigastric veins (from the external iliac veins) enter the posterior rectus sheath and course cranially above the umbilicus as the superior epigastric veins and then anastomose with the internal thoracic veins that drain into the subclavian veins (see Fig. 4-3).

The superficial veins can become enlarged during portal hypertension, when the venous flow through the liver is compromised. Important **portosystemic anastomoses** between the portal system and caval system can allow venous blood to gain access to the caval veins (both deep and superficial veins) to assist in returning blood to the heart.

Variations in the venous pattern and in the number of veins and their size are common, so it is best to understand the major venous channels and realize that smaller veins often are more variable.

Hepatic Portal System of Veins

The hepatic portal system of veins drains the abdominal GI tract and two of its accessory organs (pancreas and gallbladder) and the spleen (immune system organ) (Fig. 4-40). This blood then collects largely in the liver, where processing of absorbed GI contents takes place. (However, most fats are absorbed by the lymphatics and returned via the thoracic duct to the venous system in the neck, at the junction of the left internal jugular and left

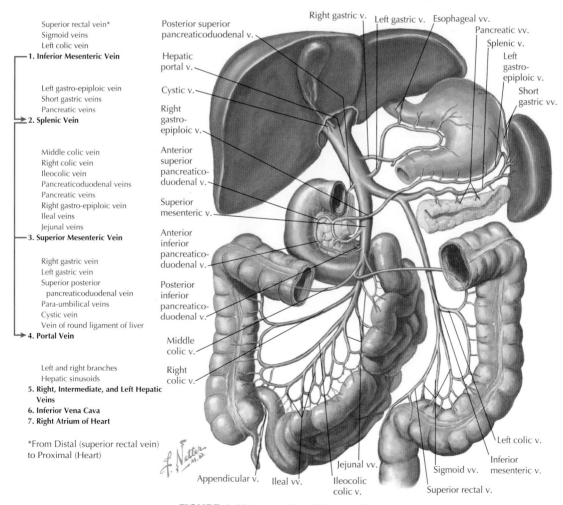

FIGURE 4-40 Hepatic Portal System of Veins.

subclavian veins.) Venous blood is returned to the liver and then collects in the **right, intermediate, and left hepatic veins (5)** and is drained into the **inferior vena cava (6)** and then the **right atrium of the heart (7)**.

The **inferior mesenteric vein (1)** essentially drains the area supplied by the inferior mesenteric artery (embryonic hindgut derivatives) and then drains into the **splenic vein (2)**. (Sometimes it also drains into the junction between the splenic and superior mesenteric vein [SMV] or into the SMV directly.) The **splenic vein (2)** drains the spleen and portions of the stomach and pancreas. The **superior mesenteric vein (3)** essentially drains the same region supplied by the superior mesenteric artery (embryonic midgut derivatives), as well as portions of the pancreas and stomach.

The **splenic vein (2)** and **superior mesenteric vein (3)** unite to form the **portal vein (4)**. The **portal vein (4)** is about 8-10 cm long and receives not only venous blood from the **splenic vein (2)** and **SMV (3)** but also smaller tributaries that drain from the stomach, para-umbilical region, and cystic duct (of the gallbladder). Just before entering the liver, the **portal vein (4)** divides into its right and left branches, one to each of the two physiologically functional lobes of the liver. Blood

leaving the liver collects into **hepatic veins (5)** and drains into the **IVC (6)** and then the **heart (7)**.

If blood cannot traverse the hepatic sinusoids (liver disease), it backs up in the portal system and causes portal hypertension. The large amount of venous blood in the portal system then must find its way back to the heart and does so by important portosystemic anastomotic connections that utilize the inferior and superior venae cavae as alternate routes to the heart. Important **portosystemic anastomoses** occur in the following regions:

- **Esophageal veins** from the portal vein that connect with the azygos system of veins draining into the SVC
- **Rectal veins** (superior rectal vein of portal system to middle and inferior rectal veins) that ultimately drain into the IVC
- **Para-umbilical veins** of the superficial abdominal wall that can drain into the tributaries of either the SVC or the IVC
- **Retroperitoneal venous connections** wherever the bowel is up against the abdominal wall and is drained by small parietal venous tributaries

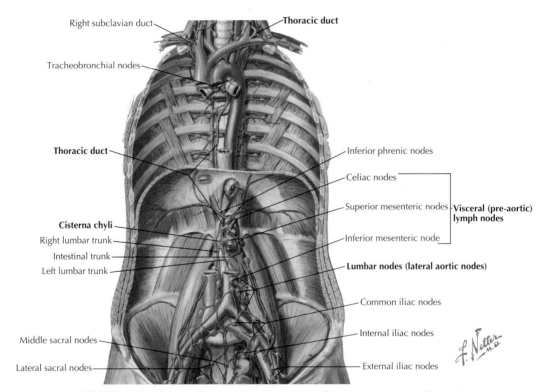

FIGURE 4-41 Abdominal Lymphatics. (From *Atlas of human anatomy*, ed 6, Plate 261.)

As with all veins, these veins can be variable in number and size, but the major venous channels are relatively constant anatomically.

Lymphatic Drainage

Lymph from the posterior abdominal wall and retroperitoneal viscera drains medially, following the arterial supply back to lumbar and visceral pre-aortic lymph nodes (Fig. 4-41). Ultimately, the lymph is collected into the **cisterna chyli** and conveyed to the venous system by the **thoracic duct.**

Innervation

Retroperitoneal visceral structures of the posterior abdominal wall (adrenal glands, kidneys, ureters) are supplied by parasympathetic fibers from the **vagus nerve** and by the **pelvic splanchnics** (S2-S4) to the distal ureters (pelvic ureters) (see Fig. 4-30). Sympathetic nerves (secretomotor) to the adrenal medulla come from the **lesser** and **least splanchnic nerves,** and sympathetic nerves to the kidneys and proximal ureters come from the **lesser** and **least splanchnic nerves** (T10-T12) and the **lumbar splanchnics** (L1-L2) (see Fig. 4-29). They synapse in the superior hypogastric plexus and superior mesenteric ganglion and send postganglionic sympathetics to the kidneys on the vasculature.

Pain afferents from all the abdominal viscera pass to the spinal cord largely by following the

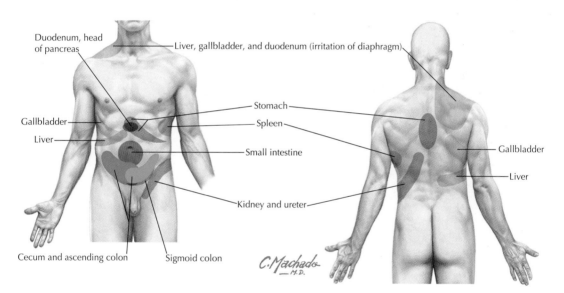

FIGURE 4-42 Sites of Visceral Referred Pain.

TABLE 4-12 Spinal Cord Levels for Visceral Referred Pain*		
ORGAN	**SPINAL CORD LEVEL**	**ANTERIOR ABDOMINAL REGION OR QUADRANT**
Stomach	T5-T9	Epigastric or left hypochondrium
Spleen	T6-T8	Left hypochondrium
Duodenum	T5-T8	Epigastric or right hypochondrium
Pancreas	T7-T9	Inferior part of epigastric
Liver or gallbladder†	T6-T9	Epigastric or right hypochondrium
Jejunum	T6-T10	Umbilical
Ileum	T7-T10	Umbilical
Cecum	T10-T11	Umbilical or right lumbar or right lower quadrant
Appendix	T10-T11	Umbilical or right inguinal or right lower quadrant
Ascending colon	T10-T12	Umbilical or right lumbar
Sigmoid colon	L1-L2	Left lumbar or left lower quadrant
Kidney	T10-L1	Lower hypochondrium or lumbar
Ureter	T11-L1	Lumbar to inguinal (loin to groin)

*These spinal cord levels are approximate. Although normal variations are common from individual to individual, these levels do show the approximate contributions.

†Irritation of the diaphragm leads to pain referred to the back (inferior scapula) and shoulder region.

thoracic and lumbar splanchnic sympathetic nerves (T5-L2). The neuronal cell bodies of these afferent fibers reside in the respective dorsal root ganglia of the spinal cord segment. Thus, visceral pain may be perceived as somatic pain over these dermatome regions, a phenomenon known clinically as **referred pain.** Pain afferents from pelvic viscera largely follow pelvic splanchnic parasympathetic nerves (S2-S4) into the cord, and the pain is largely confined to the pelvic region. Common sites of referred visceral pain are shown in Figure 4-42 and summarized in Table 4-12.

Somatic nerves of the posterior abdominal wall are derived from the **lumbar plexus**, which is composed of the ventral rami of L1-L4 (often with a small contribution from T12) (Fig. 4-43). The branches of the lumbar plexus are summarized in Table 4-13.

TABLE 4-13 Branches of Lumbar Plexus

NERVE	FUNCTION AND INNERVATION
Subcostal (T12)	Last thoracic nerve; courses inferior to 12th rib
Iliohypogastric (L1)	Motor and sensory; above pubis and posterolateral buttocks
Ilio-inguinal (L1)	Motor and sensory; sensory to inguinal region
Genitofemoral (L1-L2)	Genital branch to cremaster muscle; femoral branch to femoral triangle
Lateral cutaneous nerve of thigh (L2-L3)	Sensory to anterolateral thigh
Femoral (L2-L4)	Motor in pelvis (to iliacus) and anterior thigh muscles; sensory to thigh and medial leg
Obturator (L2-L4)	Motor to adductor muscles in thigh; sensory to medial thigh
Accessory obturator	Inconstant (10%); motor to pectineus muscle

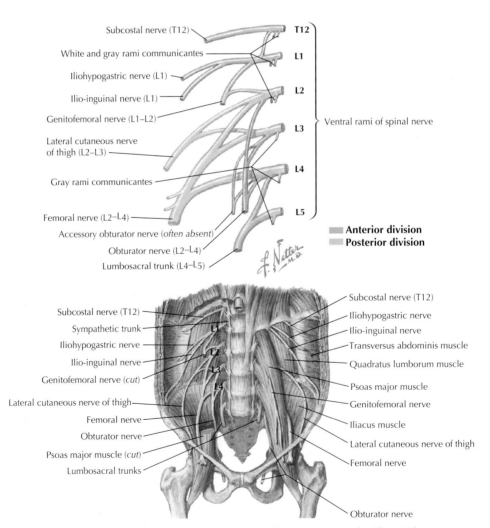

FIGURE 4-43 Lumbar Plexus. (From *Atlas of human anatomy,* ed 6, Plate 485.)

7. EMBRYOLOGY

Summary of Gut Development

The embryonic gut begins as a midline endoderm-lined tube that is divided into **foregut, midgut,** and **hindgut** regions, each giving rise to adult visceral structures with a segmental vascular supply and autonomic innervation (Fig. 4-44 and Table 4-14). Knowing this pattern of distribution related to the three embryonic gut regions will help you better organize your thinking about the abdominal viscera and their neurovascular supply.

The gut undergoes a series of rotations and differential growth that ultimately contributes to the postnatal disposition of the abdominal GI tract (see Fig. 4-44). This sequence of events can be summarized as follows:

- The **stomach** rotates 90 degrees clockwise on its longitudinal axis so that the left side of the gut tube now faces anteriorly.
- As the stomach rotates, the **duodenum** swings to the right into its familiar C-shaped configuration and becomes largely retroperitoneal.
- The **midgut** forms an initial primary intestinal loop by rotating 180 degrees counterclockwise around the axis of the SMA (which supplies blood to the midgut) and,

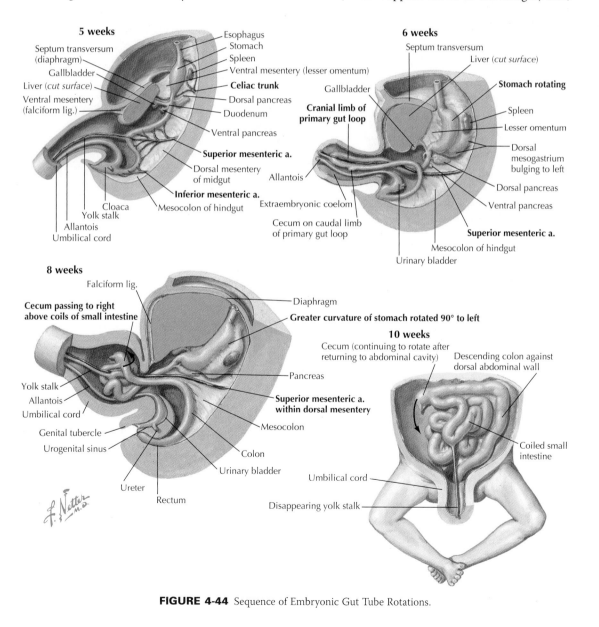

FIGURE 4-44 Sequence of Embryonic Gut Tube Rotations.

Congenital Megacolon

Congenital megacolon results from the failure of **neural crest cells** to migrate distally along the colon (usually the sigmoid colon and rectum). This leads to an aganglionic segment that lacks both **Meissner's submucosal plexus** and **Auerbach's myenteric plexus.** Distention proximal to the aganglionic region may occur shortly after birth or may cause symptoms in early childhood. Surgical repair involves prolapse and eversion of the segment.

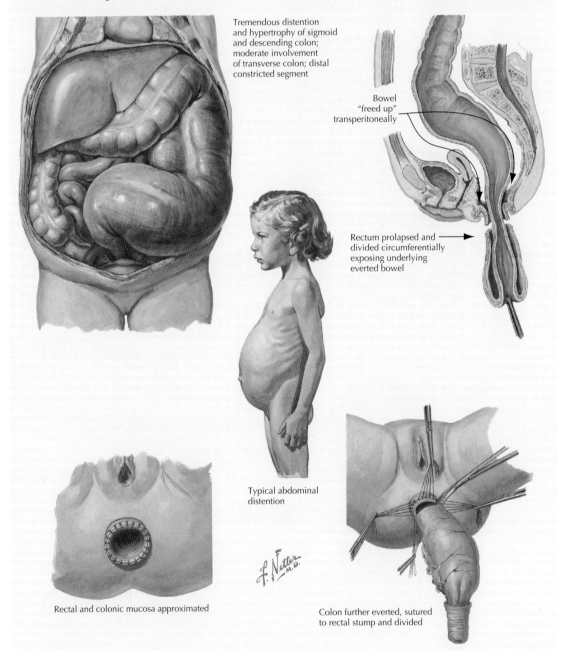

Tremendous distention and hypertrophy of sigmoid and descending colon; moderate involvement of transverse colon; distal constricted segment

Bowel "freed up" transperitoneally

Rectum prolapsed and divided circumferentially exposing underlying everted bowel

Typical abdominal distention

Rectal and colonic mucosa approximated

Colon further everted, sutured to rectal stump and divided

TABLE 4-14 Summary of Embryonic Gut Development

	FOREGUT	MIDGUT	HINDGUT
Organs	Stomach Liver Gallbladder Pancreas Spleen 1st half of duodenum	2nd half of duodenum Jejunum Ileum Cecum Ascending colon Two thirds of transverse colon	Left one third of transverse colon Descending colon Sigmoid colon Rectum
Arteries	Celiac trunk: Splenic Left gastric Common hepatic	Superior mesenteric: Ileocolic Right colic Middle colic	Inferior mesenteric: Left colic Sigmoid branches Superior rectal
Ventral mesentery	Lesser omentum Falciform ligament Coronary/triangular ligaments	None	None
Dorsal mesentery	Gastrosplenic ligament Splenorenal ligament Gastrocolic ligament Greater omentum and omental apron	Meso-intestine Meso-appendix Transverse mesocolon	Sigmoid mesocolon
Nerve Supply			
Parasympathetic	Vagus	Vagus	Pelvic splanchnics (S2-S4)
Sympathetic	Thoracic splanchnics (T5-T11)	Thoracic splanchnics (T11-T12)	Lumbar splanchnics (L1-L2)

because of its fast growth, herniates out into the umbilical cord (6 weeks).

- By the 10th week, the gut loop returns into the abdominal cavity and completes its rotation with a 90-degree swing to the right lower quadrant.
- Thus, the midgut loop completes a 270-degree rotation about the axis of the SMA and undergoes significant differential growth to form the small intestine and proximal portions of the large intestine (see Table 4-14).
- The **hindgut** then develops into the remainder of the large intestine and proximal rectum, supplied by the IMA, and ending in the cloaca (Latin for "sewer").

Liver, Gallbladder, and Pancreas Development

During the third week of development, an endodermal outpocketing of the foregut gives rise to the **hepatic diverticulum** (Fig. 4-45). Further development of this diverticulum gives rise to the liver, the biliary duct system, and the gallbladder. The liver cells (hepatocytes) are endodermal derivatives. A short time later, two **pancreatic buds** (ventral and dorsal) originate as endodermal outgrowths of the duodenum. As the duodenum swings to the right during rotation of the stomach, the ventral pancreatic bud (which will form part of the pancreatic head and the uncinate process)

swings around posteriorly and fuses with the dorsal bud to form the union of the two pancreatic ducts (main and accessory ducts) and buds. This fused pancreas embraces the SMV and SMA, which are in relationship to these developing embryonic buds (see Figs. 4-20 and 4-45). The endoderm of the pancreas gives rise to the exocrine and endocrine cells of the organ, whereas the connective tissue stroma is formed by mesoderm.

Urinary System Development

Initially, retroperitoneal intermediate mesoderm differentiates into the nephrogenic (kidney) tissue and forms the following (Fig. 4-46):

- **Pronephros**, which degenerates
- **Mesonephros** with its mesonephric duct, which functions briefly before degenerating
- **Metanephros,** the definitive kidney tissue (nephrons and loop of Henle) into which the **ureteric bud** (an outgrowth of the mesonephric duct) grows and differentiates into the ureter, renal pelvis, calices, and collecting ducts

By differential growth and some migration, the kidney "ascends" from the sacral region, first with its hilum directed anteriorly and then medially, until it reaches its adult location (Fig. 4-47). Around the 12th week, the kidney becomes

Text continued on p. 212.

Clinical Focus 4-25

Meckel's Diverticulum

Meckel's diverticulum is the most common developmental anomaly of the bowel and results from failure of the vitelline (yolk stalk) duct to involute once the gut loop has reentered the abdominal cavity. It is often referred to as the "syndrome of twos" for the following reasons:

- It occurs in approximately 2% of the population.
- It is about 2 inches (5 cm) long.
- It is located about 2 feet from the ileocecal junction.
- It often contains at least two types of mucosa.

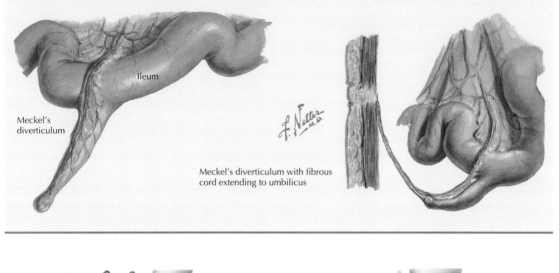

1. Bud formation

2. Beginning rotation of common duct and of ventral pancreas

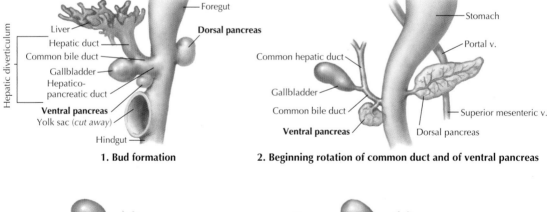

3. Rotation completed but fusion has not yet taken place

4. Fusion of ventral and dorsal pancreas and union of ducts

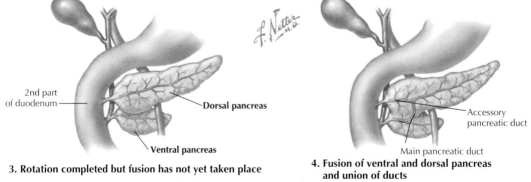

FIGURE 4-45 Development of Hepatic Diverticulum and Pancreas.

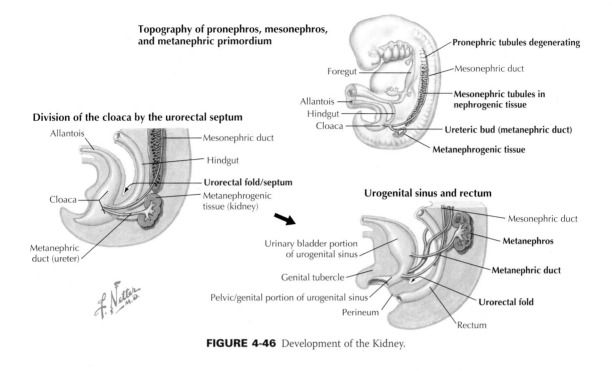

Topography of pronephros, mesonephros, and metanephric primordium

Pronephric tubules degenerating

Foregut

Mesonephric duct

Allantois

Mesonephric tubules in nephrogenic tissue

Hindgut

Cloaca

Ureteric bud (metanephric duct)

Metanephrogenic tissue

Division of the cloaca by the urorectal septum

Allantois

Mesonephric duct

Hindgut

Cloaca

Urorectal fold/septum

Metanephrogenic tissue (kidney)

Metanephric duct (ureter)

Urogenital sinus and rectum

Mesonephric duct

Metanephros

Urinary bladder portion of urogenital sinus

Metanephric duct

Genital tubercle

Pelvic/genital portion of urogenital sinus

Urorectal fold

Perineum

Rectum

FIGURE 4-46 Development of the Kidney.

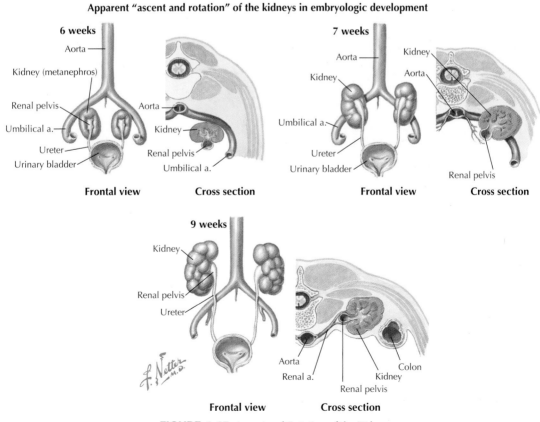

Apparent "ascent and rotation" of the kidneys in embryologic development

6 weeks

Aorta

Kidney (metanephros)

Renal pelvis

Umbilical a.

Ureter

Urinary bladder

Aorta

Kidney

Renal pelvis

Umbilical a.

Frontal view   **Cross section**

7 weeks

Aorta

Kidney

Kidney

Aorta

Umbilical a.

Ureter

Urinary bladder

Renal pelvis

Frontal view   **Cross section**

9 weeks

Kidney

Renal pelvis

Ureter

Aorta

Renal a.

Renal pelvis

Kidney

Colon

Frontal view   **Cross section**

FIGURE 4-47 Ascent and Rotation of the Kidney.

Congenital Malrotation of the Colon

Many congenital lesions of the GI tract cause intestinal obstruction, which commonly results from malrotation of the midgut, atresia, volvulus, meconium ileus, or imperforate anus. Vomiting, absence of stool, and abdominal distention characterize the clinical picture. Intestinal obstruction can be life threatening, requiring surgical intervention. The corrective procedure for congenital malrotation with volvulus of the midgut is illustrated.

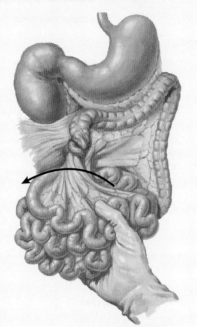

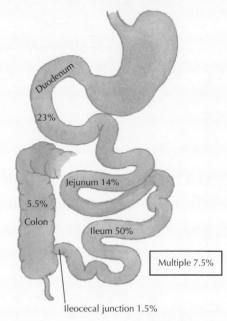

Duodenum

23%

Jejunum 14%

5.5%
Colon

Ileum 50%

Multiple 7.5%

Ileocecal junction 1.5%

1. Small intestine pulled downward to expose clockwise twist and strangulation at apex of incompletely anchored mesentery; unwinding is done in counterclockwise direction (arrow)

Approximate regional incidence (gross)

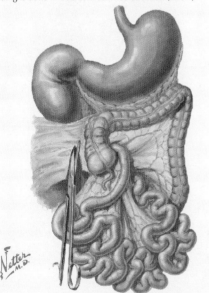

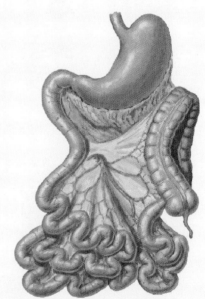

2. Volvulus unwound; peritoneal band compressing duodenum is being divided

3. Complete release of obstruction; duodenum descends toward root of superior mesenteric artery; cecum drops away to left

Clinical Focus 4-27

Renal Fusion

The term *renal fusion* refers to various common defects in which the two kidneys fuse to become one. The horseshoe kidney, in which developing kidneys fuse (usually the lower lobes) anterior to the aorta, often lies low in the abdomen and is the most common kind of fusion. Fused kidneys are close to the midline, have multiple renal arteries, and are malrotated. Obstruction, stone formation, and infection are potential complications.

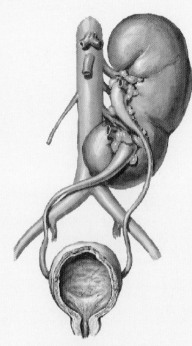

Simple crossed ectopia with fusion

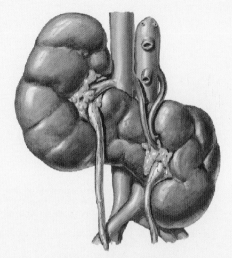

S-shaped or sigmoid kidney

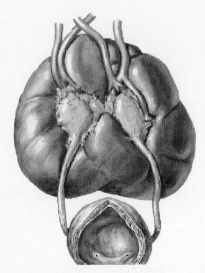

Pelvic cake or lump kidney

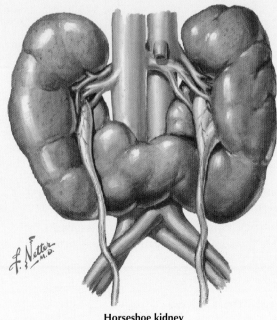

Horseshoe kidney

Clinical Focus 4-28

Pheochromocytoma

Although pheochromocytomas are relatively rare neoplasms composed largely of adrenal medullary cells, which secrete excessive amounts of catecholamines, they can occur elsewhere throughout the body associated with the sympathetic chain or at other sites where **neural crest cells** typically migrate. Common clinical features of pheochromocytoma include the following:

- Vasoconstriction and elevated blood pressure
- Headache, sweating, and flushing
- Anxiety, nausea, tremor, and palpitations or chest pain

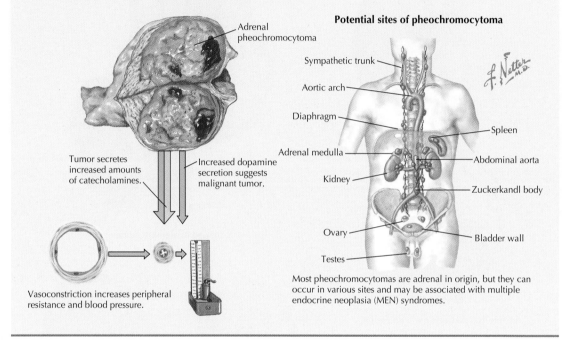

Adrenal pheochromocytoma

Tumor secretes increased amounts of catecholamines.

Increased dopamine secretion suggests malignant tumor.

Vasoconstriction increases peripheral resistance and blood pressure.

Potential sites of pheochromocytoma

Sympathetic trunk

Aortic arch

Diaphragm

Spleen

Adrenal medulla

Abdominal aorta

Kidney

Zuckerkandl body

Ovary

Bladder wall

Testes

Most pheochromocytomas are adrenal in origin, but they can occur in various sites and may be associated with multiple endocrine neoplasia (MEN) syndromes.

functional as the fetus swallows amniotic fluid, urinates into the amniotic cavity, and continually recycles fluid in this manner. Toxic fetal wastes, however, are removed through the placenta into the maternal circulation.

Adrenal (Suprarenal) Gland Development

The adrenal cortex develops from mesoderm, whereas the adrenal medulla forms from neural crest cells, which migrate into the cortex and aggregate in the center of the gland. The cells of the medulla are essentially the postganglionic neurons of the sympathetic division of the ANS, but secrete mainly epinephrine and some norepinephrine into the blood as neuroendocrine cells.

Clinical Focus

Available Online

4-29 Acute Abdomen: Visceral Etiology

4-30 Irritable Bowel Syndrome

4-31 Acute Pyelonephritis

4-32 Causes and Consequences of Portal Hypertension

Additional figures available online (see inside front cover for details).

Challenge Yourself Questions

1. Which of the following statements accurately describes why the umbilicus can be an important clinical landmark?

    A. Level of aortic bifurcation
    B. Level of L4 vertebra
    C. Level of transverse colon
    D. Level of T10 dermatome
    E. Level of third part of duodenum

2. Clinically, which of the following statements regarding an indirect inguinal hernia is false?

    A. Can be a congenital hernia.
    B. Enters the deep inguinal ring.
    C. Herniates lateral to the inferior epigastric vessels.
    D. Lies within the internal spermatic fascia.
    E. Passes through the inguinal triangle.

3. A 42-year-old obese woman comes to the clinic with episodes of severe right hypochondrial pain, usually associated with eating a fatty meal. A history of gallstones suggests that she is experiencing cholecystitis (gallbladder inflammation). Which of the following nerves carries the visceral pain associated with this condition?

    A. Greater splanchnic
    B. Intercostal
    C. Phrenic
    D. Pelvic splanchnic
    E. Vagus

4. The metastatic spread of stomach (gastric) cancer through lymphatics would most likely travel first to which of the following lymph nodes?

    A. Celiac
    B. Inferior mesenteric
    C. Inferior phrenic
    D. Lumbar
    E. Superior mesenteric

5. A 51-year-old woman with a history of alcohol abuse is diagnosed with cirrhosis of the liver and portal hypertension. In addition to esophageal varices, she presents with rectal varices. Which of the following portosystemic anastomoses is most likely responsible for these rectal varices?

    A. Inferior mesenteric vein to inferior rectal veins
    B. Left gastric veins to inferior rectal veins
    C. Portal vein to the middle and inferior rectal veins
    D. Superior mesenteric vein to superior rectal veins
    E. Superior rectal vein to the middle and inferior rectal veins

6. A patient presents with acute abdominal pain and fever. Examination of her abdomen reveals fluid (ascites) within the lesser sac, which is now draining into the greater peritoneal sac. Which of the following pathways accounts for the seepage of fluid from the lesser to the greater sac?

    A. Epiploic foramen
    B. Left paracolic gutter
    C. Posterior fornix
    D. Right paracolic gutter
    E. Vesico-uterine pouch

7. A 59-year-old man presents with deep epigastric pain. A CT scan of the abdomen reveals a pancreatic tumor that partially envelops a large artery. Which of the following arteries is most likely involved?

    A. Common hepatic
    B. Gastroduodenal
    C. Left gastric
    D. Middle colic
    E. Superior mesenteric

Multiple-choice and short-answer review questions available online; see inside front cover for details.

8. A kidney stone (calculus) passing from the kidney to the urinary bladder can become lodged at several sites along its pathway to the bladder, leading to "loin-to-groin" pain. One common site of obstruction can occur about halfway down the pathway of the ureter where it crosses which of the following structures?

   A. Common iliac vessels
   B. Lumbosacral trunk
   C. Major renal calyx
   D. Renal pelvis
   E. Sacro-iliac joint

9. An obese 46-year-old woman presents in the clinic with right upper quadrant pain for the past 48 hours, jaundice for the last 24 hours, nausea, and acute bouts of severe pain (biliary colic) after she tries to eat a meal. A diagnosis of cholelithiasis (gallstones) is made. Which of the following structures is most likely obstructed by the stone?

   A. Common bile duct
   B. Cystic duct
   C. Main pancreatic duct
   D. Right hepatic duct
   E. Thoracic duct

10. A gunshot wound to the spine of a 29-year-old man severs the lower portion of his spinal cord at about the L3-L4 level, resulting in loss of some of the central parasympathetic control of his bowel. Which of the following portions of the gastrointestinal tract is most likely affected?

    A. Ascending colon
    B. Descending colon
    C. Ileum
    D. Jejunum
    E. Transverse colon

11. If access to several arterial arcades supplying the distal ileum is required, which of the following layers of peritoneum would a surgeon need to enter to reach these vessels?

    A. Greater omentum and lesser omentum
    B. Greater omentum and mesentery
    C. Greater omentum and transverse mesocolon
    D. Parietal peritoneum and greater omentum
    E. Parietal peritoneum and mesentery
    F. Parietal peritoneum and transverse mesocolon

12. Clinically, inflammation in which of the following organs is *least* likely to present as periumbilical pain?

    A. Ascending colon
    B. Descending colon
    C. Duodenum
    D. Ileum
    E. Jejunum

13. During abdominal surgery, resection of a portion of the descending colon necessitates the sacrifice of a nerve lying on the surface of the psoas major muscle. Which of the following nerves would *most* likely be sacrificed?

    A. Femoral
    B. Genitofemoral
    C. Ilio-inguinal
    D. Lateral cutaneous nerve of thigh
    E. Subcostal

14. At autopsy it is discovered that the deceased had three ureters, one on the left side and two on the right. The condition was apparently nonsymptomatic. Which of the following embryonic events might account for the presence of two ureters on one side?

    A. Duplication of the mesonephric duct
    B. Early splitting of the ureteric bud
    C. Failure of the mesonephros to form
    D. Failure of the urorectal septum to form
    E. Persistent allantois

For each of the clinical descriptions below (15-20), select the organ from the list (A-P) that is most likely responsible.

(A)	Adrenal gland	**(I)**	Kidney
(B)	Appendix	**(J)**	Liver
(C)	Ascending colon	**(K)**	Pancreas
(D)	Descending colon	**(L)**	Rectum
(E)	Duodenum	**(M)**	Sigmoid colon
(F)	Gallbladder	**(N)**	Spleen
(G)	Ileum	**(O)**	Stomach
(H)	Jejunum	**(P)**	Transverse colon

____ 15. This retroperitoneal structure is often a site of ulceration.

____ 16. Volvulus in this segment of the bowel may also constrict its vascular supply by the inferior mesenteric artery.

____ 17. Inflammation of this structure may begin as diffuse periumbilical pain, but as the affected structure contacts the parietal peritoneum, the pain becomes acute and well localized to the right lower quadrant, often necessitating surgical resection.

___ 18. A sliding or axial hernia is the most common type of hiatal hernia and involves this structure.

___ 19. The failure of the vitelline duct to involute (occurs in about 2% of the population) during embryonic development leads to a persistent diverticulum on this structure.

___ 20. During embryonic development, this structure forms from both a dorsal and a ventral bud, which then fuse into a single structure.

Answers to Challenge Yourself Questions

1. **D.** The umbilicus denotes the T10 dermatome, just one of several key dermatome points. The shoulder is C5, the middle finger C7, the nipple T4, the inguinal region L1, the knee L4, and the second toe L5. The S1-S2 dermatomes then run up the back side of the leg and thigh.

2. **E.** The inguinal (Hesselbach's) triangle is demarcated medially by the rectus sheath, superolaterally by the inferior epigastric vessels, and inferomedially by the inguinal ligament. A hernia that does not pass down the inguinal canal but rather herniates through this triangle is considered a direct inguinal hernia. Direct inguinal hernias also are referred to as acquired hernias.

3. **A.** General visceral pain, in this case from the gallbladder, travels back to the CNS via the sympathetic pathway and the greater splanchnic nerve (T5-T9). The sensory neuronal cell bodies reside in the dorsal root ganglia associated with these spinal cord levels.

4. **A.** The lymphatic drainage will parallel the venous drainage and/or arterial supply. The celiac nodes, therefore, will receive the bulk of the lymphatic drainage from the stomach. Other adjacent nodes may also be involved, but not to the same degree as the celiac nodes.

5. **E.** The superior rectal veins (portal drainage) of the inferior mesenteric vein would communicate with the middle rectal veins, which drain into the internal iliac veins (systemic circulation into the IVC via the common iliac veins). The middle rectal and inferior rectal veins (drain into the pudendal veins, a systemic route ultimately to the IVC) also communicate and can form rectal varices in portal hypertension. Thus, venous blood flow would go from portal tributaries (superior rectal veins) into the caval (systemic) tributaries (middle and inferior rectal veins) in an effort to return blood back to the heart.

6. **A.** The epiploic foramen (of Winslow) connects the lesser sac (omental bursa), a cul-de-sac space posterior to the stomach, with the greater sac (remainder of the abdominopelvic cavity).

7. **E.** The superior mesenteric artery passes between the neck and the uncinate process of the pancreas and then anterior to the third portion of the duodenum.

8. **A.** The ureter crosses the common iliac vessels about halfway on its journey to the urinary bladder. It is slightly stretched and its lumen narrowed as it crosses these vessels, so a calculus can become lodged at this point. This site also is close to the pelvic brim.

9. **A.** The common bile duct is probably obstructed, causing the pain and jaundice. Blockage of the cystic duct may not be associated with jaundice, and obstruction of the main pancreatic duct would probably cause pancreatitis.

10. **B.** All the other portions of his bowel that are listed are innervated by the vagus nerve and its parasympathetic nerve fibers (innervates foregut and midgut embryonic derivatives of the bowel). Only the descending colon is a hindgut embryonic derivative and it receives parasympathetic efferents from the S2-S4 pelvic splanchnic nerves.

11. **E.** The surgeon would need to incise the parietal peritoneum to enter the abdominal cavity, move the apron of the greater omentum aside, and then incise the mesentery of the small bowel to access the arterial arcades.

12. **C.** The duodenum, especially its proximal portion, would present largely as epigastric pain. The other portions of the bowel would be more likely to present with periumbilical pain.

13. **B.** The genitofemoral nerve is almost always found lying on the anterior surface of the psoas major muscle.

14. **B.** Most likely this is the result of an early division of the ureteric bud, which ultimately gives rise to the ureters, renal pelvis, calices, and collecting ducts.

15. **E.** The first part of the duodenum is prone to ulcers (peptic ulcers) and is largely retroperitoneal. Ulcerative colitis may also occur in

some portions of the retroperitoneal large bowel but not as commonly as duodenal peptic ulcers.

16. M. Volvulus, or a twisting, of the bowel is most common in the small bowel (supplied by the superior mesenteric artery) but in the large bowel it is most common in the sigmoid colon. The inferior mesenteric artery supplies the distal portion of the transverse, descending, and sigmoid colon and the proximal rectum.

17. B. This is the "classic" presentation of appendicitis. The pain localizes to the lower left quadrant once the somatic pain fibers of the peritoneal wall are stimulated. This point is called "McBurney's point" and is about two thirds the distance from the umbilicus to the right anterior superior iliac spine.

18. O. A hiatal hernia is a herniation of a portion of the stomach through a widened space between the muscular right crus of the diaphragm that forms the esophageal hiatus. Sliding (also called axial or rolling) hernias account for the vast majority of hiatal hernias.

19. G. This diverticulum is called a "Meckel's diverticulum" and is the most common developmental anomaly of the bowel. It occurs about 2 feet from the ileocecal junction and is a diverticulum of the distal ileum (midgut derivative).

20. K. The pancreas develops as a fusion of a ventral and a dorsal bud. With the rotation of the duodenum, the ventral bud "flips" over and fuses with the larger dorsal bud, forming part of the head and uncinate process of the pancreas.

Pelvis and Perineum

1. INTRODUCTION

The bowl-shaped pelvic cavity is continuous superiorly with the abdomen and bounded inferiorly by the perineum, the region between the thighs. The bones of the pelvic girdle demarcate the following two regions:

- **Greater or false pelvis:** the lower portion of the abdomen that lies between the flared iliac crests.
- **Lesser or true pelvis:** demarcated by the pelvic brim, sacrum, and coccyx, and contains the pelvic viscera.

The pelvis contains the terminal gastrointestinal tract and urinary system and the internal reproductive organs. The perineum lies below the "pelvic diaphragm," or muscles that form the pelvic floor, and contains the external genitalia. Our review of the pelvis and perineum focuses on the musculoskeletal structures that support the pelvis and then examines the viscera, blood supply, and innervation of these two regions.

2. SURFACE ANATOMY

Key landmarks of the surface anatomy of the pelvis and perineum include the following (Fig. 5-1):

- **Umbilicus:** site that marks the T10 dermatome, that lies at the level of the intervertebral disc between L3 and L4; can lie slightly lower in infants or morbidly obese individuals and higher in late pregnancy.
- **Iliac crest:** rim of the ilium that lies at approximately the L4 level; also the approximate level of the bifurcation of the abdominal aorta into its two common iliac branches.

- **Anterior superior iliac spine:** superior attachment point for the inguinal ligament.
- **Inguinal ligament:** ligament formed by the aponeurosis of the external abdominal oblique muscle; forms a line of demarcation separating the lower abdominopelvic region from the thighs.
- **Pubic tubercle:** the inferior attachment point of the inguinal ligament.
- **Posterior superior iliac spine:** often seen as a "dimpling" of the skin just above the intergluteal (natal) cleft; often more obvious in females.

The surface anatomy of the perineum is reviewed later.

3. MUSCULOSKELETAL ELEMENTS

Bony Pelvic Girdle

The pelvic girdle is the attachment point of the lower limb to the body's trunk. (The pectoral girdle is its counterpart for the attachment of the upper limb.) The bones of the pelvis include the following (Fig. 5-2):

- **Right and left pelvic bones (coxal or hip bones):** fusion of three separate bones—the **ilium, ischium,** and **pubis**—that join in the **acetabulum** (cup-shaped surface where pelvis articulates with head of femur).
- **Sacrum:** fusion of the five sacral vertebrae; the two pelvic bones articulate with the sacrum posteriorly.
- **Coccyx:** terminal end of the vertebral column; a remnant of our embryonic tail (see also Table 2-2).

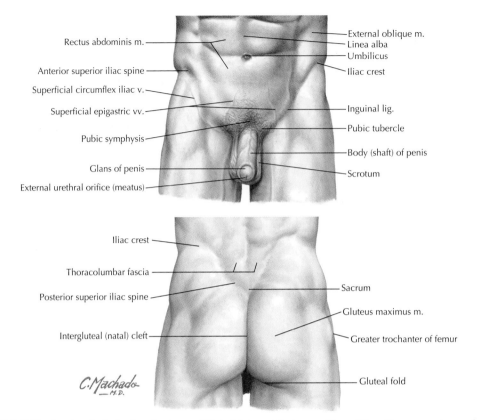

FIGURE 5-1 Key Landmarks in Surface Anatomy of Male Pelvis and Perineum. (From *Atlas of human anatomy*, ed 6, Plate 329.)

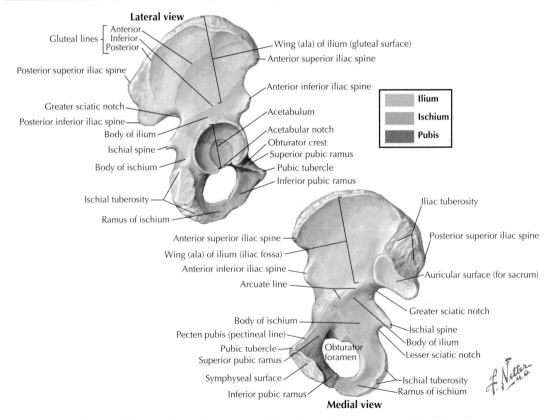

FIGURE 5-2 Right Pelvic (Coxal) Bone. (From *Atlas of human anatomy*, ed 6, Plate 473.)

Pelvic Fractures

Clinically, the term *pelvic fractures* is used to describe fractures of the pelvic ring and does not typically include *acetabular fractures*, which are a separate type of fracture, usually from high-impact falls or automobile crashes. Pelvic fractures may be high or low impact; high-impact fractures often involve significant bleeding and may be life threatening. Pelvic ring fractures are classified as *stable*, involving only one side of the ring, or *unstable*, involving both parts of the pelvic ring.

Stable pelvic ring fractures

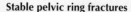

Fracture usually requires no treatment other than care in sitting; inflatable ring helpful.

Transverse fracture of the sacrum that is minimally displaced

Fracture of iliac wing from direct blow

Fracture of ipsilateral pubic and ischial ramus requires only symptomatic treatment with short-term bed rest and limited activity with walker- or crutch-assisted ambulation for 4 to 6 weeks.

Unstable pelvic fractures

Open book fracture. Disruption of symphysis pubis with wide anterior separation of pelvic ring. Anterior sacro-iliac ligaments are torn, with slight opening of sacro-iliac joints. Intact posterior sacro-iliac ligaments prevent vertical migration of the pelvis.

Straddle fracture. Double break in continuity of anterior pelvic ring causes instability but usually little displacement. Visceral (especially genito-urinary) injury likely.

Vertical shear fracture. Upward and posterior dislocation of sacro-iliac joint and fracture of both pubic rami on same side result in upward shift of hemipelvis. Note also fracture of transverse process of L5 vertebra, avulsion of ischial spine, and stretching of sacral nerves.

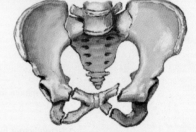

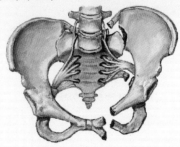

The pelvis protects the pelvic viscera, supports the weight of the body, aids in ambulation by swinging side to side in a rotary movement at the lumbosacral articulation, provides for muscle attachments, and provides a bony support for the lower birth canal. The **pelvic inlet** is the circular opening where the lower abdominal cavity is continuous with the pelvic cavity; the promontory of the sacrum protrudes into this opening and is its posterior midline margin (Fig. 5-3). The **pelvic outlet** is diamond shaped and bounded by the pubic symphysis anteriorly, the pubic arches, the inferior pubic rami and ischial rami, the sacrotuberous ligament, and the coccyx. The perineum is enclosed by these boundaries and lies below the pelvic floor (see Fig. 5-17).

The pelvic girdle forms a stable articulation to support the transfer of weight from the trunk to the lower limb. Weight is transferred from the lumbar vertebral column to the sacrum, across the sacro-iliac joints to the coxal (pelvic or hip) bones, and then to the femur (thigh bone). The joints and ligaments reflect this stability (Fig. 5-3 and Table 5-1). The sacro-iliac ligaments are strong, and the posterior sacro-iliac ligament, posterior to the articular joints, is one of the strongest ligaments in the body and supports its entire weight (see Chapter 2).

Anatomical differences in the female bony pelvis reflect the adaptations for childbirth. The differences from the male pelvis include the following:

- The bones of the female pelvis usually are smaller, lighter, and thinner.
- The pelvic inlet is oval in the female and heart shaped in the male.
- The female pelvic outlet is larger because of everted ischial tuberosities.
- The female pelvic cavity is wider and shallower.
- The female pubic arch is larger and wider.
- The greater sciatic notch is wider in females.
- The female sacrum is shorter and wider.
- The obturator foramen is oval or triangular in the female and round in the male.

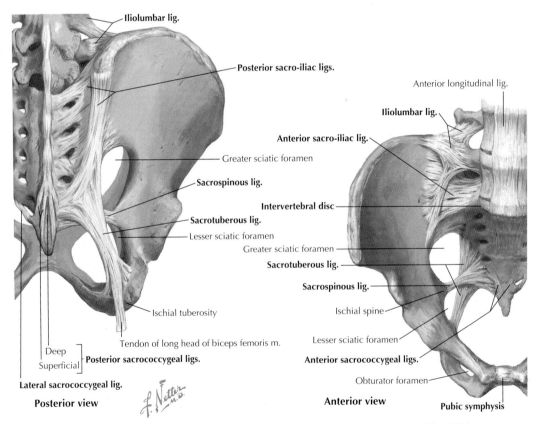

FIGURE 5-3 Bony Pelvis and Ligaments. (From *Atlas of human anatomy*, ed 6, Plate 333.)

TABLE 5-1 Joints and Ligaments of the Pelvis

LIGAMENT	ATTACHMENT	COMMENT
Lumbosacral Joint*		
Intervertebral disc	Between L5 and sacrum	Allows little movement
Iliolumbar	Transverse process of L5 to crest of ilium	Can be involved in avulsion fracture
Sacro-iliac (Plane Synovial) Joint		
Sacro-iliac	Sacrum to ilium	Allows little movement; consists of **posterior** (strong), **anterior** (provides rotational stability), and **interosseous** (strongest) ligaments
Sacrococcygeal (Symphysis) Joint		
Sacrococcygeal	Between coccyx and sacrum	Allows some movement; consists of anterior, posterior, and lateral ligaments; contains intervertebral disc between S5 and Co1
Pubic Symphysis		
Pubic	Between pubic bones	Allows some movement, fibrocartilage disc
Accessory Ligaments		
Sacrotuberous	Iliac spines and sacrum to ischial tuberosity	Provides vertical stability
Sacrospinous	Ischial spine to sacrum and coccyx	Divides sciatic notch into greater and lesser sciatic foramina

*Other ligaments include those binding any two vertebrae and facet joints.

The female pelvis may assume variable shapes, as follows:

- **Gynecoid:** normal, and most common form in Caucasian women.
- **Android:** a masculine pelvic type.
- **Platypelloid:** foreshortened in the antero-posterior dimension and wider in the transverse dimension.
- **Anthropoid:** resembling the pelvis of an anthropoid ape, with a greatly elongated anteroposterior dimension and a shortened transverse dimension.

Various asymmetric shapes may also result from scoliosis, poliomyelitis, fractures, and other pathologies.

Muscles of the Pelvis

The muscles of the true pelvis line its lateral wall and form a floor over the pelvic outlet. (The pelvic inlet is demarcated by the pelvic brim.) Two muscles line the lateral wall (obturator internus and piriformis) and attach to the femur (see Table 6-5), and two muscles form the floor, or **pelvic diaphragm** (levator ani and coccygeus) (Fig. 5-4 and Table 5-2). The **levator ani muscle** consists of

TABLE 5-2 Muscles of the Pelvis

MUSCLE	PROXIMAL ATTACHMENT (ORIGIN)	DISTAL ATTACHMENT (INSERTION)	INNERVATION	MAIN ACTIONS
Obturator internus	Pelvic aspect of obturator membrane and pelvic bones	Greater trochanter of femur	Nerve to obturator internus (L5-S1)	Rotates extended thigh laterally; abducts flexed thigh at hip
Piriformis	Anterior surface of 2nd to 4th sacral segments and sacrotuberous ligament	Greater trochanter of femur	Ventral rami of S1-S2	Rotates extended thigh laterally; abducts flexed thigh; stabilizes hip joint
Levator ani	Body of pubis, tendinous arch of obturator fascia, and ischial spine	Perineal body, coccyx, anococcygeal raphe, walls of prostate or vagina, rectum, and anal canal	Ventral rami of S3-S4, perineal nerve	Supports pelvic viscera; raises pelvic floor
Coccygeus (ischiococcygeus)	Ischial spine and sacrospinous ligament	Inferior sacrum and coccyx	Ventral rami of S4-S5	Supports pelvic viscera; draws coccyx forward

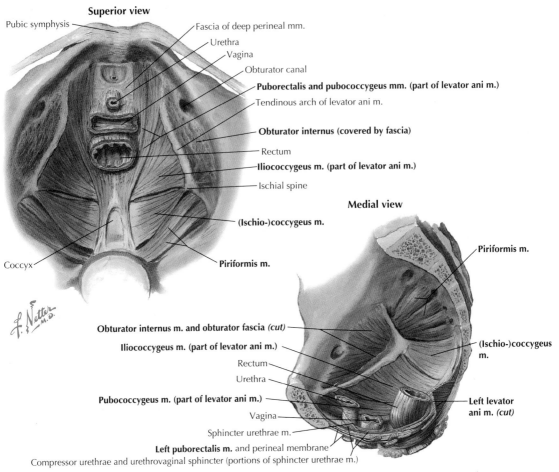

FIGURE 5-4 Muscles of the Female Pelvis. (From *Atlas of human anatomy*, ed 6, Plate 336.)

three muscle groups intermingled to form a single sheet of muscle (iliococcygeus, pubococcygeus, and puborectalis). The levator ani muscle is an important support structure for the pelvic viscera in bipeds (upright-walking humans) and helps maintain closure of the vagina and rectum. Bipedalism places greater pressure on the lower pelvic floor, and the coccygeus and levator ani muscles have been "co-opted" for a different use than originally intended in most land-dwelling quadruped mammals. Thus, the muscles once used to tuck the tail between the hind legs (coccygeus) and wag the tail (levator ani) now subserve a support function as we have evolved as bipeds and have lost our tail.

4. VISCERA

Distal Gastrointestinal Tract

In both genders the distal gastrointestinal tract passes into the pelvis as the **rectum** and **anal canal**. The rectosigmoid junction superiorly lies at about the level of the S3 vertebra, and the rectum extends inferiorly to become the anal canal just below the coccyx (Fig. 5-5). As the rectum passes through the pelvic diaphragm, it bends posteriorly at the **anorectal flexure** and becomes the anal canal. The anorectal flexure helps maintain fecal continence through the muscle tone maintained by the puborectalis portion of the levator ani muscle. During defecation this flexure straightens, and fecal matter can then move into the anal canal. Superiorly, the rectum is covered on its anterolateral surface with peritoneum, which gradually covers only the anterior surface, while the distal portion of the rectum descends below the peritoneal cavity (subperitoneal) to the anorectal flexure. Features of the rectum and anal canal are summarized in Table 5-3.

Distal Urinary Tract

The distal elements of the urinary tract lie within the pelvis and include the following (Fig. 5-6):

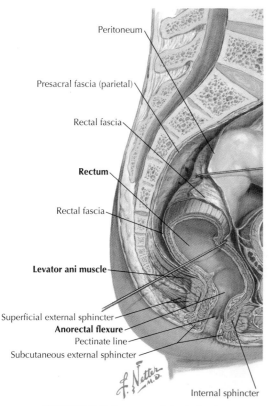

Peritoneum

Presacral fascia (parietal)

Rectal fascia

Rectum

Rectal fascia

Levator ani muscle

Superficial external sphincter
Anorectal flexure
Pectinate line
Subcutaneous external sphincter

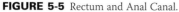

Internal sphincter

FIGURE 5-5 Rectum and Anal Canal.

TABLE 5-3 Features of the Rectum and Anal Canal	
STRUCTURE	**CHARACTERISTICS**
Pelvic diaphragm	Consists of levator ani and coccygeus muscles; supports pelvic viscera
Internal sphincter	Smooth muscle anal sphincter
Pectinate line	Demarcates visceral (above) from somatic (below) portions of anal canal by type of epithelium, innervation, and embryology
External sphincter	Skeletal muscle sphincter (subcutaneous, superficial, and deep)

and the **spongy** portion (15 cm) traverses the corpus spongiosum on the ventral aspect of the penis.

Females have an external urethral sphincter composed of skeletal muscle under voluntary control and innervated by the somatic nerve fibers in the **pudendal nerve** (S2-S4). Males have the following urethral sphincters:

- **Internal sphincter:** smooth-muscle involuntary sphincter at the neck of the bladder and innervated by sympathetic fibers from L1 to L2; during ejaculation, it contracts and prevents semen from entering the urinary bladder.
- **External sphincter:** skeletal muscle voluntary sphincter surrounding the membranous urethra and innervated by the somatic nerve fibers in the **pudendal nerve** (S2-S4).

Micturition (urination/voiding) occurs by the following sequence of events:

- Normally, the sympathetic fibers relax the bladder wall and constrict the internal urethral sphincter (smooth muscle around the bladder neck, present only in males), thus inhibiting emptying.
- Micturition is initiated by the stimulation of stretch receptors (afferents enter the spinal cord via the pelvic splanchnic nerves, S2-S4) located in the detrusor (smooth) muscle of the bladder when it begins to fill.
- Parasympathetic efferents (pelvic splanchnics) induce a reflex contraction of the detrusor muscle and relaxation of the

- **Distal ureters:** pass retroperitoneally into the pelvic inlet and are crossed anteriorly by the uterine artery in females and the ductus deferens in males before terminating in the urinary bladder. The ureter enters the bladder and passes obliquely through the smooth muscle wall; this arrangement provides for a sphincter-like action.
- **Urinary bladder:** lies behind the pubic symphysis in a subperitoneal position; holds up to 800 mL of urine (less in women and even less during pregnancy), and contains a smooth triangular area internally between the openings of the two ureters and the single urethral opening inferiorly, the **trigone of the bladder.** The smooth muscle of the bladder wall is the **detrusor muscle.**
- **Urethra:** short in the female (3-4 cm) and contains two small **para-urethral mucous glands** (Skene's glands) at its aperture; longer in the male (20 cm) and divided into the prostatic, membranous, and spongy portions. The **prostatic** portion (about 3 cm) traverses the prostate gland, the **membranous** portion (2 cm) traverses the external urethral sphincter (skeletal muscle),

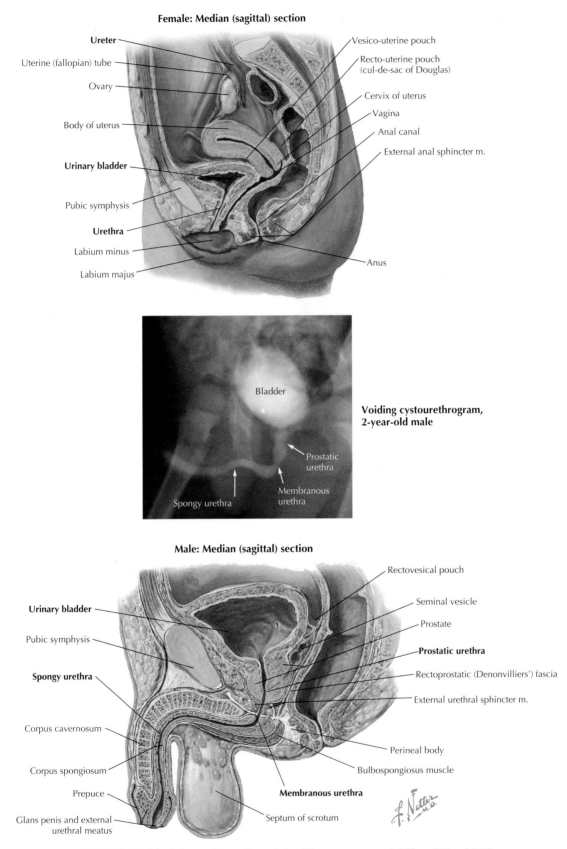

Female: Median (sagittal) section

Ureter

Uterine (fallopian) tube

Ovary

Body of uterus

Urinary bladder

Pubic symphysis

Urethra

Labium minus

Labium majus

Vesico-uterine pouch

Recto-uterine pouch
(cul-de-sac of Douglas)

Cervix of uterus

Vagina

Anal canal

External anal sphincter m.

Anus

Bladder

**Voiding cystourethrogram,
2-year-old male**

Prostatic
urethra

Membranous
urethra

Spongy urethra

Male: Median (sagittal) section

Urinary bladder

Pubic symphysis

Spongy urethra

Corpus cavernosum

Corpus spongiosum

Prepuce

Glans penis and external
urethral meatus

Rectovesical pouch

Seminal vesicle

Prostate

Prostatic urethra

Rectoprostatic (Denonvilliers') fascia

External urethral sphincter m.

Perineal body

Bulbospongiosus muscle

Membranous urethra

Septum of scrotum

FIGURE 5-6 Distal Urinary Tract. (From *Atlas of human anatomy*, ed 6, Plates 340 and 344.)

Clinical Focus 5-2

Urinary Tract Infections

Urinary tract infection (UTI) is more common in females, likely directly related to their shorter urethra, urinary tract trauma, and exposure to pathogens in an environment conducive for growth and propagation. As illustrated, a number of other risk factors also may precipitate infections in either gender. *Escherichia coli* is the usual pathogen involved. UTI may lead to urethritis, cystitis (bladder inflammation), and pyelonephritis. Symptoms of cystitis include the following:

- Dysuria
- Frequency of urination
- Urgency of urination
- Suprapubic discomfort and tenderness
- Hematuria (less common)

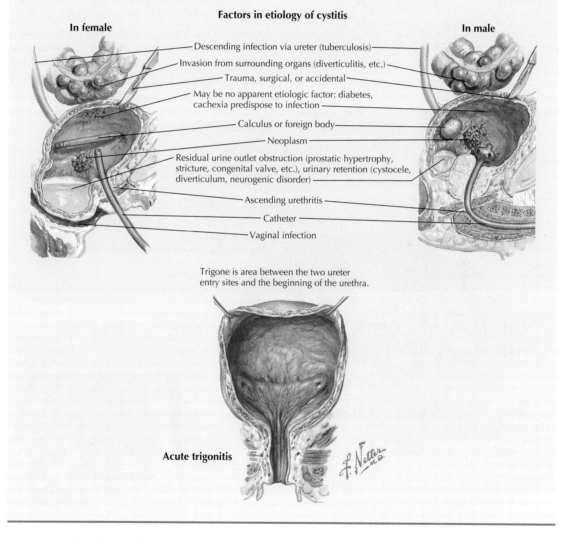

Factors in etiology of cystitis

In female

In male

Descending infection via ureter (tuberculosis)

Invasion from surrounding organs (diverticulitis, etc.)

Trauma, surgical, or accidental

May be no apparent etiologic factor: diabetes, cachexia predispose to infection

Calculus or foreign body

Neoplasm

Residual urine outlet obstruction (prostatic hypertrophy, stricture, congenital valve, etc.), urinary retention (cystocele, diverticulum, neurogenic disorder)

Ascending urethritis

Catheter

Vaginal infection

Trigone is area between the two ureter entry sites and the beginning of the urethra.

Acute trigonitis

internal sphincter (males only), enhancing the urge to void.
- When appropriate (and sometimes not!), somatic efferents via the pudendal nerve (S2-S4) cause voluntary relaxation of the external urethral sphincter, and the bladder begins to empty.

- When complete, the external urethral sphincter contracts (in males the bulbospongiosus muscle contracts to expel the last few drops of urine from the spongy urethra), and the detrusor muscle relaxes under sympathetic control.

Female Pelvic Reproductive Viscera

The female pelvic reproductive viscera include the midline **uterus** and **vagina** and the adnexa (paired **ovaries** and **uterine tubes**).

The **uterus** is pear shaped, about 7 to 8 cm long, and exhibits a body (fundus and isthmus) and cervix. While the uterine cavity looks triangular in coronal section (see Fig. 5-8), in sagittal section it appears only as a thin slit (Fig. 5-6, *top*). The normal position of the uterus is in an anteflexed (anteverted) position and lies almost in the horizontal plane. A double sheet of peritoneum (actually a mesentery) called the **broad ligament** envelops the ovaries, uterine tubes, and uterus (Figs. 5-7 and 5-8). During embryonic development the ovaries are pulled into the pelvis by a fibromuscular band (homologue of the male gubernaculum). This **ovarian ligament** attaches the inferomedial pole of the ovary to the uterus, then reflects anterolaterally off the uterus as the **round ligament of the uterus,** enters the deep inguinal ring, courses down the inguinal canal, and ends in the labia majora of the perineum as a fibrofatty mass. Features of the female pelvic reproductive viscera are summarized in Table 5-4.

The **vagina,** about 8 to 9 cm long, is a fibromuscular tube that surrounds the uterine cervix and passes inferiorly through the pelvic floor to open in the vestibule (area enclosed by the labia minora). Because the uterine cervix projects into the superoanterior aspect of the vagina, a continuous gutter surrounds the cervical opening, shallower anteriorly and deeper posteriorly, forming the anterior, lateral, and posterior fornices.

The **ovaries** are almond-shaped female gonads 3 to 4 cm long (but smaller in older women) attached to the broad ligament by its mesovarium portion. The ovary is suspended between two attachments: laterally to the pelvic wall by the **suspensory ligament of the ovary** (contains the ovarian vessels, lymphatics, and autonomic nerve fibers) and medially to the uterus by the **ovarian ligament.**

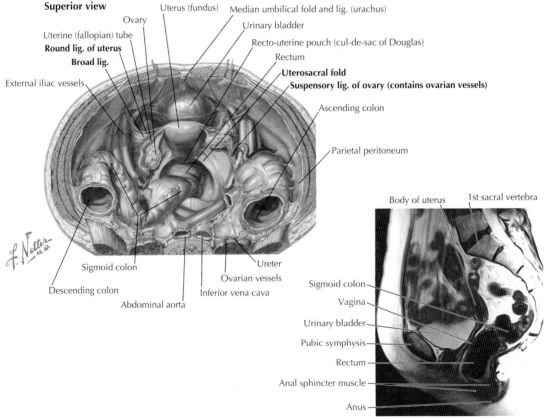

FIGURE 5-7 Peritoneal Relationships of the Female Pelvic Viscera. (From *Atlas of human anatomy,* ed 6, Plate 345; MR image from Kelley LL, Petersen C: *Sectional anatomy for imaging professionals,* Philadelphia, Mosby, 2007.)

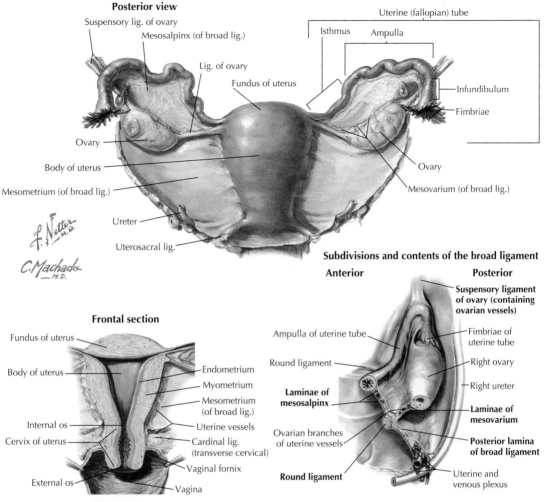

FIGURE 5-8 Uterus and Adnexa. (From *Atlas of human anatomy*, ed 6, Plates 352 and 353.)

TABLE 5-4 Features of the Female Pelvic Viscera

STRUCTURE	CHARACTERISTICS
Urinary bladder	Covered by peritoneum
Uterus	Consists of a body (fundus and isthmus) and cervix; supported by pelvic diaphragm and ligaments; enveloped in broad ligament
Ovaries	Suspended between suspensory ligament of ovary (contains ovarian vessels, nerves, and lymphatics) and ovarian ligament (tethered to uterus)
Uterine tubes (fallopian tubes)	Courses in mesosalpinx of broad ligament and consists of fimbriated end (collects ovulated ova), infundibulum, ampulla, isthmus, and intrauterine portions
Vagina	Fibromuscular tube that includes the fornix, a superior recess around protruding uterine cervix
Rectum	Distal retroperitoneal portion of large intestine
Vesico-uterine pouch	Peritoneal recess between bladder and uterus
Recto-uterine pouch (of Douglas)	Peritoneal recess between rectum and uterus and lowest point in female pelvis
Broad ligament	Peritoneal fold that suspends uterus and uterine tubes; includes mesovarium (enfolds ovary), mesosalpinx (enfolds uterine tube), and mesometrium (remainder of ligament)
Round ligament of uterus	Reflects off uterus and keeps uterus anteverted and anteflexed; passes into inguinal canal and ends as fibrofatty mass in labia majora
Transverse cervical (cardinal or Mackenrodt's) ligaments	Fibrous condensations of subperitoneal pelvic fascia that support uterus
Uterosacral ligaments	Extend from sides of cervix to sacrum, support uterus, and lie beneath peritoneum (form uterosacral fold)

Clinical Focus 5-3

Stress Incontinence in Women

Involuntary loss of urine after an increase in intraabdominal pressure is often associated with a weakening of the support structures of the pelvic floor, including the following:

- Medial and lateral pubovesical ligaments
- Pubovesical fascia at the urethrovesical junction (blends with the perineal membrane and body)
- Levator ani (provides support at the urethrovesical junction)
- Functional integrity of the urethral sphincter

Common predisposing factors for stress incontinence include multiparity, obesity, chronic cough, and heavy lifting.

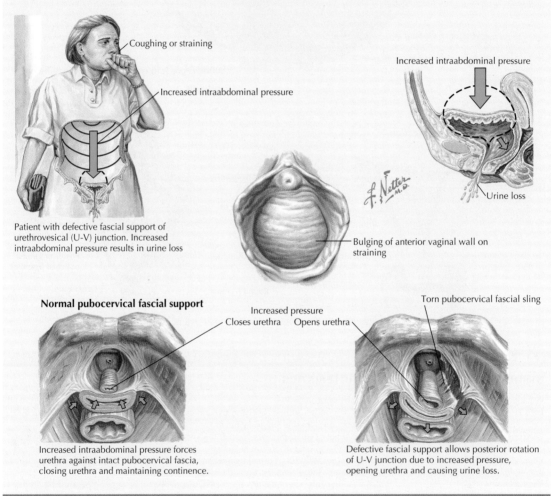

Coughing or straining

Increased intraabdominal pressure

Increased intraabdominal pressure

Urine loss

Patient with defective fascial support of urethrovesical (U-V) junction. Increased intraabdominal pressure results in urine loss

Bulging of anterior vaginal wall on straining

Normal pubocervical fascial support

Increased pressure
Closes urethra   Opens urethra

Torn pubocervical fascial sling

Increased intraabdominal pressure forces urethra against intact pubocervical fascia, closing urethra and maintaining continence.

Defective fascial support allows posterior rotation of U-V junction due to increased pressure, opening urethra and causing urine loss.

The **uterine tubes** (fallopian tubes), about 10 cm long, are suspended in the mesosalpinx portion of the broad ligament and are subdivided into four parts:

- **Infundibulum:** fimbriated, expanded distal portion that opens at the ostium into the peritoneal cavity and lies close to the ovary.

- **Ampulla:** wide portion of the tube lying between the infundibulum and the isthmus; the usual site of fertilization.
- **Isthmus:** proximal, narrow, straight, and thickened portion of the tube that joins the body of the uterus.
- **Intramural portion:** traverses the uterine wall to open into the uterine cavity.

Clinical Focus 5-4

Uterine Prolapse

Uterine prolapse may occur when the support structures of the uterus, especially the cardinal ligaments, uterosacral ligaments, and levator ani muscle, are weakened.

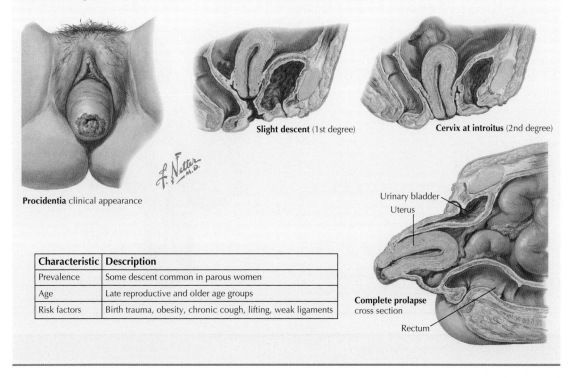

Slight descent (1st degree)

Cervix at introitus (2nd degree)

Procidentia clinical appearance

Urinary bladder

Uterus

Complete prolapse cross section

Rectum

Characteristic	Description
Prevalence	Some descent common in parous women
Age	Late reproductive and older age groups
Risk factors	Birth trauma, obesity, chronic cough, lifting, weak ligaments

Clinical Focus 5-5

Cervical Carcinoma

Approximately 85% to 90% of cervical carcinomas are squamous cell carcinomas, whereas 10% to 15% are adenocarcinomas. Most carcinomas occur near the external cervical os, where the cervical epithelium changes from simple columnar to stratified squamous epithelium (the transformation zone). The most common cause of cervical carcinoma is contraction of human papillomavirus (HPV) during sexual intercourse.

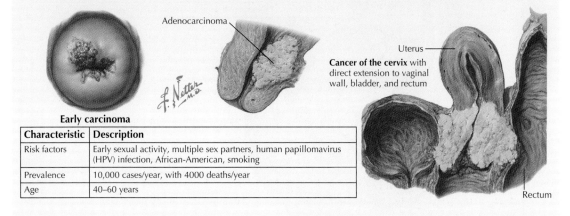

Adenocarcinoma

Uterus

Cancer of the cervix with direct extension to vaginal wall, bladder, and rectum

Early carcinoma

Rectum

Characteristic	Description
Risk factors	Early sexual activity, multiple sex partners, human papillomavirus (HPV) infection, African-American, smoking
Prevalence	10,000 cases/year, with 4000 deaths/year
Age	40–60 years

Clinical Focus 5-6

Uterine Leiomyomas (Fibroids)

Leiomyomas are benign tumors of smooth muscle and connective tissue cells of the myometrium of the uterus. These "fibroids" are firm and can range in size from 1 to 20 cm. The composite drawing shows various sizes and sites of potential leiomyomas.

Composite summary of sizes and sites

Characteristic	Description
Prevalence	30% of all women; 40–50% of women older than 50 years; most common benign tumor in women
Risk factors	Nulliparity, early menarche, African-American (4- to 10-fold increase)
Growth	Stimulated by estrogen, oral contraceptives, epidermal growth factor

Clinical Focus 5-7

Endometriosis

Endometriosis is a progressive benign condition characterized by ectopic foci of endometrial tissue, called *implants*, that grow in the pelvis—on the ovaries and in the recto-uterine pouch, uterine ligaments, and uterine tubes—or in the peritoneal cavity. As with the uterine lining, these estrogen-sensitive ectopic implants can grow and then break down and bleed in cycle with the woman's normal menstrual cycle.

Characteristic	Description
Prevalence	5–10% of all women; 30–50% of infertility patients
Age	25–45 years
Causes	Genetic, menstrual backflow through tubes, lymphatic or vascular spread, metaplasia of coelomic epithelium
Risk factors	Obstructive anomalies (cervical or vaginal outflow pathway)

Possible sites of distribution of endometriosis

Uterine Endometrial Carcinoma

Endometrial carcinoma is the most common malignancy of the female reproductive tract. It often occurs between the ages of 55 and 65 years, and risk factors include the following:

- Obesity (increased estrogen synthesis from fat cells without concomitant progesterone synthesis)
- Estrogen replacement therapy without concomitant progestin
- Breast or colon cancer
- Early menarche or late menopause (prolonged estrogen stimulation)
- Chronic anovulation
- No prior pregnancies or periods of breastfeeding
- Diabetes

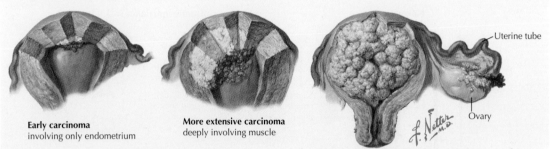

Early carcinoma involving only endometrium

More extensive carcinoma deeply involving muscle

— Uterine tube
Ovary

Extensive carcinoma invading full thickness of myometrium and escaping through tube to implant on ovary

Chronic Pelvic Inflammatory Disease

Recurrent or chronic infections of the uterine tubes or other adnexa (uterine appendages) result in cystic dilation (hydrosalpinx) and can account for approximately 40% of female infertility cases. Chronic pelvic inflammatory disease (PID) can cause scarring, causing problems with fertility, pelvic pain, or tubal (ectopic) pregnancy. The most affected age group is 15 to 25 years of age, and risk factors include the following:

- Early sexual activity
- Failure to use condoms
- Multiple sexual partners
- Sexually transmitted diseases (STDs)

Unilateral or bilateral adnexal masses are usually sausage shaped and may be palpable.

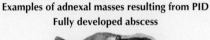
Examples of adnexal masses resulting from PID
Fully developed abscess

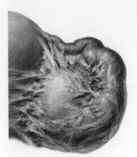
Pathogenesis of tubo-ovarian abscess
Adherence of tube and infection of ruptured follicle (corpus luteum)

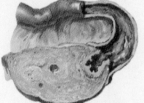
PID: hydrosalpinx (dilation of uterine tube)

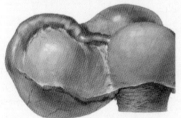
Large tubo-ovarian cyst

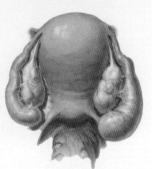
Small and moderate-sized hydrosalpinx

Dysfunctional Uterine Bleeding

Dysfunctional uterine bleeding (DUB) involves an irregular cycle or intermenstrual bleeding (painless) with no clinically identifiable cause. The etiology and pathogenesis are extensive and include local uterine, ovarian, or adnexal disorders, as well as systemic and pregnancy-related disorders. Hormonal imbalance is a common cause.

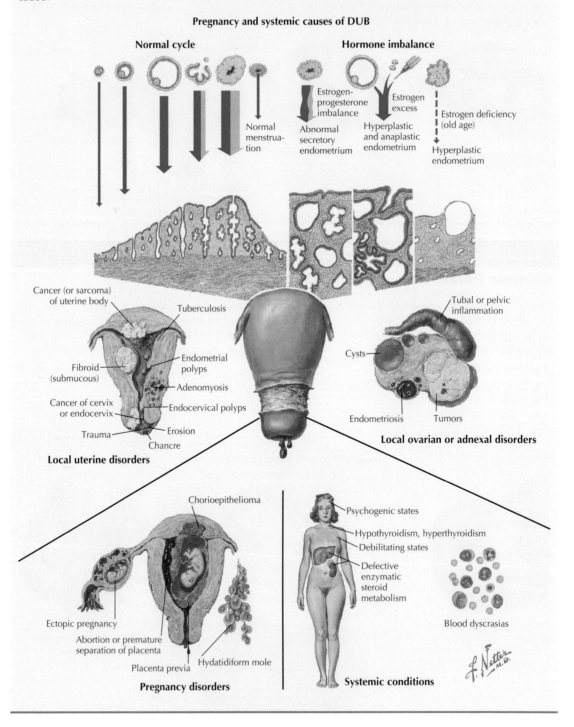

Pregnancy and systemic causes of DUB

Normal cycle

Hormone imbalance

Estrogen-progesterone imbalance

Estrogen excess

Estrogen deficiency (old age)

Normal menstrua-tion

Abnormal secretory endometrium

Hyperplastic and anaplastic endometrium

Hyperplastic endometrium

Cancer (or sarcoma) of uterine body

Tuberculosis

Endometrial polyps

Fibroid (submucous)

Adenomyosis

Cancer of cervix or endocervix

Endocervical polyps

Trauma

Erosion

Chancre

Local uterine disorders

Tubal or pelvic inflammation

Cysts

Endometriosis

Tumors

Local ovarian or adnexal disorders

Chorioepithelioma

Psychogenic states

Hypothyroidism, hyperthyroidism

Debilitating states

Defective enzymatic steroid metabolism

Ectopic pregnancy

Abortion or premature separation of placenta

Placenta previa

Hydatidiform mole

Blood dyscrasias

Pregnancy disorders

Systemic conditions

Ectopic Pregnancy

Ectopic pregnancy involves implantation of a blastocyst outside the uterine cavity, most often in the fallopian tube. Because of the potential medical danger of an ectopic pregnancy, the pregnancy is usually terminated medically (if detected early enough) or surgically (often laparoscopically).

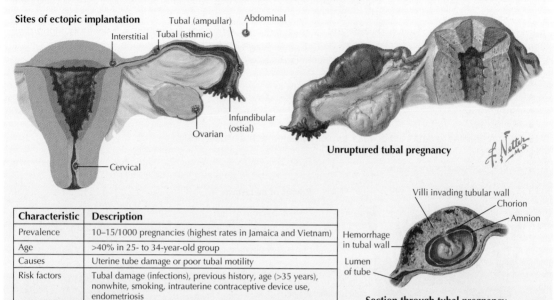

Sites of ectopic implantation

Interstitial — Tubal (isthmic) — Tubal (ampullar) — Abdominal

Ovarian — Infundibular (ostial)

Cervical

Unruptured tubal pregnancy

Villi invading tubular wall — Chorion — Amnion

Hemorrhage in tubal wall

Lumen of tube

Section through tubal pregnancy

Characteristic	Description
Prevalence	10–15/1000 pregnancies (highest rates in Jamaica and Vietnam)
Age	>40% in 25- to 34-year-old group
Causes	Uterine tube damage or poor tubal motility
Risk factors	Tubal damage (infections), previous history, age (>35 years), nonwhite, smoking, intrauterine contraceptive device use, endometriosis

Assisted Reproduction

Approximately 10% to 15% of infertile couples may benefit from various assisted reproductive strategies.

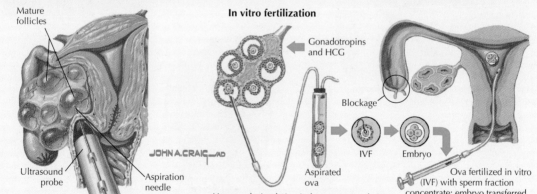

Mature follicles

In vitro fertilization

Gonadotropins and HCG

Blockage

IVF — Embryo

Ultrasound probe — Aspiration needle

Aspirated ova

Ova fertilized in vitro (IVF) with sperm fraction concentrate; embryo transferred directly into uterus, bypassing tubal occlusion

In superovulating ovary, ova harvested from mature follicles transvaginally with ultrasound-guided needle

Hormonal stimulation induces superovulation; ova aspirated from mature follicles

Technique	Definition
Artificial insemination	Use of donor sperm
GIFT	Gamete intrafallopian transfer
IUI	Intrauterine insemination (partner's or donor's sperm)
IVF/ET	In vitro fertilization with embryo transfer to uterine cavity (illustrated)
ZIFT	In vitro fertilization with zygote transfer to fallopian tube

Clinical Focus 5-13

Ovarian Cancer

Ovarian cancer is the most lethal cancer of the female reproductive tract. From 85% to 90% of all malignancies occur from the surface epithelium, with cancerous cells often breaking through the capsule and seeding the peritoneal surface, invading the adjacent pelvic organs, or seeding the omentum, mesentery, and intestines. Additionally, the cancer cells spread via the venous system to the lungs (ovarian vein and inferior vena cava) and liver (portal system) and via lymphatics. Risk factors include the following:

- Family history of ovarian cancer
- High-fat diet
- Age
- Nulliparity
- Early menarche or late menopause (prolonged estrogen stimulation)
- White race
- Higher socioeconomic status

Routes of metastases

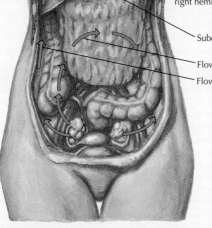

Transdiaphragmatic communication of pleural and abdominal lymphatic vessels results in pleural effusion.

Malignant cells in peritoneal fluid embolize to lymphatic vessels of right hemidiaphragm.

Subdiaphragmatic cell flow

Flow over omentum

Flow along paracolic gutters

Occlusion of lymphatic vessels causes ascites.

Para-aortic nodes

Pelvic nodes

Lymphatic spread primarily to pelvic and para-aortic lymph node chains

Peritoneal seeding of free-floating malignant cells most common mode of spread

JOHN A.CRAIG─AD

Parenchymal pulmonary metastasis

Parenchymal hepatic metastasis

Spread via portal v.

Spread via ovarian v.

Hematogenous spread primarily to lung via ovarian v. and vena cava and to liver via portal venous system

Male Pelvic Reproductive Viscera

The male pelvic reproductive viscera include the **prostate gland** and paired **seminal vesicles.** These structures lie in a subperitoneal position and are in close association with the urethra (Fig. 5-9). The testes descend into the scrotum late in human prenatal development and are connected to the seminal vesicles by the **ductus (vas) deferens**, which ascends in the scrotum, passes through the inguinal canal, and then courses retroperitoneally to join the duct of the seminal vesicles (ejaculatory ducts) (Table 5-5).

The **testes** are paired gonads about the size of a chestnut with the following features (Fig. 5-10):

- During descent of the testes into the scrotum, a pouch of peritoneum called the **tunica vaginalis** attaches to the anterior and lateral aspect of the testes (has visceral and parietal layers).
- Testes are encased within a thick capsule, the **tunica albuginea.**
- Testes are divided into lobules that contain **seminiferous tubules.**
- The seminiferous tubules are lined with germinal epithelium that gives rise to spermatozoa.
- Testes drain spermatozoa into the **rete testes** (straight tubules) and **efferent ductules** of the epididymis.
- Sperm mature and are stored in the **epididymis,** a long coiled tube about 23 feet in length.

It is within the seminiferous tubules that spermatogenesis occurs. The testis is divided into about 250 lobules, each containing one to four seminiferous tubules, each about 50 cm (20 inches) long on average at full length. The complete cycle of spermatogenesis takes about 74 days and 12 more days for the sperm to mature and

TABLE 5-5 Features of the Male Pelvic Viscera	
STRUCTURE	**CHARACTERISTICS**
Urinary bladder	Lies retroperitoneal and has detrusor muscle (smooth muscle) lining its walls
Prostate gland	Walnut-sized gland with five lobes (anterior, middle, posterior, right lateral, left lateral); middle lobe prone to benign hypertrophy and surrounds prostatic urethra
Seminal vesicles	Lobulated glands whose ducts join ductus deferens to form ejaculatory duct; secretes alkaline seminal fluid
Rectum	Distal portion of large intestine that is retroperitoneal
Rectovesical pouch	Recess between bladder and rectum
Testes	Develop in retroperitoneal abdominal wall and descend into scrotum
Epididymis	Consists of head, body, and tail and functions in maturation and storage of sperm
Ductus (vas) deferens	Passes in spermatic cord through inguinal canal to join duct of seminal vesicles (ejaculatory duct)

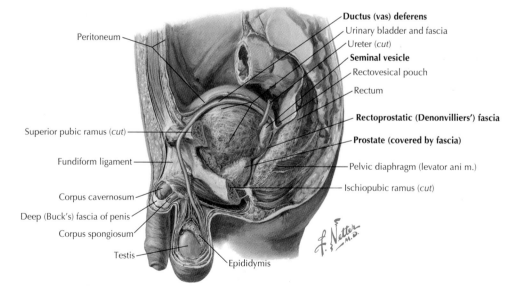

Peritoneum

Superior pubic ramus (*cut*)

Fundiform ligament

Corpus cavernosum

Deep (Buck's) fascia of penis

Corpus spongiosum

Testis

Epididymis

Ductus (vas) deferens

Urinary bladder and fascia

Ureter (*cut*)

Seminal vesicle

Rectovesical pouch

Rectum

Rectoprostatic (Denonvilliers') fascia

Prostate (covered by fascia)

Pelvic diaphragm (levator ani m.)

Ischiopubic ramus (*cut*)

FIGURE 5-9 Male Reproductive Viscera. (From *Atlas of human anatomy,* ed 6, Plate 344.)

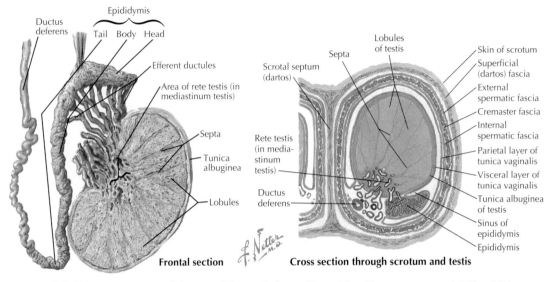

FIGURE 5-10 Testis, Epididymis, and Ductus Deferens. (From *Atlas of human anatomy*, ed 6, Plate 368.)

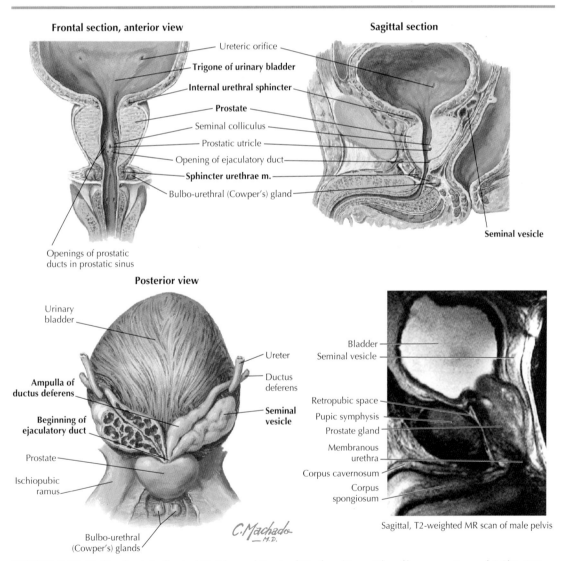

FIGURE 5-11 Bladder, Prostate, Seminal Vesicles, and Proximal Urethra. (From *Atlas of human anatomy*, ed 6, Plate 362; MR image from Weber E, Vilensky J, Carmichael M: *Netter's concise radiologic anatomy*, Philadelphia, Saunders, 2009.)

pass through the epididymis. About 300 million sperm cells are produced daily in the human testis.

The ductus deferens is 40 to 45 cm long and joins the ducts of the seminal vesicles to form the **ejaculatory ducts,** which empty into the **prostatic urethra,** the first portion of the male urethra leaving the urinary bladder (Fig. 5-11; see Fig. 5-9 and Table 5-5). The **seminal vesicles** have the following features:

- Contribute fluid to the ejaculate; produce about 70% of the ejaculate volume.
- Produce a viscous and alkaline fluid that nourishes the spermatozoa and protects them from the acidic environment of the female vagina.

The **prostate** is a walnut-sized gland that surrounds the proximal urethra and has the following features:

- Contributes fluid to the ejaculate; produces about 20% of the ejaculate volume.
- Produces a thin, milky, slightly alkaline fluid that helps to liquefy coagulated semen after it is deposited in the vagina; contains citric acid, proteolytic enzymes, sugars, phosphate, and various ions.

About 3 to 5 mL of semen and 100 million sperm/mL are present in each ejaculation. The pH is between 7 and 8.

Clinical Focus 5-14

Vasectomy

Vasectomy offers birth control with a failure rate below that of the pill, condom, intrauterine device, and tubal ligation. It can be performed as an office procedure with a local anesthetic. (Approximately 500,000 are performed each year in the United States.) One approach uses a small incision on each side of the scrotum to isolate the vas deferens; another uses a small puncture (no incision) in the scrotal skin to isolate both the right and left vas. The muscular vas is identified, and a small segment is isolated between two small metal clips or sutures. The isolated segment is resected, the clipped ends of the vas are cauterized, and the incision is closed (or, in the nonincisional approach, the puncture wound is left unsutured).

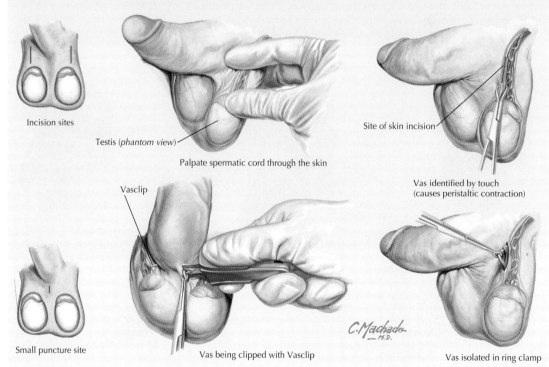

Incision sites

Testis (phantom view)

Palpate spermatic cord through the skin

Site of skin incision

Vas identified by touch
(causes peristaltic contraction)

Vasclip

Small puncture site

Vas being clipped with Vasclip

Vas isolated in ring clamp

Testicular Cancer

Testicular tumors are heterogeneous neoplasms, with 95% arising from germ cells and almost all malignant. Of the germ cell tumors, 60% show mixed histologic features, and 40% show a single histologic pattern. Surgical resection usually is performed using an inguinal approach (radical inguinal orchiectomy) to avoid spread of the cancer to the adjacent scrotal tissues.

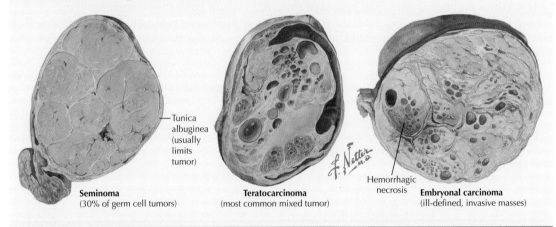

Tunica albuginea (usually limits tumor)

Seminoma
(30% of germ cell tumors)

Teratocarcinoma
(most common mixed tumor)

Hemorrhagic necrosis

Embryonal carcinoma
(ill-defined, invasive masses)

Hydrocele and Varicocele

The most common cause of scrotal enlargement is *hydrocele,* an excessive accumulation of serous fluid within the tunica vaginalis (usually a potential space). An infection in the testis or epididymis, trauma, or a tumor may lead to hydrocele, or it may be idiopathic.

Varicocele is an abnormal dilation and tortuosity of the pampiniform venous plexus. Almost all varicoceles are on the left side, perhaps because the left testicular vein drains into the left renal vein, which has a slightly higher pressure, rather than into the larger inferior vena cava, as the right testicular vein does. A varicocele is evident at physical examination when a patient stands, but it usually resolves when the patient is recumbent.

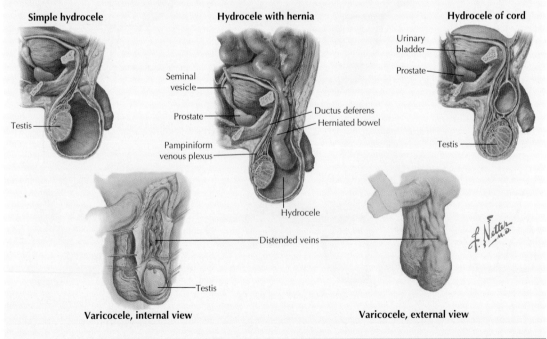

Simple hydrocele

Hydrocele with hernia

Hydrocele of cord

Urinary bladder

Prostate

Seminal vesicle

Prostate

Ductus deferens

Herniated bowel

Testis

Pampiniform venous plexus

Testis

Hydrocele

Distended veins

Testis

Varicocele, internal view

Varicocele, external view

Clinical Focus 5-17

Transurethral Resection of the Prostate

Benign prostatic hypertrophy (BPH) occurs in about 20% of men by age 40, increasing with age to 90% of males older than 80. BPH is really a nodular *hyperplasia,* not hypertrophy, and results from proliferation of epithelial and stromal tissues, often in the periurethral area. This growth can lead to urinary urgency, decreased stream force, frequency, and nocturia. Symptoms may necessitate transurethral resection of the prostate (TURP), in which the obstructing periurethral part of the gland is removed using a resectoscope. Although relatively rare, several surgical complications are illustrated.

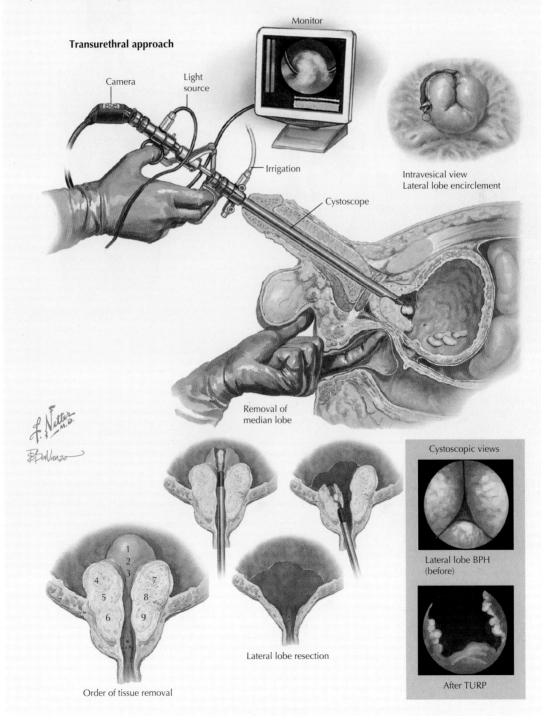

Transurethral approach

Monitor

Camera

Light source

Irrigation

Intravesical view
Lateral lobe encirclement

Cystoscope

Removal of
median lobe

Order of tissue removal

Lateral lobe resection

Cystoscopic views

Lateral lobe BPH
(before)

After TURP

Clinical Focus 5-18

Prostatic Carcinoma

Prostatic carcinoma is the most common visceral cancer in males and the second leading cause of death in men older than 50, after lung cancer. Primary lesions invade the prostatic capsule, then spread along the ejaculatory ducts into the space between the seminal vesicles and bladder. The pelvic lymphatics and rich venous drainage of the prostate (prostatic venous plexus) facilitate metastatic spread to distant sites.

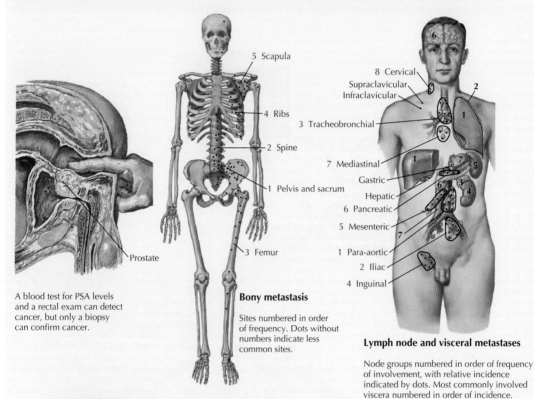

A blood test for PSA levels and a rectal exam can detect cancer, but only a biopsy can confirm cancer.

Prostate

5 Scapula

4 Ribs

2 Spine

1 Pelvis and sacrum

3 Femur

Bony metastasis

Sites numbered in order of frequency. Dots without numbers indicate less common sites.

8 Cervical
Supraclavicular
Infraclavicular

3 Tracheobronchial

7 Mediastinal

Gastric

Hepatic

6 Pancreatic

5 Mesenteric

1 Para-aortic

2 Iliac

4 Inguinal

Lymph node and visceral metastases

Node groups numbered in order of frequency of involvement, with relative incidence indicated by dots. Most commonly involved viscera numbered in order of incidence.

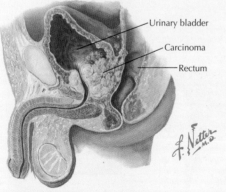

Urinary bladder

Carcinoma

Rectum

Extension of carcinoma into bladder, peritoneum, and rectal wall

Characteristic	Description
Site	90% arise in outer glands (adenocarcinomas) and are palpable by digital rectal examination
Metastases	Regional pelvic lymph nodes, bone, seminal vesicles, bladder, and periurethral zones
Etiology	Hormonal (androgens), genetic, environmental factors
Prevalence	Increased in African-Americans and Scandinavians, few in Japan

Pelvic Fascia

The pelvic (endopelvic) fascia is the extraperitoneal layer just deep to the peritoneum that covers the lateral pelvic walls. The pelvic fascia covers the bladder, uterus, upper portion of the vagina, rectum, and anterior and lateral prostate. This fascia envelops the neurovascular bundles and condenses around the pelvic viscera, forming significant support structures, especially in the female. The major fascial condensations in the female include the following (Fig. 5-12):

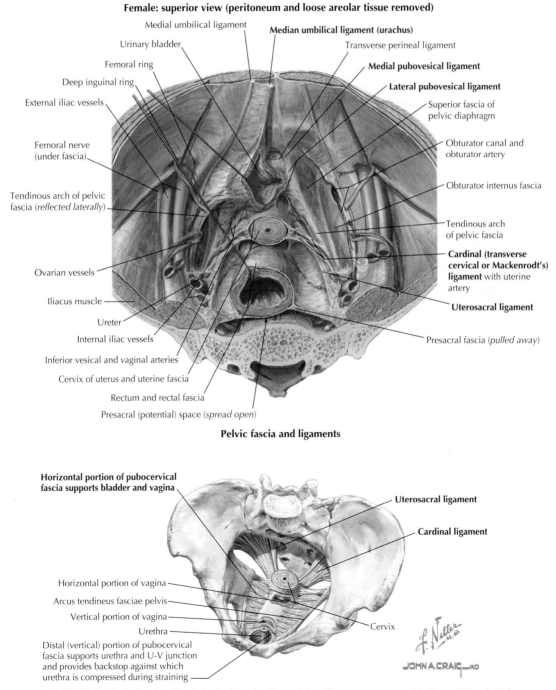

Female: superior view (peritoneum and loose areolar tissue removed)

Medial umbilical ligament
Median umbilical ligament (urachus)
Urinary bladder
Transverse perineal ligament
Femoral ring
Medial pubovesical ligament
Deep inguinal ring
Lateral pubovesical ligament
External iliac vessels
Superior fascia of pelvic diaphragm
Femoral nerve (under fascia)
Obturator canal and obturator artery
Obturator internus fascia
Tendinous arch of pelvic fascia (*reflected laterally*)
Tendinous arch of pelvic fascia
Cardinal (transverse cervical or Mackenrodt's) ligament with uterine artery
Ovarian vessels
Uterosacral ligament
Iliacus muscle
Ureter
Internal iliac vessels
Inferior vesical and vaginal arteries
Presacral fascia (*pulled away*)
Cervix of uterus and uterine fascia
Rectum and rectal fascia
Presacral (potential) space (*spread open*)

Pelvic fascia and ligaments

Horizontal portion of pubocervical fascia supports bladder and vagina
Uterosacral ligament
Cardinal ligament
Horizontal portion of vagina
Arcus tendineus fasciae pelvis
Vertical portion of vagina
Urethra
Cervix
Distal (vertical) portion of pubocervical fascia supports urethra and U-V junction and provides backstop against which urethra is compressed during straining

JOHN A.CRAIG—AD

FIGURE 5-12 Endopelvic Fascia in the Female. (From *Atlas of human anatomy*, ed 6, Plates 343 and 351.)

- **Median umbilical ligament:** midsagittal anterior ligament in both genders that extends to the umbilicus (a remnant of the embryonic urachus).
- **Medial pubovesical ligament:** connects the bladder to the pubis in both genders.
- **Lateral ligament of the bladder (pubovesical):** provides lateral support that conveys the superior vesical vessels supplying the bladder in both genders.
- **Pubocervical ligaments:** fascial condensations that course from the cervix to the anterior pelvic wall, passing on either side of the female bladder.
- **Transverse cervical ligaments:** provide important posterolateral support of the uterus and upper vagina and convey the uterine vessels; also called cardinal, lateral cervical, or Mackenrodt's ligaments.
- **Uterosacral ligaments:** fascial condensations that course from the cervix posteriorly to the pelvic walls.
- **Rectovaginal septum:** fascial condensations between the rectum and vagina.

The same ligaments that support the female urinary bladder also support the male bladder. Males have a condensation called the **prostatic fascia** that surrounds the anterolateral aspect of the prostate gland, envelops the prostatic venous plexus, and extends posteriorly to envelop the prostatic arteries and nerve plexus (**rectoprostatic septum (fascia)** or Denonvilliers' fascia; see Fig. 5-9).

The peritoneum of the pelvis forms the following structures (see Figs. 5-7 and 5-9):

- Covers the pelvic viscera in both genders and forms the **broad ligament** in females.
- Forms the **median umbilical** (urachus) **fold** and the **medial umbilical folds** (remnants of the fetal umbilical arteries) in both genders.
- Forms the **vesico-uterine** and **recto-uterine** (pouch of Douglas) **pouches** in females.
- Forms the **rectovesical pouch** in males.
- Forms the **uterosacral fold** in females and the **vesicosacral fold** in males.

5. BLOOD SUPPLY

The arterial supply to the pelvis arises from the paired **internal iliac arteries,** which not only supply the pelvis but also send branches into the perineum, the gluteal region, and the medial thigh. The arteries in the female pelvis are shown in Figure 5-13 and summarized in Table 5-6.

The arteries in the male are similar, except that the uterine, vaginal, and ovarian branches are replaced by arteries to the ductus deferens (from a vesical branch), the prostatic artery (from the inferior vesical artery), and the testicular arteries (from the abdominal aorta). Significant variability exists for these arteries, so they are best identified and named for the structure they supply. Corresponding veins, usually multiple, course with each of these arterial branches and drain into the **internal iliac vein** directly or into other larger veins. (Multiple connections among veins are common.) Extensive venous plexuses are associated with the bladder, rectum, vagina, uterus, and prostate, referred to as the **pelvis plexus of veins.** The veins surrounding the rectum form an important portosystemic anastomosis via the superior rectal (portal system) vein and the middle and inferior rectal (caval system) veins (see Figs. 4-26 and 5-19).

Overview of Pelvic and Perineal Arteries

The aorta bifurcates at about the L4 vertebral level into the **common iliac artery (1)** (right and left branches), which then bifurcates into the **internal iliac artery (2)** and the **external iliac artery (3)** at about the L5-S1 intervertebral level. The external iliac artery passes inferiorly to the thigh, where it becomes the femoral artery after passing deep to the inguinal ligament (Fig. 5-14).

The **internal iliac artery (2)** provides branches to the sacrum, the obturator artery to the medial compartment of the thigh (adductor muscles of hip), the gluteal arteries to the gluteal muscles, and a partially patent umbilical artery (becomes the medial umbilical ligament as it approaches the anterior abdominal wall). The internal iliac also gives rise to arteries to the urinary bladder (the vesical artery, usually from the umbilical artery), the uterus and vagina in females, and the middle rectal artery to the rectum (with vaginal and prostatic branches, depending on the sex).

The **internal pudendal artery** passes out the greater sciatic foramen and around the sacrospinous ligament and enters the pudendal canal through the lesser sciatic foramen to pass forward and inferiorly to the perineum. The internal pudendal artery supplies the skin, external genitalia, and

Right paramedian section: lateral view

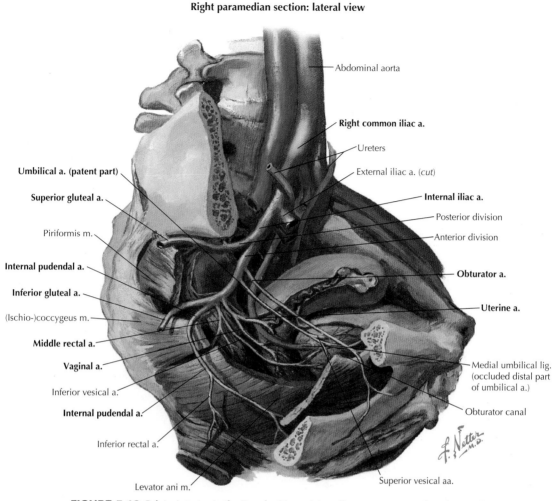

- Abdominal aorta
- Right common iliac a.
- Ureters
- External iliac a. (*cut*)
- Internal iliac a.
- Posterior division
- Anterior division
- Obturator a.
- Uterine a.
- Medial umbilical lig. (occluded distal part of umbilical a.)
- Obturator canal
- Superior vesical aa.

- Umbilical a. (patent part)
- Superior gluteal a.
- Piriformis m.
- Internal pudendal a.
- Inferior gluteal a.
- (Ischio-)coccygeus m.
- Middle rectal a.
- Vaginal a.
- Inferior vesical a.
- Internal pudendal a.
- Inferior rectal a.
- Levator ani m.

FIGURE 5-13 Pelvic Arteries in the Female. (From *Atlas of human anatomy*, ed 6, Plate 380.)

TABLE 5-6 Branches (Divisions) of the Female Pelvic Arteries

ARTERIAL BRANCH*	COURSE AND STRUCTURES SUPPLIED
Common iliac	Divides into external (to thigh) and internal (to pelvis) iliac
Internal iliac	Divides into posterior division (P) and anterior division (A)
Iliolumbar (P)	To iliacus muscle (iliac artery), psoas, quadratus lumborum, and spine (lumbar artery)
Lateral sacral (P)	To piriformis muscle and sacrum (meninges and nerves)
Superior gluteal (P)	Between lumbosacral trunk and S1 nerves, through greater sciatic foramen and to gluteal region
Inferior gluteal (A)	Between S1 or S2 and S2 or S3 to gluteal region
Internal pudendal (A)	To perineal structures through greater sciatic foramen and into lesser sciatic foramen to perineum
Umbilical (A)	Gives rise to superior vesical artery to bladder and becomes medial umbilical ligament when it reaches anterior abdominal wall
Obturator (A)	Passes into medial thigh via obturator foramen (with obturator nerve)
Uterine (A)	Runs over levator ani muscle and ureter to reach uterus (may give rise to vesical arteries)
Vaginal (A)	From internal iliac or uterine, passes to vagina
Middle rectal (A)	To lower rectum and superior part of anal canal
Ovarian	From abdominal aorta, runs in suspensory ligament of ovary
Superior rectal	Continuation of inferior mesenteric artery to rectum
Median sacral	From aortic bifurcation, unpaired artery to sacrum and coccyx (caudal artery)

*A, Branch of anterior trunk; P, branch of posterior trunk.

Aortic Bifurcation*
1. **Common Iliac Artery (right and left)**

2. **Internal Iliac Artery**
　Iliolumbar Artery
　Lateral Sacral Arteries
　Obturator Artery
　　Pubic branch
　　Acetabular branch
　　Ant. and post. branches
　Superior Gluteal Artery
　　Superficial and deep branches
　Inferior Gluteal Artery
　　Artery to sciatic nerve
　Umbilical Artery (patent part)
　　Artery to ductus deferens
　　Ureteric branches
　　Superior vesical arteries
　Inferior Vesical Artery
　　Prostatic branches (male)
　Uterine Artery (female)
　　Helicine branches
　　Vaginal branches
　　Ovarian branches
　　Tubal branch
　Vaginal Artery
　Middle Rectal Artery
　　Vaginal (female) and prostatic
　　　(male) branches
　Internal Pudendal Artery
　　Inferior rectal artery
　　Perineal artery
　　Labial (female) and scrotal (male) branches
　　Urethral artery
　　Artery of bulb (vestibule-female;
　　　penis-male)
　　Dorsal artery of clitoris (female) and
　　　penis
　　Deep artery of clitoris and penis

3. **External Iliac Artery**
　Inferior epigastric artery
　　Obturator branch
　　Cremasteric artery (male)
　Deep circumflex artery
　　Ascending branch

*Proximal (aortic bifurcation)
to Distal (internal pudendal artery)

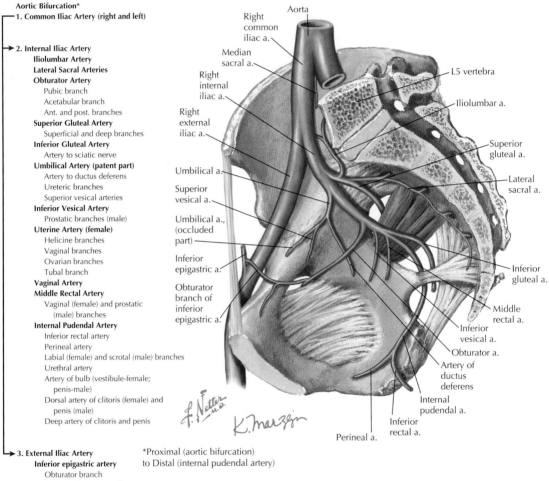

FIGURE 5-14 Arteries of Pelvis and Perineum in the Male. (From *Atlas of human anatomy,* ed 6, Plate 382.)

muscles of the perineum (anal and urogenital triangle).

Some anatomists divide the branches of the internal iliac artery into anterior and posterior trunks for descriptive purposes. The posterior branches are the iliolumbar, lateral sacral, and superior gluteal arteries; all the other major arteries are from the anterior trunk.

The veins of the pelvis and perineum course with the arteries and generally have the same names. They drain largely back into the **internal iliac vein,** common iliac vein, inferior vena cava, and then to the heart. Important **portosystemic anastomoses** occur between the superior rectal vein (from the inferior mesenteric vein of the portal system) and the middle (internal iliac vein) and inferior (internal pudendal vein) rectal veins of the caval system (Fig. 5-19).

6. LYMPHATICS

Much of the lymphatic drainage of the pelvis parallels the venous drainage and drains into lymph nodes along the internal iliac vessels (Fig. 5-15 and

Table 5-7). The major exception is the drainage from the ovaries and the adjacent uterine tubes and upper uterus, and from the testes and scrotal structures, which flows directly back to the aortic (lumbar) nodes of the midabdomen. Because some lymph from the uterus may drain along the round ligament of the uterus to the inguinal nodes,

TABLE 5-7 Pelvic Lymphatics	
LYMPH NODES	**DRAINAGE**
Superficial inguinal	Receive lymph from perineum (and lower limb and lower abdomen) and deep pelvic viscera and drain lymph to external iliac nodes
Deep inguinal	Receive lymph from perineum (and lower limb) and drain lymph to external iliac nodes
Internal iliac	Receive lymph from pelvic viscera and drain lymph along iliac nodes, ultimately to reach aortic (lumbar) nodes
External iliac	Convey lymph along iliac nodes to reach aortic (lumbar) nodes
Gonadal lymphatics	Drain lymph from gonads directly to aortic (lumbar) nodes

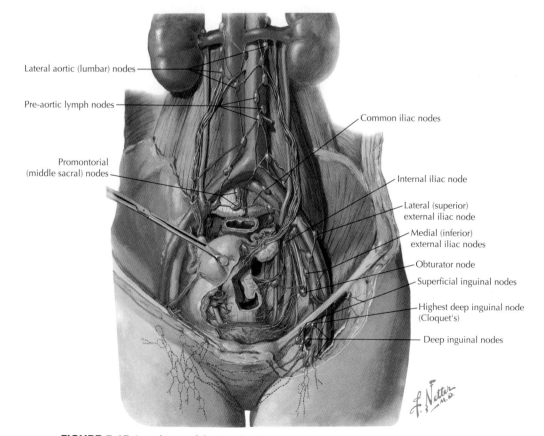

FIGURE 5-15 Lymphatics of the Female Pelvis. (From *Atlas of human anatomy*, ed 6, Plate 384.)

physicians must be aware that uterine cancer could spread to these nodes as well as the external iliac nodes.

7. INNERVATION

The skin and skeletal muscle of the pelvis are innervated by the somatic division of the peripheral nervous system. The muscle innervation is reviewed in Table 5-2 and is derived from the ventral rami of the **sacral** (L4-S4) and **coccygeal plexus**. Although most of the sacral plexus is involved in innervation of the gluteal muscles and muscles of the lower limb, several small twigs innervate the pelvic musculature (nerve to the obturator internus and nerves to the pelvic diaphragm) and the perineum, which is supplied by the **pudendal nerve** (S2-S4). **Somatic afferent fibers** convey pain, touch, and temperature from the skin, skeletal muscle, and joints via nerves from these plexuses to the same relative spinal cord levels.

The smooth muscle and glands of the pelvis are innervated by the autonomic division of the peripheral nervous system via the **pelvic splanchnics** (S2-S4; parasympathetic) and the **lumbar and sacral splanchnics** (L1-L2; sympathetic) (Fig. 5-16 and Table 5-8).

The **parasympathetic efferent fibers** generally do the following:

- Vasodilate.
- Contract the bladder's detrusor smooth muscle.
- Stimulate engorgement of the erectile tissues.
- Modulate the enteric nervous system's control of the distal bowel (from splenic flexure to rectum).
- Inhibit contraction of both the male internal urethral sphincter for urination and the internal anal sphincter for defecation in both genders.

The **sympathetic efferent fibers** generally do the following:

- Vasoconstrict and/or maintain vasomotor tone.
- Increase secretion from sweat glands.
- Contract the male internal urethral sphincter and the internal anal sphincters in both genders.

TABLE 5-8 Summary of Pelvic Nerves

NERVE	INNERVATION
Lumbar splanchnics	From L1 to L2 or L3: sympathetics to hypogastric plexus (superior and inferior) to innervate hindgut derivatives and pelvic reproductive viscera
Sacral splanchnics	From L1 to L2 or L3: sympathetics to inferior hypogastric plexus that first travel down sympathetic chain before synapsing in plexus
Pelvic splanchnics	From S2 to S4: parasympathetics to inferior hypogastric plexus to innervate hindgut derivatives and pelvic reproductive viscera
Inferior hypogastric plexus	Plexus of nerves (splanchnics) and ganglia where sympathetic and parasympathetic preganglionic fibers synapse
Pudendal nerve	From S2 to S4: somatic nerve that innervates skin and skeletal muscle of pelvic diaphragm and perineum (from sacral plexus)

- Through smooth muscle contraction, move the sperm along the male reproductive tract and stimulate secretion from the seminal vesicles and prostate.
- Stimulate secretion from the greater vestibular (Bartholin's) glands in females and the bulbo-urethral (Cowper's) glands in males, along with minor lubricating glands associated with the reproductive tract in both genders.

Visceral afferent fibers convey pelvic sensory information (largely pain) via both the sympathetic fibers (to the upper lumbar spinal cord [L1-L2] or lower thoracic levels [T11-T12]) and parasympathetic fibers (to the S2-S4 levels of the spinal cord).

8. FEMALE PERINEUM

The perineum is a diamond-shaped region between the thighs and is divided descriptively into an anterior **urogenital triangle** and a posterior **anal triangle** (Fig. 5-17). The boundaries of the perineum include the following:

- Pubic symphysis anteriorly
- Ischial tuberosities laterally (lateral margins are demarcated by the ischiopubic rami anteriorly and the sacrotuberous ligaments posteriorly; see Fig. 5-3.)

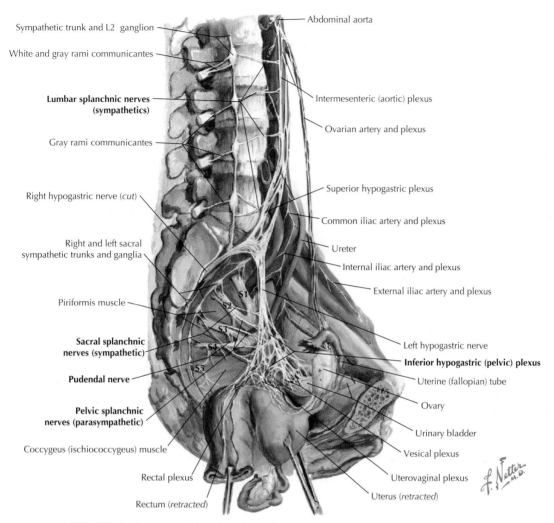

Sympathetic trunk and L2 ganglion
White and gray rami communicantes
Lumbar splanchnic nerves (sympathetics)
Gray rami communicantes
Right hypogastric nerve (*cut*)
Right and left sacral sympathetic trunks and ganglia
Piriformis muscle
Sacral splanchnic nerves (sympathetic)
Pudendal nerve
Pelvic splanchnic nerves (parasympathetic)
Coccygeus (ischiococcygeus) muscle
Rectal plexus
Rectum (*retracted*)

Abdominal aorta
Intermesenteric (aortic) plexus
Ovarian artery and plexus
Superior hypogastric plexus
Common iliac artery and plexus
Ureter
Internal iliac artery and plexus
External iliac artery and plexus
Left hypogastric nerve
Inferior hypogastric (pelvic) plexus
Uterine (fallopian) tube
Ovary
Urinary bladder
Vesical plexus
Uterovaginal plexus
Uterus (*retracted*)

S1 S2 S3 S4 S5

FIGURE 5-16 Nerves of the Pelvic Cavity. (From *Atlas of human anatomy*, ed 6, Plate 390.)

Regions (triangles) of perineum: surface topography

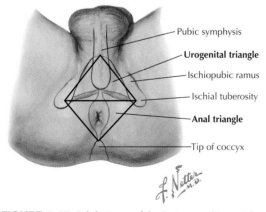

Pubic symphysis
Urogenital triangle
Ischiopubic ramus
Ischial tuberosity
Anal triangle
Tip of coccyx

FIGURE 5-17 Subdivisions of the Perineum. (From *Atlas of human anatomy*, ed 6, Plate 358.)

- Coccyx posteriorly
- Roof formed largely by levator ani muscle

Anal Triangle (Both Genders)

The key feature of the anal triangle is the anal opening and the **external anal sphincter,** which has the following attachments (Fig. 5-18):

- Subcutaneous part: just beneath the skin
- Superficial part: attaches to the perineal body and coccyx
- Deep part: surrounds the anal canal

Similar to the skin and all the skeletal muscles of the perineum, the external anal sphincter is innervated by the **pudendal nerve** (S2-S4) (inferior rectal branches; see Fig. 5-23) from the sacral

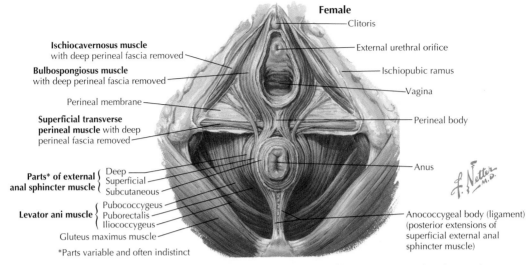

Female

- Clitoris
- Ischiocavernosus muscle with deep perineal fascia removed
- Bulbospongiosus muscle with deep perineal fascia removed
- Perineal membrane
- Superficial transverse perineal muscle with deep perineal fascia removed
- External urethral orifice
- Ischiopubic ramus
- Vagina
- Perineal body
- Parts* of external anal sphincter muscle { Deep, Superficial, Subcutaneous
- Levator ani muscle { Pubococcygeus, Puborectalis, Iliococcygeus
- Gluteus maximus muscle
- Anus
- Anococcygeal body (ligament) (posterior extensions of superficial external anal sphincter muscle)

*Parts variable and often indistinct

FIGURE 5-18 Muscles of the Female Perineum. (From *Atlas of human anatomy,* ed 6, Plate 373.)

plexus and supplied by the **internal pudendal artery** (rectal branches), a branch of the internal iliac artery in the pelvis (see Figs. 5-13 and 5-14). The venous drainage of the lower rectum and anal canal provides an important portosystemic anastomosis between the superior rectal vein (portal system) and the median sacral vein and middle and inferior rectal branches (caval system) (Fig. 5-19 and Table 5-9).

The anal canal and external anal sphincter are flanked on either side by a wedge-shaped fat-filled space called the **ischio-anal** (ischiorectal) **fossa** (Fig. 5-20). This space allows for the expansion of the anal canal during defecation and accommodates the fetus during childbirth. The ischio-anal fossa can become infected (e.g., glandular, abrasive lesions, boils), and because the two fossae communicate posterior to the anal canal, the infection can easily spread from side to side or, in extreme cases, burst through the levator ani and infect the pelvis.

Urogenital Triangle

The urogenital triangle is divided into a **superficial pouch,** containing the external genitalia and associated skeletal muscles, and a **deep pouch,** largely occupied by the urethrovaginalis–skeletal muscle sphincter complex surrounding the urethra and vaginal apertures. Superior to the deep pouch lies the levator ani muscle, with an intervening anterior extension of the ischio-anal fossae (fat) separating the deep pouch and muscle.

TABLE 5-9 Rectal Portosystemic Anastomoses

VEIN	COURSE AND STRUCTURES DRAINED
Superior rectal	Tributary of inferior mesenteric vein (portal system)
Middle rectal	Drains into internal iliac, vesical, or uterine (female) veins, draining pelvic diaphragm, rectum, and proximal anal canal
Inferior rectal	Drains into internal pudendal vein from external anal sphincter
Median sacral	Drains into the common iliac vein from the sacrum, coccyx and rectum

The female external genitalia (vulva) are shown in Figure 5-21 and summarized in Table 5-10.

The **perineal body** (central tendon of the perineum) is an important fibromuscular support region lying just beneath the skin midway between the two ischial tuberosities and an important attachment point for the perineal muscles, especially the urethrovaginalis complex in women, and the levator ani superiorly (see Fig. 5-21).

The deep perineal pouch contains the following (Fig. 5-22):

- **Urethra:** extends from the bladder, runs through the deep pouch, and opens into the vestibule.
- **Vagina:** distal portion passes through the deep pouch and opens into the vestibule.

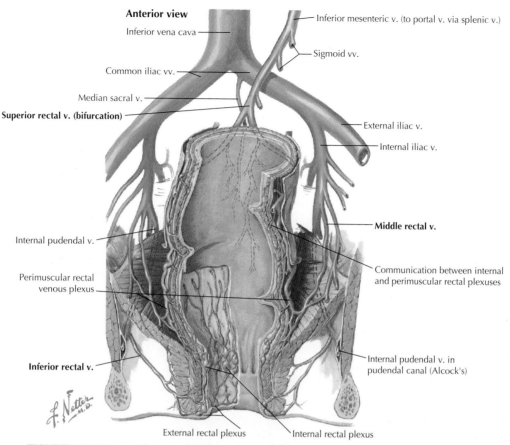

Anterior view
Inferior vena cava
Inferior mesenteric v. (to portal v. via splenic v.)
Sigmoid vv.
Common iliac vv.
Median sacral v.
Superior rectal v. (bifurcation)
External iliac v.
Internal iliac v.
Internal pudendal v.
Middle rectal v.
Perimuscular rectal venous plexus
Communication between internal and perimuscular rectal plexuses
Inferior rectal v.
Internal pudendal v. in pudendal canal (Alcock's)
External rectal plexus
Internal rectal plexus

FIGURE 5-19 Veins of the Rectum and Anal Canal. (From *Atlas of human anatomy,* ed 6, Plate 377.)

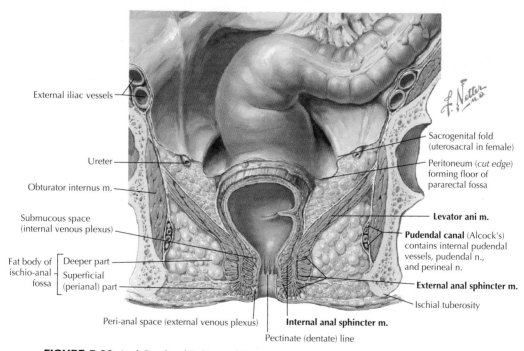

External iliac vessels
Sacrogenital fold (uterosacral in female)
Ureter
Peritoneum (*cut edge*) forming floor of pararectal fossa
Obturator internus m.
Levator ani m.
Submucous space (internal venous plexus)
Pudendal canal (Alcock's) contains internal pudendal vessels, pudendal n., and perineal n.
Fat body of ischio-anal fossa — Deeper part
Superficial (perianal) part
External anal sphincter m.
Ischial tuberosity
Peri-anal space (external venous plexus)
Internal anal sphincter m.
Pectinate (dentate) line

FIGURE 5-20 Anal Canal and Ischio-anal Fossae. (From *Atlas of human anatomy,* ed 6, Plate 370.)

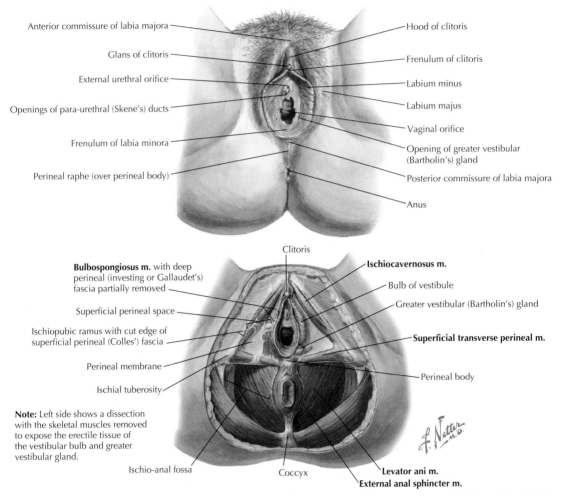

FIGURE 5-21 Female Perineum and Superficial Perineal Pouch. (From *Atlas of human anatomy*, ed 6, Plates 354 and 356.)

TABLE 5-10 Features of the Female External Genitalia

STRUCTURE	CHARACTERISTICS
Mons pubis	Anterior fatty eminence overlying pubic symphysis
Anterior labial commissure	Site where two labia majora meet anteriorly
Labia majora	Folds of pigmented skin, mainly fat and sebaceous glands; in the adult, covered with pubic hair externally but smooth and pink on internal aspect
Clitoris	Erectile tissue, distinguished by midline glans covered with prepuce (foreskin), body, and two crura (corpora cavernosa) that extend along ischiopubic rami, and covered by ischiocavernosus muscles
Labia minora	Fat-free hairless pink skin folds that contain some erectile tissue; course anteriorly to form frenulum and prepuce of clitoris; posteriorly, unite to form frenulum of labia minora (fourchette)
Vestibule	Space surrounded by labia minora that contains openings of urethra, vagina, and vestibular glands
Greater vestibular glands	Paired mucous glands lying posterior to bulbs of vestibule that produce secretions during arousal
Bulbs of vestibule	Paired erectile tissues lying deep and lateral to labia minora that flank vaginal and urethral openings and extend anteriorly to form small connection to glans of clitoris; covered by bulbospongiosus skeletal muscle
Posterior labial commissure	Site where two labia majora meet posteriorly; overlies perineal body

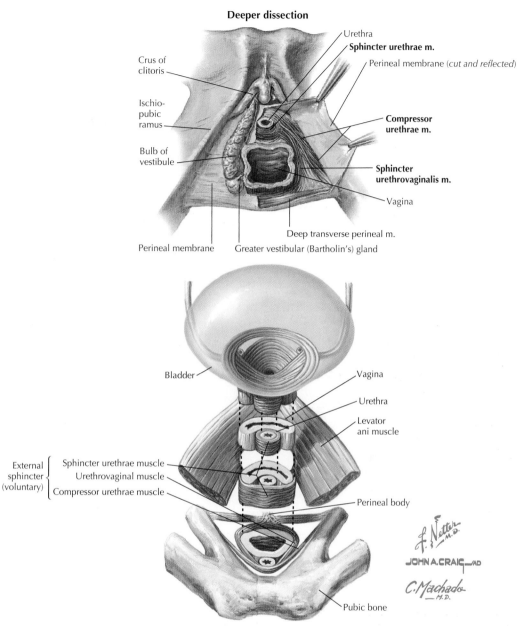

FIGURE 5-22 Female Perineum and Urethrovaginalis Sphincter Complex. (From *Atlas of human anatomy,* ed 6, Plates 347 and 356.)

- **External urethral sphincter:** skeletal muscle sphincter
- **Compressor urethrae:** two thin skeletal muscle bands that extend from the ischiopubic rami and fuse in the midline around the anterior aspect of the urethra.
- **Sphincter urethrovaginalis muscle:** extends from the perineal body around the lateral sides of the vagina and fuses in the midline around the anterior aspect of the urethra.

- **Deep transversus perineal muscles:** extend from the ischial tuberosities and rami to the perineal body; stabilize the perineal body.

These structures, along with their respective neurovascular bundles, lie between the **perineal membrane** (thick fascial sheath) and the fascia covering the inferior aspect of the levator ani muscle. The neurovascular components include the following (Fig. 5-23):

- **Pudendal nerve:** passes out the greater sciatic foramen around the sacrospinous ligament and into the lesser sciatic foramen to enter the **pudendal (Alcock's) canal;** represents the somatic innervation (S2-S4) of the skin and skeletal muscles of the perineum; includes the inferior rectal (anal), perineal, labial, and dorsal clitoral branches.
- **Internal pudendal artery:** arises from the internal iliac artery, passes out the greater sciatic foramen around the sacrospinous ligament and into the lesser sciatic foramen to enter the pudendal (Alcock's) canal, and distributes to the perineum as the inferior rectal, perineal, labial, artery of the bulb, and dorsal clitoral branches.

9. MALE PERINEUM

The boundaries of the perineum and the anal triangle in both genders are discussed in the previous section; this section focuses on the male urogenital triangle. The urogenital triangle is divided into a **superficial pouch** containing the external genitalia and associated skeletal muscles and a **deep pouch** largely occupied by the external urethral sphincter surrounding the membranous urethra.

The male external genitalia are shown in Figure 5-24 and summarized in Table 5-11.

The bulb and crura form the root of the penis, whereas the **corpus spongiosum** and the two **corpora cavernosa** compose the shaft of the

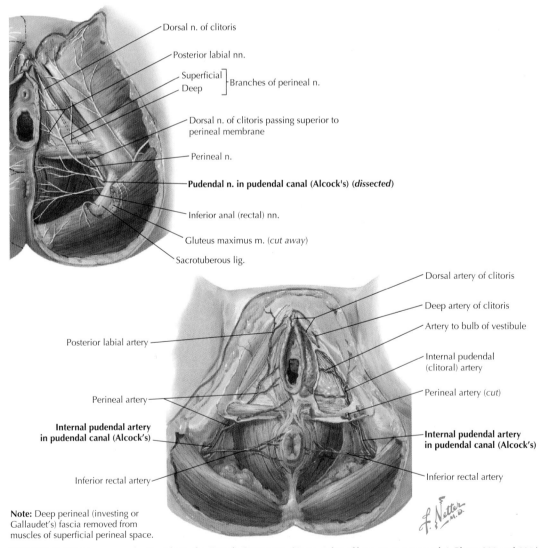

Dorsal n. of clitoris

Posterior labial nn.

Superficial ⎤
Deep ⎦ Branches of perineal n.

Dorsal n. of clitoris passing superior to perineal membrane

Perineal n.

Pudendal n. in pudendal canal (Alcock's) (*dissected*)

Inferior anal (rectal) nn.

Gluteus maximus m. (*cut away*)

Sacrotuberous lig.

Dorsal artery of clitoris

Deep artery of clitoris

Artery to bulb of vestibule

Posterior labial artery

Internal pudendal (clitoral) artery

Perineal artery (*cut*)

Perineal artery

Internal pudendal artery in pudendal canal (Alcock's)

Internal pudendal artery in pudendal canal (Alcock's)

Inferior rectal artery

Inferior rectal artery

Note: Deep perineal (investing or Gallaudet's) fascia removed from muscles of superficial perineal space.

FIGURE 5-23 Neurovascular Supply to the Female Perineum. (From *Atlas of human anatomy,* ed 6, Plates 382 and 391.)

Hemorrhoids

Hemorrhoids are symptomatic varicose dilations of submucosal veins that protrude into the anal canal and can extend through the anal opening (external hemorrhoid). Hemorrhoids can bleed, causing the blood to pool and clot, yielding a "thrombosed" hemorrhoid.

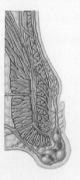

Origin below dentate line
(external plexus)

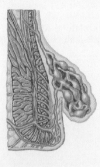

Origin above dentate line
(internal plexus)

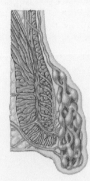

Origin above and below dentate line
(internal and external plexus)

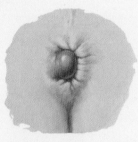

Thrombosed external hemorrhoid

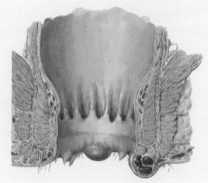

External hemorrhoids and skin tabs

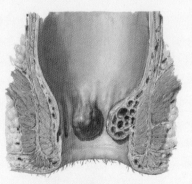

Internal hemorrhoids

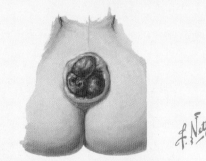

Prolapsed "rosette" of internal hemorrhoids

Characteristic	Description
Types	Internal: dilations of veins of internal rectal plexus; External: dilations of veins of external rectal plexus Mixed: combination of internal and external
Prevalence	50–80% of all Americans; more common after pregnancy
Signs and symptoms	Perianal swelling, itching, pain, rectal bleeding, constipation, hematochezia, inflammation
Risk factors	Pregnancy, obesity, chronic cough, constipation, heavy lifting, sedentary work or lifestyle, hepatic disease, colon malignancy, portal hypertension, anal intercourse

Clinical Focus 5-20

Episiotomy

Occasionally, if there is danger of tearing of the perineal body during childbirth, the physician may perform an incision called an episiotomy to enlarge the vaginal opening to accommodate the head of the fetus. The incision is easier to repair and heals better than a tear. Episiotomies usually are either directly in the midline through the perineal body or posterolateral, to avoid the perineal body.

Posterolateral Approach
(one of two approaches normally used, posterolateral (shown here) or median)

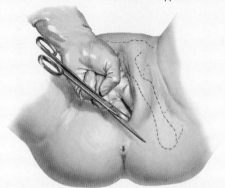

A. Scissors are directed from the midline to the tuberosity

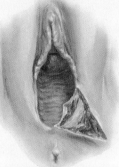

B. Incision in the bulbospongiosus muscle

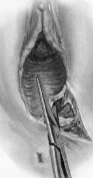

C. Division of the vaginal mucosa

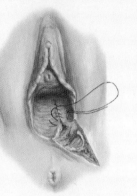

D. Continuous suture of vaginal mucosa

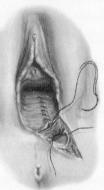

E. Inverted crown suture in perineal body

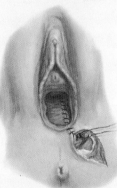

F. Running suture under hymen and continued in skin after approximation of perineal body

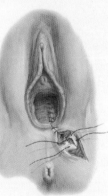

G. Closure of bulbospongiosus and fascia

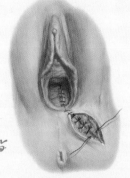

H. Closure of superficial tissues of perineum

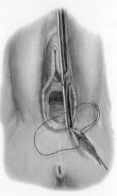

I. Subcuticular stitch in superficial fascia approximating the skin

Sexually Transmitted Diseases

Human papillomavirus (HPV) and *Chlamydia trachomatis* infections are the two most common STDs in the United States. HPV infections (>90% benign) are characterized in both genders by warty lesions caused most often by serotypes 6 and 11. The virus is typically spread by skin-to-skin contact; the incubation period is 3 weeks to 8 months. HPV is highly associated with cervical cancer in women. Chlamydial infection is the most common bacterial STD, with antibodies present in up to 40% of all sexually active women (which suggests prior infection). Infected structures include the urethra, cervix, greater vestibular glands, and uterine tubes in females and the urethra, epididymis, and prostate in males.

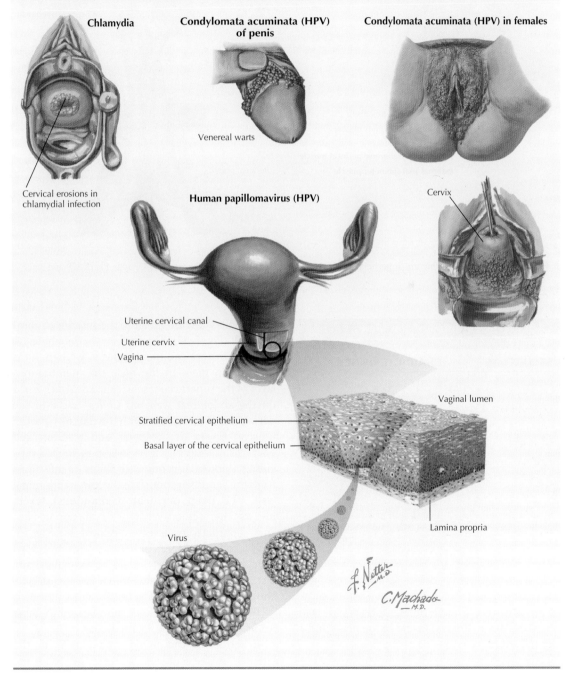

Chlamydia

Condylomata acuminata (HPV) of penis

Condylomata acuminata (HPV) in females

Venereal warts

Cervical erosions in chlamydial infection

Human papillomavirus (HPV)

Cervix

Uterine cervical canal

Uterine cervix

Vagina

Vaginal lumen

Stratified cervical epithelium

Basal layer of the cervical epithelium

Lamina propria

Virus

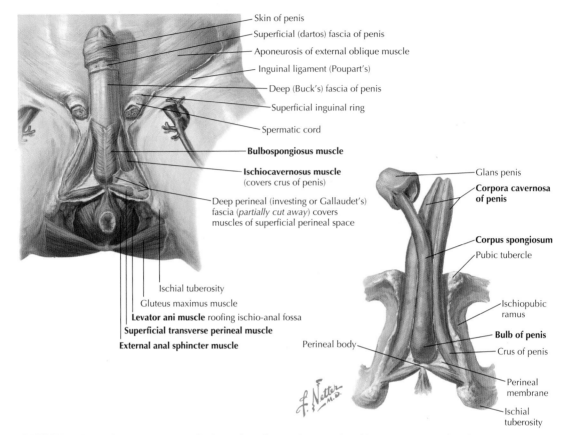

FIGURE 5-24 Male Perineum, Superficial Pouch, and Penis. (From *Atlas of human anatomy*, ed 6, Plates 359 and 360.)

TABLE 5-11 Features of the Male External Genitalia	
STRUCTURE	**CHARACTERISTICS**
Bulb of penis	Erectile tissue anchored to perineal membrane; proximal part of corpus spongiosum; covered by bulbospongiosus skeletal muscle
Crura of penis	Paired erectile tissues attached to pubic arch that form proximal part of corpora cavernosa of penis; covered by ischiocavernosus skeletal muscles
Superficial transverse perineal muscle	Thin skeletal muscle extending from ischial tuberosity to perineal body; stabilizes perineal body

penis. They are bound tightly together by the **investing deep (Buck's) fascia** of the penis and a **superficial (dartos) fascia** of the penis.

The superficial fascia (subcutaneous tissue) of the perineum includes a fatty and membranous layer (Colles' fascia) similar to the anterior abdominal wall (Fig. 5-25). The fatty layer contributes to the labia majora and mons pubis in women but is minimal in men. In the male the membranous layer of the superficial fascia (called *Scarpa's fascia* on the abdominal wall but *Colles' fascia* in the perineum) is continuous with the **dartos** (smooth muscle) **fascia** of the penis and scrotum and envelops the superficial perineal pouch, thus providing a potential conduit for fluids or infections from the superficial pouch to the lower abdominal wall. The **deep perineal (Gallaudet's) fascia** invests the ischiocavernosus, bulbospongiosus, and superficial transverse perineal muscles in both genders and is continuous with the deep (Buck's) fascia of the penis and the deep investing fascia of the external abdominal oblique muscle and rectus sheath (see Fig. 5-24).

Features of the penis are summarized in Table 5-12 and illustrated in Figure 5-26.

Erection of the penis (and clitoris in the female) and ejaculation involve the following sequence of events:

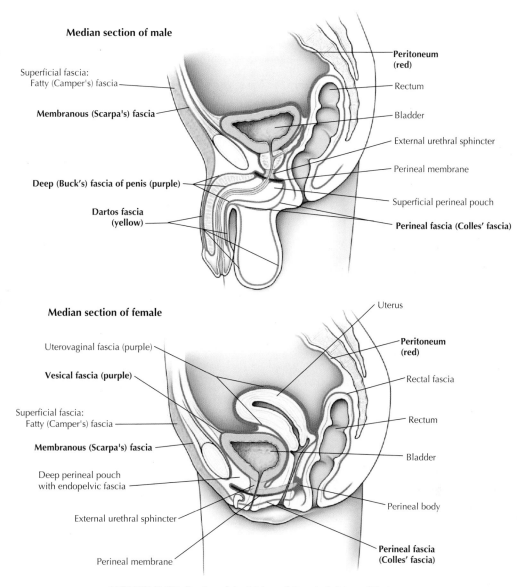

Median section of male

Superficial fascia:
Fatty (Camper's) fascia

Membranous (Scarpa's) fascia

Deep (Buck's) fascia of penis (purple)

**Dartos fascia
(yellow)**

Peritoneum
(red)

Rectum

Bladder

External urethral sphincter

Perineal membrane

Superficial perineal pouch

Perineal fascia (Colles' fascia)

Median section of female

Uterovaginal fascia (purple)

Vesical fascia (purple)

Superficial fascia:
Fatty (Camper's) fascia

Membranous (Scarpa's) fascia

Deep perineal pouch
with endopelvic fascia

External urethral sphincter

Perineal membrane

Uterus

**Peritoneum
(red)**

Rectal fascia

Rectum

Bladder

Perineal body

**Perineal fascia
(Colles' fascia)**

FIGURE 5-25 Fasciae of the Male and Female Pelvis and Perineum.

1. Friction and sexual stimulation evoke the excitation of parasympathetic fibers (pelvic splanchnics S2-S4), which leads to relaxation of the cavernous vessels and engorgement of the erectile tissue with blood.
2. Sympathetic fibers then initiate contraction of the smooth muscle of the epididymal ducts, ductus deferens, seminal vesicles, and prostate, in that order.
3. Sperm and the seminal and prostatic secretions enter the prostatic urethra and combine with secretions of the bulbo-urethral and penile urethral glands (semen). (The seminal vesicles

provide 70% of the seminal fluid volume and produce a viscous alkaline fluid that nourishes and protects the sperm from the acidic environment of the vaginal tract.)
4. Under sympathetic stimulation (L1-L2), the internal urethral sphincter contracts to prevent ejaculation into the urinary bladder. Through rhythmic contractions of the bulbospongiosus muscle and somatic stimulation from the pudendal nerve, the semen moves along the spongy urethra with help from parasympathetic stimulation of urethral smooth muscle and is ejaculated (orgasm).

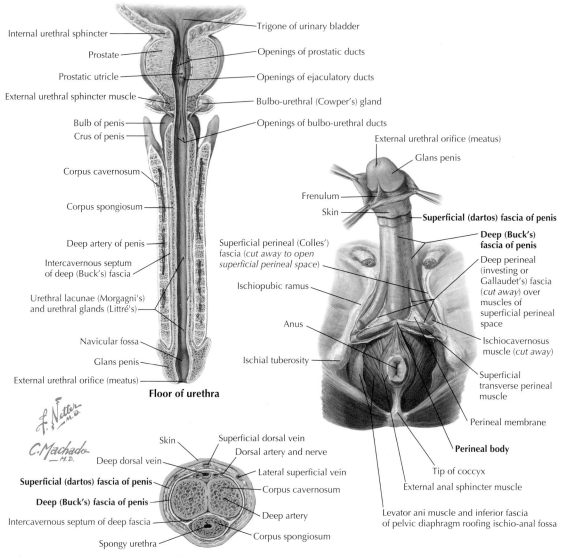

Floor of urethra

Section through body of penis

FIGURE 5-26 Penis and Urethra. (From *Atlas of human anatomy*, ed 6, Plates 359, 360, and 363.)

TABLE 5-12 Features of the Penis			
STRUCTURE	**CHARACTERISTICS**	**STRUCTURE**	**CHARACTERISTICS**
Root of penis	Composed of bulb (proximal part of corpus spongiosum) and two crura (proximal part of corpora cavernosa)	Prepuce (foreskin)	Thin, double layer of skin that extends over most of glans penis*
Body of penis	Covered by skin, dartos fascia, and deep (Buck's) fascia of penis, which envelops the corpora cavernosa and corpus spongiosum, which contains spongy urethra	Suspensory ligament	Deep fascia that extends from dorsum of penis to pubic symphysis
		Fundiform ligament	Subcutaneous tissue that extends from dartos fascia superiorly to midline linea alba (see Fig. 5-9)
Glans penis	Expanded distal end of corpus spongiosum where spongy urethra expands (navicular fossa) and opens externally (external urethral meatus)		

*Male circumcision removes foreskin to expose glans.

Urethral Trauma in the Male

Although rare, direct trauma to the corpora cavernosa can occur. Rupture of the thick tunica albuginea usually involves the deep fascia of the penis (Buck's fascia), and blood can extravasate quickly, causing penile swelling. Urethral rupture is more common and involves one of three mechanisms:

- External trauma or a penetrating injury
- Internal injury (caused by a catheter, instrument, or foreign body)
- Spontaneous rupture (caused by increased intraurethral pressure or periurethral inflammation)

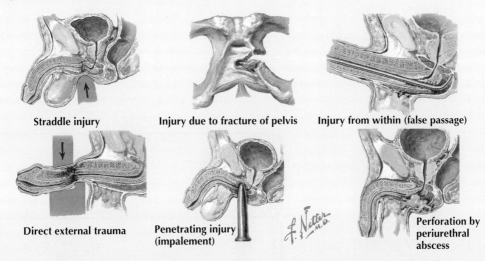

Straddle injury **Injury due to fracture of pelvis** **Injury from within (false passage)**

Direct external trauma **Penetrating injury (impalement)** **Perforation by periurethral abscess**

Urine Extravasation in the Male

Rupture of the male urethra can lead to urine extravasation into various pelvic or perineal spaces that are largely limited by the fascial planes.

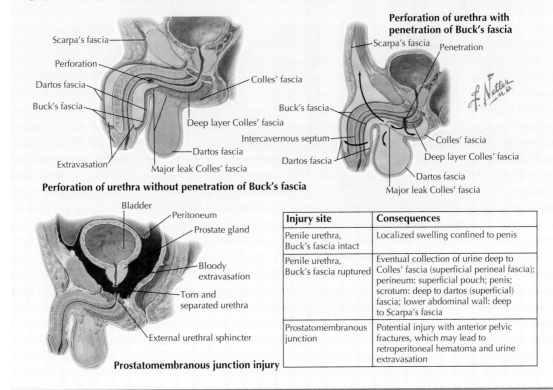

Perforation of urethra without penetration of Buck's fascia

- Scarpa's fascia
- Perforation
- Dartos fascia
- Buck's fascia
- Colles' fascia
- Deep layer Colles' fascia
- Extravasation
- Dartos fascia
- Major leak Colles' fascia

Perforation of urethra with penetration of Buck's fascia

- Scarpa's fascia
- Penetration
- Buck's fascia
- Intercavernous septum
- Dartos fascia
- Colles' fascia
- Deep layer Colles' fascia
- Dartos fascia
- Major leak Colles' fascia

Prostatomembranous junction injury

- Bladder
- Peritoneum
- Prostate gland
- Bloody extravasation
- Torn and separated urethra
- External urethral sphincter

Injury site	Consequences
Penile urethra, Buck's fascia intact	Localized swelling confined to penis
Penile urethra, Buck's fascia ruptured	Eventual collection of urine deep to Colles' fascia (superficial perineal fascia); perineum: superficial pouch; penis; scrotum: deep to dartos (superficial) fascia; lower abdominal wall: deep to Scarpa's fascia
Prostatomembranous junction	Potential injury with anterior pelvic fractures, which may lead to retroperitoneal hematoma and urine extravasation

Erectile Dysfunction

Erectile dysfunction (ED) is an inability to achieve and maintain penile erection sufficient for sexual intercourse. Its occurrence increases with age, and some of the probable causes are illustrated. Normal erectile function occurs when a sexual stimulus causes the release of nitric oxide from nerve endings and endothelial cells of the corpora cavernosa, thus relaxing the smooth muscle tone of the vessels and increasing blood flow into the erectile tissues. As the erectile tissue becomes engorged with blood, it compresses the veins in the tunica albuginea so that the blood remains in the cavernous bodies. The available drugs to treat ED aid in relaxing the smooth muscle of the blood vessels of the erectile tissues. Erectile dysfunction can also occur from damage to the nerves innervating the perineum (e.g., a complication of prostatic surgery). Afferent impulses conveying stimulation/arousal sensations are conveyed by the pudendal nerve (S2-S4, somatic fibers), whereas the autonomic efferent innervation of the cavernous vasculature is via the pelvic splanchnics (S2-S4, parasympathetic fibers).

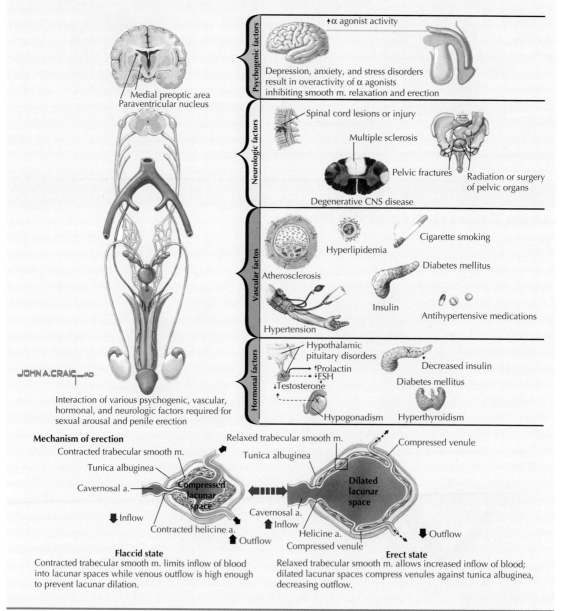

Psychogenic factors

↑α agonist activity

Depression, anxiety, and stress disorders result in overactivity of α agonists inhibiting smooth m. relaxation and erection

Neurologic factors

Spinal cord lesions or injury

Multiple sclerosis

Pelvic fractures

Radiation or surgery of pelvic organs

Degenerative CNS disease

Vascular factors

Hyperlipidemia

Cigarette smoking

Atherosclerosis

Diabetes mellitus

Insulin

Antihypertensive medications

Hypertension

Hormonal factors

Hypothalamic pituitary disorders

↑Prolactin
↓FSH
↓Testosterone

Decreased insulin

Diabetes mellitus

Hypogonadism   Hyperthyroidism

Medial preoptic area
Paraventricular nucleus

JOHN A.CRAIG—AD

Interaction of various psychogenic, vascular, hormonal, and neurologic factors required for sexual arousal and penile erection

Mechanism of erection

Contracted trabecular smooth m.

Tunica albuginea

Cavernosal a.

Compressed lacunar space

↓Inflow

Contracted helicine a.

↑Outflow

Relaxed trabecular smooth m.

Tunica albuginea

Compressed venule

Dilated lacunar space

Cavernosal a.

↑Inflow

Helicine a.

Compressed venule

↓Outflow

Flaccid state
Contracted trabecular smooth m. limits inflow of blood into lacunar spaces while venous outflow is high enough to prevent lacunar dilation.

Erect state
Relaxed trabecular smooth m. allows increased inflow of blood; dilated lacunar spaces compress venules against tunica albuginea, decreasing outflow.

The deep perineal space in males includes the following (Fig. 5-27):

- **Membranous urethra:** a continuation of the prostatic urethra.
- **Deep transversus perineal muscles:** extend from the ischial tuberosities and rami to the perineal body; stabilize the perineal body.
- **Bulbo-urethral glands:** their ducts pass from the deep pouch to enter the proximal part of the spongy urethra; provide a mucus-like secretion that lubricates the spongy urethra.
- **External urethral sphincter:** skeletal muscle that encircles the membranous urethra, is under voluntary control (via the pudendal nerve), and extends superiorly

over the anterior aspect of the prostate gland but does not possess sphincter action on the gland.

These structures, along with their respective neurovascular bundles, lie between the **perineal membrane** (thick fascial sheath) and the fascia covering the inferior aspect of the levator ani muscle. The neurovascular components include the following:

- **Pudendal nerve:** passes out the greater sciatic foramen with the internal pudendal vessels, around the sacrospinous ligament, and into the lesser sciatic foramen to enter the **pudendal (Alcock's) canal;** provides the somatic innervation (S2-S4) of the skin and skeletal muscles of the perineum and

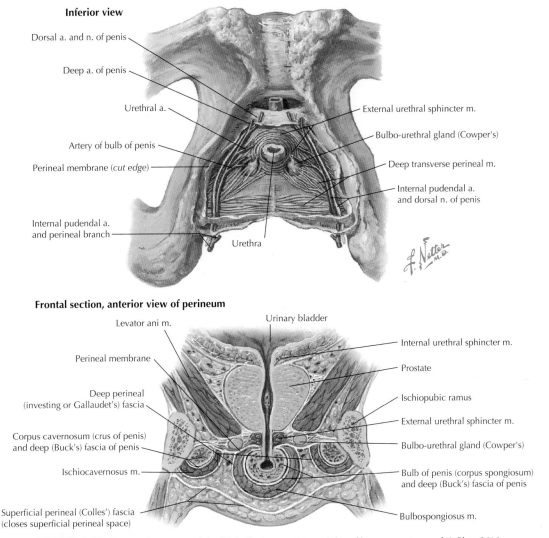

Inferior view

Dorsal a. and n. of penis

Deep a. of penis

Urethral a.

Artery of bulb of penis

Perineal membrane (*cut edge*)

Internal pudendal a. and perineal branch

External urethral sphincter m.

Bulbo-urethral gland (Cowper's)

Deep transverse perineal m.

Internal pudendal a. and dorsal n. of penis

Urethra

Frontal section, anterior view of perineum

Levator ani m.

Urinary bladder

Perineal membrane

Deep perineal (investing or Gallaudet's) fascia

Corpus cavernosum (crus of penis) and deep (Buck's) fascia of penis

Ischiocavernosus m.

Superficial perineal (Colles') fascia (closes superficial perineal space)

Internal urethral sphincter m.

Prostate

Ischiopubic ramus

External urethral sphincter m.

Bulbo-urethral gland (Cowper's)

Bulb of penis (corpus spongiosum) and deep (Buck's) fascia of penis

Bulbospongiosus m.

FIGURE 5-27 Deeper Structures of the Male Perineum. (From *Atlas of human anatomy*, ed 6, Plate 361.)

includes the inferior rectal (anal), perineal, scrotal, and dorsal nerves of the penis.

- **Internal pudendal artery:** arises from the internal iliac artery; passes out the greater sciatic foramen with the pudendal nerve, around the sacrospinous ligament, and into the lesser sciatic foramen to enter the pudendal (Alcock's) canal and distribute to the perineum as the inferior rectal, perineal, scrotal, and dorsal arteries of the penis as well as the artery of the bulb.

10. EMBRYOLOGY

Development of the Reproductive Organs

The reproductive systems of the female and male develop from undifferentiated primordia and follow the sexual differentiation of each gender based on the genetic makeup of the embryo (XX for females and XY for males). In females, mesonephric ducts degenerate while the **paramesonephric ducts** develop into the uterine tubes,

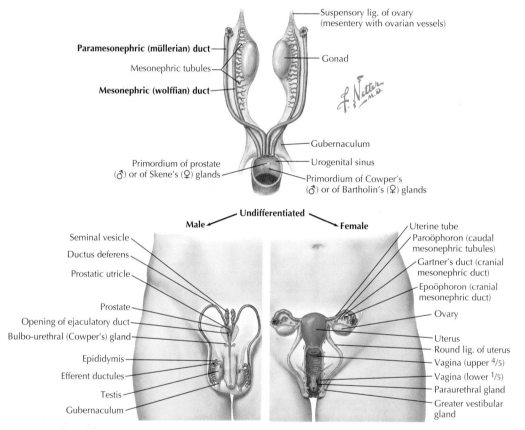

FIGURE 5-28 Derivation of the Reproductive Organs. (From *Atlas of human anatomy*, ed 6, Plate 344.)

TABLE 5-13 Derivatives of the Urogenital System

MALE	FEMALE	MALE	FEMALE
From Urogenital Sinus		**From Mesonephric Duct and Tubules**	
Urinary bladder	Urinary bladder	Efferent ductules	Degenerates
Urethra (except navicular fossa)	Urethra	Duct of epididymis	(Ureter, renal pelvis,
		Ductus deferens	calices, and collecting
Prostatic utricle	Lower vagina	Ejaculatory duct	tubules in both genders)
Prostate	Urethral and paraurethral glands	Seminal vesicles	
		From Paramesonephric Duct	
Bulbo-urethral glands	Greater vestibular glands	Degenerates	Uterine tubes, uterus, upper vagina

uterus, and upper portion of the vagina (Fig. 5-28 and Table 5-13). In males the **mesonephric ducts** persist and become the ductus deferens, ejaculatory ducts, and seminal vesicles.

Development of the External Genitalia

The female and male external genitalia develop from the **genital tubercle** (the phallic structures), paired **urogenital folds**, and **labioscrotal folds** (Fig. 5-29 and Table 5-14). Initially these tissues are undifferentiated, but after 10 weeks recognizable external genital features associated with each sex begin to form.

TABLE 5-14 Homologues of the External Genitalia

MALE	FEMALE
From Genital Tubercle/Phallus	
Penis	Clitoris
Glans penis	Glans clitoridis
Corpora cavernosum penis	Corpora cavernosa clitoridis
Corpus spongiosum penis	Bulb of vestibule
From Urogenital Folds	
Ventral raphe of penis	Labia minora
Most of the penile urethra	
Perineal raphe	Perineal raphe
Perianal tissue (and external sphincter)	Perianal tissue (and external anal sphincter)
From Labioscrotal Folds	
Scrotum	Labia majora
From Gubernaculum	
Gubernaculum testis	Ovarian ligament
	Round ligament of uterus

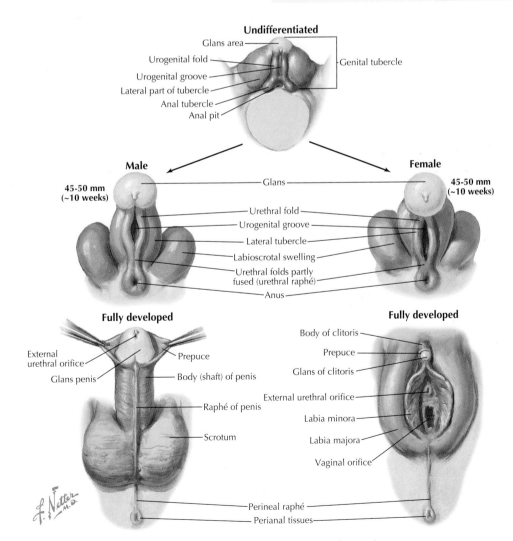

FIGURE 5-29 Development of the External Genitalia.

Clinical Focus 5-25

Hypospadias and Epispadias

Hypospadias and epispadias are congenital anomalies of the penis. *Hypospadias* is much more common (1 in 300 male births) and is characterized by failure of fusion of the urogenital folds, which normally seal the penile (spongy) urethra within the penis. The defect occurs on the ventral aspect of the penis (corpus spongiosum). Hypospadias may be associated with inguinal hernias and undescended testes. Epispadias is rare (1 in 30,000 male births) and is characterized by a urethral orifice on the dorsal aspect of the penis.

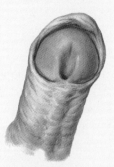

Glanular hypospadias

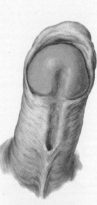

Penile hypospadias

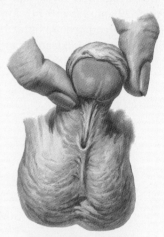

Penoscrotal hypospadias
(with chordee)

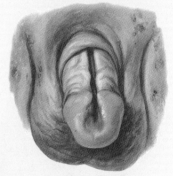

Scrotal hypospadias
(bifid scrotum, chordee)

Complete epispadias

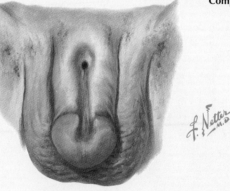

Penile epispadias

Clinical Focus 5-26

Uterine Anomalies

Incomplete fusion of the distal paramesonephric (müllerian) ducts can lead to septation of the uterus or partial or complete duplication of the uterus (bicornuate uterus). The prevalence is up to 3% for *septate* uterine anomalies but only about 0.1% for *bicornuate* anomalies. If only one paramesonephric duct persists and develops, a *unicornuate* uterus results. These conditions seem to be transmitted by a polygenic or multifactorial pattern and carry a higher risk for recurrent spontaneous abortions (15-25%), premature labor, uterine pain, breech or transverse deliveries, and dysmenorrhea.

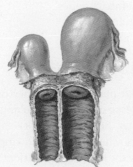
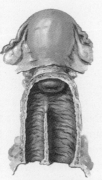
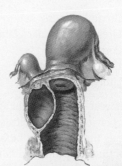

Complete septum
(with double uterus and double vagina)

Partial septum

Rudimentary second vagina
(without external opening, forming cyst)

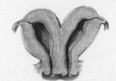
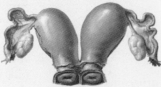
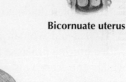

Bicornuate uterus with complete septum
(double cervix)

Double uterus

Bicornuate uterus

Septate uterus

Partial septum

Unicornuate uterus

Clinical Focus

Available Online

5-27 Ovarian Tumors

Additional figures available online (see inside front cover for details).

Challenge Yourself Questions

1. Cancer of the uterine cervix reaches an advanced stage and disseminates anteriorly. Which of the following structures is *most likely* to be involved in the spread of the tumor?

    A. Broad ligament
    B. Greater vestibular glands
    C. Perineal body
    D. Urinary bladder
    E. Uterine artery

2. A 14-year-old woman in an automobile crash has pelvic trauma. Ultrasound examination reveals that she has a bicornuate uterus with a complete septum and double cervix. Which of the following developmental events *best* accounts for this condition?

    A. Absence of a mesonephric duct on one side
    B. Division of the urogenital sinus
    C. Duplication of the gubernaculum
    D. Malfusion of the distal paramesonephric ducts
    E. Incomplete folding of the urogenital folds

3. A 41-year-old woman presents in the clinic with a uterine prolapse (cervix at introitus) in which the cervix is visible at the vaginal opening. She has delivered seven healthy children. Which of the following structures is the most important support structure of the uterus?

    A. Broad ligament
    B. Deep transverse perineal muscles
    C. Pubocervical ligaments
    D. Rectovaginal fascial condensations
    E. Transverse cervical ligaments

4. A 44-year-old woman is diagnosed with metastatic ovarian cancer. Which of the following lymph nodes will be the first to harbor disseminated ovarian cancer cells?

    A. Aortic (lumbar) nodes
    B. Deep inguinal nodes
    C. External iliac nodes
    D. Internal iliac nodes
    E. Superficial inguinal nodes

5. A 69-year-old man with a history of atherosclerotic disease and heavy smoking tells his physician that he is "impotent." Significant narrowing of which of the following arteries is most likely the cause of this patient's erectile dysfunction?

    A. External iliac
    B. Inferior epigastric
    C. Internal pudendal
    D. Lateral sacral
    E. Vas deferens

6. A 73-year-old woman is admitted to the hospital with significant abdominal ascites. When she sits upright on the side of her bed, the intraperitoneal fluid accumulates in her pelvis. Which of the following sites represents the lowest extent of the female abdominopelvic cavity where this fluid will collect?

    A. Left paracolic gutter
    B. Pararectal fossa
    C. Presacral space
    D. Recto-uterine pouch
    E. Vesico-uterine pouch

Multiple-choice and short-answer review questions available online; see inside front cover for details.

7. A male driver has sustained severe trauma to the pelvic region in a motor vehicle crash, resulting in a tearing of the prostatomembranous urethral junction (a tear just superior to the external urethral sphincter). Blood and urine from this injury would collect in which of the following spaces?

   A. Anterior lower abdominal wall deep to Scarpa's (membranous layer of superficial) fascia
   B. Beneath the deep (Buck's) fascia of the penis
   C. Beneath the superficial perineal (Colles') fascia
   D. Deep to the dartos fascia of the scrotum and penis
   E. Subperitoneal (retroperitoneal)

8. After an automobile crash the teenage male driver presents to the emergency department with pelvic fractures and paralysis of his urinary bladder. Which of the following nerves was (were) most likely injured and caused this patient's condition?

   A. Ilio-inguinal
   B. Lumbar splanchnics
   C. Pelvic splanchnics
   D. Pudendal
   E. Superior hypogastric

9. Biopsy of the inguinal lymph nodes reveals metastatic cancer. Which of the following pelvic structures is drained by these nodes?

   A. Distal rectum
   B. Proximal anal canal
   C. Ovaries
   D. Urinary bladder
   E. Uterine body

10. During surgery deep within the pelvis, the surgeon clamps the transverse cervical (cardinal) ligaments and the uterine arteries to provide hemostasis for a female patient. Which of the following structures lies close to these structures and must be preserved?

    A. Internal iliac artery
    B. Obturator nerve
    C. Pudendal nerve
    D. Superior gluteal nerve
    E. Ureter

11. Sexual arousal and orgasm employ a coordinated regulatory effort mediated by somatic and autonomic nerves, as well as by endocrine and central nervous system input. During male ejaculation, which of the following nerves contract the internal urethral sphincter and prevent the semen from entering the urinary bladder?

    A. Least splanchnic
    B. Lumbosacral trunk
    C. Pelvic splanchnics
    D. Pudendal
    E. Sacral splanchnics

12. The dissemination of cancer cells from the left testis would enter the testicular veins and then first enter which of the following veins?

    A. Inferior mesenteric
    B. Inferior vena cava
    C. Left inferior epigastric
    D. Left internal iliac
    E. Left internal pudendal
    F. Left renal

13. A forensic pathologist is asked to characterize the bony pelvis of an unidentified and largely decomposed human body. The pathologist identifies the bone as coming from a female. Which of the following pelvic features is unique to the female pelvis?

    A. The greater sciatic notch is narrow.
    B. The ischial tuberosities are inverted.
    C. The obturator foramen is round.
    D. The pelvic inlet is heart shaped.
    E. The pubic arch is wider.

For each of the descriptions below (14-20), select the muscle from the list (A-M) that is most closely associated.

(A) Bulbospongiosus
(B) Cremaster
(C) Compressor urethrae
(D) Coccygeus
(E) Detrusor
(F) External anal sphincter
(G) External urethral sphincter
(H) Gluteus maximus
(I) Internal urethral sphincter
(J) Ischiocavernosus
(K) Levator ani
(L) Obturator internus
(M) Piriformis

___ 14. This muscle is actually a derivative of one of the abdominal wall muscles.

___ 15. Trauma injuring the pelvic splanchnic nerves would compromise this muscle's ability to contract.

___ 16. The integrity of this muscle is critical for support of the pelvic viscera.

___ 17. Contraction of this muscle expels the last few drops of urine from the male urethra.

___ 18. An abscess in the ischio-anal fossa is limited in its spread superiorly by this muscle.

___ 19. Ventral rami of S2-S4 exit the anterior sacral foramina and then pass directly over (superficial to) this muscle.

___ 20. Trauma to the L1-L2 sympathetic outflow would result in the inability to contract this muscle.

Answers to Challenge Yourself Questions

1. D. The urinary bladder is directly anterior to the uterine cervix, lying just deep to the vesico-uterine pouch.

2. D. Incomplete fusion of the distal parameso-nephric (mullerian) ducts can lead to septation of the uterus, resulting in a partial or complete duplication of the uterus.

3. E. The transverse cervical (cardinal or Macken-rodt's) ligaments are fibrous condensations of the subperitoneal pelvic fascia and are the most important of the supporting structures for the uterus.

4. A. The ovaries descend into the pelvis from their original embryonic origin from the abdominal urogenital ridge. They drag their vessels (ovarian artery from aorta and ovarian veins draining into the IVC on the right and left renal and then IVC on the left) with them. Thus, the lymphatic drainage courses back to the lumbar (aortic) nodes (the same is true for the male testes).

5. C. The internal pudendal arteries give rise to the arteries of the bulb of the penis and the corpora cavernosa, which supply the erectile tissues. Narrowing of these vessels by athero-sclerosis can be just one of several problems that may lead to erectile dysfunction (ED).

6. D. The space between the rectum and uterus, called the recto-uterine pouch (of Douglas), is the lowest point in the female abdominopel-vic cavity in the upright position. Fluids within the cavity will eventually percolate down and collect in this space.

7. E. This rupture occurs before the prostatic urethra is completely surrounded by the external urethral sphincter, so blood and urine would collect primarily in the subperito-neal space beneath the pelvic floor. Excessive fluids in this space will allow it to expand superiorly and stretch the peritoneal floor of the pelvis.

8. C. The pelvic splanchnic nerves arise from the S2-S4 spinal nerves and convey the pregan-glionic parasympathetic fibers that innervate the urinary bladder. Those fibers destined to innervate the bladder enter the inferior hypo-gastric plexus of nerves and then enter the vesical plexus on the bladder wall where they synapse on their postganglionic parasympa-thetic neurons.

9. E. While most of the listed structures do not drain to the inguinal nodes, some lymph can track along the broad ligament of the uterus and enter the inguinal nodes. First, one must eliminate the possibility of perineal cancer, cancer of the distal anal canal, and cancer of the lower limb before focusing on the uterus.

10. E. The ureters pass just inferior to the uterine vessels ("water flows under the bridge") and must be identified before anything in this region is clamped and/or incised.

11. E. The sacral splanchnic nerves convey pregan-glionic sympathetic fibers to the inferior hypogastric plexus, where they synapse and send postganglionic fibers to innervate the internal urethral sphincter at the neck of the male urinary bladder (females do not have an internal urethral sphincter).

12. F. The cancer cells from the left testis would course along the testicular vein(s) to the left renal vein and then into the IVC. On the right side, the right testicular vein drains directly into the IVC.

13. E. The easiest way to identify the female pelvis is by the width of the pubic arch. Most of the adaptations that differentiate the female from the male pelvis pertain to its relationship to childbirth.

14. B. As the testis descends through the inguinal canal, it becomes covered by three layers of spermatic fascia. The middle spermatic fascia is the cremasteric fascia or muscle, and is derived from the internal abdominal oblique muscle. The cremaster muscle is innervated by the genital branch of the genitofemoral nerve.

15. E. The pelvic splanchnic nerves (parasympathetics) would innervate a smooth muscle and the only smooth muscle in the list that is innervated by them, resulting in contraction, is the detrusor muscle of the bladder wall. Contraction of this muscle empties the urinary bladder and is under parasympathetic control.

16. K. The levator ani is one of two muscles comprising the pelvic diaphragm (the other one is the coccygeus), and is itself really the amalgam of three separate but closely associated muscles (the puborectalis, pubococcygeus, and iliococcygeus) that is commonly referred to as the levator ani.

17. A. Contraction of the bulbospongiosus muscle following voiding helps evacuate the remaining urine in the penile urethra.

18. K. The levator ani muscle is the "roof" of the ischio-anal fossa and extends up the sides to contact the obturator internus muscle. This fossa is largely filled with fat; however, infections in this area can spread anteriorly, superior to the deep perineal pouch.

19. M. The ventral rami of S2-S4 lie on the surface of the piriformis muscle and join L4-S1 to form the sciatic nerve (L4-S3), which then exits the pelvic cavity via the greater sciatic foramen and enters the gluteal region.

20. I. The internal urethral sphincter is one of two smooth muscles in the list (the other is the detrusor) and the only one innervated by the sympathetic nerves of the ANS. This muscle contracts during ejaculation, thus preventing the semen from entering the urinary bladder.

Lower Limb

1. INTRODUCTION

As with the upper limb in Chapter 7, this chapter approaches our study of the lower limb by organizing its anatomical structures into functional compartments. The thigh and leg each are organized into three functional compartments, with their respective muscles and neurovascular bundles. The lower limb subserves the following important functions and features:

- Supports the weight of the body, and transfers that support to the axial skeleton across the hip and sacro-iliac joints.
- The hip and knee joints lock into position when standing still in anatomical position, adding stability and balance to the transfer of weight and conserving the muscles' energy; this allows one to stand erect for prolonged periods.
- Functions in locomotion through the process of walking (our gait).
- Anchored to the axial skeleton by the pelvic girdle, which allows for less mobility but significantly more stability than the pectoral girdle of the upper limb.

Be sure to review the movements of the lower limb as described in Chapter 1 (see Fig. 1-3). Note the terms *dorsiflexion* (extension) and *plantarflexion* (flexion), and *inversion* (supination) and *eversion* (pronation), which are unique to the movements of the ankle.

2. SURFACE ANATOMY

The components of the lower limb include the gluteal region, thigh, leg, and foot. The key surface landmarks include the following (Fig. 6-1):

- **Inguinal ligament:** the folded, inferior edge of the external abdominal oblique aponeurosis that separates the abdominal region from the thigh (Poupart's ligament).
- **Greater trochanter:** the point of the hip and attachment site for several gluteal muscles.
- **Quadriceps femoris:** the muscle mass of the anterior thigh, composed of four muscles—rectus femoris and three vastus muscles—that extend the leg at the knee.
- **Patella:** the kneecap; largest sesamoid bone in the body.
- **Popliteal fossa:** the region posterior to the knee.
- **Gastrocnemius muscles:** the muscle mass that forms the calf.
- **Calcaneal (Achilles) tendon:** the prominent tendon of several calf muscles.
- **Small saphenous vein:** drains blood from the lateral dorsal venous arch and posterior leg (calf) into the popliteal vein posterior to the knee.
- **Great saphenous vein:** drains blood from the medial dorsal venous arch, leg, and thigh into the femoral vein just inferior to the inguinal ligament.

Superficial veins drain blood toward the heart and communicate with deep veins that parallel the arteries of the lower limb. When vigorous muscle contraction compresses the deep veins, venous blood is shunted into superficial veins and returned to the heart. All these veins have valves to aid in the venous return to the heart.

Corresponding cutaneous nerves are terminal sensory branches of major lower limb nerves that arise from lumbar (L1-L4) and sacral (L4-S4) plexuses (Fig. 6-2). Note that the gluteal region has

Anterior view

Posterior view

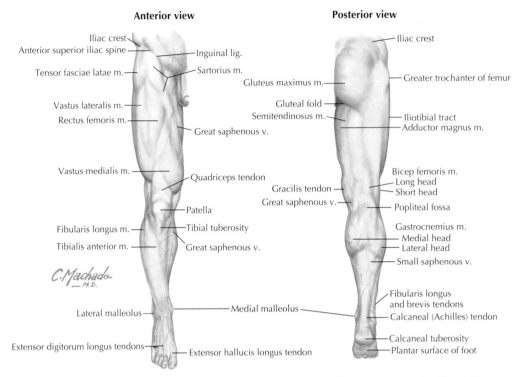

FIGURE 6-1 Surface Anatomy of the Lower Limb. (From *Atlas of human anatomy*, ed 6, Plate 468.)

Anterior view

Posterior view

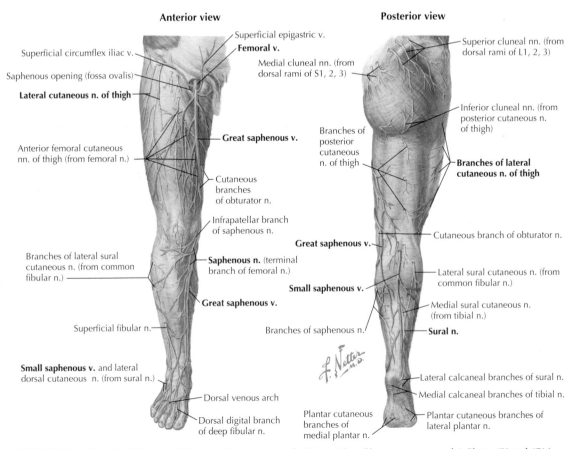

FIGURE 6-2 Superficial Veins and Nerves of the Lower Limb. (From *Atlas of human anatomy*, ed 6, Plates 470 and 471.)

Clinical Focus 6-1

Deep Venous Thrombosis

Although deep venous (or deep vein) thrombosis (DVT) may occur anywhere in the body, veins of the lower limb are most often involved. Three cardinal events account for the pathogenesis and risk of DVT: stasis, venous wall injury, and hypercoagulability. (See also Clinical Focus 3-7, Pulmonary Embolism.)

Clinical risk factors for DVT include the following:

- Postsurgical immobility
- Vessel trauma
- Infection
- Paralysis
- Malignancy
- Pregnancy

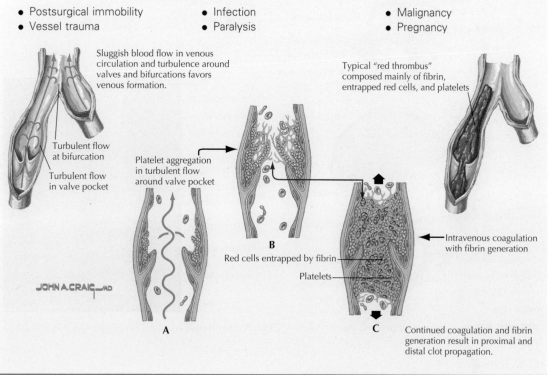

Sluggish blood flow in venous circulation and turbulence around valves and bifurcations favors venous formation.

Typical "red thrombus" composed mainly of fibrin, entrapped red cells, and platelets

Turbulent flow at bifurcation

Turbulent flow in valve pocket

Platelet aggregation in turbulent flow around valve pocket

JOHN A.CRAIG__AD

B

Red cells entrapped by fibrin

Platelets

Intravenous coagulation with fibrin generation

A   C

Continued coagulation and fibrin generation result in proximal and distal clot propagation.

---

superior, middle, and inferior cluneal nerves, and the thigh has posterior, lateral, anterior, and medial cutaneous nerves. The leg has lateral sural, superficial fibular, saphenous, and sural cutaneous nerves (named from the lateral leg to the posterior leg). The **sural nerve** on the posterior leg parallels the small saphenous vein, and the **saphenous nerve** (terminal portion of the femoral nerve) parallels the great saphenous vein from the medial ankle to the level of the knee.

3. HIP

Bones and Joints of the Pelvic Girdle and Hip

The pelvic girdle is the attachment point of the lower limb to the body's trunk and axial skeleton. The *pectoral girdle* is its counterpart for the attachment of the upper limb. The sacro-iliac ligaments

(posterior, anterior, and interosseous) are among the strongest ligaments in the body and support its entire weight, almost pulling the sacrum into the pelvis. Note that the pelvis (sacrum and coxal bones) in anatomical position is tilted forward such that the pubic symphysis and the anterior superior iliac spines lie in the same vertical plane, placing great stress on the sacro-iliac joints and ligaments (see Figs. 5-3 and 6-3). In fact, the body's center of gravity when standing upright lies just anterior to the S2 vertebra of the fused sacrum.

The bones of the pelvis include the following (Fig. 6-3 and Table 6-1):

- **Right and left pelvic bones (coxal or hip bones):** the fusion of three separate bones called the ilium, ischium, and pubis, which join each other in the acetabulum (cup-shaped feature for articulation of the head of the femur).

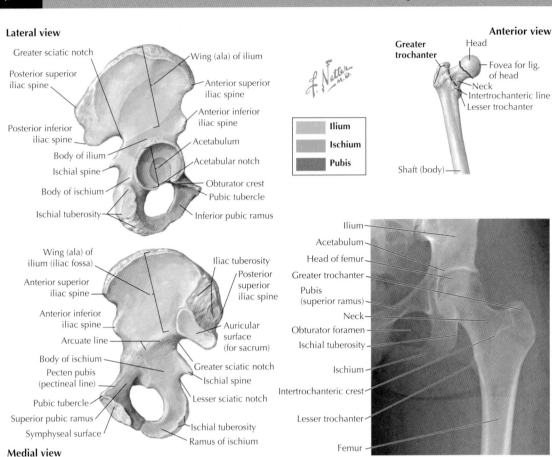

FIGURE 6-3 Features of the Pelvis and Proximal Femur. (From *Atlas of human anatomy,* ed 6, Plates 473, 475, and 476.)

TABLE 6-1 Features of the Pelvis and Proximal Femur

FEATURE	CHARACTERISTICS
Coxal (Hip) Bone	
	Fusion of three bones on each side to form the pelvis, which articulates with the sacrum to form the pelvic girdle
Ilium	Body fused to ischium and pubis, all meeting in the acetabulum (socket for articulation with femoral head) Ala (wing): weak spot of ilium
Ischium	Body fused with other two bones; ramus fused with pubis
Pubis	Body fused with other two bones; ramus fused with ischium
Femur (Proximal)	
Long bone	Longest bone in the body and very strong
Head	Point of articulation with acetabulum of coxal bone
Neck	Common fracture site
Greater trochanter	Point of the hip; attachment site for several gluteal muscles
Lesser trochanter	Attachment site of iliopsoas tendon (strong hip flexor)

- **Sacrum:** the fusion of the five sacral vertebrae; the two pelvic bones articulate with the sacrum posteriorly.
- **Coccyx:** the terminal end of the vertebral column, and a remnant of our embryonic tail.

Additionally, the proximal femur (thigh bone) articulates with the pelvis at the acetabulum (see Fig. 6-3 and Table 6-1).

The hip joint is a classic ball-and-socket synovial joint that affords great stability, provided by both its bony anatomy and its strong ligaments (Fig. 6-4 and Table 6-2). As with most large joints, there is a rich vascular anastomosis around the hip joint, contributing a blood supply not only to the hip but also to the associated muscles (Fig. 6-5 and Table 6-3).

The other features of the pelvic girdle and its stabilizing lumbosacral and sacro-iliac joints are illustrated and summarized in Chapter 5.

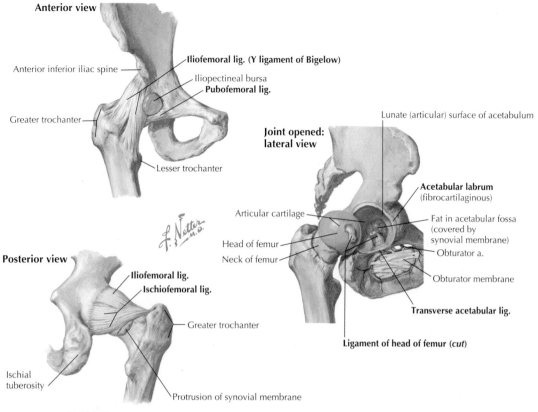

FIGURE 6-4 Hip Joint and Its Ligaments. (From *Atlas of human anatomy*, ed 6, Plate 474.)

TABLE 6-2 Ligaments of the Hip Joint (Multiaxial Synovial Ball and Socket)

LIGAMENT	ATTACHMENT	COMMENT
Capsular	Acetabular margin to femoral neck	Encloses femoral head and part of neck; acts in flexion, extension, abduction, adduction, medial and lateral rotation, and circumduction
Iliofemoral	Iliac spine and acetabulum to intertrochanteric line	Forms inverted Y (of Bigelow); limits hyperextension and lateral rotation; the stronger ligament
Ischiofemoral	Acetabulum to femoral neck posteriorly	Limits extension and medial rotation; the weaker ligament
Pubofemoral	Pubic ramus to lower femoral neck	Limits extension and abduction
Labrum	Acetabulum	Fibrocartilage, deepens socket
Transverse acetabular	Acetabular notch inferiorly	Cups acetabulum to form a socket for femoral head
Ligament of head of femur	Acetabular notch and transverse ligament to femoral head	Artery to femoral head runs in ligament

TABLE 6-3 Arteries of the Hip Joint

ARTERY	COURSE AND STRUCTURES SUPPLIED	ARTERY	COURSE AND STRUCTURES SUPPLIED
Medial circumflex	Usually arises from deep artery of thigh; branches supply femoral head and neck; passes posterior to iliopsoas muscle tendon	Acetabular branch	Arises from obturator artery; runs in ligament of head of femur; supplies femoral head
Lateral circumflex	Usually arises from deep artery of the thigh	Gluteal branches (superior and inferior)	Form anastomoses with medial and lateral femoral circumflex branches

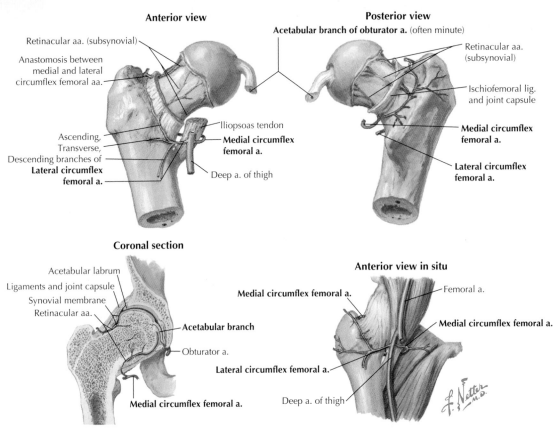

Anterior view

Retinacular aa. (subsynovial)

Anastomosis between medial and lateral circumflex femoral aa.

Ascending, Transverse, Descending branches of **Lateral circumflex femoral a.**

Iliopsoas tendon

Medial circumflex femoral a.

Deep a. of thigh

Posterior view

Acetabular branch of obturator a. (often minute)

Retinacular aa. (subsynovial)

Ischiofemoral lig. and joint capsule

Medial circumflex femoral a.

Lateral circumflex femoral a.

Coronal section

Acetabular labrum

Ligaments and joint capsule

Synovial membrane

Retinacular aa.

Acetabular branch

Obturator a.

Lateral circumflex femoral a.

Medial circumflex femoral a.

Anterior view in situ

Medial circumflex femoral a.

Femoral a.

Medial circumflex femoral a.

Deep a. of thigh

FIGURE 6-5 Arteries of the Hip Joint. (From *Atlas of human anatomy,* ed 6, Plate 491.)

Clinical Focus 6-2

Congenital Hip Dislocation

In the United States, 1.5 in 1000 infants are born with congenital hip dislocation. With early diagnosis and treatment, about 96% of affected children have normal hip function. Girls are affected more often than boys. About 60% of affected children are firstborns, which may suggest that unstretched uterine and abdominal walls limit fetal movement. Ortolani's test of hip abduction confirms the diagnosis.

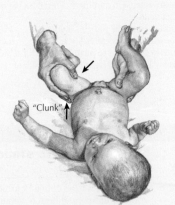

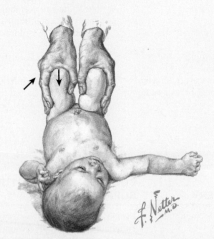

Ortolani's (reduction) test
With baby relaxed and content on firm surface, hips and knees flexed to 90°. Hips examined one at a time. Examiner grasps baby's thigh with middle finger over greater trochanter and lifts thigh to bring femoral head from its dislocated posterior position to opposite the acetabulum. Simultaneously, thigh gently abducted, reducing femoral head into acetabulum. In positive finding, examiner senses reduction by palpable, nearly audible "clunk."

Barlow's (dislocation) test
Reverse of Ortolani's test. If femoral head is in acetabulum at time of examination, Barlow's test is performed to discover any hip instability. Baby's thigh grasped as shown and adducted with gentle downward pressure. Dislocation is palpable as femoral head slips out of acetabulum. Diagnosis confirmed with Ortolani's test.

Clinical Focus 6-3

Pelvic Fractures

Pelvic fractures involve fractures that are, by definition, limited to the pelvic ring (pelvis and sacrum), whereas *acetabular* fractures (caused by high-impact trauma such as falls and automobile crashes) are described and classified separately. *Stable* pelvic fractures involve only one side of the pelvic ring, whereas *unstable* fractures involve two portions of the pelvic ring and/or ligamentous disruption. Excessive bleeding, nerve injury, and soft tissue damage (muscle and viscera) may accompany pelvic fractures.

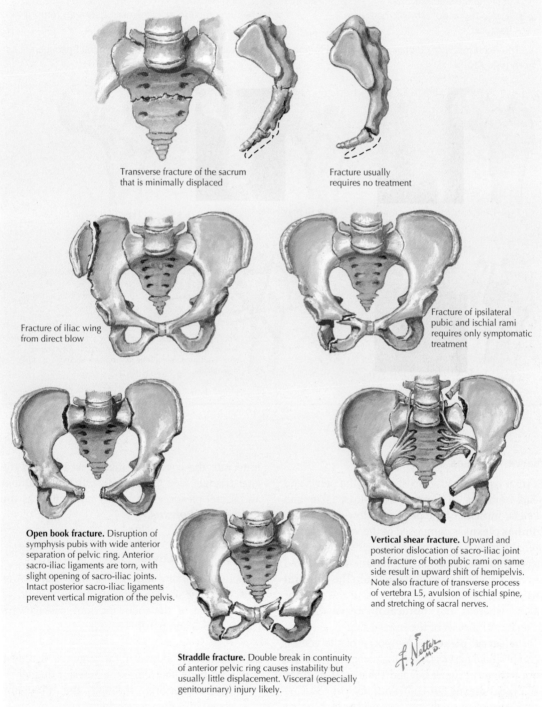

Transverse fracture of the sacrum that is minimally displaced

Fracture usually requires no treatment

Fracture of iliac wing from direct blow

Fracture of ipsilateral pubic and ischial rami requires only symptomatic treatment

Open book fracture. Disruption of symphysis pubis with wide anterior separation of pelvic ring. Anterior sacro-iliac ligaments are torn, with slight opening of sacro-iliac joints. Intact posterior sacro-iliac ligaments prevent vertical migration of the pelvis.

Vertical shear fracture. Upward and posterior dislocation of sacro-iliac joint and fracture of both pubic rami on same side result in upward shift of hemipelvis. Note also fracture of transverse process of vertebra L5, avulsion of ischial spine, and stretching of sacral nerves.

Straddle fracture. Double break in continuity of anterior pelvic ring causes instability but usually little displacement. Visceral (especially genitourinary) injury likely.

Clinical Focus 6-4

Intracapsular Femoral Neck Fracture

Femoral neck fractures are common injuries. In young persons the fracture often results from trauma; in elderly people the cause is often related to osteoporosis and associated with a fall. The Garden classification identifies four fracture types:

- I: impaction of superior portion of femoral neck (incomplete fracture)
- II: nondisplaced fracture (complete fracture)
- III: partial displacement between femoral head and neck
- IV: complete displacement between femoral head and neck

    The occurrence of complications related to nonunion and avascular necrosis of the femoral head increases from type I to IV.

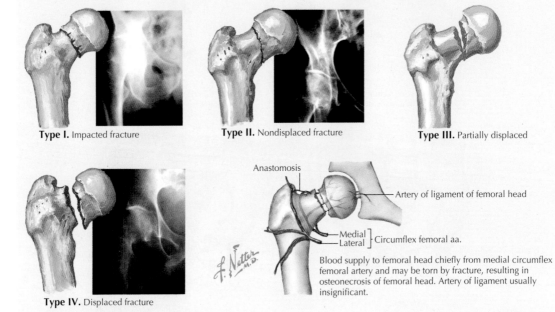

Type I. Impacted fracture

Type II. Nondisplaced fracture

Type III. Partially displaced

Type IV. Displaced fracture

Anastomosis

Artery of ligament of femoral head

Medial
Lateral } Circumflex femoral aa.

Blood supply to femoral head chiefly from medial circumflex femoral artery and may be torn by fracture, resulting in osteonecrosis of femoral head. Artery of ligament usually insignificant.

Nerve Plexuses

Several nerve plexuses exist within the pelvis and send branches to somatic structures (skin and skeletal muscle) of the pelvis and lower limb. The **lumbar plexus** is composed of the ventral rami of spinal nerves L1-L4, which give rise to two large nerves, the femoral and obturator nerves, and several smaller branches (Fig. 6-6). The **femoral nerve** (L2-L4) innervates muscles of the anterior thigh, whereas the **obturator nerve** (L2-L4) innervates muscles of the medial thigh.

    The **sacral plexus** is composed of the ventral rami of spinal nerves L4-S4. Its major branches are summarized in Figure 6-7 and Table 6-4. The small **coccygeal plexus** has contributions from S4-Co1 and gives rise to small anococcygeal branches that

innervate the coccygeus muscle and skin of the anal triangle (see Chapter 5). Often the lumbar and sacral plexuses are simply referred to as the *lumbosacral plexus*.

Access to the Lower Limb

Structures passing out of or into the lower limb from the abdominopelvic cavity may do so through one of the following four passageways (see Figs. 5-3 and 6-10):

- Anteriorly between the inguinal ligament and bony pelvis into the anterior thigh
- Anteroinferiorly through the obturator canal into the medial thigh

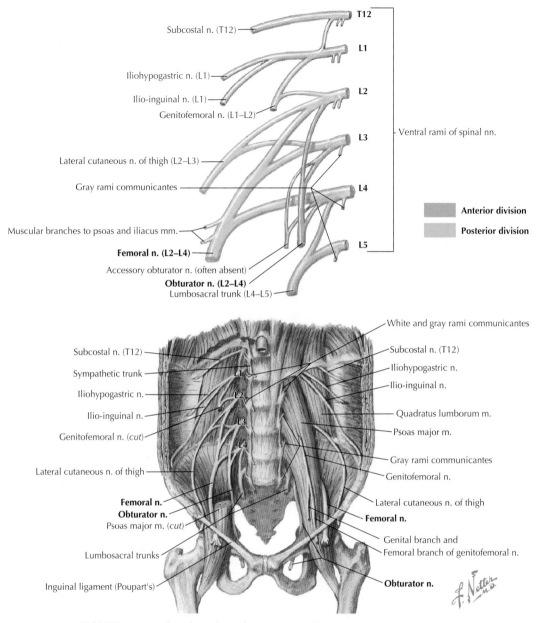

FIGURE 6-6 Lumbar Plexus (L1-L4). (From *Atlas of human anatomy,* ed 6, Plate 485.)

TABLE 6-4 Major Branches of the Sacral Plexus

DIVISION AND NERVE	INNERVATION	DIVISION AND NERVE	INNERVATION
Anterior		**Posterior**	
Pudendal	Supplies motor and sensory innervation to perineum (S2-S4)	Superior gluteal	Innervates several gluteal muscles (L4-S1)
Tibial	Innervates posterior thigh muscles, posterior leg muscles, and foot; forms the sciatic nerve (largest nerve in body) with common fibular nerve	Inferior gluteal	Innervates gluteus maximus muscle (L5-S2)
		Common fibular	Portion of sciatic nerve (with tibial) that innervates lateral and anterior muscle compartments of leg

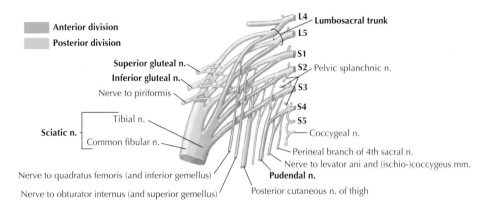

Anterior division
Posterior division

L4 **Lumbosacral trunk**
L5
S1
Superior gluteal n.
Inferior gluteal n.
S2 Pelvic splanchnic n.
Nerve to piriformis
S3
S4
S5
Tibial n.
Sciatic n.
Common fibular n.
Coccygeal n.
Perineal branch of 4th sacral n.
Nerve to levator ani and (ischio-)coccygeus mm.
Nerve to quadratus femoris (and inferior gemellus)
Pudendal n.
Nerve to obturator internus (and superior gemellus)
Posterior cutaneous n. of thigh

Topography: medial and slightly anterior view of hemisected pelvis

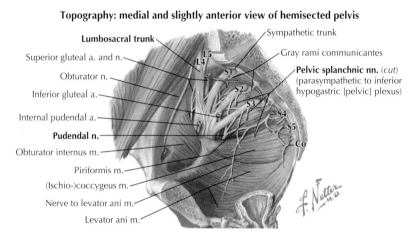

Lumbosacral trunk
Sympathetic trunk
Superior gluteal a. and n.
L5
L4
Gray rami communicantes
Obturator n.
S1
Pelvic splanchnic nn. (*cut*)
(parasympathetic to inferior
hypogastric [pelvic] plexus)
S2
Inferior gluteal a.
S3
Internal pudendal a.
S4
S5
Pudendal n.
Co
Obturator internus m.
Piriformis m.
(Ischio-)coccygeus m.
Nerve to levator ani m.
Levator ani m.

FIGURE 6-7 Sacral and Coccygeal Plexuses. (From *Atlas of human anatomy,* ed 6, Plate 486.)

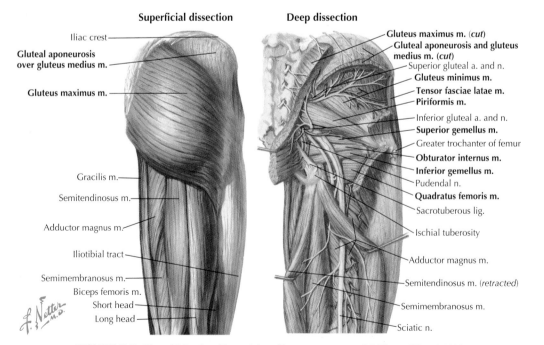

Superficial dissection   **Deep dissection**

Iliac crest
**Gluteal aponeurosis
over gluteus medius m.**
Gluteus maximus m.
Gracilis m.
Semitendinosus m.
Adductor magnus m.
Iliotibial tract
Semimembranosus m.
Biceps femoris m.
Short head
Long head

Gluteus maximus m. (*cut*)
**Gluteal aponeurosis and gluteus
medius m.** (*cut*)
Superior gluteal a. and n.
Gluteus minimus m.
Tensor fasciae latae m.
Piriformis m.
Inferior gluteal a. and n.
Superior gemellus m.
Greater trochanter of femur
Obturator internus m.
Inferior gemellus m.
Pudendal n.
Quadratus femoris m.
Sacrotuberous lig.
Ischial tuberosity
Adductor magnus m.
Semitendinosus m. (*retracted*)
Semimembranosus m.
Sciatic n.

FIGURE 6-8 Gluteal Muscles. (From *Atlas of human anatomy,* ed 6, Plates 482 and 489.)

- Posterolaterally through the greater sciatic foramen into the gluteal region
- Posterolaterally through the lesser sciatic foramen from the gluteal region into the perineum (via the pudendal [Alcock's] canal)

4. GLUTEAL REGION

Muscles

The muscles of the gluteal (buttock) region are arranged into superficial and deep groups, as follows (Fig. 6-8 and Table 6-5):

- Superficial muscles include the three gluteal muscles and the tensor fasciae latae laterally.
- Deep muscles act on the hip, primarily as lateral rotators of the thigh at the hip, and assist in stabilizing the hip joint.

The **gluteus maximus muscle** is one of the strongest muscles in the body in absolute terms and is a powerful extensor of the thigh at the hip (Fig. 6-8). It is especially important in extending the hip when rising from a squatting or sitting position, and when climbing stairs. The gluteus

TABLE 6-5 Gluteal Muscles

MUSCLE	PROXIMAL ATTACHMENT (ORIGIN)	DISTAL ATTACHMENT (INSERTION)	INNERVATION	MAIN ACTIONS
Gluteus maximus	Ilium posterior to posterior gluteal line, dorsal surface of sacrum and coccyx, and sacrotuberous ligament	Most fibers end in iliotibial tract that inserts into lateral condyle of tibia; some fibers insert on gluteal tuberosity of femur	Inferior gluteal nerve (L5-S2)	Extends flexed thigh at the hip and assists in its lateral rotation; abducts and assists in raising trunk from flexed position
Gluteus medius	Lateral surface of ilium	Lateral surface of greater trochanter of femur	Superior gluteal nerve (L4-S1)	Abducts and medially rotates thigh at hip; steadies pelvis on limb when opposite limb is raised
Gluteus minimus	Lateral surface of ilium	Anterior surface of greater trochanter of femur	Superior gluteal nerve (L4-S1)	Abducts and medially rotates thigh at hip; steadies pelvis on limb when opposite limb is raised
Tensor fasciae latae	Anterior superior iliac spine and anterior iliac crest	Iliotibial tract that attaches to lateral condyle of tibia	Superior gluteal nerve (L4-L5)	Abducts, medially rotates, and flexes thigh at hip; helps to keep knee extended
Piriformis	Anterior surface of sacrum and sacrotuberous ligament	Superior border of greater trochanter of femur	Branches of ventral rami (L5-S2)	Laterally rotates extended thigh at hip and abducts flexed thigh at hip; steadies femoral head in acetabulum
Obturator internus	Pelvic surface of obturator membrane and surrounding bones	Medial surface of greater trochanter of femur	Nerve to obturator internus (L5-S2)	Laterally rotates extended thigh at hip and abducts flexed thigh at hip; steadies femoral head in acetabulum
Gemelli, superior and inferior	*Superior:* ischial spine *Inferior:* ischial tuberosity	Medial surface of greater trochanter of femur	*Superior gemellus:* same nerve supply as obturator internus *Inferior gemellus:* same nerve supply as quadratus femoris	Laterally rotate extended thigh at the hip and abducts flexed thigh at the hip; steady femoral head in acetabulum
Quadratus femoris	Lateral border of ischial tuberosity	Quadrate tubercle on intertrochanteric crest of femur	Nerve to quadratus femoris (L4-S1)	Laterally rotates thigh at hip; steadies femoral head in acetabulum

Clinical Focus 6-5

Pressure (Decubitus) Ulcers

Pressure ulcers (bedsores) are common complications in patients confined to beds or wheelchairs. They form when soft tissue is compressed between a bony eminence (e.g., greater trochanter) and the bed or wheelchair. Comatose, paraplegic, or debilitated patients cannot sense discomfort caused by pressure from prolonged contact with hard surfaces. Common ulcer sites are shown in the figure, with more than half associated with the pelvic girdle (sacrum, iliac crest, ischium, and greater trochanter of femur). The four stages of these ulcers are as follows:

- **Stage I:** Changes in skin temperature, consistency, or sensation; persistent redness
- **Stage II:** Partial-thickness skin loss, similar to an abrasion with a shallow crater or blister
- **Stage III:** Full-thickness skin loss with subcutaneous tissue damage and a deep crater
- **Stage IV:** Full-thickness skin loss with necrosis or damage to muscle, bone, or adjacent structures

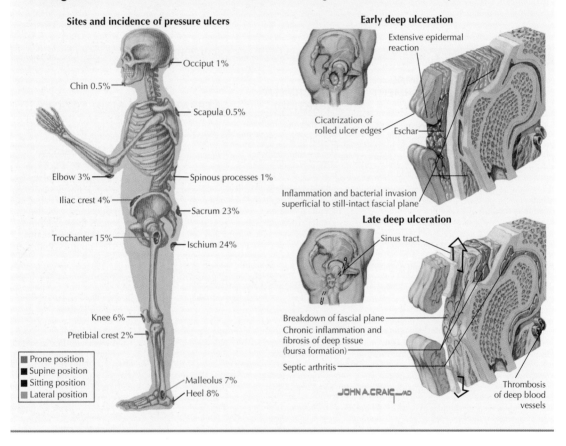

maximus also stabilizes and laterally rotates the hip joint. The **gluteus medius** and **gluteus minimus muscles** are primarily abductors and medial rotators of the thigh at the hip, steadying the pelvis over the lower limb when the opposite lower limb is raised off the ground (see Fig. 6-34).

The **tensor fasciae latae muscle** abducts, medially rotates, and stabilizes the extended knee.

The deep fascia of the thigh (fascia lata) is especially thickened laterally and is known as the *iliotibial tract*. Both the tensor fasciae latae and most of the gluteus maximus muscles insert into this tract and help stabilize the hip and knee extension when standing. People may shift their weight from one lower limb to the other and stabilize the limb they are standing on by placing tension on this iliotibial tract.

Iliotibial Tract (Band) Syndrome

Iliotibial tract syndrome is common in runners and presents as lateral knee pain, often in the midrange of flexion, between 20 and 70 degrees of knee flexion. The iliotibial tract, often referred to as "iliotibial band" by clinicians, rubs across the lateral femoral condyle, and this pain also may be associated with more proximal pain from greater trochanteric bursitis.

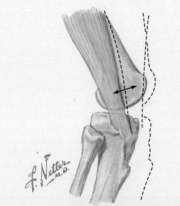

Iliotibial Tract Friction Syndrome
As knee flexes and extends, iliotibial tract glides back and forth over lateral femoral epicondyle, causing friction

Neurovascular Structures

The nerves innervating the gluteal muscles arise from the **sacral plexus** (see Figs. 6-7 and 6-8 and Tables 6-4 and 6-5) and gain access to the gluteal region largely by passing through the greater sciatic foramen. The blood supply to this region is via the **superior** and **inferior gluteal arteries,** which are branches of the internal iliac artery in the pelvis (see also Fig. 5-13 and Table 5-6) and also gain access to the gluteal region via the greater sciatic foramen. These neurovascular elements pass in the plane deep to the gluteus medius muscle (superior gluteal neurovascular bundle) or deep to the gluteus maximus muscle (inferior gluteal neurovascular structures). Also passing through the gluteal region is the largest nerve in the body, the **sciatic nerve** (L4-S3), which exits the greater sciatic foramen, passes through or more often inferior to the piriformis muscle, and enters the posterior thigh passing deep to the long head of the biceps femoris muscle (see Fig. 6-8).

The **internal pudendal artery** and **pudendal nerve** (a somatic nerve, S2-S4) pass out of the greater sciatic foramen, wrap around the sacrospinous ligament, and reenter the lesser sciatic foramen to gain access to the pudendal (Alcock's) canal (see Figs. 5-22 and 6-8). The pudendal nerve innervates the skeletal muscle and skin of the perineum (see Table 6-4). The internal pudendal artery is the major blood supply to the perineum and external genitalia.

5. THIGH

The thigh is the region of the lower limb between the hip and knee. As you learn the anatomical arrangement of the thigh and leg, organize your study around the functional muscular compartments. The thigh is divided into three muscular compartments: an anterior (extensor) compartment, a medial (adductor) compartment, and a posterior (flexor) compartment by intermuscular septae.

Bones

The **femur,** the longest bone in the body, is the bone of the thigh. It is slightly bowed anteriorly and runs slightly diagonally, lateral to medial, from the hip to the knee (Fig. 6-9 and Table 6-6). Proximally the femur articulates with the pelvis, and distally it articulates with the **tibia** and the **patella** (kneecap), which is the largest sesamoid bone in the body. The proximal femur is supplied with blood from the medial and lateral femoral circumflex branches of the deep femoral artery (see Fig. 6-13), an acetabular branch of the obturator artery, and by anastomotic branches of the inferior gluteal

TABLE 6-6 Features of the Femur	
STRUCTURE	**CHARACTERISTICS**
Long bone	Longest bone in the body; very strong
Head	Point of articulation with acetabulum of coxal bone
Neck	Common fracture site
Greater trochanter	Point of hip; attachment site for several gluteal muscles
Lesser trochanter	Attachment site of iliopsoas tendon (strong hip flexor)
Distal condyles	Medial and lateral (smaller) sites that articulate with tibial condyles
Patella	Sesamoid bone (largest) embedded in quadriceps femoris tendon

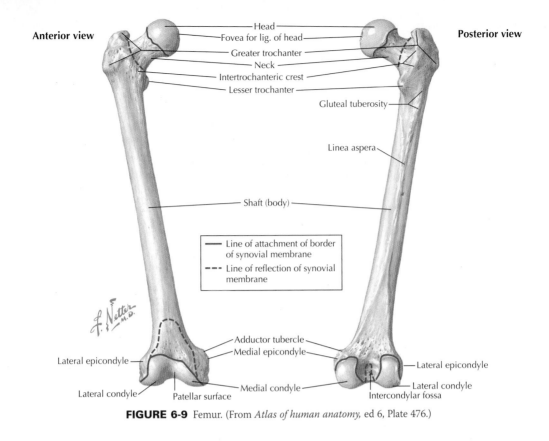

FIGURE 6-9 Femur. (From *Atlas of human anatomy,* ed 6, Plate 476.)

Fractures of the Shaft and Distal Femur

Femoral shaft fractures occur in all age groups but are especially common in young and elderly persons. Spiral fractures usually occur from torsional forces rather than direct forces. Fractures of the distal femur are divided into two groups depending on whether the joint surface is involved. If reduction and fixation of intraarticular fractures are not satisfactory, osteoarthritis is a common posttraumatic complication.

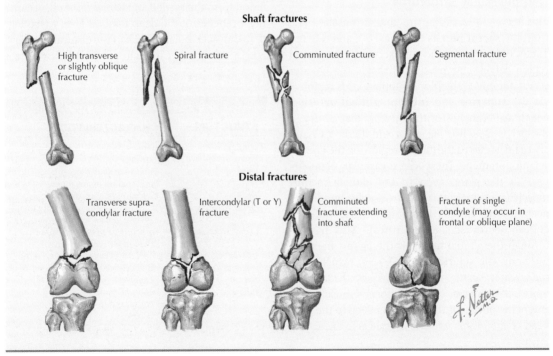

Shaft fractures

High transverse or slightly oblique fracture

Spiral fracture

Comminuted fracture

Segmental fracture

Distal fractures

Transverse supra-condylar fracture

Intercondylar (T or Y) fracture

Comminuted fracture extending into shaft

Fracture of single condyle (may occur in frontal or oblique plane)

artery. The shaft and distal femur is supplied by femoral nutrient arteries and by anastomotic branches of the popliteal artery, the distal continuation of the femoral artery posterior to the knee.

Anterior Compartment Thigh Muscles, Vessels, and Nerves

Muscles of the anterior compartment exhibit the following characteristics (Figs. 6-10 and 6-11 and Table 6-7):

- Include the quadriceps muscles, which attach to the patella by the quadriceps femoris tendon and to the tibia by the patellar ligament (clinicians often refer to this ligament as the "patellar tendon").
- Are primarily extensors of the leg at the knee.
- Two can secondarily flex the thigh at the hip (sartorius and rectus femoris).
- Are innervated by the **femoral nerve.**
- Are supplied by the femoral artery and its deep (femoral) artery of the thigh.

Additionally, the psoas major and iliacus muscles (which form the iliopsoas) pass from the posterior abdominal wall to the anterior thigh by passing deep to the inguinal ligament to insert on the lesser trochanter of the femur. These muscles act jointly as powerful flexors of the thigh at the hip joint (Table 6-7; see also Fig. 4-32).

Medial Compartment Thigh Muscles, Vessels, and Nerves

Muscles of the medial compartment exhibit the following characteristics (see Figs. 6-10 and 6-11 and Table 6-8):

- Are primarily adductors of the thigh at the hip.
- Most can secondarily flex and/or rotate the thigh.
- Are largely innervated by the **obturator nerve.**
- Are supplied by the obturator artery and deep (femoral) artery of the thigh.

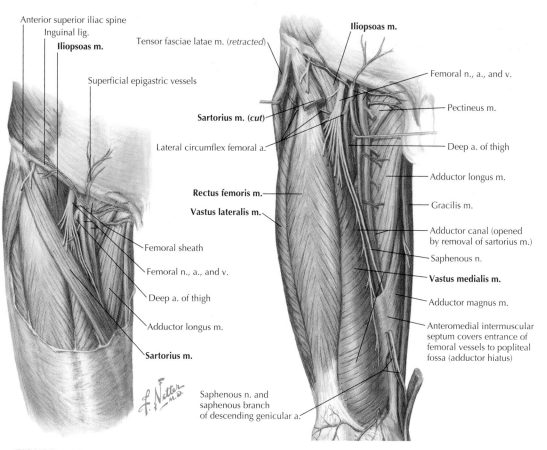

FIGURE 6-10 Anterior Compartment Thigh Muscles and Nerves. (From *Atlas of human anatomy,* ed 6, Plate 487.)

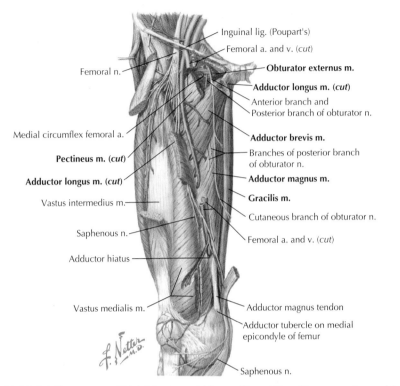

Inguinal lig. (Poupart's)

Femoral a. and v. (*cut*)

Femoral n.

Obturator externus m.

Adductor longus m. (*cut*)

Anterior branch and
Posterior branch of obturator n.

Medial circumflex femoral a.

Adductor brevis m.

Branches of posterior branch
of obturator n.

Pectineus m. (*cut*)

Adductor magnus m.

Adductor longus m. (*cut*)

Gracilis m.

Vastus intermedius m.

Cutaneous branch of obturator n.

Saphenous n.

Femoral a. and v. (*cut*)

Adductor hiatus

Vastus medialis m.

Adductor magnus tendon

Adductor tubercle on medial
epicondyle of femur

Saphenous n.

FIGURE 6-11 Medial Compartment Thigh Muscles and Nerves. (From *Atlas of human anatomy,* ed 6, Plate 488.)

TABLE 6-7 Anterior Compartment Thigh Muscles

MUSCLE	PROXIMAL ATTACHMENT (ORIGIN)	DISTAL ATTACHMENT (INSERTION)	INNERVATION	MAIN ACTIONS
Psoas major (iliopsoas)	Sides of T12-L5 vertebrae and discs between them; transverse processes of all lumbar vertebrae	Lesser trochanter of femur	Ventral rami of lumbar nerves (L1-L3)	Acts jointly with iliacus in flexing thigh at hip joint and in stabilizing hip joint
Iliacus (iliopsoas)	Iliac crest, iliac fossa, ala of sacrum, and anterior sacro-iliac ligaments	Tendon of psoas major, lesser trochanter, and femur	Femoral nerve (L2-L3)	Acts jointly with psoas major in flexing thigh at hip joint and in stabilizing hip joint
Sartorius	Anterior superior iliac spine and superior part of notch inferior to it	Superior part of medial surface of tibia	Femoral nerve (L2-L3)	Flexes, abducts, and laterally rotates thigh at hip joint; flexes knee joint
Quadriceps Femoris				
Rectus femoris	Anterior inferior iliac spine and ilium superior to acetabulum	Base of patella and by patellar ligament to tibial tuberosity	Femoral nerve (L2-L4)	Extends leg at knee joint; also steadies hip joint and helps iliopsoas to flex thigh at hip
Vastus lateralis	Greater trochanter and lateral lip of linea aspera of femur	Base of patella and by patellar ligament to tibial tuberosity	Femoral nerve (L2-L4)	Extends leg at knee joint
Vastus medialis	Intertrochanteric line and medial lip of linea aspera of femur	Base of patella and by patellar ligament to tibial tuberosity	Femoral nerve (L2-L4)	Extends leg at knee joint
Vastus intermedius	Anterior and lateral surfaces of femoral shaft	Base of patella and by patellar ligament to tibial tuberosity	Femoral nerve (L2-L4)	Extends leg at knee joint

TABLE 6-8 Medial Compartment Thigh Muscles

MUSCLE	PROXIMAL ATTACHMENT (ORIGIN)	DISTAL ATTACHMENT (INSERTION)	INNERVATION	MAIN ACTIONS
Pectineus	Superior ramus of pubis	Pectineal line of femur, just inferior to lesser trochanter	Femoral nerve; may receive a branch from obturator nerve	Adducts and flexes thigh at hip; assists with medial rotation of thigh
Adductor longus	Body of pubis inferior to pubic crest	Middle third of linea aspera of femur	Obturator nerve (L2-L4)	Adducts thigh at hip
Adductor brevis	Body and inferior ramus of pubis	Pectineal line and proximal part of linea aspera of femur	Obturator nerve (L2-L4)	Adducts thigh at hip and, to some extent, flexes it
Adductor magnus	Inferior ramus of pubis, ramus of ischium, and ischial tuberosity	*Adductor part:* gluteal tuberosity, linea aspera, medial supracondylar line. *Hamstring part:* adductor tubercle of femur	*Adductor part:* obturator nerve *Hamstring part:* tibial part of sciatic nerve	Adducts thigh at hip *Adductor part:* also flexes thigh at hip *Hamstring part:* extends thigh
Gracilis	Body and inferior ramus of pubis	Superior part of medial surface of tibia	Obturator nerve (L2-L3)	Adducts thigh at hip; flexes leg at knee and helps to rotate it medially
Obturator externus	Margins of obturator foramen and obturator membrane	Trochanteric fossa of femur	Obturator nerve (L2-L3)	Rotates thigh laterally at hip; steadies femoral head in acetabulum

Clinical Focus 6-8

Thigh Muscle Injuries

Muscle injuries are common and may include pulled muscles (muscle "strain," actually a partial tearing of a muscle-tendon unit) from overstretching, or actual muscle tears, which can cause significant focal bleeding. Groin injuries usually involve muscles of the medial compartment, especially the adductor longus. Because the hamstring muscles cross two joints and are actively used in walking and running, they can become pulled or torn if not adequately stretched and loosened before vigorous use. Likewise, a "charley horse" is a muscle pain or stiffness often felt in the quadriceps muscles of the anterior compartment or in the hamstrings. Additionally, quadriceps muscle tears and tendon disruptions can occur, especially in athletes (see images).

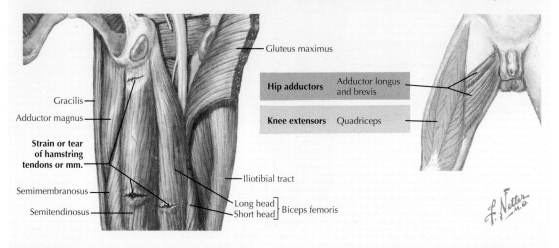

The pectineus muscle, while residing in the medial compartment, is largely innervated by the femoral nerve, although it also may receive a branch from the obturator nerve. The adductor magnus, being an exceptionally large and powerful muscle, also receives some innervation via the tibial portion of the sciatic nerve, which runs in the posterior compartment of the thigh.

Posterior Compartment Thigh Muscles, Vessels, and Nerves

Muscles of the posterior compartment exhibit the following characteristics (Fig. 6-12 and Table 6-9; see Fig. 6-8):

- Are largely flexors of the leg at the knee and extensors of the thigh at the hip (except the short head of the biceps femoris muscle).
- Are collectively referred to as the *hamstrings;* can also rotate the knee and are attached proximally to the ischial tuberosity (except the short head of biceps femoris).

- Are innervated by the **tibial division of the sciatic nerve** (except short head of biceps femoris, which is innervated by common fibular division).
- Are supplied by the deep (femoral) artery of the thigh and the femoral artery.

Femoral Triangle

The **femoral triangle** is located on the anterosuperior aspect of the thigh and is bound by the following structures (see Fig. 6-10):

- **Inguinal ligament:** forms the base of the triangle.
- **Sartorius muscle:** forms the lateral boundary.
- **Adductor longus muscle:** forms the medial boundary.

Inferiorly, a fascial sleeve extends from the apex of the femoral triangle and is continuous with the **adductor (Hunter's) canal;** the femoral vessels

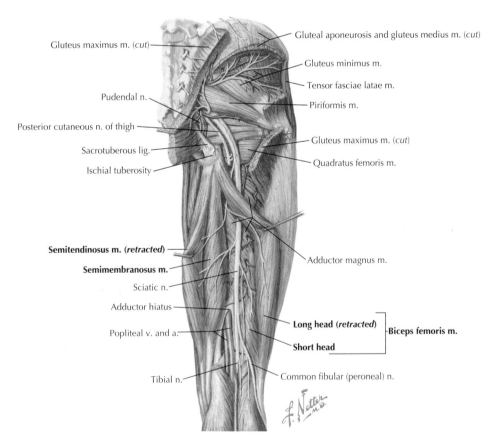

FIGURE 6-12 Posterior Compartment Thigh Muscles and Nerves. (From *Atlas of human anatomy,* ed 6, Plate 489.)

TABLE 6-9 Posterior Compartment Thigh Muscles

MUSCLE	PROXIMAL ATTACHMENT (ORIGIN)	DISTAL ATTACHMENT (INSERTION)	INNERVATION	MAIN ACTIONS
Semitendinosus	Ischial tuberosity	Medial surface of superior part of tibia	Tibial division of sciatic nerve (L5-S2)	Extends thigh at hip; flexes leg at knee and rotates it medially; with flexed hip and knee, extends trunk
Semimembranosus	Ischial tuberosity	Posterior part of medial condyle of tibia	Tibial division of sciatic nerve (L5-S2)	Extends thigh at hip; flexes leg at knee and rotates it medially; with flexed hip and knee, extends trunk
Biceps femoris	*Long head:* ischial tuberosity *Short head:* linea aspera and lateral supracondylar line of femur	Lateral side of head of fibula; tendon at this site split by fibular collateral ligament of knee	*Long head:* tibial division of sciatic nerve (L5-S2) *Short head:* common fibular division of sciatic nerve (L5-S2)	Flexes leg at knee and rotates it laterally; extends thigh at hip (e.g., when starting to walk)

Clinical Focus 6-9

Diagnosis of Hip, Buttock, and Back Pain

Athletically active individuals may report hip pain when the injury may actually be related to the lumbar spine (herniated disc), buttocks (bursitis or hamstring injury), or pelvic region (intrapelvic disorder). Careful follow-up should examine all potential causes of the pain to determine whether it is referred and thus originates from another source.

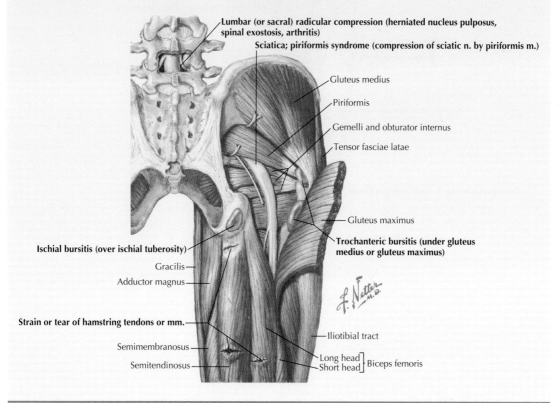

Lumbar (or sacral) radicular compression (herniated nucleus pulposus, spinal exostosis, arthritis)

Sciatica; piriformis syndrome (compression of sciatic n. by piriformis m.)

Gluteus medius

Piriformis

Gemelli and obturator internus

Tensor fasciae latae

Gluteus maximus

Trochanteric bursitis (under gluteus medius or gluteus maximus)

Ischial bursitis (over ischial tuberosity)

Gracilis

Adductor magnus

Strain or tear of hamstring tendons or mm.

Semimembranosus

Semitendinosus

Iliotibial tract

Long head
Short head } Biceps femoris

course through this canal and become the popliteal vessels posterior to the knee. The femoral triangle contains the femoral nerve and vessels as they pass beneath the inguinal ligament and gain access to the anterior thigh (see Fig. 6-10). Within this triangle is a fascial sleeve called the **femoral sheath,** a continuation of transversalis fascia and iliac fascia of the abdomen, that contains the femoral artery and vein and medially the lymphatics. Laterally the femoral nerve lies within the femoral triangle but outside this femoral sheath. The most medial portion of the femoral sheath is called the **femoral canal** and contains the lymphatics that drain through the **femoral ring** and into the external iliac lymph nodes. The femoral canal and ring are a weak point and the site for femoral hernias. The femoral ring is narrow, and consequently, femoral hernias may be difficult to reduce and may be prone to strangulation.

Femoral Artery

The femoral artery supplies the tissues of the thigh and then descends into the adductor canal to gain access to the popliteal fossa (Fig. 6-13 and Table 6-10). The superomedial aspect of the thigh also

TABLE 6-10 Key Arteries of the Thigh	
ARTERY	**COURSE AND STRUCTURES SUPPLIED**
Obturator	Arises from internal iliac artery (pelvis); has anterior and posterior branches; passes through obturator foramen
Femoral	Continuation of external iliac artery with numerous branches to perineum, hip, thigh, and knee
Deep artery of thigh	Arises from femoral artery; supplies hip and thigh

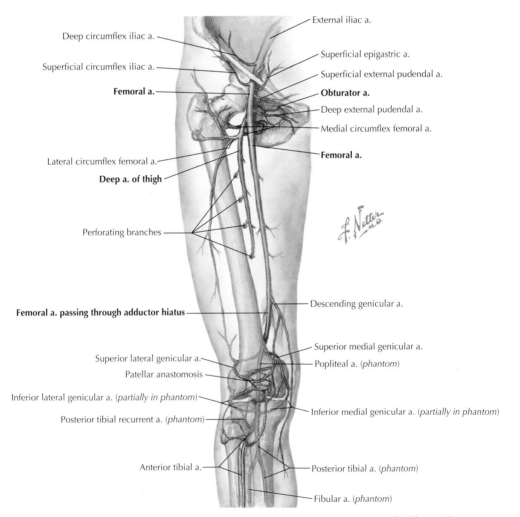

FIGURE 6-13 Key Arteries of the Thigh. (From *Atlas of human anatomy,* ed 6, Plate 499.)

Clinical Focus 6-10

Revascularization of the Lower Limb

Peripheral vascular disease and claudication can usually be managed medically by reducing the associated risk factors. However, patients who are refractory to medical management have the following invasive options:

- Percutaneous angioplasty: balloon dilation (with or without an endovascular stent) for recanalization of a stenosed artery (percutaneous revascularization)
- Surgical bypass: bypassing a diseased segment of the artery with a graft (1-3% operative mortality)

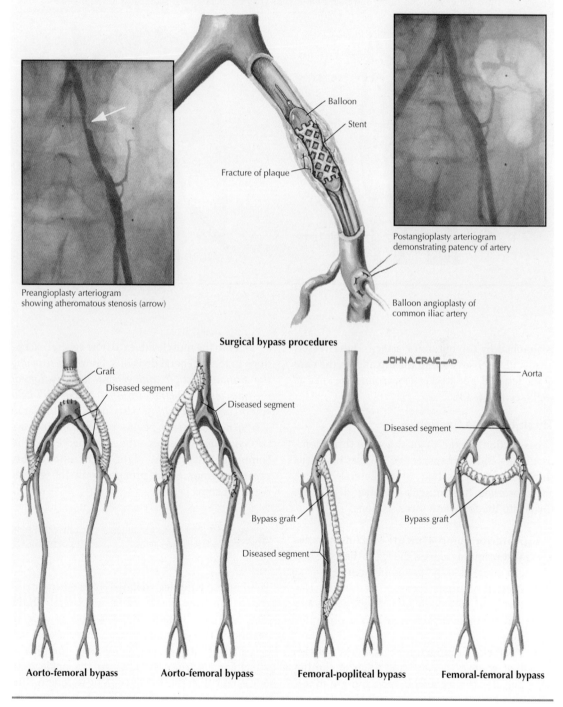

Balloon

Stent

Fracture of plaque

Preangioplasty arteriogram
showing atheromatous stenosis (arrow)

Postangioplasty arteriogram
demonstrating patency of artery

Balloon angioplasty of
common iliac artery

Surgical bypass procedures

JOHN A. CRAIG—AD

Graft

Diseased segment

Diseased segment

Aorta

Diseased segment

Bypass graft

Bypass graft

Diseased segment

Diseased segment

Aorto-femoral bypass   **Aorto-femoral bypass**   **Femoral-popliteal bypass**   **Femoral-femoral bypass**

Clinical Focus 6-11

Femoral Pulse and Vascular Access

The femoral pulse is felt at about the midpoint of the inguinal ligament. The femoral artery at this point lies directly over or just medial to the femoral head, just lateral to the femoral vein and about a finger's breadth medial to the femoral nerve (see Figs. 6-10 and 6-13). The femoral artery and vein may be used to gain access to major vessels of the limbs, abdominopelvic cavity, and thorax (e.g., catheter threaded through femoral artery and into aorta for coronary artery angiography and angioplasty). Similarly, the larger veins of the inferior vena cava and the right side of the heart and pulmonary veins may be accessed through the femoral vein.

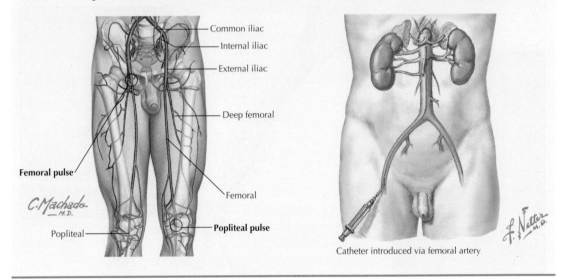

Catheter introduced via femoral artery

---

is supplied by the obturator artery. These vessels form anastomoses around the hip and, in the case of the femoral-popliteal artery, around the knee as well (see Fig. 6-13).

Thigh in Cross Section

Cross sections of the thigh show the three compartments and their respective muscles and neurovascular elements (Fig. 6-14). Lateral, medial, and posterior intermuscular septae divide the thigh into the following three sections:

- **Anterior compartment:** contains muscles that primarily extend the leg at the knee and are innervated by the femoral nerve.
- **Medial compartment:** contains muscles that primarily adduct the thigh at the hip and are innervated largely by the obturator nerve.
- **Posterior compartment:** contains muscles that primarily extend the thigh at the hip and flex the leg at the knee and are innervated by the sciatic nerve (tibial portion).

Refer to the muscle tables to note several exceptions to these general divisions. However, *learning the primary action and general innervation of the muscles by functional compartments will help you organize your study.* Also, note that the large sciatic nerve usually begins to separate into its two component nerves—the tibial nerve and the common fibular nerve—in the thigh, although this separation may occur proximally in the gluteal region in some cases.

6. LEG

Bones

The bones of the leg (defined as knee to ankle) are the medially placed **tibia** and lateral **fibula** (Fig. 6-15 and Table 6-11). The tibia is weight-bearing in the leg, and the two bones are joined by a fibrous interosseous membrane. The tibia is subcutaneous from the knee to the ankle (our shin) and vulnerable to injury along its length. The fibula functions primarily for muscle attachments,

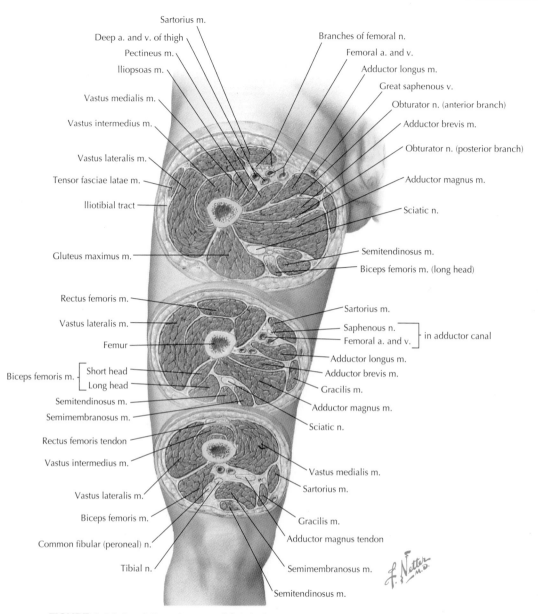

FIGURE 6-14 Serial Cross Sections of the Thigh. (From *Atlas of human anatomy*, ed 6, Plate 492.)

TABLE 6-11 Features of the Tibia and Fibula			
FEATURE	**CHARACTERISTICS**	**FEATURE**	**CHARACTERISTICS**
Tibia		Medial malleolus	Prominence on medial aspect of ankle
Long bone	Large, weight-bearing bone		
Proximal facets	Large plateau for articulation with femoral condyles	**Fibula**	
Tibial tuberosity	Insertion site for patellar ligament	Long bone	Slender bone, primarily for muscle attachment
Inferior articular surface	Surface for cupping talus at ankle joint	Neck	Possible damage to common fibular nerve if fracture occurs here

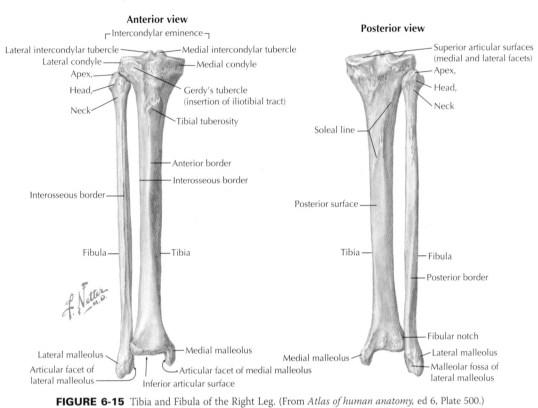

Anterior view

Intercondylar eminence

Lateral intercondylar tubercle — — Medial intercondylar tubercle
Lateral condyle — — Medial condyle
Apex, —
Head, — — Gerdy's tubercle
Neck — (insertion of iliotibial tract)

— Tibial tuberosity

— Anterior border
— Interosseous border

Interosseous border —

Fibula — — Tibia

Lateral malleolus — — Medial malleolus
Articular facet of — — Articular facet of medial malleolus
lateral malleolus — Inferior articular surface

Posterior view

— Superior articular surfaces
(medial and lateral facets)
— Apex,
— Head,
— Neck

Soleal line —

Posterior surface —

Tibia — — Fibula
— Posterior border

— Fibular notch
Medial malleolus — — Lateral malleolus
— Malleolar fossa of
lateral malleolus

FIGURE 6-15 Tibia and Fibula of the Right Leg. (From *Atlas of human anatomy*, ed 6, Plate 500.)

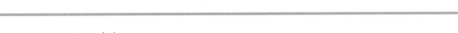

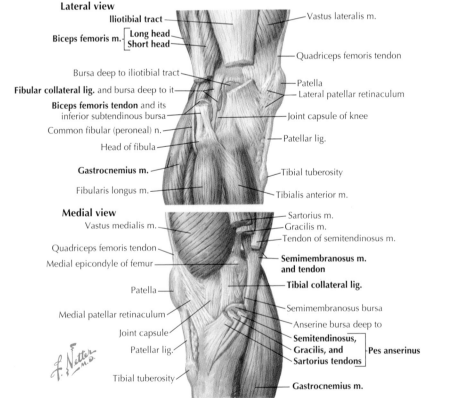

Lateral view

Iliotibial tract — — Vastus lateralis m.
Biceps femoris m. [**Long head**
Short head] — — Quadriceps femoris tendon

Bursa deep to iliotibial tract —
Fibular collateral lig. and bursa deep to it — — Patella
Biceps femoris tendon and its — Lateral patellar retinaculum
inferior subtendinous bursa —
Common fibular (peroneal) n. — — Joint capsule of knee
Head of fibula — — Patellar lig.

Gastrocnemius m. —
Fibularis longus m. — — Tibial tuberosity
— Tibialis anterior m.

Medial view
Vastus medialis m. — — Sartorius m.
— Gracilis m.
Quadriceps femoris tendon — — Tendon of semitendinosus m.
Medial epicondyle of femur — **Semimembranosus m.**
and tendon

Patella — **Tibial collateral lig.**

Medial patellar retinaculum — — Semimembranosus bursa
Joint capsule — — Anserine bursa deep to
Patellar lig. — **Semitendinosus,**
Gracilis, and] Pes anserinus
Sartorius tendons
Tibial tuberosity — — **Gastrocnemius m.**

FIGURE 6-16 Muscle Tendon Support of the Knee. (From *Atlas of human anatomy*, ed 6, Plate 493.)

forms part of the ankle joint, and acts as a pulley for the fibularis longus and fibularis brevis muscle tendons.

Knee Joint

The knee is the most sophisticated joint in the body and the largest of the synovial joints. It participates in flexion, extension, and some gliding and rotation when flexed. With full extension, the femur rotates medially on the tibia, the supporting ligaments tighten, and the knee is locked into position. The knee consists of the articulation between the femur and the tibia (biaxial condylar synovial joint) and between the patella and the femur.

Features of the knee joint are shown in Figures 6-16 (muscle tendon support), 6-17 and 6-19 (ligaments), 6-18 (radiographs), and 6-19 (bursae) and are summarized in Tables 6-12 and 6-13. Because

of the number of muscle-tendon units running across the knee joint, several bursae protect the underlying structures from friction (Fig. 6-19). The first four of the bursae listed in Table 6-14 also communicate with the synovial cavity of the knee joint. The vascular supply to the knee primarily arises from genicular branches of the popliteal artery, the inferior continuation of the femoral artery (Fig. 6-13).

The innervation to the knee joint is via articular branches from the femoral, obturator, tibial, and common fibular nerves.

The proximal (superior) tibiofibular joint is a plane synovial joint between the fibular head and the lateral condyle of the tibia (Fig. 6-20). The joint is stabilized by a wider and stronger anterior ligament and a narrow weaker posterior ligament; this joint allows for some minimal gliding movement.

Text continued on p. 305.

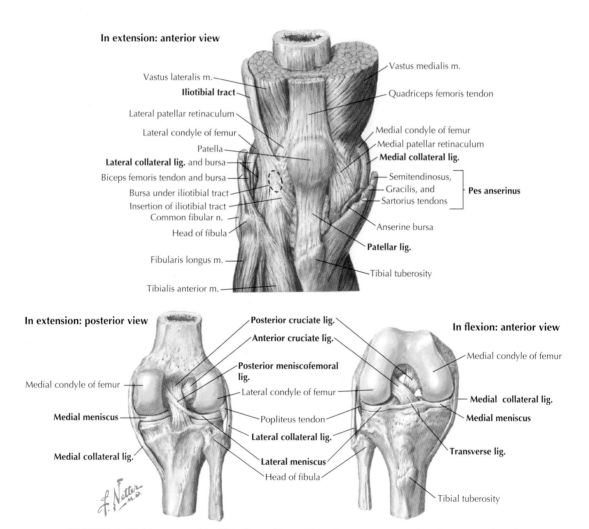

FIGURE 6-17 Ligaments of the Right Knee. (From *Atlas of human anatomy*, ed 6, Plates 494 and 496.)

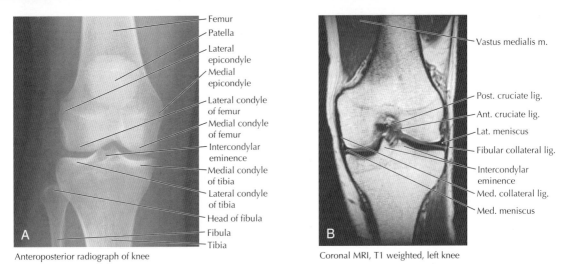

Femur
Patella
Lateral epicondyle
Medial epicondyle
Lateral condyle of femur
Medial condyle of femur
Intercondylar eminence
Medial condyle of tibia
Lateral condyle of tibia
Head of fibula
Fibula
Tibia

Anteroposterior radiograph of knee

Vastus medialis m.
Post. cruciate lig.
Ant. cruciate lig.
Lat. meniscus
Fibular collateral lig.
Intercondylar eminence
Med. collateral lig.
Med. meniscus

Coronal MRI, T1 weighted, left knee

FIGURE 6-18 Radiograph and MR Image of Knee. (**A** from *Atlas of human anatomy*, ed 6, Plate 497; **B** from Bo W et al: *Basic atlas of sectional anatomy*, ed 4, Philadelphia, Saunders, 2007.)

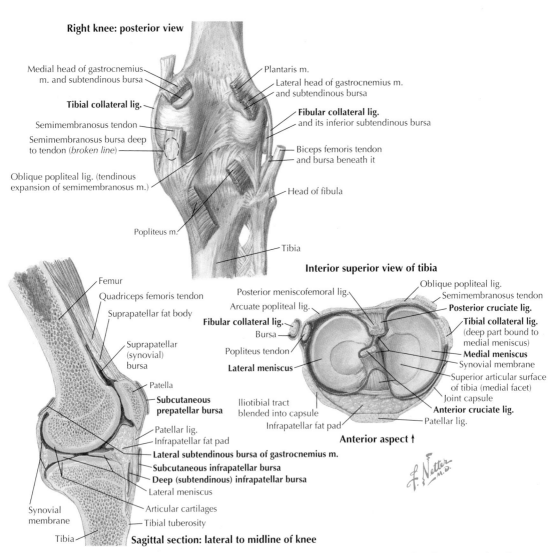

Right knee: posterior view

Medial head of gastrocnemius m. and subtendinous bursa
Tibial collateral lig.
Semimembranosus tendon
Semimembranosus bursa deep to tendon (*broken line*)
Oblique popliteal lig. (tendinous expansion of semimembranosus m.)
Popliteus m.

Plantaris m.
Lateral head of gastrocnemius m. and subtendinous bursa
Fibular collateral lig. and its inferior subtendinous bursa
Biceps femoris tendon and bursa beneath it
Head of fibula
Tibia

Interior superior view of tibia

Femur
Quadriceps femoris tendon
Suprapatellar fat body
Suprapatellar (synovial) bursa
Patella
Subcutaneous prepatellar bursa
Patellar lig.
Infrapatellar fat pad
Lateral subtendinous bursa of gastrocnemius m.
Subcutaneous infrapatellar bursa
Deep (subtendinous) infrapatellar bursa
Lateral meniscus
Synovial membrane
Articular cartilages
Tibial tuberosity
Tibia

Posterior meniscofemoral lig.
Arcuate popliteal lig.
Fibular collateral lig.
Bursa
Popliteus tendon
Lateral meniscus
Iliotibial tract blended into capsule
Infrapatellar fat pad

Oblique popliteal lig.
Semimembranosus tendon
Posterior cruciate lig.
Tibial collateral lig. (deep part bound to medial meniscus)
Medial meniscus
Synovial membrane
Superior articular surface of tibia (medial facet)
Joint capsule
Anterior cruciate lig.
Patellar lig.

Anterior aspect †

Sagittal section: lateral to midline of knee

FIGURE 6-19 Knee Joint Ligaments and Bursae. (From *Atlas of human anatomy*, ed 6, Plates 495 and 498.)

TABLE 6-12 Muscle Tendon Support of the Knee

MUSCLE AND TENDON	COMMENT
Lateral Aspect	
Biceps femoris	Posterolateral support, attaching to fibular head
Gastrocnemius (lateral)	Support somewhat more posteriorly
Iliotibial tract	Lateral support and stabilization
Popliteus	Located posterolaterally beneath the fibular collateral ligament
Medial Aspect	
Semimembranosus	Posteromedial support
Gastrocnemius (medial)	Support somewhat more posteriorly
Pes anserinus	Semitendinosus, gracilis, and sartorius (looks like a goose's foot) tendons, attaching to medial tibial condyle

TABLE 6-14 Features of the Knee Joint Bursae

BURSA	LOCATION
Suprapatellar	Between quadriceps tendon and femur
Popliteus	Between popliteus tendon and lateral tibial condyle
Anserine	Between pes anserinus and tibia and tibial collateral ligament
Subtendinous	Deep to heads of the gastrocnemius muscles
Semimembranosus	Deep to the tendon of the semimembranosus muscle
Prepatellar	Between skin and patella
Subcutaneous infrapatellar	Between skin and tibia
Deep infrapatellar	Between patellar ligament and tibia

TABLE 6-13 Ligaments of the Knee

LIGAMENT	ATTACHMENT	COMMENT
Knee (Biaxial Condylar Synovial) Joint		
Capsule	Surrounds femoral and tibial condyles and patella	Is fibrous, weak (offers little support); flexion, extension, some gliding and medial rotation
Extracapsular Ligaments		
Tibial collateral	Medial femoral epicondyle to medial tibial condyle	Limits extension and abduction of leg; attached to medial meniscus
Fibular collateral	Lateral femoral epicondyle to fibular head	Limits extension and adduction of leg; overlies popliteus tendon
Patellar	Patella to tibial tuberosity	Acts in extension of quadriceps tendon
Arcuate popliteal	Fibular head to capsule	Passes over popliteus muscle
Oblique popliteal	Semimembranosus tendon to posterior knee	Limits hyperextension and lateral rotation
Intracapsular Ligaments		
Medial meniscus	Interarticular area of tibia, lies over medial facet, attached to tibial collateral	Is semicircular (C-shaped); acts as cushion; often torn
Lateral meniscus	Interarticular area of tibia, lies over lateral facet	Is more circular and smaller than medial meniscus; acts as cushion
Anterior cruciate	Anterior intercondylar tibia to lateral femoral condyle	Prevents posterior slipping of femur on tibia; torn in hyperextension
Posterior cruciate	Posterior intercondylar tibia to medial femoral condyle	Prevents anterior slipping of femur on tibia; shorter and stronger than anterior cruciate
Transverse	Anterior aspect of menisci	Binds and stabilizes menisci
Posterior meniscofemoral (of Wrisberg)	Posterior lateral meniscus to medial femoral condyle	Is strong
Patellofemoral (Biaxial Synovial Saddle) Joint		
Quadriceps tendon	Muscles to superior patella	Is part of extension mechanism
Patellar	Patella to tibial tuberosity	Acts in extension of quadriceps tendon; patella stabilized by medial and lateral ligament (retinaculum) attachment to tibia and femur

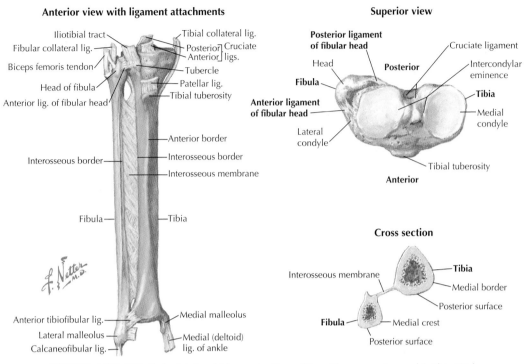

Anterior view with ligament attachments

- Iliotibial tract
- Fibular collateral lig.
- Biceps femoris tendon
- Head of fibula
- Anterior lig. of fibular head
- Tibial collateral lig.
- Posterior ⎤ Cruciate
- Anterior ⎦ ligs.
- Tubercle
- Patellar lig.
- Tibial tuberosity
- Anterior border
- Interosseous border
- Interosseous border
- Interosseous membrane
- Fibula
- Tibia
- Anterior tibiofibular lig.
- Lateral malleolus
- Calcaneofibular lig.
- Medial malleolus
- Medial (deltoid) lig. of ankle

Superior view

- Posterior ligament of fibular head
- Head
- Fibula
- Anterior ligament of fibular head
- Lateral condyle
- Posterior
- Cruciate ligament
- Intercondylar eminence
- Tibia
- Medial condyle
- Tibial tuberosity
- Anterior

Cross section

- Interosseous membrane
- Fibula
- Medial crest
- Posterior surface
- Tibia
- Medial border
- Posterior surface

FIGURE 6-20 Tibiofibular Joint and Ligaments. (From *Atlas of human anatomy*, ed 6, Plate 501.)

Clinical Focus 6-12

Multiple Myeloma

Multiple myeloma, a tumor of plasma cells, is the most malignant type of primary bone tumor. This painful tumor is sensitive to radiation therapy, and newer chemotherapeutic agents and bone marrow transplantation offer hope for improved survival. Fever, weight loss, fatigue, anemia, thrombocytopenia, and renal failure are associated with this cancer, which usually occurs in middle age.

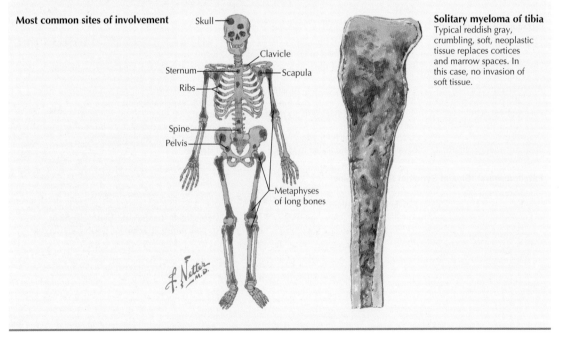

Most common sites of involvement

- Skull
- Clavicle
- Sternum
- Scapula
- Ribs
- Spine
- Pelvis
- Metaphyses of long bones

Solitary myeloma of tibia
Typical reddish gray, crumbling, soft, neoplastic tissue replaces cortices and marrow spaces. In this case, no invasion of soft tissue.

Clinical Focus 6-13

Tibial Fractures

Six types of tibial plateau fractures are recognized, most of which involve the lateral tibial condyle (plateau). Most result from direct trauma and, because they involve the articular surface, must be stabilized. Fractures of the tibial shaft are the most common fractures of a long bone. Because the tibia is largely subcutaneous along its medial border, many of these fractures are open injuries. Often, both tibia and fibula are fractured.

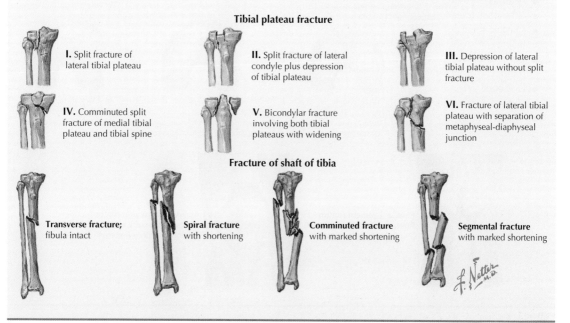

Tibial plateau fracture

I. Split fracture of lateral tibial plateau

II. Split fracture of lateral condyle plus depression of tibial plateau

III. Depression of lateral tibial plateau without split fracture

IV. Comminuted split fracture of medial tibial plateau and tibial spine

V. Bicondylar fracture involving both tibial plateaus with widening

VI. Fracture of lateral tibial plateau with separation of metaphyseal-diaphyseal junction

Fracture of shaft of tibia

Transverse fracture; fibula intact

Spiral fracture with shortening

Comminuted fracture with marked shortening

Segmental fracture with marked shortening

Clinical Focus 6-14

Deep Tendon Reflexes

A brisk tap to a partially stretched muscle tendon near its point of insertion elicits a deep tendon (muscle stretch) reflex (DTR) that is dependent on the following:

- Intact afferent (sensory) nerve fibers
- Normal functional synapses in the spinal cord at the appropriate level
- Intact efferent (motor) nerve fibers
- Normal functional neuromuscular junctions on the tapped muscle
- Normal muscle fiber functioning (contraction)

Characteristically, the DTR usually involves only several spinal cord segments (and their afferent and efferent nerve fibers). If a pathologic process is involved at the level tested, the reflex may be weak or absent, requiring further testing to determine where along the pathway the lesion occurred. For the lower limb, you should know the following segmental levels for the DTR:

- **Patellar ligament (tendon) reflex L3 and L4**
- **Calcaneal tendon reflex S1 and S2**

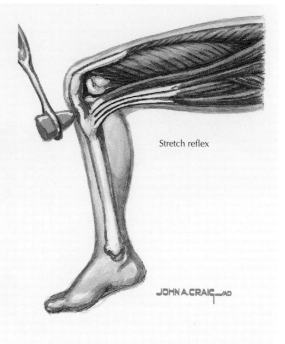

Stretch reflex

Patellar Injuries

Subluxation of the patella, usually laterally, is a fairly common occurrence, especially in adolescent girls and young women. It often presents with tenderness along the medial patellar aspect and atrophy of the quadriceps tendon, especially the oblique portion medially derived from the vastus medialis. Patellar ligament rupture usually occurs just inferior to the patella as a result of direct trauma in younger people. Quadriceps tendon rupture occurs mostly in older individuals, from either minor trauma or age-related degenerative changes, including the following:

- Arthritis
- Arteriosclerosis
- Chronic renal failure
- Corticosteroid therapy
- Diabetes
- Hyperparathyroidism
- Gout

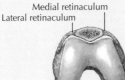
Medial retinaculum
Lateral retinaculum

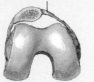
Medial retinaculum stretched

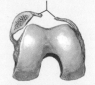
Medial retinaculum torn

Skyline view. Normally, patella rides in groove between medial and lateral femoral condyles.

In subluxation, patella deviates laterally because of weakness of vastus medialis muscle and tightness of lateral retinaculum.

In dislocation, patella is displaced completely out of intercondylar groove.

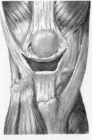
Patellar ligament rupture
Rupture of patellar ligament at inferior margin of patella

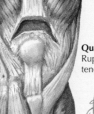
Quadriceps tendon rupture
Rupture of quadriceps femoris tendon at superior margin of patella

Rupture of the Anterior Cruciate Ligament

Rupture of the anterior cruciate ligament (ACL) is a common athletic injury usually related to sharp turns, when the knee is twisted while the foot is firmly on the ground. The patient may hear a popping sound and feel a tearing sensation associated with acute pain. Joint stability can be assessed by using the Lachman and anterior drawer tests. With an ACL injury, the tibia moves anteriorly (the ACL normally limits knee hyperextension) in the anterior drawer test and back and forth in the Lachman test.

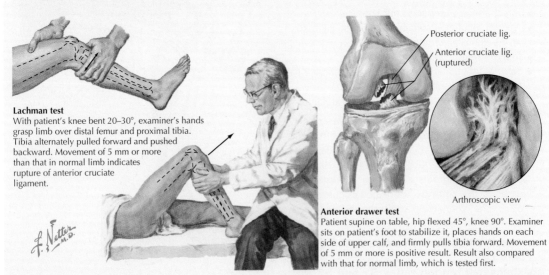

Posterior cruciate lig.

Anterior cruciate lig. (ruptured)

Lachman test
With patient's knee bent 20–30°, examiner's hands grasp limb over distal femur and proximal tibia. Tibia alternately pulled forward and pushed backward. Movement of 5 mm or more than that in normal limb indicates rupture of anterior cruciate ligament.

Arthroscopic view

Anterior drawer test
Patient supine on table, hip flexed 45°, knee 90°. Examiner sits on patient's foot to stabilize it, places hands on each side of upper calf, and firmly pulls tibia forward. Movement of 5 mm or more is positive result. Result also compared with that for normal limb, which is tested first.

Sprains of the Knee Ligaments

Ligament injuries (sprains) of the knee are common in athletes and can be characterized as:

- First degree: stretched ligament with little or no tearing
- Second degree: partial tearing of the ligament with joint laxity
- Third degree: complete rupture of the ligament, resulting in an unstable joint

Damage to the tibial collateral ligament may also involve a tear of the medial meniscus, as the meniscus is attached to the ligament. The "unhappy triad"—tears of these structures and the ACL—is usually the result of a direct blow to the lateral aspect of the knee with the foot on the ground.

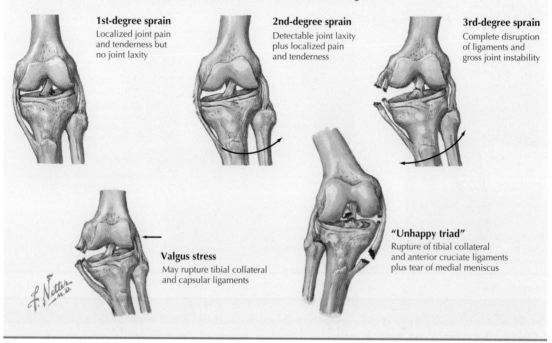

1st-degree sprain
Localized joint pain and tenderness but no joint laxity

2nd-degree sprain
Detectable joint laxity plus localized pain and tenderness

3rd-degree sprain
Complete disruption of ligaments and gross joint instability

Valgus stress
May rupture tibial collateral and capsular ligaments

"Unhappy triad"
Rupture of tibial collateral and anterior cruciate ligaments plus tear of medial meniscus

Tears of the Meniscus

The fibrocartilaginous menisci are often torn when the knee undergoes a twisting injury. Patients complain of pain at the joint line, and the involved knee "gives way" when flexed or extended. Rupture of the tibial collateral ligament often involves a tear of the medial meniscus because the ligament and meniscus are attached.

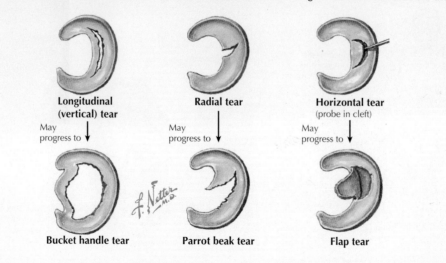

Longitudinal (vertical) tear
May progress to

Radial tear
May progress to

Horizontal tear
(probe in cleft)
May progress to

Bucket handle tear

Parrot beak tear

Flap tear

Osgood-Schlatter Disease

Osgood-Schlatter disease (OSD) is a partial avulsion of the tibial tuberosity. During normal fetal development, the tuberosity develops as a distinct anterior segment of the epiphysis of the proximal tibia. After birth, this segment develops its own growth plate composed mostly of fibrocartilage instead of hyaline cartilage, the fibrocartilage perhaps serving as a means to handle the tensile stress placed on the tuberosity by the patellar ligament. The tuberosity normally ossifies and joins with the tibial epiphysis, but in OSD, repetitive stress on the tuberosity may cause it to separate (avulse) from the tibia. The avulsed fragment continues to grow, with the intervening space filled with new bone or fibrous connective tissue, so that the tibial tuberosity is enlarged. At times, a painful prominence occurs. OSD is usually more common in children who engage in vigorous physical activity than in less active children.

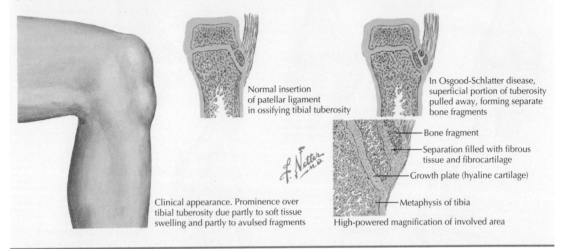

Normal insertion of patellar ligament in ossifying tibial tuberosity

In Osgood-Schlatter disease, superficial portion of tuberosity pulled away, forming separate bone fragments

Bone fragment

Separation filled with fibrous tissue and fibrocartilage

Growth plate (hyaline cartilage)

Metaphysis of tibia

Clinical appearance. Prominence over tibial tuberosity due partly to soft tissue swelling and partly to avulsed fragments

High-powered magnification of involved area

Osteoarthritis of the Knee

As with arthritis of the hip, osteoarthritis of the knee is a painful condition associated with activity, although other causes may also precipitate painful episodes, including changes in the weather. Stiffness after inactivity and decreased range of motion are common. With time, subluxation of the knee may occur with a varus (bowleg) deformity.

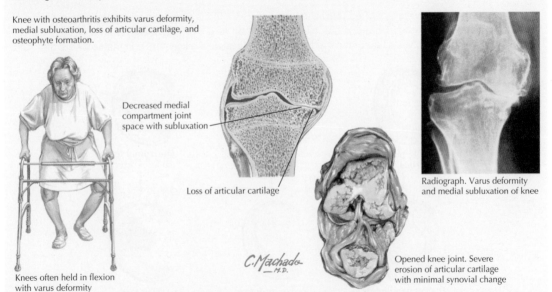

Knee with osteoarthritis exhibits varus deformity, medial subluxation, loss of articular cartilage, and osteophyte formation.

Decreased medial compartment joint space with subluxation

Loss of articular cartilage

Radiograph. Varus deformity and medial subluxation of knee

Opened knee joint. Severe erosion of articular cartilage with minimal synovial change

Knees often held in flexion with varus deformity

Clinical Focus 6-21

Septic Bursitis and Arthritis

Humans have more than 150 bursae in their subcutaneous tissues. With increased irritation, these bursae, which are lined with synovium and contain synovial fluid, produce more fluid until significant swelling and bacterial infection occur. The result is septic bursitis, characterized by the following:

- Heat over the affected area
- Swelling
- Local tenderness
- Limited range of motion

Septic arthritis occurs when infection gains entry to the joint space. If initial therapy fails, surgical debridement and lengthy antibiotic treatment may be needed.

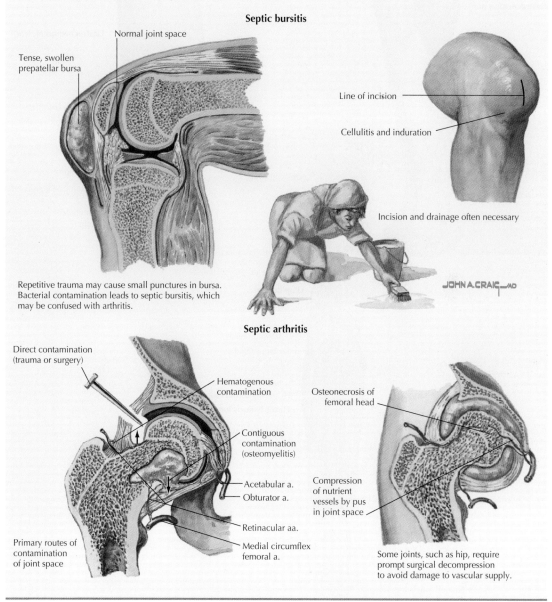

Septic bursitis

Normal joint space

Tense, swollen prepatellar bursa

Line of incision

Cellulitis and induration

Incision and drainage often necessary

Repetitive trauma may cause small punctures in bursa. Bacterial contamination leads to septic bursitis, which may be confused with arthritis.

JOHN A. CRAIG—MD

Septic arthritis

Direct contamination (trauma or surgery)

Hematogenous contamination

Osteonecrosis of femoral head

Contiguous contamination (osteomyelitis)

Acetabular a.

Obturator a.

Compression of nutrient vessels by pus in joint space

Retinacular aa.

Primary routes of contamination of joint space

Medial circumflex femoral a.

Some joints, such as hip, require prompt surgical decompression to avoid damage to vascular supply.

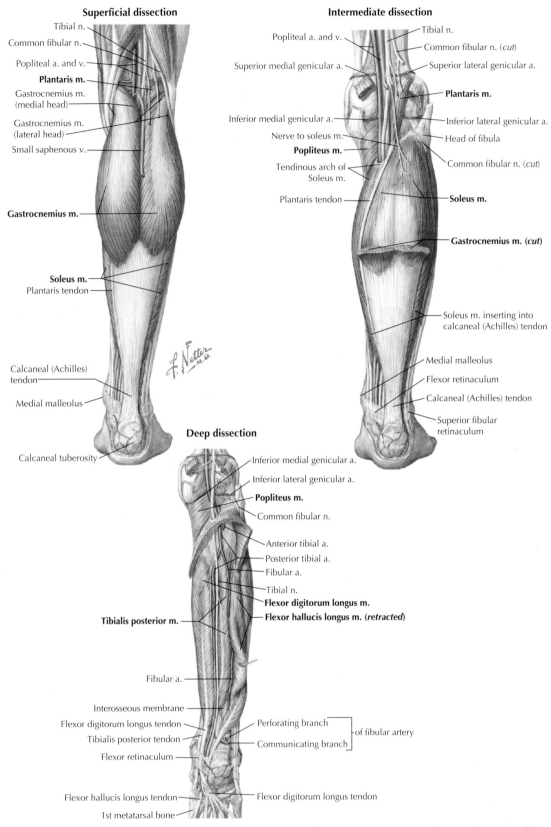

Superficial dissection

Tibial n.
Common fibular n.
Popliteal a. and v.
Plantaris m.
Gastrocnemius m. (medial head)
Gastrocnemius m. (lateral head)
Small saphenous v.

Gastrocnemius m.

Soleus m.
Plantaris tendon

Calcaneal (Achilles) tendon
Medial malleolus

Calcaneal tuberosity

Intermediate dissection

Popliteal a. and v.
Superior medial genicular a.

Inferior medial genicular a.
Nerve to soleus m.
Popliteus m.
Tendinous arch of Soleus m.
Plantaris tendon

Tibial n.
Common fibular n. (*cut*)
Superior lateral genicular a.
Plantaris m.
Inferior lateral genicular a.
Head of fibula
Common fibular n. (*cut*)
Soleus m.

Gastrocnemius m. (*cut*)

Soleus m. inserting into calcaneal (Achilles) tendon
Medial malleolus
Flexor retinaculum
Calcaneal (Achilles) tendon
Superior fibular retinaculum

Deep dissection

Inferior medial genicular a.
Inferior lateral genicular a.
Popliteus m.
Common fibular n.
Anterior tibial a.
Posterior tibial a.
Fibular a.
Tibial n.
Flexor digitorum longus m.
Flexor hallucis longus m. (*retracted*)

Tibialis posterior m.

Fibular a.

Interosseous membrane
Flexor digitorum longus tendon
Tibialis posterior tendon
Flexor retinaculum

Perforating branch
Communicating branch
} of fibular artery

Flexor hallucis longus tendon
1st metatarsal bone
Flexor digitorum longus tendon

FIGURE 6-21 Posterior Compartment Leg Muscles (Superficial and Deep Group), Vessels, and Nerves. (From *Atlas of human anatomy,* ed 6, Plates 503 to 505.)

Popliteal Fossa

The popliteal fossa is a "diamond-shaped" region behind the knee and contains the popliteal vessels and the tibial and common fibular nerves (Fig. 6-21). This fossa marks the transition region between the thigh and the leg, where the vascular components of the thigh pass to the flexor side of the knee joint. (At most joints, the neurovascular bundles pass on the flexor side of the joint.) The

superior margins of this diamond-shaped fossa are formed medially by the distal portions of the semitendinosus and semimembranosus muscles and laterally by the distal end of the long head of the biceps femoris muscle. The lower margins of the diamond are formed medially by the medial head of the gastrocnemius muscle and laterally by the plantaris and lateral head of the gastrocnemius muscles (see Figs. 6-12 and 6-21). The small

---

Clinical Focus 6-22
Shin Splints

Shin splints cause pain along the inner distal two thirds of the tibial shaft. The syndrome is common in athletes. The primary cause is repetitive pulling of the tibialis posterior tendon as one pushes off the foot during running. Stress on the muscle occurs at its attachment to the tibia and interosseous membrane. Chronic conditions can produce periostitis and bone remodeling or can lead to stress fractures. Pain usually begins as soreness after running that worsens and then occurs while walking or climbing stairs.

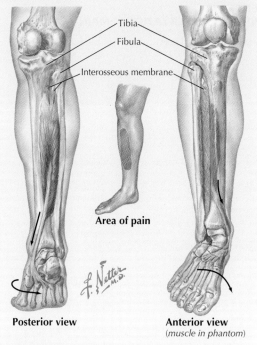

Tibia

Fibula

Interosseous membrane

Area of pain

Posterior view   **Anterior view**
                          (muscle in phantom)

Tibialis posterior muscle originates at posterior surface of tibia, interosseous membrane, and fibula and inserts on undersurface of navicular bone, cuboid, all three cuneiform bones, and 2nd, 3rd, and 4th metatarsal bones. Upper arrows indicate direction of excessive traction of tendon on tibial periosteum and interosseous membrane caused by hypereversion (lower arrows).

Clinical Focus 6-23
Osteosarcoma of the Tibia

Osteosarcoma is the most common malignant bone tumor of mesenchymal origin. It is more common in males and usually occurs before 30 years of age, often in the distal femur or proximal tibia. Other sites include the proximal humerus, proximal femur, and pelvis. Most tumors appear in the metaphysis of long bones at areas of greatest growth. The tumors often invade cortical bone in this region because of its rich vascular supply and then infiltrate surrounding soft tissue. These tumors are aggressive and require immediate attention.

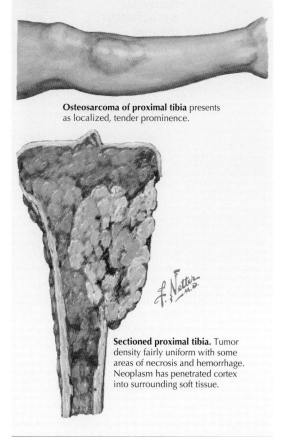

Osteosarcoma of proximal tibia presents as localized, tender prominence.

Sectioned proximal tibia. Tumor density fairly uniform with some areas of necrosis and hemorrhage. Neoplasm has penetrated cortex into surrounding soft tissue.

saphenous vein courses subcutaneously upward toward the knee in the midline of the calf and drains into the popliteal vein (see Fig. 6-2).

Posterior Compartment Leg Muscles, Vessels, and Nerves

The posterior compartment leg muscles are arranged into a superficial group (gastrocnemius, plantaris, soleus) and a deep group (remaining posterior compartment muscles). These muscles exhibit the following general features (Fig. 6-21 and Table 6-15):

- Are primarily flexors of the foot at the ankle (plantarflexion) and flexors of the toes.
- Several can flex the leg at the knee or invert the foot.
- Are innervated by the **tibial nerve.**
- Are supplied by the posterior tibial artery (the popliteal artery divides into the anterior and posterior tibial arteries) with some supply from the fibular artery (a branch of the posterior tibial artery).

Anterior Compartment Leg Muscles, Vessels, and Nerves

The muscles of the anterior compartment exhibit the following features (Fig. 6-22 and Table 6-16):

- Are primarily extensors of the foot at the ankle (dorsiflexion) and extensors of the toes.
- Several can invert the foot, and one muscle (fibularis tertius) can weakly evert the foot.
- Are innervated by the **deep fibular nerve** (the common fibular nerve divides into the superficial and deep branches).
- Are supplied by the anterior tibial artery.

Lateral Compartment Leg Muscles, Vessels, and Nerves

The two muscles of the lateral compartment exhibit the following features (Fig. 6-23 and Table 6-17):

- Are primarily able to evert the foot, and can weakly plantarflex the foot at the ankle.

TABLE 6-15 Posterior Compartment Leg Muscles and Nerves

MUSCLE	PROXIMAL ATTACHMENT (ORIGIN)	DISTAL ATTACHMENT (INSERTION)	INNERVATION	MAIN ACTIONS
Gastrocnemius	*Lateral head:* lateral aspect of lateral condyle of femur *Medial head:* popliteal surface of femur, superior to medial condyle	Posterior surface of calcaneus via calcaneal tendon	Tibial nerve (S1-S2)	Plantarflexes foot at ankle; raises heel during walking; flexes leg at knee joint
Soleus	Posterior aspect of head of fibula, superior fourth of posterior surface of fibula, soleal line and medial border of tibia	Posterior surface of calcaneus via calcaneal tendon	Tibial nerve (S1-S2)	Plantarflexes foot at ankle; steadies leg on foot
Plantaris	Inferior end of lateral supracondylar line of femur and oblique popliteal ligament	Posterior surface of calcaneus via calcaneal tendon	Tibial nerve (L5-S1)	Weakly assists gastrocnemius in plantarflexing foot at ankle and flexing knee
Popliteus	Lateral condyle of femur and lateral meniscus	Posterior surface of tibia, superior to soleal line	Tibial nerve (L4-S1)	Weakly flexes leg at knee and unlocks it (rotates femur)
Flexor hallucis longus	Inferior two thirds of posterior surface of fibula and inferior interosseous membrane	Base of distal phalanx of great toe (big toe)	Tibial nerve (L5-S2)	Flexes great toe at all joints and plantarflexes foot at ankle; supports longitudinal arches of foot
Flexor digitorum longus	Medial part of posterior surface of tibia inferior to soleal line, and from fascia covering tibialis posterior	Bases of distal phalanges of lateral four digits	Tibial nerve (L5-S1)	Flexes lateral four digits and plantarflexes foot at ankle; supports longitudinal arches of foot
Tibialis posterior	Interosseous membrane, posterior surface of tibia inferior to soleal line, and posterior surface of fibula	Tuberosity of navicular, cuneiform, and cuboid and bases of metatarsals 2, 3, and 4	Tibial nerve (L4-L5)	Plantarflexes foot at ankle and inverts foot

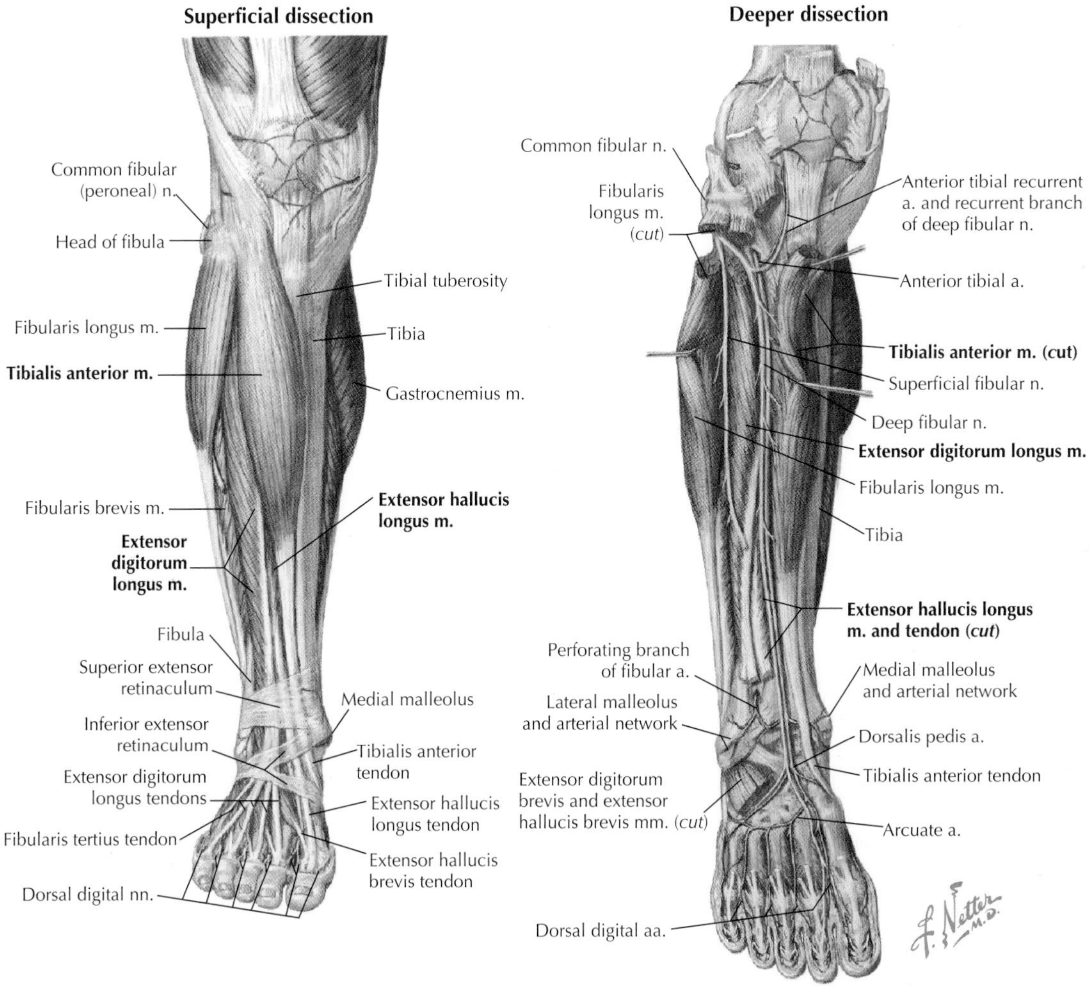

Superficial dissection   Deeper dissection

FIGURE 6-22 Anterior Compartment Leg Muscles, Vessels, and Nerves. (From *Atlas of human anatomy,* ed 6, Plates 507 and 508.)

TABLE 6-16 Anterior Compartment Leg Muscles and Nerves

MUSCLE	PROXIMAL ATTACHMENT (ORIGIN)	DISTAL ATTACHMENT (INSERTION)	INNERVATION	MAIN ACTIONS
Tibialis anterior	Lateral condyle and superior half of lateral tibia and interosseous membrane	Medial and inferior surfaces of medial cuneiform and base of 1st metatarsal	Deep fibular nerve (L4-L5)	Dorsiflexes foot at ankle and inverts foot
Extensor hallucis longus	Middle part of anterior surface of fibula and interosseous membrane	Dorsal aspect of base of distal phalanx of great toe	Deep fibular nerve (L5-S1)	Extends great toe and dorsiflexes foot at ankle
Extensor digitorum longus	Lateral condyle of tibia and superior ¾ of anterior surface of interosseous membrane and fibula	Middle and distal phalanges of lateral four digits	Deep fibular nerve (L5-S1)	Extends lateral four digits and dorsiflexes foot at ankle
Fibularis tertius	Inferior third of anterior surface of fibula and interosseous membrane	Dorsum of base of 5th metatarsal	Deep fibular nerve (L5-S1)	Dorsiflexes foot at ankle and aids in eversion of foot

TABLE 6-17 Lateral Compartment Leg Muscles and Nerves

MUSCLE	PROXIMAL ATTACHMENT (ORIGIN)	DISTAL ATTACHMENT (INSERTION)	INNERVATION	MAIN ACTIONS
Fibularis longus	Head and superior ⅔ of lateral surface of fibula	Base of 1st metatarsal and medial cuneiform	Superficial fibular nerve (L5-S2)	Everts foot and weakly plantarflexes foot at ankle
Fibularis brevis	Inferior ⅔ of lateral surface of fibula	Dorsal surface of tuberosity on lateral side of 5th metatarsal	Superficial fibular nerve (L5-S2)	Everts foot and weakly plantarflexes foot at ankle

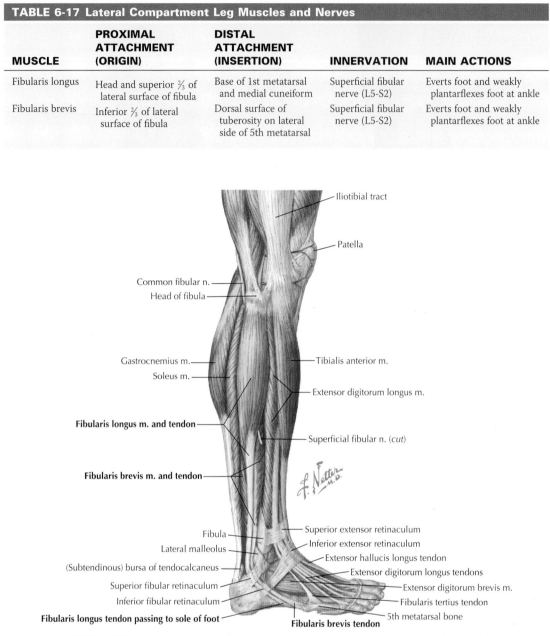

FIGURE 6-23 Lateral Compartment Leg Muscles. (From *Atlas of human anatomy,* ed 6, Plate 506.)

- Are innervated by the **superficial fibular nerve.**
- Are supplied by the fibular artery, a branch of the posterior tibial artery (see Fig. 6-21).

Leg in Cross Section

The interosseous membrane and intermuscular septae divide the leg into three compartments. The posterior compartment is further subdivided into the superficial and deep compartments.

Moreover, the leg is ensheathed in a tight deep fascia, and some of the underlying muscle fibers actually attach to this fascial sleeve. The compartments may be summarized as follows (Fig. 6-24):

- **Posterior compartment:** muscles that plantarflex and invert the foot at the ankle and flex the toes, are innervated by the tibial nerve, and are supplied largely by the posterior tibial artery.

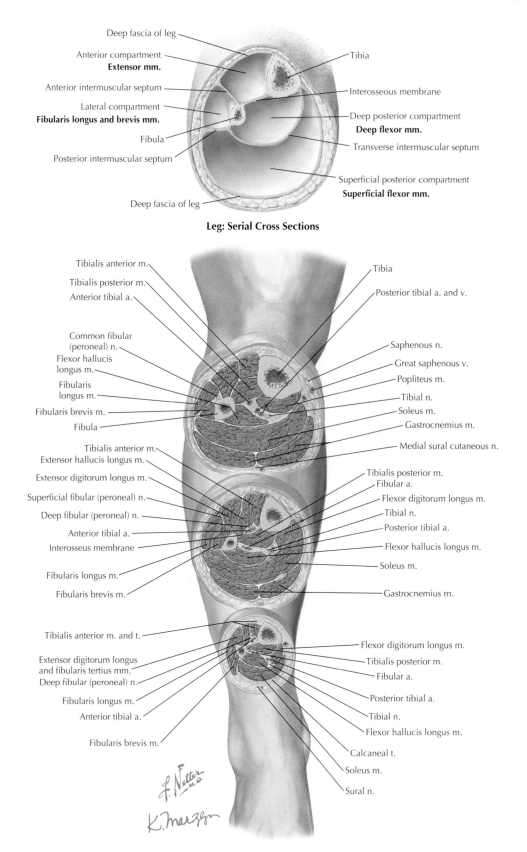

Leg: Serial Cross Sections

FIGURE 6-24 Cross Section of the Right Leg. (From *Atlas of human anatomy,* ed 6, Plate 510.)

Genu Varum and Valgum

The knee of a standing patient should look symmetric and level. The tibia normally has a slight valgus angulation compared with the femur. *Valgus* is used to describe the bone distal to the examined joint; a *valgus angulation* refers to a slight lateral angle. Excessive valgus angulation is called *genu valgum,* or knock-knee, and an excessive varus angulation is called *genu varum,* or bowleg. These deformities occur in growing children and are often related to rickets, skeletal dysplasia, or trauma. Most resolve without treatment.

Two brothers, younger (left) with bowleg (genu varum), older (right) with knock-knee (genu valgum).

Exertional Compartment Syndromes

Anterior (tibial) compartment syndrome (or anterior or lateral shin splints) occurs from excessive contraction of anterior compartment muscles; pain over these muscles radiates down the ankle and dorsum of the foot overlying the extensor tendons. *Lateral compartment syndrome* occurs in people with excessively mobile ankle joints in which hypereversion irritates the lateral compartment muscles. These conditions are usually chronic, and expansion of the compartment may lead to nerve and vessel compression. In the acute syndrome (rapid, unrelenting expansion), the compartment may have to be opened surgically (fasciotomy) to relieve pressure. The **five Ps** of acute anterior compartment syndrome are:

- Pain
- Pallor
- Paresis (footdrop, caused by compression of deep fibular nerve)
- Paresthesia
- Pulselessness (variable)

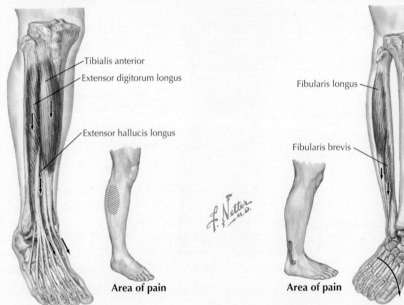

Anterior compartment syndrome

Tibialis anterior
Extensor digitorum longus
Extensor hallucis longus

Area of pain

Lateral compartment syndrome

Fibularis longus
Fibularis brevis

Area of pain

Clinical Focus 6-26

Achilles Tendinitis and Bursitis

Tendinitis of the calcaneal (Achilles) tendon is a painful inflammation that often occurs in runners who run on hills or uneven surfaces. Repetitive stress on the tendon occurs as the heel strikes the ground and when plantarflexion lifts the foot and toes. Tendon rupture is a serious injury, and the avascular tendon heals slowly. Retrocalcaneal bursitis, an inflammation of the subtendinous bursa between the overlying tendon and the calcaneus, presents as a tender area just anterior to the tendon attachment.

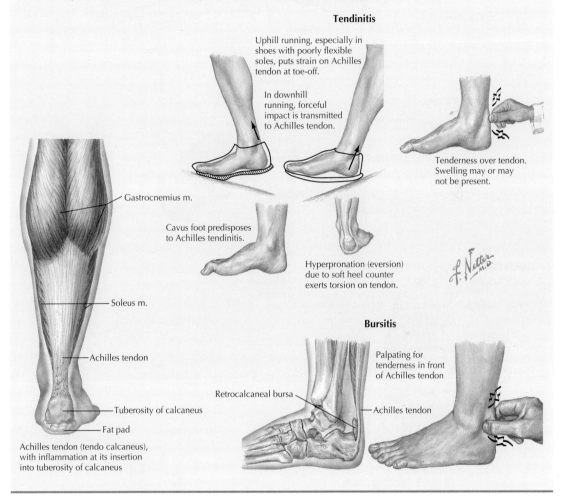

Tendinitis

Uphill running, especially in shoes with poorly flexible soles, puts strain on Achilles tendon at toe-off.

In downhill running, forceful impact is transmitted to Achilles tendon.

Tenderness over tendon. Swelling may or may not be present.

Gastrocnemius m.

Cavus foot predisposes to Achilles tendinitis.

Hyperpronation (eversion) due to soft heel counter exerts torsion on tendon.

Soleus m.

Bursitis

Achilles tendon

Palpating for tenderness in front of Achilles tendon

Retrocalcaneal bursa

Achilles tendon

Tuberosity of calcaneus

Fat pad

Achilles tendon (tendo calcaneus), with inflammation at its insertion into tuberosity of calcaneus

- **Anterior compartment:** muscles that dorsiflex (extend) and invert/evert the foot at the ankle and extend the toes, are innervated by the deep fibular nerve, and are supplied by the anterior tibial artery.
- **Lateral compartment:** muscles that evert the foot at the ankle and weakly plantarflex, are innervated by the superficial fibular nerve, and are supplied by the fibular artery.

7. ANKLE AND FOOT

Bones and Joints

The ankle connects the foot to the leg and is composed of seven **tarsal bones** arranged in a proximal group (talus and calcaneus), intermediate group (navicular), and distal group (cuboid and three cuneiforms). The foot includes five **metatarsals** and the five digits and their **phalanges** (Figs. 6-25 and 6-26 and Table 6-18).

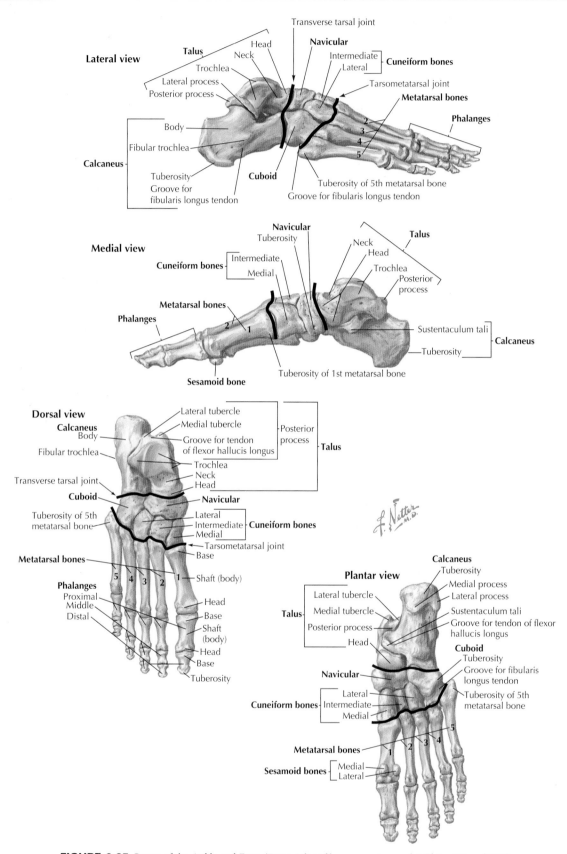

FIGURE 6-25 Bones of the Ankle and Foot. (From *Atlas of human anatomy,* ed 6, Plates 511 and 512.)

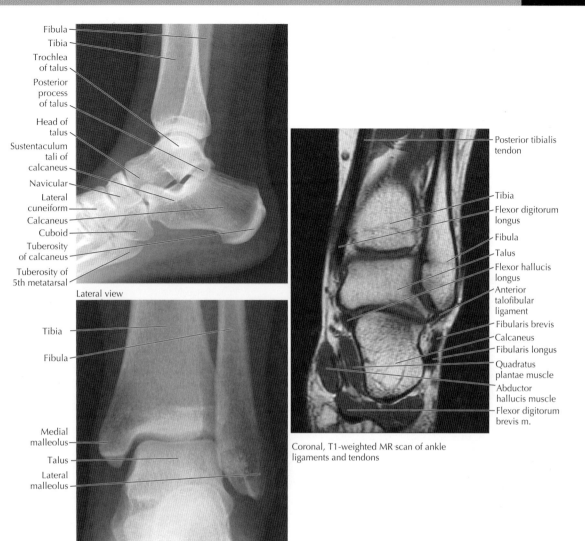

Fibula
Tibia
Trochlea of talus
Posterior process of talus
Head of talus
Sustentaculum tali of calcaneus
Navicular
Lateral cuneiform
Calcaneus
Cuboid
Tuberosity of calcaneus
Tuberosity of 5th metatarsal

Lateral view

Tibia
Fibula

Medial malleolus
Talus
Lateral malleolus

Anterior view

Posterior tibialis tendon
Tibia
Flexor digitorum longus
Fibula
Talus
Flexor hallucis longus
Anterior talofibular ligament
Fibularis brevis
Calcaneus
Fibularis longus
Quadratus plantae muscle
Abductor hallucis muscle
Flexor digitorum brevis m.

Coronal, T1-weighted MR scan of ankle ligaments and tendons

FIGURE 6-26 Radiographs of the Ankle. (Left images from *Atlas of human anatomy,* ed 6, Plate 531; right image from Kelley LL, Petersen C: *Sectional anatomy for imaging professionals,* Philadelphia, Mosby, 2007.)

TABLE 6-18 Features of the Bones of the Ankle and Foot

STRUCTURE	CHARACTERISTICS	STRUCTURE	CHARACTERISTICS
Talus (ankle bone)*	Transfers weight from tibia to foot; no muscle attachment	Groove	For fibularis longus tendon
		*Cuneiforms**	Three wedge-shaped bones
Trochlea	Articulates with tibia and fibula	**Metatarsals**	
Head	Articulates with navicular bone	Numbered 1 to 5, from great toe to little toe	Possess base, shaft, and head
Calcaneus (heel bone)*	Articulates with talus superiorly and cuboid anteriorly		Fibularis brevis tendon inserts on 5th metatarsal
Sustentaculum tali	Medial shelf that supports talar head	Two sesamoid bones	Associated with flexor hallucis brevis tendons
*Navicular**	Boat shaped, between talar head and three cuneiforms	**Phalanges**	
		Three for each digit except great toe	Possess base, shaft, and head
Tuberosity	If large, can cause medial pain in tight-fitting shoe		Termed *proximal, middle,* and *distal*
*Cuboid**	Most lateral tarsal bone		Stubbed 5th toe common injury

*Tarsal bones.

The ankle (talocrural) joint is a uniaxial synovial hinge joint between the talus and the tibia (inferior surface and medial malleolus) and fibula (lateral malleolus). This combination forms a mortise that is then covered by the capsule of the joint and reinforced medially and laterally by ligaments. The ankle joint functions primarily in **plantarflexion** and **dorsiflexion.** Intertarsal, tarsometatarsal, intermetatarsal, metatarsophalangeal, and interphalangeal joints complete the ankle and foot joint complex (Fig. 6-27 and Table 6-19). A variety of movements are possible at these joints, and the ankle and foot can provide a stable but flexible platform for standing, walking, and running. Because of the shape of the talus (the anterior portion of its superior articular aspect is wider), the ankle is more stable when dorsiflexed than when plantarflexed.

The bones of the foot do not lie in a flat plane but are arranged to form the following structures (see Fig. 6-25):

TABLE 6-19 Features of the Joints and Ligaments of the Ankle and Foot

LIGAMENT	ATTACHMENT	COMMENT
Distal Tibiofibular (Fibrous [Syndesmosis]) Joint		
Anterior tibiofibular	Anterior distal tibia and fibula	Runs obliquely
Posterior tibiofibular	Posterior distal tibia and fibula	Is weaker than anterior ligament
Inferior transverse	Medial malleolus to fibula	Is deep continuation of posterior ligament
Talocrural (Uniaxial Synovial Hinge [Ginglymus]) Joint		
Capsule	Tibia and fibula to talus	Functions in plantarflexion and dorsiflexion
Medial (deltoid)	Medial malleolus to talus, calcaneus, and navicular	Limits eversion of foot; maintains medial long arch; has four parts
Lateral (collateral)	Lateral malleolus to talus and calcaneus	Is weak and often sprained; resists inversion of foot; has three parts
Intertarsal Joints (Next Three Joints)		
Talocalcaneal (Subtalar Plane Synovial) Joints		
Capsule	Margins of articulation	Functions in inversion and eversion
Talocalcaneal	Talus to calcaneus	Has medial, lateral, and posterior parts
Interosseous talocalcaneal	Talus to calcaneus	Is strong; binds bones together
Talocalcaneonavicular (Partial Ball-and-Socket Synovial) Joint		
Capsule	Encloses part of joint	Functions in gliding and rotational movements
Plantar calcaneonavicular	Sustentaculum tali to navicular	Is strong plantar support for head of talus (called *spring ligament*)
Dorsal talonavicular	Talus to navicular	Is dorsal support to talus
Calcaneocuboid (Plane Synovial) Joint		
Capsule	Encloses joint	Functions in inversion and eversion
Calcaneocuboid	Calcaneus to cuboid	Are dorsal, plantar (short plantar, strong), and long plantar ligaments
Tarsometatarsal (Plane Synovial) Joints		
Capsule	Encloses joint	Functions in gliding or sliding movements
Tarsometatarsal	Tarsals to metatarsals	Are dorsal, plantar, interosseous ligaments
Intermetatarsal (Plane Synovial) Joints		
Capsule	Base of metatarsals	Provides little movement, supports transverse arch
Intermetatarsal	Adjacent metatarsals	Are dorsal, plantar, interosseous ligaments
Deep transverse	Adjacent metatarsals	Connect adjacent heads
Metatarsophalangeal (Multiaxial Condyloid Synovial) Joints		
Capsule	Encloses joint	Functions in flexion, extension, some abduction and adduction, and circumduction
Collateral	Metatarsal heads to base of proximal phalanges	Are strong ligaments
Plantar (plates)	Plantar side of capsule	Are part of weight-bearing surface
Interphalangeal (Uniaxial Hinge Synovial) Joints		
Capsule	Encloses each joint	Functions in flexion and extension
Collateral	Head of one to base of other	Support the capsule
Plantar (plates)	Plantar side of capsule	Support the capsule

Cuboideonavicular, cuneonavicular, intercuneiform, and cuneocuboid joints: dorsal, plantar, and interosseous ligaments are present, but little movement occurs at these joints, and they have little clinical significance.

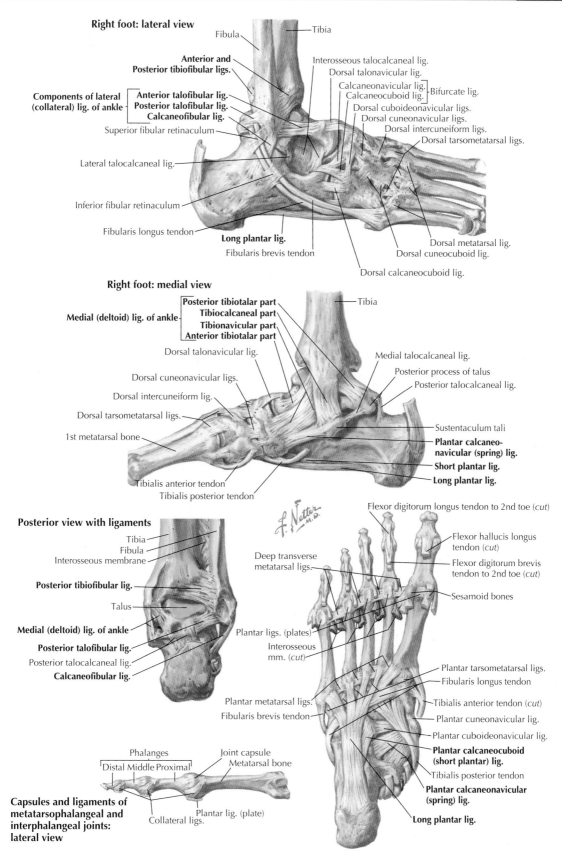

Right foot: lateral view

Fibula
Tibia
Anterior and Posterior tibiofibular ligs.
Interosseous talocalcaneal lig.
Dorsal talonavicular lig.
Calcaneonavicular lig.
Calcaneocuboid lig.
Bifurcate lig.
Components of lateral (collateral) lig. of ankle
Anterior talofibular lig.
Posterior talofibular lig.
Calcaneofibular lig.
Dorsal cuboideonavicular ligs.
Dorsal cuneonavicular ligs.
Dorsal intercuneiform ligs.
Dorsal tarsometatarsal ligs.
Superior fibular retinaculum
Lateral talocalcaneal lig.
Inferior fibular retinaculum
Fibularis longus tendon
Long plantar lig.
Fibularis brevis tendon
Dorsal metatarsal lig.
Dorsal cuneocuboid lig.
Dorsal calcaneocuboid lig.

Right foot: medial view

Medial (deltoid) lig. of ankle
Posterior tibiotalar part
Tibiocalcaneal part
Tibionavicular part
Anterior tibiotalar part
Tibia
Dorsal talonavicular lig.
Medial talocalcaneal lig.
Posterior process of talus
Posterior talocalcaneal lig.
Dorsal cuneonavicular ligs.
Dorsal intercuneiform lig.
Dorsal tarsometatarsal ligs.
1st metatarsal bone
Sustentaculum tali
Plantar calcaneo-navicular (spring) lig.
Short plantar lig.
Long plantar lig.
Tibialis anterior tendon
Tibialis posterior tendon

f. Netter m.d.

Flexor digitorum longus tendon to 2nd toe (cut)
Flexor hallucis longus tendon (cut)
Deep transverse metatarsal ligs.
Flexor digitorum brevis tendon to 2nd toe (cut)
Sesamoid bones

Posterior view with ligaments
Tibia
Fibula
Interosseous membrane
Posterior tibiofibular lig.
Talus
Medial (deltoid) lig. of ankle
Posterior talofibular lig.
Posterior talocalcaneal lig.
Calcaneofibular lig.
Plantar ligs. (plates)
Interosseous mm. (cut)
Plantar metatarsal ligs.
Fibularis brevis tendon
Plantar tarsometatarsal ligs.
Fibularis longus tendon
Tibialis anterior tendon (cut)
Plantar cuneonavicular lig.
Plantar cuboideonavicular lig.
Plantar calcaneocuboid (short plantar) lig.
Tibialis posterior tendon
Plantar calcaneonavicular (spring) lig.
Long plantar lig.

Phalanges
Distal Middle Proximal
Joint capsule
Metatarsal bone
Capsules and ligaments of metatarsophalangeal and interphalangeal joints: lateral view
Collateral ligs.
Plantar lig. (plate)

FIGURE 6-27 Joints and Ligaments of the Ankle and Foot. (From _Atlas of human anatomy_, ed 6, Plates 514 and 515.)

Clinical Focus 6-27

Footdrop

An inability to dorsiflex the foot at the ankle resulting in a foot that cannot be raised is characterized as footdrop. A patient with footdrop must raise the knee during the swing phase of gait to avoid dragging the affected foot on the ground or to avoid tripping. This distinctive gait pattern is called "steppage" gait, and at the end of the swing phase, the foot slaps down to the ground. Typically, footdrop results from injury to the common fibular nerve or deep fibular nerve. The common fibular nerve is vulnerable to injury because it lies superficially beneath the skin where the nerve passes around the fibular neck (coffee table or car bumper height). This nerve also may be affected by a herniated disc that compresses the L5 nerve root (L4-L5 herniated disc; see Chapter 2).

Clinical Focus 6-28

Ankle Sprains

Most ankle sprains involve an inversion injury when the foot is plantarflexed, placing stress on the components of the lateral collateral ligament (see Fig. 6-27). Often the severity of the injury occurs from anterior to posterior, involving first the anterior talofibular ligament, then the calcaneofibular ligament, and finally, if especially severe, the posterior talofibular ligament. The anterior drawer test, in which the tibia is held steady while the heel is pulled anteriorly with the foot in about 10 to 20° of plantarflexion, will confirm the injury to the anterior talofibular ligament if the translation of the foot anteriorly is excessive compared to the uninjured contralateral ankle.

A. Anterior Drawer Test for Instability of Ankle (Test for tear of anterior talofibular ligament)
Examiner applies backward pressure on lower tibia causing anterior subluxation of talus (foot firmly fixed by other hand).

B. Talar-Tilt Sign (Test for tear of calcaneofibular and anterior talofibular ligaments)
Examiner firmly rotates foot in varus. Tear of calcaneofibular ligament permits excessive mobility in this direction (leg firmly fixed by other hand).

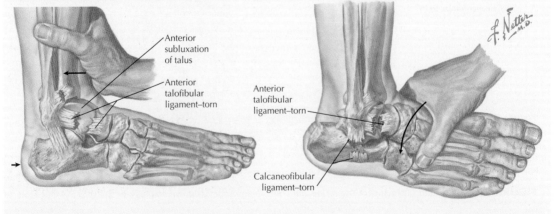

Anterior subluxation of talus

Anterior talofibular ligament–torn

Anterior talofibular ligament–torn

Calcaneofibular ligament–torn

Clinical Focus 6-29

Ankle Fractures

Ankle fractures are common in all age groups and may be grouped according to the Lauge-Hansen classification into the following four types with subdivided stages (pronation is eversion; supination is inversion):

- Supination-adduction (SA): stages I and II; usually stable (I-IV reflect sequence of occurrence)
- Supination–external rotation (SER): stages I to IV; usually unstable or displaced
- Pronation-abduction (PA): stages I to III; perfect symmetrical mortise reduction needed
- Pronation–external rotation (PER): stages I to IV; must also correct fibular length

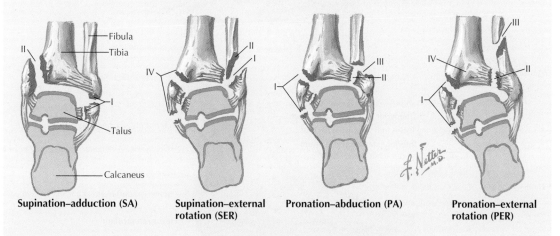

| Supination–adduction (SA) | Supination–external rotation (SER) | Pronation–abduction (PA) | Pronation–external rotation (PER) |

- **Longitudinal arch:** extends from the posterior calcaneus to the metatarsal heads; is higher medially (medial longitudinal arch) than laterally (lateral longitudinal arch).
- **Transverse arch:** extends from medial to lateral across the cuboid, cuneiforms, and base of the metatarsals; is higher medially than laterally.

These arches are supported by muscles and ligaments. Supporting muscles include the tibialis anterior, tibialis posterior, and fibularis longus. Ligaments include the plantar calcaneonavicular (spring) ligament, plantar calcaneocuboid (short plantar) ligament, and long plantar ligament. The plantar aponeurosis also provides some support.

Synovial sheaths provide protection and lubrication for muscle tendons passing from the leg to the foot. Various fibrous bands (retinacula) tether the tendons at the ankle (Fig. 6-28):

- **Flexor retinaculum:** medial malleolus to calcaneus (plantarflexor tendons)
- **Extensor retinaculum:** superior and inferior bands (dorsiflexor tendons)

- **Fibular retinacula:** superior and inferior bands (fibularis tendons of the lateral compartment)

Muscles, Vessels, and Nerves of the Dorsum of the Foot

The dorsum of the foot consists of two intrinsic muscles, the extensor digitorum brevis and the extensor hallucis brevis. These muscles function to extend the toes and are supplied by the anterior tibial artery from the leg via its **dorsalis pedis branch** (Fig. 6-29). A **dorsal venous arch** drains most of the blood from the foot, ultimately carrying the blood to the medially located great saphenous vein or laterally and posteriorly to the small saphenous vein (see Fig. 6-2). The deep fibular nerve, passing from the leg into the foot, innervates the two intrinsic muscles on the dorsum of the foot (see Fig. 6-29).

Muscles, Vessels, and Nerves of the Sole of the Foot

The sole of the foot is protected by a thick layer of the deep fascia called the **plantar aponeurosis,** which extends from the calcaneal tuberosity to

Lateral view

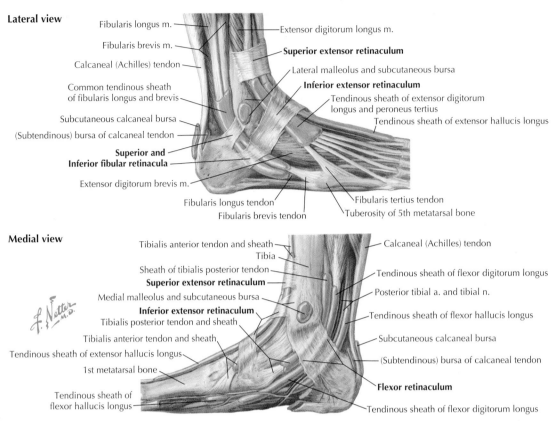

Fibularis longus m.

Fibularis brevis m.

Calcaneal (Achilles) tendon

Common tendinous sheath of fibularis longus and brevis

Subcutaneous calcaneal bursa

(Subtendinous) bursa of calcaneal tendon

Superior and Inferior fibular retinacula

Extensor digitorum brevis m.

Fibularis longus tendon

Fibularis brevis tendon

Extensor digitorum longus m.

Superior extensor retinaculum

Lateral malleolus and subcutaneous bursa

Inferior extensor retinaculum

Tendinous sheath of extensor digitorum longus and peroneus tertius

Tendinous sheath of extensor hallucis longus

Fibularis tertius tendon

Tuberosity of 5th metatarsal bone

Medial view

Tibialis anterior tendon and sheath

Tibia

Sheath of tibialis posterior tendon

Superior extensor retinaculum

Medial malleolus and subcutaneous bursa

Inferior extensor retinaculum

Tibialis posterior tendon and sheath

Tibialis anterior tendon and sheath

Tendinous sheath of extensor hallucis longus

1st metatarsal bone

Tendinous sheath of flexor hallucis longus

Calcaneal (Achilles) tendon

Tendinous sheath of flexor digitorum longus

Posterior tibial a. and tibial n.

Tendinous sheath of flexor hallucis longus

Subcutaneous calcaneal bursa

(Subtendinous) bursa of calcaneal tendon

Flexor retinaculum

Tendinous sheath of flexor digitorum longus

FIGURE 6-28 Tendon Sheaths and Retinacula of the Ankle. (From *Atlas of human anatomy,* ed 6, Plate 516.)

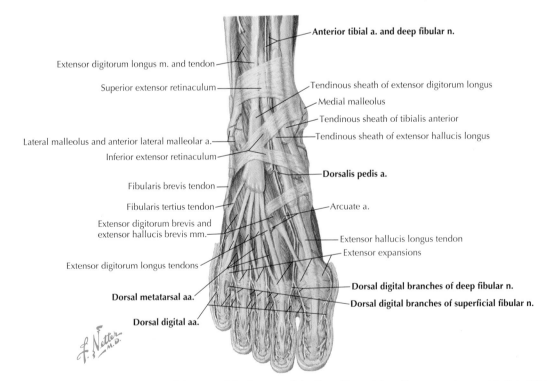

Anterior tibial a. and deep fibular n.

Extensor digitorum longus m. and tendon

Superior extensor retinaculum

Lateral malleolus and anterior lateral malleolar a.

Inferior extensor retinaculum

Fibularis brevis tendon

Fibularis tertius tendon

Extensor digitorum brevis and extensor hallucis brevis mm.

Extensor digitorum longus tendons

Dorsal metatarsal aa.

Dorsal digital aa.

Tendinous sheath of extensor digitorum longus

Medial malleolus

Tendinous sheath of tibialis anterior

Tendinous sheath of extensor hallucis longus

Dorsalis pedis a.

Arcuate a.

Extensor hallucis longus tendon

Extensor expansions

Dorsal digital branches of deep fibular n.

Dorsal digital branches of superficial fibular n.

FIGURE 6-29 Muscles, Nerves, and Arteries of the Dorsum of the Foot. (From *Atlas of human anatomy,* ed 6, Plate 517.)

Rotational Fractures

Most ankle injuries are caused by twisting, so that the talus rotates in the frontal plane and impinges on either the lateral or medial malleolus. This causes it to fracture and places tension on supporting ligaments of the opposite side. The following three types are recognized:

- **Type A:** Medial rotation of the talus
- **Type B:** Lateral rotation of the talus
- **Type C:** Injury extends proximally, with torn tibiofibular ligament and interosseous membrane (a variant is the Maisonneuve fracture)

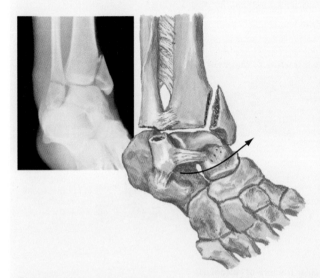

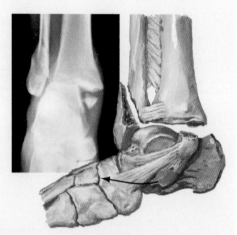

Type A. Avulsion fracture of lateral malleolus and shear fracture of medial malleolus caused by medial rotation of talus. **Tibiofibular ligaments intact.**

Type B. Shear fracture of lateral malleolus and small avulsion fracture of medial malleolus caused by lateral rotation of talus. **Tibiofibular ligaments intact or only partially torn.**

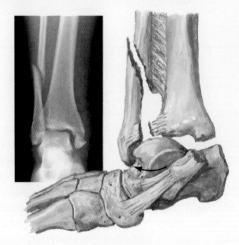

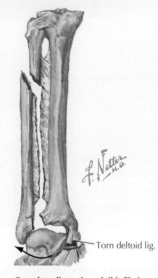

Torn deltoid lig.

Type C. **Disruption of tibiofibular ligaments** with diastasis of syndesmosis caused by external rotation of talus. Force transmitted to fibula results in oblique fracture at higher level. In this case, avulsion of medial malleolus has also occurred.

Maisonneuve fracture. Complete disruption of tibiofibular syndesmosis with diastasis caused by external rotation of talus and transmission of force to proximal fibula, resulting in high fracture of fibula. **Interosseous membranes torn longitudinally.**

Fractures of the Calcaneus

Calcaneal fractures (the most common tarsal fracture) are extraarticular or intraarticular. Extraarticular fractures include the following:

- **Anterior process fracture:** stress on the bifurcate ligament caused by landing on an adducted plantarflexed foot
- **Avulsion fracture of the calcaneal tuberosity:** sudden forceful contraction of the gastrocnemius and soleus muscles
- **Fracture of the sustentaculum tali:** jumping and landing on an inverted foot
- **Fracture of the body:** jumping and landing on a heel

About 75% of all calcaneal fractures are intraarticular (forceful landing on a heel); the talus is "driven" down into the calcaneus, which cannot withstand the force because it is cancellous bone.

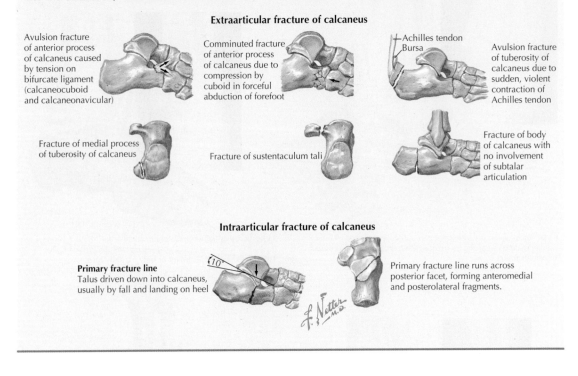

Extraarticular fracture of calcaneus

Avulsion fracture of anterior process of calcaneus caused by tension on bifurcate ligament (calcaneocuboid and calcaneonavicular)

Comminuted fracture of anterior process of calcaneus due to compression by cuboid in forceful abduction of forefoot

Achilles tendon
Bursa

Avulsion fracture of tuberosity of calcaneus due to sudden, violent contraction of Achilles tendon

Fracture of medial process of tuberosity of calcaneus

Fracture of sustentaculum tali

Fracture of body of calcaneus with no involvement of subtalar articulation

Intraarticular fracture of calcaneus

Primary fracture line
Talus driven down into calcaneus, usually by fall and landing on heel

Primary fracture line runs across posterior facet, forming anteromedial and posterolateral fragments.

individual bands of fascia that attach to the toes anteriorly (Fig. 6-30).

Beneath the plantar aponeurosis, the intrinsic muscles of the foot are arranged into four layers, shown in sequence in Figures 6-31, 6-32, and 6-33 and Tables 6-20, 6-21, and 6-22. These muscles functionally assist the long muscle tendons that pass from the leg into the foot. The **lumbrical muscles** and the **interosseus muscles** have the same actions as their counterparts in the hand. The lumbricals flex the metatarsophalangeal joints and extend the interphalangeal joints via the extensor hood. The plantar interossei adduct (**PAD**) the digits (2-4) and help flex the metatarsophalangeal joints, while the dorsal interossei abduct (**DAB**) the digits and help flex the metatarsophalangeal joints. All these intrinsic muscles of the sole are innervated by the **medial** or **lateral plantar nerves** (from the tibial nerve) (Tables 6-20, 6-21, and 6-22) and are supplied with blood from the **medial** and **lateral plantar arteries** (from the posterior tibial artery). Pulses may be palpated between the medial malleolus and the heel (posterior tibial artery) and on the dorsum of the foot just lateral to the extensor hallucis longus tendon (dorsalis pedis artery).

Text continued on p. 330.

Superficial dissection

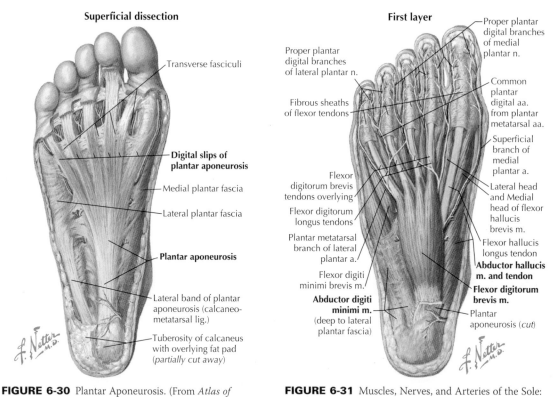

Transverse fasciculi

Digital slips of plantar aponeurosis

Medial plantar fascia

Lateral plantar fascia

Plantar aponeurosis

Lateral band of plantar aponeurosis (calcaneo-metatarsal lig.)

Tuberosity of calcaneus with overlying fat pad (*partially cut away*)

First layer

Proper plantar digital branches of medial plantar n.

Proper plantar digital branches of lateral plantar n.

Fibrous sheaths of flexor tendons

Common plantar digital aa. from plantar metatarsal aa.

Superficial branch of medial plantar a.

Flexor digitorum brevis tendons overlying

Flexor digitorum longus tendons

Lateral head and Medial head of flexor hallucis brevis m.

Plantar metatarsal branch of lateral plantar a.

Flexor hallucis longus tendon

Abductor hallucis m. and tendon

Flexor digiti minimi brevis m.

Flexor digitorum brevis m.

Abductor digiti minimi m. (deep to lateral plantar fascia)

Plantar aponeurosis (*cut*)

FIGURE 6-30 Plantar Aponeurosis. (From *Atlas of human anatomy*, ed 6, Plate 519.)

FIGURE 6-31 Muscles, Nerves, and Arteries of the Sole: First Layer. (From *Atlas of human anatomy*, ed 6, Plate 520.)

Second layer

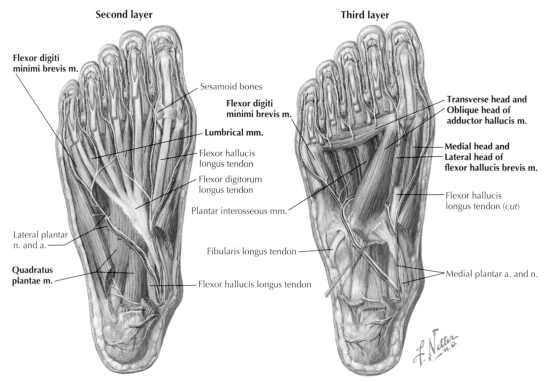

Flexor digiti minimi brevis m.

Sesamoid bones

Flexor digiti minimi brevis m.

Lumbrical mm.

Flexor hallucis longus tendon

Flexor digitorum longus tendon

Plantar interosseous mm.

Lateral plantar n. and a.

Quadratus plantae m.

Fibularis longus tendon

Flexor hallucis longus tendon

Third layer

Transverse head and Oblique head of adductor hallucis m.

Medial head and Lateral head of flexor hallucis brevis m.

Flexor hallucis longus tendon (*cut*)

Medial plantar a. and n.

FIGURE 6-32 Muscles, Nerves, and Arteries of the Sole: Second and Third Layers. (From *Atlas of human anatomy*, ed 6, Plates 521 and 522.)

TABLE 6-20 Muscles of the Sole: First Layer

MUSCLE	PROXIMAL ATTACHMENT (ORIGIN)	DISTAL ATTACHMENT (INSERTION)	INNERVATION	MAIN ACTIONS
Abductor hallucis	Medial tubercle of tuberosity of calcaneus, flexor retinaculum, and plantar aponeurosis	Medial side of base of proximal phalanx of 1st digit	Medial plantar nerve (S2-S3)	Abducts and flexes great toe
Flexor digitorum brevis	Medial tubercle of tuberosity of calcaneus, plantar aponeurosis, and intermuscular septa	Both sides of middle phalanges of lateral four digits	Medial plantar nerve (S2-S3)	Flexes lateral four digits
Abductor digiti minimi	Medial and lateral tubercles of tuberosity of calcaneus, plantar aponeurosis, and intermuscular septa	Lateral side of base of proximal phalanx of 5th digit	Lateral plantar nerve (S2-S3)	Abducts and flexes little toe

TABLE 6-21 Muscles of the Sole: Second and Third Layers

MUSCLE	PROXIMAL ATTACHMENT (ORIGIN)	DISTAL ATTACHMENT (INSERTION)	INNERVATION	MAIN ACTIONS
Quadratus plantae	Medial surface and lateral margin of plantar surface of calcaneus	Posterolateral margin of tendon of flexor digitorum longus	Lateral plantar nerve (S1-S3)	Assist flexor digitorum longus in flexing lateral four digits
Lumbricals	Tendons of flexor digitorum longus	Medial aspect of dorsal expansion over lateral four digits	*Medial one:* medial plantar nerve *Lateral three:* lateral plantar nerve	Flex metatarsophalangeal joints and extend interphalangeal joints of lateral four digits
Flexor hallucis brevis	Plantar surfaces of cuboid and lateral cuneiforms	Both sides of base of proximal phalanx of 1st digit	Medial plantar nerve (S1-S2)	Flexes proximal phalanx of great toe
Adductor hallucis	*Oblique head:* bases of metatarsals 2-4 *Transverse head:* plantar ligaments of metatarsophalangeal joints of digits 3-5	Tendons of both heads attach to lateral side of base of proximal phalanx of 1st digit	Deep branch of lateral plantar nerve (S2-S3)	Adducts great toe; assists in maintaining transverse arch of foot
Flexor digiti minimi brevis	Base of 5th metatarsal	Lateral base of proximal phalanx of 5th digit	Superficial branch of lateral plantar nerve (S2-S3)	Flexes proximal phalanx of little toe, thereby assisting with its flexion

TABLE 6-22 Muscles of the Sole: Fourth Layer

MUSCLE	PROXIMAL ATTACHMENT (ORIGIN)	DISTAL ATTACHMENT (INSERTION)	INNERVATION	MAIN ACTIONS
Plantar interossei (three muscles)	Bases and medial sides of metatarsals 3-5	Medial sides of bases of proximal phalanges of digits 3-5	Lateral plantar nerve (S2-S3)	Adduct digits 2-4, flex metatarsophalangeal joints, and extend phalanges
Dorsal interossei (four muscles)	Adjacent sides of metatarsals 1-5	*First:* medial side of proximal phalanx of second digit *Second to fourth:* lateral sides of digits 2-4	Lateral plantar nerve (S2-S3)	Abduct digits 2-4, flex metatarsophalangeal joints, and extend phalanges

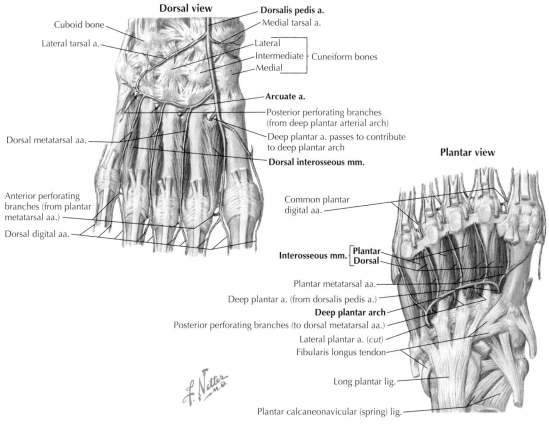

Dorsal view

Cuboid bone

Lateral tarsal a.

Dorsalis pedis a.

Medial tarsal a.

Lateral
Intermediate } Cuneiform bones
Medial

Arcuate a.

Posterior perforating branches
(from deep plantar arterial arch)

Deep plantar a. passes to contribute
to deep plantar arch

Dorsal metatarsal aa.

Dorsal interosseous mm.

Plantar view

Anterior perforating
branches (from plantar
metatarsal aa.)

Dorsal digital aa.

Common plantar
digital aa.

Interosseous mm. [**Plantar** / **Dorsal**]

Plantar metatarsal aa.

Deep plantar a. (from dorsalis pedis a.)

Deep plantar arch

Posterior perforating branches (to dorsal metatarsal aa.)

Lateral plantar a. (*cut*)

Fibularis longus tendon

Long plantar lig.

Plantar calcaneonavicular (spring) lig.

FIGURE 6-33 Muscles and Arteries of the Sole: Fourth Layer. (From *Atlas of human anatomy,* ed 6, Plate 523.)

Clinical Focus 6-32

Congenital Clubfoot

Congenital clubfoot (congenital equinovarus) is a structural defect in which the entire foot is plantarflexed (equinus) and the hindfoot and forefoot are inverted (varus). This deformity has a strong genetic link; males are more frequently affected, but females often have a more severe deformity. The bones not only are misaligned with each other but also may have an abnormal shape and size. Thus, after correction, the true clubfoot is smaller than normal. Management may be conservative or may require splinting, casting, or even surgery.

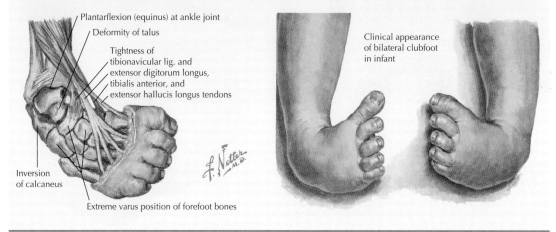

Plantarflexion (equinus) at ankle joint

Deformity of talus

Tightness of
tibionavicular lig. and
extensor digitorum longus,
tibialis anterior, and
extensor hallucis longus tendons

Clinical appearance
of bilateral clubfoot
in infant

Inversion
of calcaneus

Extreme varus position of forefoot bones

Metatarsal and Phalangeal Injuries

Direct trauma to the foot can result in fractures of the metatarsals and phalanges. These fractures can usually be treated with immobilization, as the fragments are often not displaced. Avulsion fractures of the fifth metatarsal are common to this bone and result from stresses placed on the **fibularis brevis tendon** during muscle contraction. Dislocation of the first metatarsal is common in athletes and ballet dancers because of repeated hyperdorsiflexion.

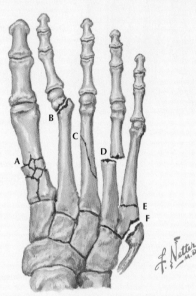

Types of fractures of metatarsal: A. comminuted fracture, B. displaced neck fracture, C. oblique fracture, D. displaced transverse fracture, E. fracture of base of 5th metatarsal, F. avulsion of tuberosity of 5th metatarsal with fibularis brevis tendon

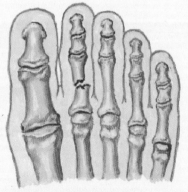

Fracture of proximal phalanx

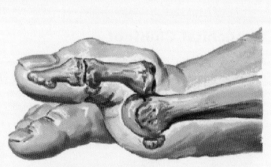

Dorsal dislocation of 1st metatarsophalangeal joint

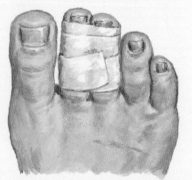

Fracture of phalanx splinted by taping to adjacent toe (buddy taping)

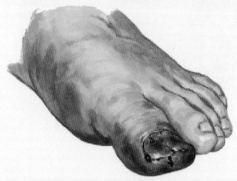

Crush injury of great toe

Plantar Fasciitis

Plantar fasciitis *(heel spur syndrome)* is the most common cause of heel pain, especially in joggers, and results from inflammation of plantar aponeurosis (fascia) at its point of attachment to the calcaneus. Generally, it is more common in females and obese persons. A bony spur may develop with plantar fasciitis, but the inflammation causes most of the pain, mediated by the medial calcaneal branch of the tibial nerve. Most patients can be managed nonsurgically, but relief from the pain may take 6 to 12 months. Exercises and orthotic devices are usually recommended in the initial course of treatment.

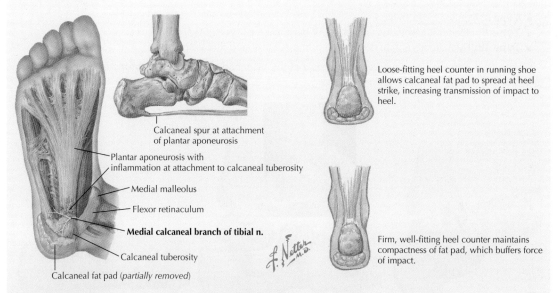

Calcaneal spur at attachment of plantar aponeurosis

Plantar aponeurosis with inflammation at attachment to calcaneal tuberosity

Medial malleolus

Flexor retinaculum

Medial calcaneal branch of tibial n.

Calcaneal tuberosity

Calcaneal fat pad *(partially removed)*

Loose-fitting heel counter in running shoe allows calcaneal fat pad to spread at heel strike, increasing transmission of impact to heel.

Firm, well-fitting heel counter maintains compactness of fat pad, which buffers force of impact.

Deformities of the Toes

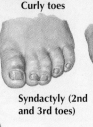

Overlapping 5th toe   **Curly toes**   **Hammertoe**

Bifid 5th toe

Syndactyly (2nd and 3rd toes)

Polydactyly (with partially cleft foot)

Defect	Comment
Overlapping fifth toe	Common familial deformity
Curly toes	Familial deformity, usually from hypoplasia or absence of intrinsic muscles of affected toes
Hammertoe	Proximal interphalangeal joint flexion deformity associated with poorly fitting shoes
Bifid fifth toe	May share common phalanx
Syndactyly	Web deformity (also occurs in the hand)
Cleft foot	Often associated with cleft hand, lip, and palate
Hallux valgus	Bunion, often in women from wearing narrow shoes
Turf toe	Hyperextension of great toe, common in football players (not shown)

Lateral head of flexor hallucis brevis m.

Metatarsus primus varus

Exostosis

10°

Subluxation
Hallux valgus

Laterally displaced lateral sesamoid

Oblique head
Transverse head   } Adductor hallucis m.

Bunion/hallux valgus

Clinical Focus 6-36

Fractures of the Talar Neck

The talar neck is the most common site for fractures of this tarsal. Injury usually results from direct trauma or landing on the foot after a fall from a great height. The foot is hyperdorsiflexed so that the neck impinges on the distal tibia. The three types of fractures are as follows:

- **Type I:** Nondisplaced fractures
- **Type II:** Neck fracture with subluxation or dislocation of the subtalar joint
- **Type III:** Neck fracture with dislocation of the subtalar and tibiotalar joints

  These fractures can lead to avascular necrosis of the talus body because most of the blood supply to the talus passes through the talar neck.

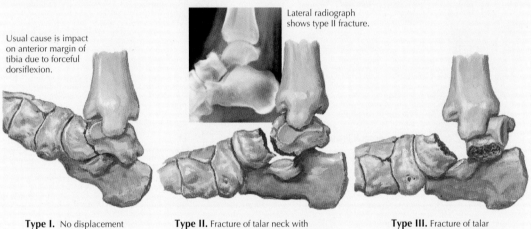

Usual cause is impact on anterior margin of tibia due to forceful dorsiflexion.

Lateral radiograph shows type II fracture.

Type I. No displacement

Type II. Fracture of talar neck with subluxation or dislocation of subtalar joint

Type III. Fracture of talar neck with dislocation of subtalar and tibiotalar joints

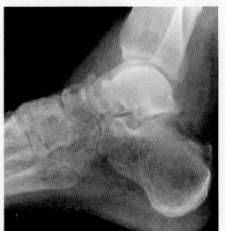

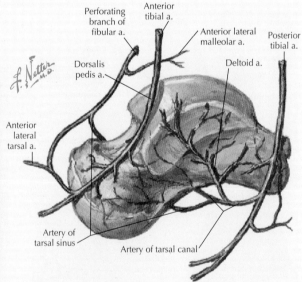

Perforating branch of fibular a.

Anterior tibial a.

Anterior lateral malleolar a.

Posterior tibial a.

Dorsalis pedis a.

Deltoid a.

Anterior lateral tarsal a.

Artery of tarsal sinus

Artery of tarsal canal

Avascular necrosis of talar body evidenced by increased density (sclerosis) compared with other tarsal bones

Because of profuse intraosseous anastomoses, avascular necrosis commonly occurs only when surrounding soft tissue is damaged, as in type II and III fractures of talar neck.

Common Foot Infections

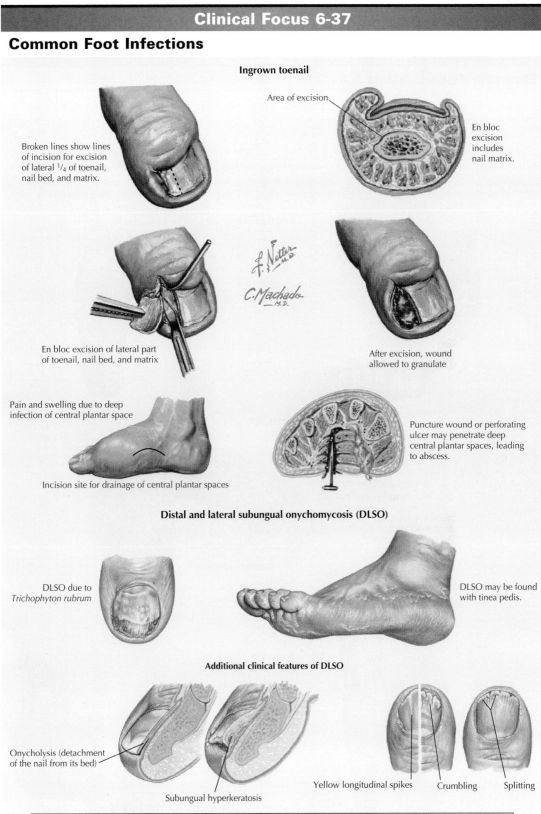

Ingrown toenail

Broken lines show lines of incision for excision of lateral ¼ of toenail, nail bed, and matrix.

Area of excision

En bloc excision includes nail matrix.

En bloc excision of lateral part of toenail, nail bed, and matrix

After excision, wound allowed to granulate

Pain and swelling due to deep infection of central plantar space

Puncture wound or perforating ulcer may penetrate deep central plantar spaces, leading to abscess.

Incision site for drainage of central plantar spaces

Distal and lateral subungual onychomycosis (DLSO)

DLSO due to *Trichophyton rubrum*

DLSO may be found with tinea pedis.

Additional clinical features of DLSO

Onycholysis (detachment of the nail from its bed)

Subungual hyperkeratosis

Yellow longitudinal spikes   Crumbling   Splitting

Condition	Comment
Ingrown toenail	Usually great toe, medial or lateral aspect; can lead to an inflamed area that becomes secondarily infected
Onychomycosis	Fungal nail infection, which makes a toenail thick and brittle
Puncture wound	Common injury; can lead to deep infection; requires check of tetanus status

Diabetic Foot Lesions

Diabetes mellitus (DM), a common complex metabolic disorder characterized by hyperglycemia, affects over 18 million people in the United States. The skin is one of many organ systems affected, especially the skin of the leg and foot. Microvascular disease may result in a decreased cutaneous blood flow. Peripheral sensory neuropathy may render the skin susceptible to injury and may blunt healing. Hyperglycemia predisposes the extremity to bacterial and fungal infection. Associated complications in the lower limb include Charcot joint (progressive destructive arthropathy caused by neuropathy), ulceration, infection, gangrene, and amputation. DM accounts for most nontraumatic foot and lower leg amputations, which total more than 80,000 per year.

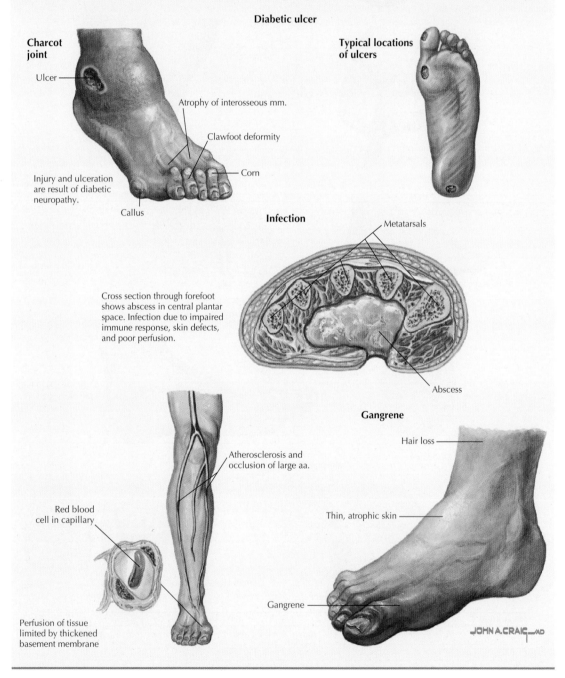

Diabetic ulcer

Charcot joint
Ulcer
Atrophy of interosseous mm.
Clawfoot deformity
Corn
Injury and ulceration are result of diabetic neuropathy.
Callus

Typical locations of ulcers

Infection
Metatarsals
Cross section through forefoot shows abscess in central plantar space. Infection due to impaired immune response, skin defects, and poor perfusion.
Abscess

Red blood cell in capillary
Atherosclerosis and occlusion of large aa.

Perfusion of tissue limited by thickened basement membrane

Gangrene
Hair loss
Thin, atrophic skin
Gangrene

JOHN A.CRAIG—AD

Arterial Occlusive Disease

Atherosclerosis can affect not only the coronary and cerebral vasculature but also the arteries that supply the kidneys, intestines, and lower limbs. The resulting arterial stenosis (narrowing) or occlusion in the leg leads to *peripheral vascular disease* (PVD), a disorder largely associated with increasing age. PVD produces symptoms of claudication, which should be a warning sign of atherosclerosis elsewhere that may produce myocardial infarction and stroke (see also Clinical Focus 6-11).

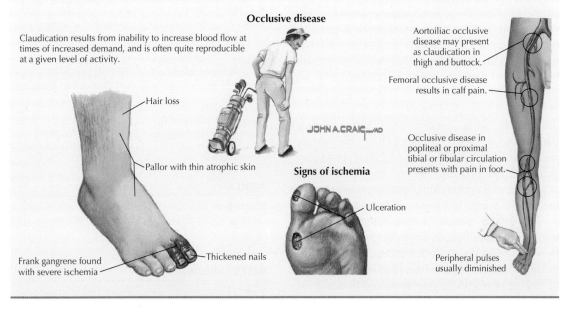

Occlusive disease

Claudication results from inability to increase blood flow at times of increased demand, and is often quite reproducible at a given level of activity.

Aortoiliac occlusive disease may present as claudication in thigh and buttock.

Femoral occlusive disease results in calf pain.

Occlusive disease in popliteal or proximal tibial or fibular circulation presents with pain in foot.

Hair loss

Pallor with thin atrophic skin

Signs of ischemia

Ulceration

Frank gangrene found with severe ischemia

Thickened nails

Peripheral pulses usually diminished

JOHN A.CRAIG—MD

Gout

Uric acid (ionized urate in plasma) is a by-product of purine metabolism and is largely eliminated from the body by renal secretion and excretion. An abnormally elevated serum urate concentration may lead to gout. Gout is caused by precipitation of sodium urate crystals within the joint's synovial or tenosynovial spaces, which produces inflammation. About 85% to 90% of clinical gout is caused by underexcretion of urate by the kidneys. The disorder may be caused by genetic or renal disease or diseases that affect renal function. Chronic gout presents with deforming arthritis that affects the hands, wrists, feet (especially the great toe), knees, and shoulders.

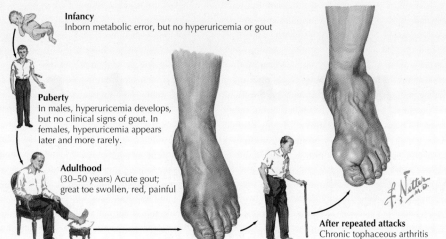

Natural history

Infancy
Inborn metabolic error, but no hyperuricemia or gout

Puberty
In males, hyperuricemia develops, but no clinical signs of gout. In females, hyperuricemia appears later and more rarely.

Adulthood
(30–50 years) Acute gout; great toe swollen, red, painful

After repeated attacks
Chronic tophaceous arthritis

8. LOWER LIMB MUSCLE SUMMARY AND GAIT

Table 6-23 summarizes the actions of major muscles on the joints. *The list is not exhaustive and highlights only major muscles responsible for each movement;* the separate muscle tables provide more detail. Realize that most joints move because of the action of multiple muscles working on that joint, and that this list only focuses on the more important of these muscles for each joint.

Gait

The gait (walking) cycle involves both a **swing phase** and a **stance phase** (when the foot is weight-bearing). Additionally, walking produces pelvic tilt and rotation, hip and knee flexion and extension, and a smoothly coordinated interaction among the pelvis, hip, knee, ankle, and foot.

The **swing phase** occurs from pre-swing toe-off (TO) position, in which the push-off of the toes occurs by the powerful plantarflexion of the ankle and the forward swing of the hips. The "ball" of the big toe, with its two sesamoid bones, provides the last push needed to accelerate into the swing phase. The foot then accelerates through the initial swing to the midswing (MSW) and terminal swing phase. (Follow the girl's right lower limb in images 5 to 7 of Figure 6-34.) When the right foot is off the ground, drooping of the pelvis (pelvic dip or tilt) to the unsupported side (right side) is prevented by the action of hip abductors, primarily the gluteus medius and minimus muscles. Paralysis of these muscles, as from polio or pelvic fractures that damage the superior gluteal nerves, can

TABLE 6-23 Summary of Actions of Major Lower Limb Muscles

HIP

Flex: iliopsoas, rectus femoris, sartorius	**Rotate medially:** gluteus medius and gluteus minimus
Extend: hamstrings, gluteus maximus	**Rotate laterally:** gluteus maximus, obturator internus, gemelli, piriformis
Abduct: gluteus medius, gluteus minimus, tensor fasciae latae	**Adduct:** adductor muscles of medial thigh

KNEE

Flex: hamstrings, gracilis, sartorius, gastrocnemius	**Rotate medially:** semitendinosus, semimembranosus
Extend: quadriceps femoris	**Rotate laterally:** biceps femoris

ANKLE

Plantarflex: gastrocnemius, soleus, tibialis posterior, flexor digitorum longus, flexor hallucis longus	**Dorsiflex:** tibialis anterior, extensor digitorum longus, extensor hallucis longus, fibularis tertius

INTERTARSAL

Evert: fibularis longus, brevis, and tertius	**Invert:** tibialis anterior and posterior

METATARSOPHALANGEAL

Flex: interossei and lumbricals	**Abduct:** dorsal interossei
Extend: extensor digitorum longus and brevis	**Adduct:** plantar interossei

INTERPHALANGEAL

Flex: flexor digitorum longus and brevis	**Extend:** extensor digitorum longus and brevis, lumbricals

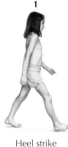 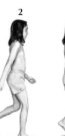 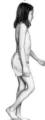 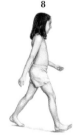

1	2	3	4	5	6	7	8
Heel strike	Foot flat	Midstance	Opposite heel strike	Pre-swing	Initial swing	Terminal swing	Heel strike

FIGURE 6-34 Phases of Gait.

TABLE 6-24 Major Muscles Involved in the Gait Cycle

GAIT CYCLE	MUSCLE ACTIONS
Toe-off (TO) to midswing (MSW)	Hip flexors accelerate the thigh, knee is flexed, and foot is dorsiflexed to clear the ground (**swing phase**).
MSW to heel strike (HS)	Knee is extended rapidly, and foot is dorsiflexed (**swing phase**).
HS to flat foot (FF)	Hip is flexed, knee is extended, and ankle is in neutral position, but foot then plantarflexes flat on the ground, and limb extensors stabilize the weight-bearing joints (**stance phase**).
FF to midstance (MST)	Body moves forward, extensors support limb while other limb is in the swing phase, and hip abductors control pelvic tilt (**stance phase**).
MST to heel-off (HO)	Body continues forward; plantarflexors contract as weight moves from heel to metatarsal heads, and hip abductors control pelvic tilt (**stance phase**).
HO to TO	Push-off as opposite heel strikes the ground, plantarflexors exert thrust, and knee flexes; foot goes into dorsiflexed position at beginning of HO to plantarflexed as toes push off at TO, and hip abductors relax while hip flexors ready for the swing phase (**stance phase**).

lead to a "gluteal or pelvic dip" and a **positive Trendelenburg sign**.

The limb then decelerates to the heel strike (HS) phase when the foot meets the ground (image 8 in Fig. 6-34). The **stance phase** occurs from the HS position, to the flat foot (FF) position, to the midstance (MST) phase, and then the heel-off (HO) (forward thrust to TO position and, correspondingly, the HS position for the opposite foot; follow the girl's right lower limb in images 1 to 4 in Fig. 6-34). Table 6-24 summarizes the major muscles involved in the gait cycle.

9. LOWER LIMB ARTERY AND VEIN SUMMARY

Arteries of the Lower Limb

The **abdominal aorta (1)** gives rise to the **left** and **right common iliac arteries (2).** These arteries divide into internal and external iliac arteries (Fig. 6-35). The internal iliac artery generally supplies the pelvis, perineum, and gluteal regions, while the **external iliac artery (3)** passes deep to the

inguinal ligament and into the thigh to become the **femoral artery (4)**. The femoral artery gives off a **deep artery of thigh (profunda femoris) (5)** and then continues inferiorly by passing through the adductor hiatus to become the **popliteal artery (6)** posterior to the knee. The popliteal artery divides in the leg to give rise to the **anterior tibial artery (7)** and **posterior tibial artery (9)**. The posterior tibial artery gives rise to the small **fibular artery (10)** and passes into the sole of the foot, where it divides into the **medial plantar artery (11)** and **lateral plantar artery (12)**. The anterior tibial artery supplies the anterior compartment of the leg, the ankle, and continues onto the dorsum of the foot as the **dorsal artery of the foot (dorsalis pedis) (8)** (Fig. 6-35).

Anastomoses occur around the hip joint, largely supplied by the deep artery of thigh with contributions from several other arteries (e.g., branch from obturator artery). The knee and ankle joints also have a rich vascular supply by genicular arteries (knee), and malleolar and tarsal arteries (ankle). Many of these arteries have small muscular branches (not listed) to supply the muscles of the limb and nutrient arteries to the adjacent bones (not named). **Arteriovenous (AV) anastomoses** are direct connections between small arteries and veins, and usually are involved in cutaneous thermoregulation.

Major pulse points of the lower limb include:

- **Femoral pulse:** just inferior to the inguinal ligament.
- **Popliteal pulse:** felt deep behind the knee (very difficult to feel).
- **Posterior tibial pulse:** on medial aspect of the ankle as it passes through the tarsal tunnel posterior to the medial malleolus.
- **Dorsalis pedis pulse** (farthest pulse from the heart): felt just lateral to the flexor hallucis longus tendon when pressed against the intermediate cuneiform bone.

In the outline of arteries, major vessels often dissected in anatomy courses include the first-order arteries (in **bold** and numbered) and their second-order major branches. Only more detailed courses in anatomy will dissect the third-order or fourth-order arteries.

Veins of the Lower Limb

Note that the venous drainage of the lower limb begins largely on the dorsum of the foot, with

1. **Abdominal Aorta***
2. **Right Common Iliac Artery/ Left Common
   Iliac Artery**
3. **Right External Iliac Artery**
4. **Femoral Artery**
   Superficial epigastric artery
   Superficial circumflex iliac artery
   Superficial external pudendal artery
   Deep external pudendal artery
   Descending genicular artery (knee)
5. **Deep Artery of Thigh**
   Medial circumflex femoral artery
   Lateral circumflex femoral artery
   Perforating aa. (muscles/bone)
6. **Popliteal Artery**
   Superior lateral and medial geniculate aa.
   Inferior lateral and medial geniculate aa.
   Genicular and patellar anastomoses
7. **Anterior Tibial Artery**
   Ant. and post. tibial recurrent aa.
   Ant. lateral and medial malleolar aa.
   Lateral malleolar network
8. **Dorsal Artery of Foot (Dorsalis Pedis)**
   Lateral and medial tarsal aa.
   Dorsal metatarsal aa.
   Dorsal digital aa.
   Deep plantar artery
9. **Posterior Tibial Artery**
   Medial malleolar aa.
   Calcaneal aa.
   Tibial nutrient artery
10. **Fibular Artery**
    Perforating branches
    Communicating branch
    Lateral malleolar artery
    Calcaneal branches
    Fibular nutrient artery
11. **Medial Plantar Artery**
    Superficial and deep branches
12. **Lateral Plantar Artery**
    Deep plantar artery
        Metatarsal and perforating aa.
        Common plantar digital aa.
            Plantar digital arteries proper
*Direction of blood flow from proximal to distal.

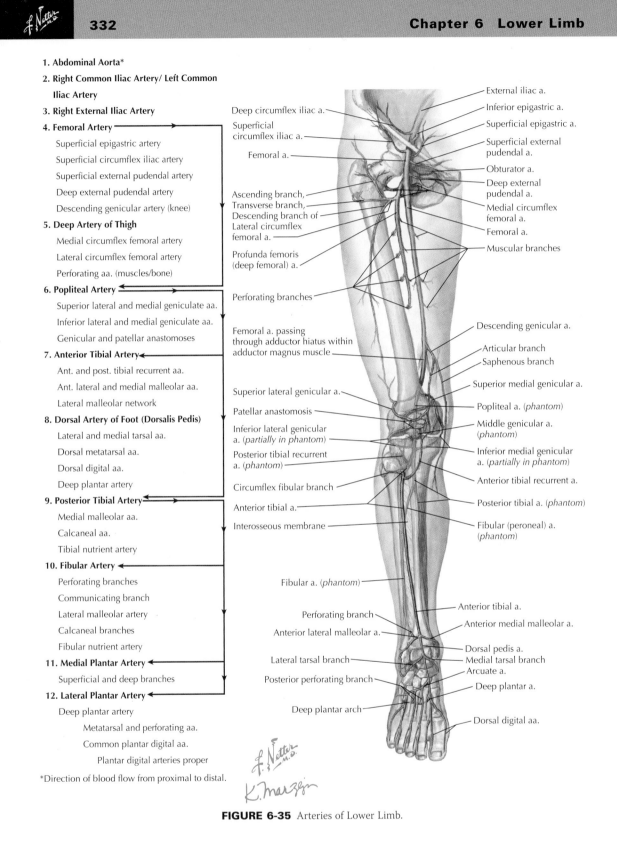

FIGURE 6-35 Arteries of Lower Limb.

2. Deep Veins

Fibular veins
Posterior tibial veins
Anterior tibial veins
Genicular veins
Sural veins

4. Popliteal Vein
  Perforating veins
  Lat. circumflex femoral veins
  Med. circumflex femoral veins
6. Deep Vein of Thigh
  (Profunda Femoris)
7. Femoral Vein
External Iliac Vein
Common Iliac Vein
Inferior Vena Cava
Heart (Right Atrium)

*Distal (foot) to Proximal (heart)

1. Superficial Veins

Plantar digital veins
Plantar metatarsal veins
Plantar venous arch
Dorsal digital veins
Dorsal metatarsal veins
Dorsal venous arch/network of foot
3. Small Saphenous Vein
Dorsal venous arch/network of foot
Ant. labial (scrotal) veins
Supf. dorsal v. clitoris (penis)
Accessory saphenous vein
Supf. epigastric vein
External pudendal vein
5. Great Saphenous Vein

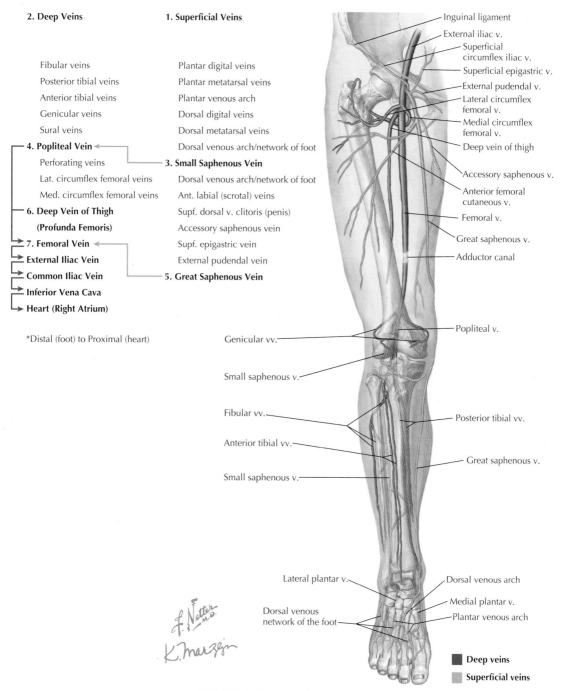

Inguinal ligament
External iliac v.
Superficial circumflex iliac v.
Superficial epigastric v.
External pudendal v.
Lateral circumflex femoral v.
Medial circumflex femoral v.
Deep vein of thigh
Accessory saphenous v.
Anterior femoral cutaneous v.
Femoral v.
Great saphenous v.
Adductor canal

Genicular vv.
Small saphenous v.
Fibular vv.
Anterior tibial vv.
Small saphenous v.

Popliteal v.
Posterior tibial vv.
Great saphenous v.

Lateral plantar v.
Dorsal venous network of the foot
Dorsal venous arch
Medial plantar v.
Plantar venous arch

■ Deep veins
■ Superficial veins

FIGURE 6-36 Veins of Lower Limb.

venous blood returning proximally in both a **superficial (1)** and **deep (2)** venous pattern (Fig. 6-36). The **small saphenous vein (3)** drains most of the foot and then this same vein and the **deep veins (2)** drain the leg, both largely terminating in the **popliteal vein (4)**. Variable connections between these veins are common, so the flow patterns should never be considered absolute; the pattern outlined details the major flow pattern from distal to proximal.

Genicular veins, draining into the popliteal vein, drain the arterial anastomosis around the knee joint. The **great saphenous vein (5)** courses up the medial aspect of the leg and medioanterior thigh to drain into the **femoral vein (7)**. The **great saphenous vein (5)** receives tributaries from the superficial perineal structures (labia and clitoris/scrotum and penis) and lower anterior abdominal wall adjacent to the inguinal region. The **deep vein of the thigh (profunda femoris) (6)** drains the deep thigh structures (muscles and bone) and is a major tributary of the **femoral vein (7)**. The

femoral vein then drains into the **external iliac vein**, which combined with the **internal iliac vein**, forms the **common iliac vein**. This then drains into the **inferior vena cava** and the **right atrium of the heart** (Fig. 6-36).

In the human body, the venous system is the compliance system, and, at rest, about 65% of the blood resides in the low-pressure venous system. Veins generally are larger than their corresponding arteries and have thinner walls; often multiple veins accompany a single artery (the body has many more veins than arteries).

10. LOWER LIMB NERVE SUMMARY

Femoral Nerve

The femoral nerve (L2-L4) innervates the muscles in the anterior compartment of the thigh, which are largely extensors of the leg at the knee (Fig. 6-37). The **patellar tendon reflex (L3-L4)**

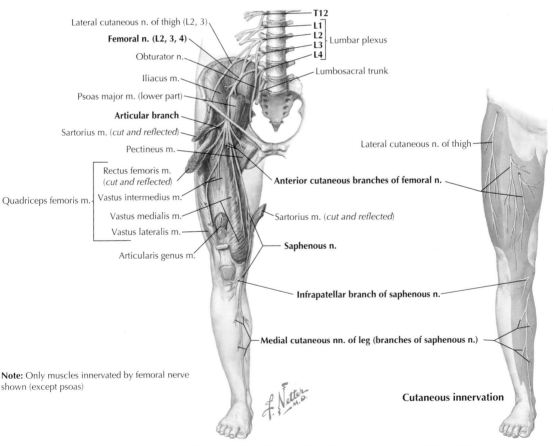

Note: Only muscles innervated by femoral nerve shown (except psoas)

FIGURE 6-37 Course of Femoral Nerve. (From *Atlas of human anatomy*, ed 6, Plate 525.)

(knee extension) tests the integrity of this nerve. Injury to this nerve can lead to an inability to fully extend the knee unless one pushes on the anterior thigh with one's hand. Major cutaneous branches include the separate lateral cutaneous nerve of the thigh and, from the femoral nerve directly, the following:

- Anterior cutaneous branches to the anterior thigh
- Saphenous nerve (terminal branch of femoral) to medial knee, leg, and ankle

Obturator Nerve

The obturator nerve (L2-L4) innervates the muscles of the medial compartment of the thigh, which are largely adductors of the thigh at the hip (Fig. 6-38). The nerve divides into anterior and posterior branches on both sides of the obturator externus and adductor brevis muscles (the anterior and posterior branches, in effect, "scissors" these two muscles). A small field of cutaneous innervation exists on the medial thigh. Injury to this nerve usually occurs inside the pelvis and can lead to weakened adduction of the thigh.

Sciatic Nerve

The sciatic nerve (L4-S3) is the largest nerve in the body and is composed of the **tibial** and **common fibular (peroneal) nerves** (Fig. 6-39). The sciatic nerve innervates muscles of the posterior compartment of the thigh (tibial component), which are largely extensors of the thigh at the hip and flexors of the leg at the knee. It also innervates all muscles below the knee, via its tibial and common fibular components.

Tibial Nerve

The tibial nerve (L4-S3), the larger of the two components of the sciatic nerve, innervates muscles of the posterior compartment of the leg and all muscles of the plantar foot (Fig. 6-40). These muscles are largely plantarflexors, and some have an inversion function. A lesion to this nerve may result in the loss of plantarflexion and weakened inversion of the foot, and thus a *shuffling gait.* The

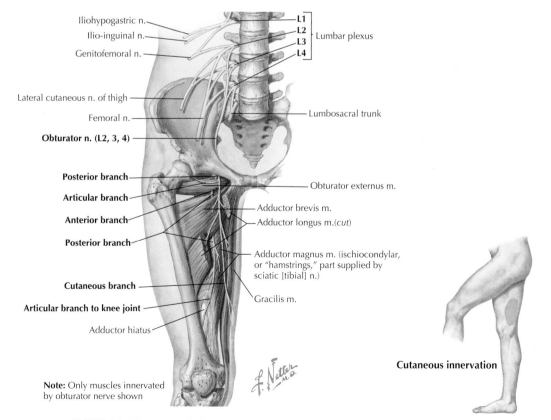

FIGURE 6-38 Course of Obturator Nerve. (From *Atlas of human anatomy*, ed 6, Plate 526.)

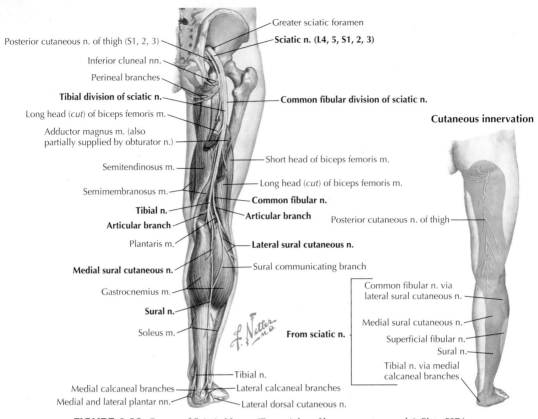

Greater sciatic foramen

Posterior cutaneous n. of thigh (S1, 2, 3)

Sciatic n. (L4, 5, S1, 2, 3)

Inferior cluneal nn.

Perineal branches

Tibial division of sciatic n.

Common fibular division of sciatic n.

Long head (*cut*) of biceps femoris m.

Adductor magnus m. (also partially supplied by obturator n.)

Cutaneous innervation

Semitendinosus m.

Short head of biceps femoris m.

Semimembranosus m.

Long head (*cut*) of biceps femoris m.

Common fibular n.

Tibial n.

Articular branch

Articular branch

Plantaris m.

Posterior cutaneous n. of thigh

Lateral sural cutaneous n.

Medial sural cutaneous n.

Sural communicating branch

Gastrocnemius m.

Common fibular n. via lateral sural cutaneous n.

Sural n.

Medial sural cutaneous n.

Soleus m.

Superficial fibular n.

Sural n.

From sciatic n.

Tibial n. via medial calcaneal branches

Tibial n.

Medial calcaneal branches

Lateral calcaneal branches

Medial and lateral plantar nn.

Lateral dorsal cutaneous n.

FIGURE 6-39 Course of Sciatic Nerve. (From *Atlas of human anatomy*, ed 6, Plate 527.)

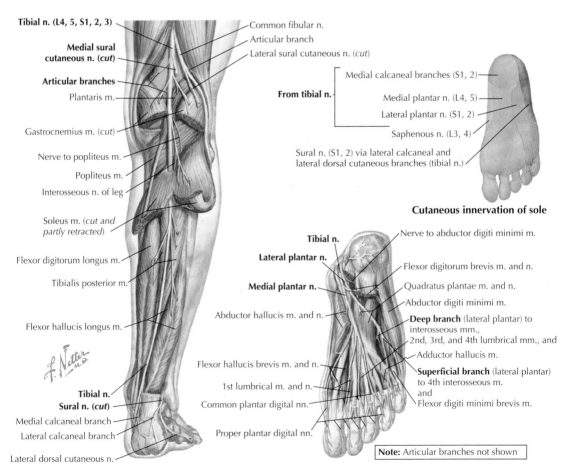

Tibial n. (L4, 5, S1, 2, 3)

Common fibular n.

Articular branch

Medial sural cutaneous n. (*cut*)

Lateral sural cutaneous n. (*cut*)

Articular branches

Medial calcaneal branches (S1, 2)

Plantaris m.

From tibial n.

Medial plantar n. (L4, 5)

Gastrocnemius m. (*cut*)

Lateral plantar n. (S1, 2)

Nerve to popliteus m.

Saphenous n. (L3, 4)

Popliteus m.

Sural n. (S1, 2) via lateral calcaneal and lateral dorsal cutaneous branches (tibial n.)

Interosseous n. of leg

Soleus m. (*cut and partly retracted*)

Cutaneous innervation of sole

Nerve to abductor digiti minimi m.

Flexor digitorum longus m.

Tibial n.

Tibialis posterior m.

Lateral plantar n.

Flexor digitorum brevis m. and n.

Medial plantar n.

Quadratus plantae m. and n.

Abductor digiti minimi m.

Abductor hallucis m. and n.

Deep branch (lateral plantar) to interosseous mm., 2nd, 3rd, and 4th lumbrical mm., and

Flexor hallucis longus m.

Adductor hallucis m.

Flexor hallucis brevis m. and n.

Superficial branch (lateral plantar) to 4th interosseous m. and

1st lumbrical m. and n.

Flexor digiti minimi brevis m.

Tibial n.

Sural n. (*cut*)

Common plantar digital nn.

Medial calcaneal branch

Proper plantar digital nn.

Lateral calcaneal branch

Note: Articular branches not shown

Lateral dorsal cutaneous n.

FIGURE 6-40 Course of Tibial Nerve. (From *Atlas of human anatomy*, ed 6, Plate 528.)

calcaneal (Achilles) tendon reflex (S1-S2) (plantarflexion) tests this nerve.

Fibular Nerve

The common fibular nerve (L4-S2) innervates muscles of the lateral compartment of the leg (everts the foot) via its superficial branch, and muscles of the anterior compartment of the leg and dorsum of the foot via its deep branch (Fig. 6-41). These muscles are largely dorsiflexors. *Footdrop* and *steppage gait* (high stepping) may occur if this nerve or its deep branch is injured (see Clinical Focus 6-27). The common fibular nerve is most vulnerable to injury as it passes around the fibular neck.

Dermatomes

The spiral dermatome pattern of the lower limb is the result of its embryonic medial rotation. Because of the stability of the hip joint, the spiral

dermatome pattern is similar to a barbershop pole. Considerable overlap and some variability in the dermatome pattern is to be expected. However, the following key dermatome regions are generally constant:

- Inguinal region: L1
- Anterior knee: L4
- Second toe: L5
- Posterior leg and thigh: S1-S2

Zones of autonomous sensory testing and spinal cord levels involved in primary movements of the joints are illustrated in Figure 6-42.

11. EMBRYOLOGY

While the upper limb rotates 90 degrees laterally, the lower limb rotates about **90 degrees medially** so that the knee and elbow are oriented

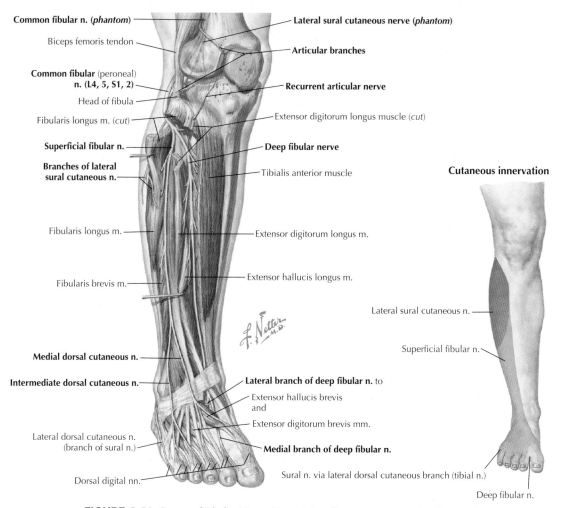

FIGURE 6-41 Course of Fibular Nerve. (From *Atlas of human anatomy*, ed 6, Plate 529.)

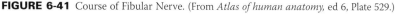

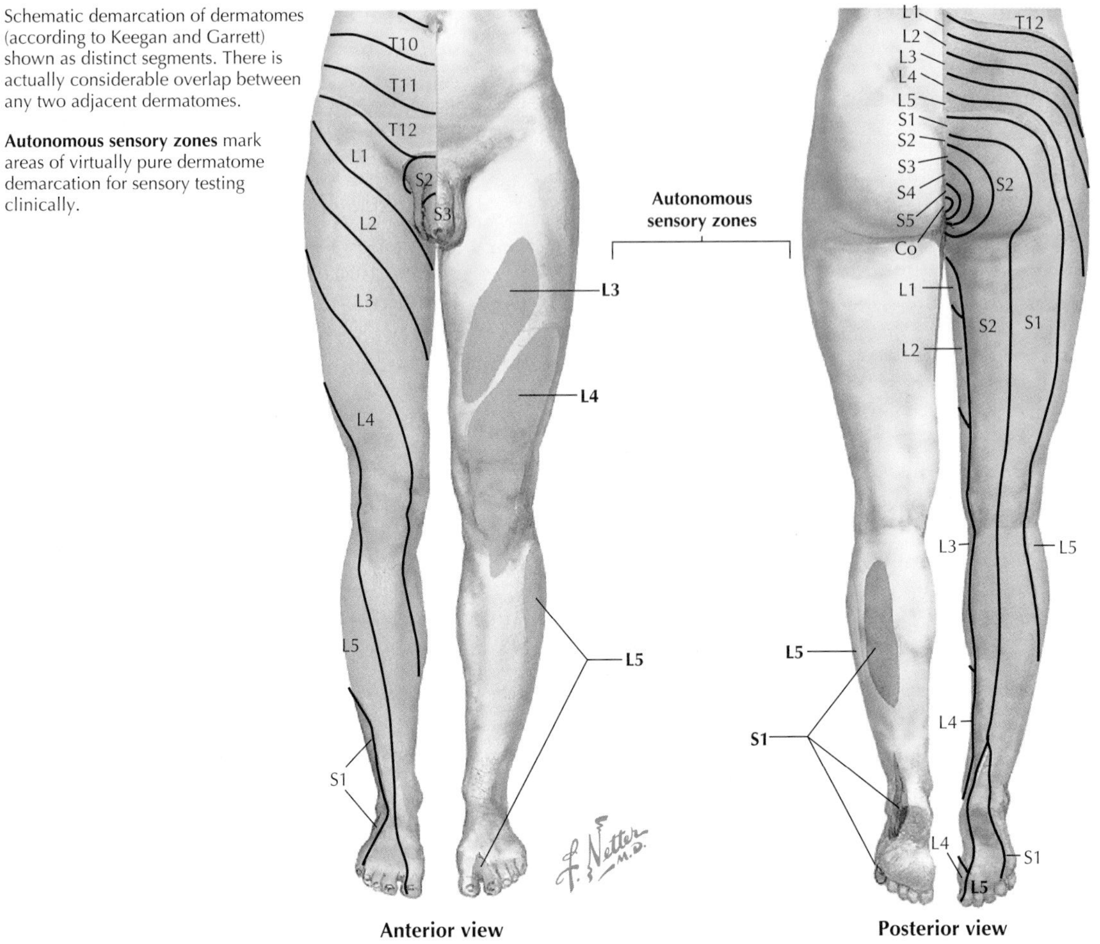

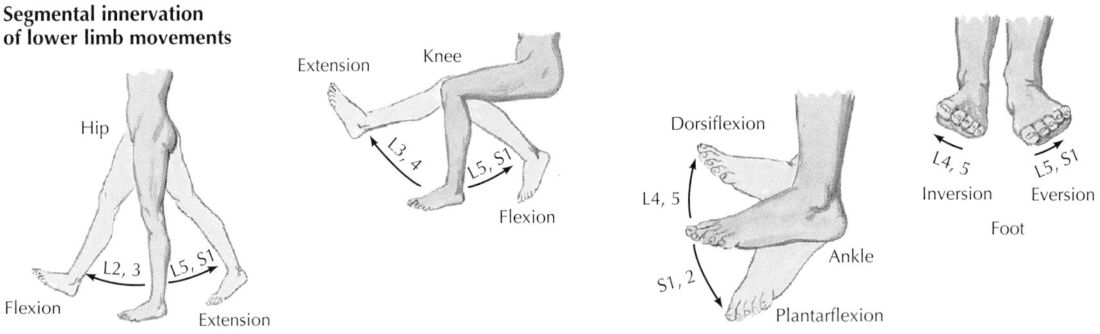

Schematic demarcation of dermatomes (according to Keegan and Garrett) shown as distinct segments. There is actually considerable overlap between any two adjacent dermatomes.
Autonomous sensory zones mark areas of virtually pure dermatome demarcation for sensory testing clinically.
T10
T11
T12
L1
L2
L3
L4
L5
S1
S2
S3
Autonomous sensory zones
L3
L4
L5
Anterior view
L1
L2
L3
L4
L5
S1
S2
S3
S4
S5
Co
T12
S2
S1
L1
L2
L3
L5
L5
S1
L4
L4
S1
L5
Posterior view

Segmental innervation of lower limb movements
Hip
Flexion
L2, 3
L5, S1
Extension
Extension
Knee
L3, 4
L5, S1
Flexion
Dorsiflexion
L4, 5
S1, 2
Ankle
Plantarflexion
L4, 5
Inversion
L5, S1
Eversion
Foot

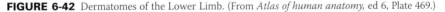

FIGURE 6-42 Dermatomes of the Lower Limb. (From *Atlas of human anatomy,* ed 6, Plate 469.)

about 180 degrees from each other (Fig. 6-43; see also Fig. 7-43). The thumb lies laterally in anatomical position, with the great toe medially. Knee, ankle, and toe flexor muscles are on the posterior aspect of the lower limb, and knee, ankle, and toe extensor muscles are on the ventral aspect. The hip is unaffected, so hip flexors are anterior and extensors are posterior. This limb rotation pattern produces a spiral (barbershop pole) arrangement of the dermatomes as one moves distally along the limb (Fig. 6-43). All the muscles of the lower limb are from **hypaxial** (hypomeres) embryonic ventral mesoderm (see Fig. 2-22) and are innervated by ventral rami and their respective lumbosacral nerves (gluteal, obturator, femoral, and sciatic).

Changes in position of limbs before birth

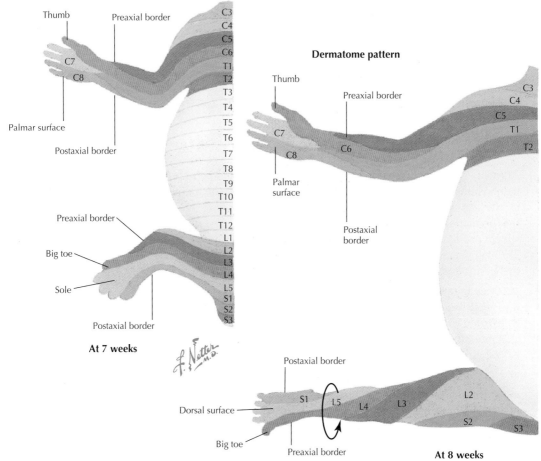

At 8 weeks. Torsion of lower limbs results in twisted or "barber pole" arrangement of their cutaneous innervation.

At 7 weeks. Upper and lower limbs have undergone 90° torsion about their long axes, but in opposite directions, so elbows point caudally and knees cranially.

Thumb   Preaxial border

C3
C4
C5
C6
T1
T2
T3
T4
T5
T6
T7
T8
T9
T10
T11
T12
L1
L2
L3
L4
L5
S1
S2
S3

C7
C8

Palmar surface

Postaxial border

Preaxial border

Big toe

Sole

Postaxial border

At 7 weeks

Dermatome pattern

Thumb

Preaxial border

C3
C4
C5
T1
T2

C7
C8

C6

Palmar surface

Postaxial border

Postaxial border

Dorsal surface

Big toe

Preaxial border

S1   L5   L4   L3   L2

S2

S3

At 8 weeks

FIGURE 6-43 Lower Limb Rotation.

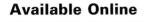

Clinical Focus

Available Online

6-41 Healing of Fractures

Additional figures available online (see inside front cover for details).

Challenge Yourself Questions

1. An elderly patient who has been minimally ambulatory is transported to the clinic with a swollen lower limb and evidence of a deep vein thrombosis. Your examination reveals a sizable clot in her small saphenous vein, and you are concerned that a thromboembolus might originate from this clot and pass to her heart and lungs. After it exits the small saphenous vein, the thromboembolus would next pass into which of the following veins on its journey to the heart?

   A. Deep femoral
   B. External iliac
   C. Femoral
   D. Great saphenous
   E. Popliteal

2. An obese 48-year-old woman presents with a painful lump in her proximal thigh, just medial to the femoral vessels. Examination reveals the herniation of some abdominal viscera, which passes under the inguinal ligament. Through which of the following openings has this hernia passed to enter her thigh?

   A. Deep inguinal ring
   B. Femoral ring
   C. Fossa ovalis
   D. Obturator canal
   E. Superficial inguinal ring

3. The hip is a stable ball-and-socket synovial joint with several strong supporting ligaments. Hip flexion exhibits a significant range of motion, but hip extension is more limited. Which of the following hip ligaments is the strongest ligament and the one that limits hip extension?

   A. Iliofemoral
   B. Ischiofemoral
   C. Ligament of head of femur
   D. Pubofemoral
   E. Transverse acetabular

4. A football player receives a blow to the lateral aspect of his weight-bearing right leg and immediately feels his knee give way. Under extreme pain, he is carried from the field and immediately examined by the team physician, who is able to move the player's right tibia forward excessively compared to the uninjured leg. Which of the following ligaments is injured?

   A. Anterior cruciate
   B. Fibular collateral
   C. Posterior cruciate
   D. Tibial collateral
   E. Transverse

5. During a routine physical exam, the physician taps a patient's patellar ligament with a reflex hammer and elicits a knee-jerk reflex. Which of the following nerves mediates this patellar reflex?

   A. Common fibular
   B. Femoral
   C. Obturator
   D. Saphenous
   E. Tibial

6. A long-distance runner is examined by her physician after complaining of pain along the anteromedial aspect of her left leg, extending from just below the knee to just above the ankle. She has been running on a hard surface and notices that the pain is especially acute as she pushes off from the ground with the affected limb. Which of the following muscles of the leg is most likely affected by this stress injury?

   A. Extensor digitorum longus
   B. Fibularis longus
   C. Gastrocnemius
   D. Popliteus
   E. Tibialis posterior

7. A stab injury to the buttocks results in the patient's inability to rise from a seated position without the use of his arms, as well as weakness in climbing stairs. A nerve injury is suspected. Which of the following muscles was most likely affected by this stab injury?

   A. Gluteus maximus
   B. Gluteus medius
   C. Obturator internus
   D. Piriformis
   E. Semitendinosus

8. An inversion ankle injury results in the tearing of two of the three major ligaments that stabilize this joint. Which of the following pairs of ligaments are most likely injured?

   A. Anterior talofibular and calcaneofibular
   B. Calcaneofibular and deltoid
   C. Deltoid and long plantar
   D. Long plantar and posterior talofibular
   E. Posterior talofibular and anterior talofibular

9. An 11-year-old boy jumps from a tree house 15 feet above the ground and lands on his feet before rolling forward, immediately feeling extreme pain in his right ankle. Radiographic examination reveals that he has broken the most frequently fractured tarsal bone in the body. Which of the following tarsal bones is most likely fractured?

   A. Calcaneus
   B. Cuboid
   C. Medial cuneiform
   D. Navicular
   E. Talus

10. A laceration across the back of the lower leg results in numbness over the site of the laceration that extends inferiorly over the heel and the lateral back of the sole. Which of the following nerves was mostly likely injured?

    A. Lateral plantar
    B. Medial plantar
    C. Saphenous
    D. Superficial fibular
    E. Sural

11. A 54-year-old man presents with an inability to fully dorsiflex his foot at the ankle, although he can invert and evert his foot. Which of the following nerves may be affected?

    A. Common fibular
    B. Deep fibular
    C. Medial plantar
    D. Superficial fibular
    E. Tibial

12. A man is seen in the clinic waiting room who enters with a "shuffling" gait and a weakened ability to plantarflex his foot. Which of the following nerve-muscle combinations is most likely involved?

    A. Deep fibular and tibialis anterior muscle
    B. Deep fibular and tibialis posterior muscle
    C. Superficial fibular and fibularis longus muscle
    D. Tibial and tibialis anterior muscle
    E. Tibial and tibialis posterior muscle

13. A first-year medical student is asked to demonstrate the location of the dorsalis pedis pulse. Which of the following landmarks would be a reliable guide for finding this artery?

    A. Lateral to the extensor hallucis longus tendon
    B. Medial to the extensor digitorum longus tendons
    C. Over the intermediate cuneiform bone
    D. Over the second metatarsal bone
    E. Web space between toes 1 and 2

14. A 38-year-old woman complains of pain in her feet when walking. Examination reveals the presence of bunions on the medial aspect of both her great (first) toes, from wearing shoes with a very narrow toe. Which of the following clinical terms is used to describe this condition?

    A. Cleft foot
    B. Genu vara
    C. Hammertoes
    D. Hallux valgus
    E. Syndactyly

15. Irritation of the knee in a cleaning lady who scrubs floors on her knees results in septic bursitis and "housemaid's knee." Which of the following bursae is most likely involved?

   A. Anserine
   B. Deep infrapatellar
   C. Prepatellar
   D. Subcutaneous infrapatellar
   E. Suprapatellar

For each condition described below (16-20), select the muscle from the list (A-N) that is most likely responsible or affected.

(A) Adductor longus   **(H)** Piriformis
(B) Biceps femoris   **(I)** Quadratus femoris
      (short head)
(C) Gluteus maximus   **(J)** Rectus femoris
(D) Gluteus medius   **(K)** Sartorius
(E) Gracilis   **(L)** Semimembranosus
(F) Obturator   **(M)** Semitendinosus
      externus
(G) Obturator   **(N)** Tensor fasciae
      internus   latae

____ 16. Pain over the lateral knee leads to a common muscle-tendon injury in runners called ITB (iliotibial tract or band) syndrome.

____ 17. A dipping of the pelvis during the stance phase of walking may occur if there is an injury to the nerves innervating this important abductor of the femur at the hip.

____ 18. Weakened flexion of the thigh and abduction at the hip, and flexion of the leg at the knee would suggest an injury to this muscle or to the nerves innervating this muscle.

____ 19. An orthopedic surgeon examining the integrity of the medial aspect of the knee palpates the tendons of the pes anserinus (goose's foot), including the tendons of the sartorius, semitendinosus, and this muscle.

____ 20. An athlete "pulls" her hamstring muscles while sprinting. Although this muscle is a muscle of the posterior compartment of the thigh and does flex the leg at the knee, it is not a true hamstring.

Answers to Challenge Yourself Questions

1. **E.** The small saphenous vein drains superiorly along the posterior aspect of the leg and then dives deeply to drain into the popliteal vein deep within the knee.

2. **B.** This woman has a femoral hernia, which gains access to the anterior thigh via the femoral ring. The femoral ring is the abdominal opening in the femoral canal.

3. **A.** The iliofemoral ligament forms an inverted "Y" (of Bigelow) configuration and is the strongest of the hip ligaments.

4. **A.** Excessive movement of the tibia forward on a fixed femur suggests rupture of the anterior cruciate ligament, which limits hyperextension. The posterior cruciate ligament is shorter and the stronger of the two cruciate ligaments.

5. **B.** Extension of the knee occurs with the contraction of the quadriceps femoris group of muscles, which are innervated by the femoral nerve (L2-L4). The patellar reflex tests the L3-L4 component of the femoral nerve.

6. **E.** The leg muscles are encased in a strong and tight crural fascia, and overuse of these muscles can lead to swelling and pain or damage to the muscles in this tight compartment. The muscle most often affected by pushing off the ground is the tibialis posterior muscle during the action of plantarflexion at the ankle.

7. **A.** The inferior gluteal nerves were probably injured and they innervate the most powerful extensor of the hip, the gluteus maximus. We use this muscle especially when climbing stairs or rising from a sitting position. One can exercise on a "stair master" and build up this muscle of the buttock ("buns of steel").

8. **A.** These two ligaments are the most susceptible to inversion injuries of the ankle. In a very severe injury, the posterior talofibular ligament also may be injured.

9. **A.** The calcaneus is a rather soft (cancellous) bone compared to the denser talus, and falls from a great height that include landing on the feet will result in the talus being driven down into the calcaneus, causing an intraarticular fracture.

10. E. The sural nerve is a cutaneous nerve (contains only somatic afferent fibers and postganglionic sympathetic fibers) and lies subcutaneously along the posterior aspect of the leg and close to the small saphenous vein. It innervates the skin of the calf, heel and posterior sole.

11. B. Since the man can evert and invert but cannot fully dorsiflex at the ankle, he most likely has injured his deep fibular nerve. If he had lost eversion alone, he would have injured the superficial fibular nerve and if dorsiflexion and eversion were weakened, then one would suspect an injury of the common fibular nerve.

12. E. The tibial nerve innervates the muscles that plantarflex the foot at the ankle. The major muscle that accomplishes this action is the tibialis posterior muscle.

13. A. The dorsalis pedis pulse can be reliably and most easily found just lateral to the extensor hallucis longus tendon (points the big toe up), where this artery can be palpated by pressing it against the underlying navicular or intermediate cuneiform bone.

14. D. Hallux valgus is the clinical term for a bunion. Bunions result from a medial angling of the distal first metatarsal (varus) coupled with a subluxation and proximal lateral displacement (valgus) of the first phalanx (big toe).

15. C. The prepatellar bursa lies right over the lower aspect of the patella and the patellar ligament when the knee is flexed. Thus, it is in the perfect position to bear the brunt of the pressure on the bended knee.

16. N. The iliotibial tract (often called "band" by clinicians) is the lower extension and insertion of the tensor fasciae latae muscle on the lateral condyle of the tibia. The IT tract rubs on the lateral epicondyle of the femur.

17. D. The gluteus medius muscle is a powerful abductor of the femur at the hip and maintains a relatively stable pelvis when the opposite foot is off the ground. The "gluteal dip" or lurch is seen when the patient stands on the injured limb and the pelvis dips on the other side when that limb is off the ground (a positive Trendelenburg sign). The gluteus medius (and minimus) cannot abduct the hip on the affected side (stance side) to prevent the dip. Usually, this denotes an injury to the superior gluteal nerves innervating the medius and minimus.

18. K. The sartorius ("tailor's") muscle flexes and abducts the hip and flexes the knee (think about the action of sitting in a chair with one thigh crossed over the other, as a "tailor" might do while stitching). Thus, it acts on both joints and is innervated by branches of the femoral nerve.

19. E. The gracilis is the third muscle of the pes anserinus (three toes of a goose's foot). These muscle tendons help to stabilize the medial aspect of the knee.

20. B. The biceps femoris (short head) is a muscle of the posterior compartment of the thigh but only flexes the leg at the knee and does not cross the hip joint and extend the thigh at the hip, like the other three "hamstring" muscles. Therefore, it is not a true hamstring muscle and not as commonly injured.

Upper Limb

1. INTRODUCTION

The upper limb is part of the **appendicular skeleton** and includes the shoulder, arm, forearm, and hand. It is continuous with the lower neck and is suspended from the trunk at the shoulder. It is anatomically and clinically convenient and beneficial to divide the limb into its functional muscle compartments and to review the nerve(s) and vessels supplying these compartments. Thus, for each component of the upper limb, this chapter focuses on organizing the clinical anatomy into functional compartments and understanding how that anatomy is ideally suited for a wide range of motion, thereby allowing us to manipulate our surrounding environment.

To prepare for your study, review the movements of the upper limb at the shoulder, elbow, wrist, and fingers in Chapter 1.

2. SURFACE ANATOMY

Much of the underlying anatomy of the upper limb can be appreciated by a careful inspection of the surface features (Fig. 7-1). The following surface features are of special note:

- **Acromion:** attachment site of the trapezius and deltoid muscles; easily palpable.
- **Clavicle:** long bone that lies subcutaneously throughout its length.
- **Olecranon:** elbow and proximal portion of the ulna.
- **Deltoid muscle:** muscle that caps the shoulder.
- **Flexor tendons:** wrist and finger flexors visible at the distal anterior forearm.
- **Extensor tendons:** wrist and finger extensors visible on the dorsum of the hand.
- **Thenar eminence:** cone of muscles at the base of the thumb.
- **Hypothenar eminence:** cone of muscles at the base of the little finger.
- **Dorsal venous network:** veins seen on the dorsum of the hand.
- **Cephalic vein:** subcutaneous vein that drains the lateral forearm and arm into the axillary vein.
- **Basilic vein:** subcutaneous vein that drains the medial forearm and distal arm into the axillary vein.
- **Median cubital vein:** subcutaneous vein that lies in the cubital fossa (anterior aspect of the elbow); often used for venipuncture.

As seen elsewhere in the body, a set of superficial and deep veins drain the upper limb. Superficial veins drain blood toward the heart and communicate with deep veins that parallel the major arteries of the upper limb (Fig. 7-2). When vigorous muscle contraction increases the blood flow to the limb and compresses the deep veins, venous blood is shunted into the superficial veins and then returned to the heart. (The veins become more prominent as the limb is being exercised, e.g., when lifting weights.) The superficial and deep veins have valves to assist in venous return. Cutaneous nerves also lie in the superficial fascia and are the terminal sensory branches of the major nerves arising from the brachial plexus (ventral rami of C5-T1 spinal levels) (Fig. 7-2).

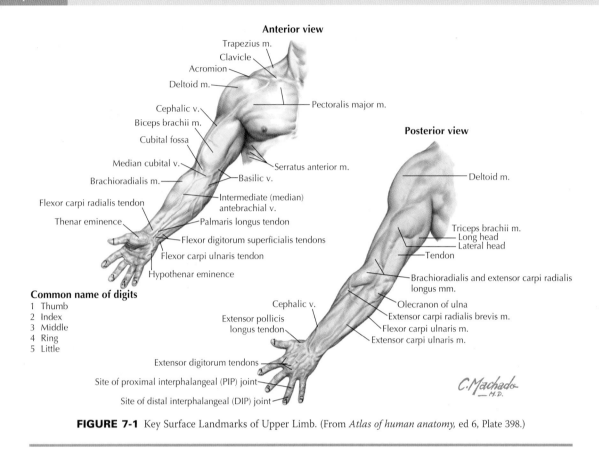

FIGURE 7-1 Key Surface Landmarks of Upper Limb. (From *Atlas of human anatomy,* ed 6, Plate 398.)

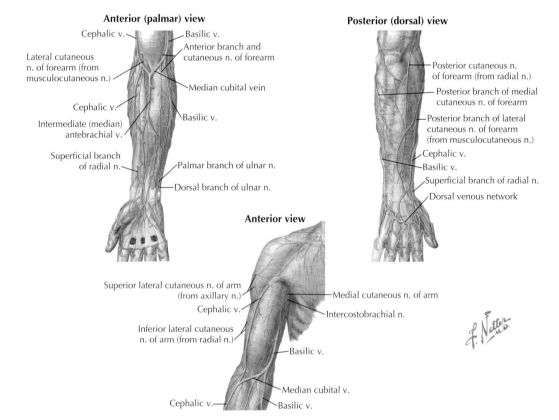

FIGURE 7-2 Superficial Veins and Nerves of Upper Limb. (From *Atlas of human anatomy,* ed 6, Plates 401 and 402.)

3. SHOULDER

Bones and Joints of Pectoral Girdle and Shoulder

The pectoral girdle is composed of the following structures:

- **Clavicle** (collar bone)
- **Scapula** (shoulder blade)

The humerus, or arm bone, articulates with the scapula and forms the shoulder joint. These bones are shown in Figure 7-3 and listed in Table 7-1. The three joints contributing to the pectoral girdle and shoulder are described in Table 7-2 (acromioclavicular and glenohumeral joints) and Table 3-2 (sternoclavicular joint).

The **sternoclavicular** and **acromioclavicular joints** of the pectoral girdle allow for a significant amount of movement of the limb and combined with the shallow ball-and-socket **glenohumeral joint** permit extension, flexion, abduction, adduction, protraction, retraction, and circumduction movements. This flexibility and

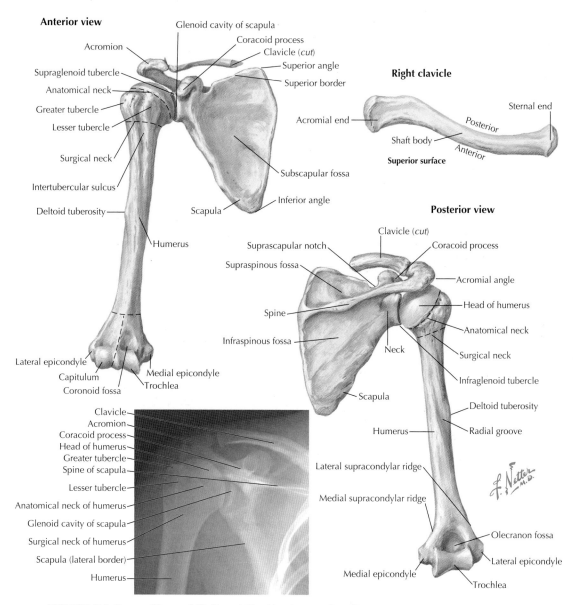

FIGURE 7-3 Bones of Pectoral Girdle and Shoulder. (From *Atlas of human anatomy*, ed 6, Plates 404 to 407.)

TABLE 7-1 Features of the Clavicle, Scapula, and Humerus

CLAVICLE	SCAPULA	HUMERUS
Cylindrical bone with slight S-shaped curve; has no medullary cavity Middle third: narrowest portion First bone to ossify, but last to fuse; formed by intramembranous ossification Most frequently fractured long bone; acts as a strut to keep limb away from trunk	Flat triangular bone Shallow glenoid cavity Attachment locations for 16 muscles Fractures relatively uncommon	Long bone Proximal head: articulates with glenoid cavity of scapula Distal medial and lateral condyles: articulate at elbow with ulna and radius Surgical neck is common fracture site, endangering axillary nerve Midshaft fracture: radial nerve vulnerable

Clinical Focus 7-1

Glenohumeral Dislocations

Almost 95% of shoulder (glenohumeral joint) dislocations occur in an anterior direction. Abduction, extension, and lateral (external) rotation of the arm at the shoulder (e.g., the throwing motion) place stress on the capsule and anterior elements of the rotator cuff (subscapularis tendon). The types of anterior dislocations include the following:

- Subcoracoid (most common)
- Subglenoid
- Subclavicular (rare)

The axillary (most often) and musculocutaneous nerves may be injured during such dislocations.

Anterior dislocation of glenohumeral joint

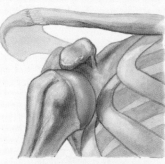
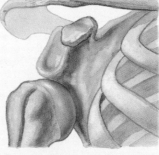
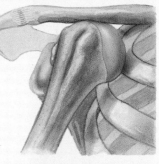

Subcoracoid dislocation   Subglenoid dislocation   Subclavicular dislocation

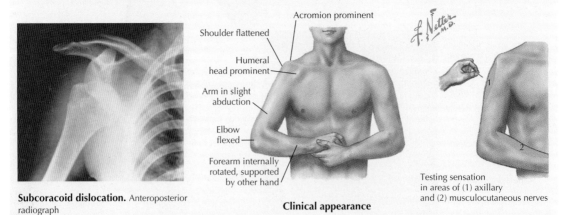

Subcoracoid dislocation. Anteroposterior radiograph

Shoulder flattened

Acromion prominent

Humeral head prominent

Arm in slight abduction

Elbow flexed

Forearm internally rotated, supported by other hand

Clinical appearance

Testing sensation in areas of (1) axillary and (2) musculocutaneous nerves

TABLE 7-2 Acromioclavicular and Glenohumeral Joints

LIGAMENT OR BURSA	ATTACHMENT	COMMENT
Acromioclavicular (Synovial Plane) Joint		
Capsule and articular disc	Surrounds joint	Allows gliding movement as arm is raised and scapula rotates
Acromioclavicular	Acromion to clavicle	
Coracoclavicular (conoid and trapezoid ligaments)	Clavicle to coracoid process	Reinforces the joint
Glenohumeral (Multiaxial Synovial Ball-and-Socket) Joint		
Capsule	Surrounds joint	Permits flexion, extension, abduction, adduction, protraction, retraction, circumduction; most common dislocated joint
Coracohumeral	Coracoid process to greater tubercle of humerus	
Glenohumeral	Supraglenoid tubercle to lesser tubercle of humerus	Composed of superior, middle, and inferior thickenings
Transverse humeral	Spans greater and lesser tubercles of humerus	Holds long head of biceps tendon in intertubercular groove
Glenoid labrum	Margin of glenoid cavity of scapula	Is fibrocartilaginous ligament that deepens glenoid cavity
Bursae		
Subacromial		Between coraco-acromial arch and suprascapular muscle
Subdeltoid		Between deltoid muscle and capsule
Subscapular		Between subscapularis tendon and scapular neck

Clinical Focus 7-2

Fracture of the Proximal Humerus

Fractures of the proximal humerus often occur from a fall on an outstretched hand or from direct trauma to the area. They are especially common in elderly persons, in whom osteoporosis is a factor. The most common site is the surgical neck of the humerus, because the bone begins to taper down at this point and is structurally weaker (see Fig. 7-3).

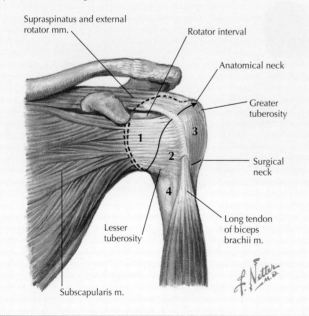

Neer four-part classification of fractures of proximal humerus. 1. Articular fragment (humeral head). 2. Lesser tuberosity. 3. Greater tuberosity. 4. Shaft. If no fragments displaced, fracture considered stable (most common) and treated with minimal external immobilization and early range-of-motion exercise. Displacement of 1 cm or angulation of 45° of one or more fragments necessitates open reduction and internal fixation or prosthetic replacement.

Clavicular Fractures

Fracture of the clavicle is quite common, especially in children. Clavicular fracture usually results from a fall on an outstretched hand or from direct trauma to the shoulder. Fractures of the medial third of the clavicle are rare (about 5%), but fractures of the middle third are common (about 80%). Fractures of the lateral third can involve coracoclavicular ligament tears.

Fractures of lateral third of clavicle

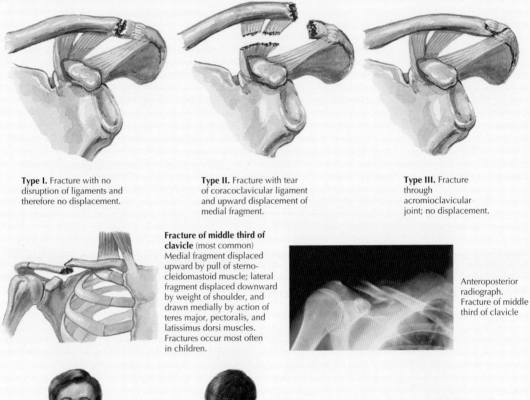

Type I. Fracture with no disruption of ligaments and therefore no displacement.

Type II. Fracture with tear of coracoclavicular ligament and upward displacement of medial fragment.

Type III. Fracture through acromioclavicular joint; no displacement.

Fracture of middle third of clavicle (most common) Medial fragment displaced upward by pull of sternocleidomastoid muscle; lateral fragment displaced downward by weight of shoulder, and drawn medially by action of teres major, pectoralis, and latissimus dorsi muscles. Fractures occur most often in children.

Anteroposterior radiograph. Fracture of middle third of clavicle

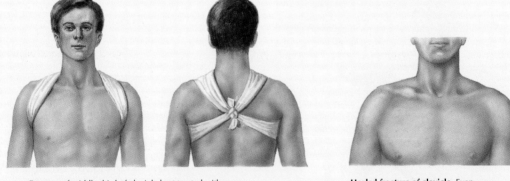

Fracture of middle third of clavicle best treated with snug figure-of-8 bandage or clavicle harness for 3 weeks or until pain subsides.

Healed fracture of clavicle. Even with proper treatment, small lump may remain.

range of movement greatly enhance our ability to interact with our environment. The tendons of the four **rotator cuff muscles** also help stabilize this shallow articulation without inhibiting the extensive range of motion at the shoulder (Fig. 7-4).

Muscles

Muscles of the shoulder include the superficial back muscles, the deltoid and teres major muscles, the four rotator cuff muscles, and the superficial muscles of the pectoral region (anterior chest wall) (Fig. 7-5 and Table 7-3). It is important to note that 16 different muscles attach to the scapula (back, limb, and neck muscles) and account for the range of movement of the scapula as the upper limb is abducted (the scapula rotates), adducted, flexed, extended, and rotated.

Note that abduction at the shoulder is initiated by the **supraspinatus muscle** up to about 15 degrees of abduction and then abduction to 90 degrees is achieved largely by the action of the **deltoid muscle.** For full elevation to 180 degrees, the scapula must laterally rotate upward (the inferior angle swings laterally) by the action of the trapezius and serratus anterior muscles, with assistance from the levator scapulae and both rhomboid muscles. In reality, abduction at the shoulder is a smooth movement, and even as one initiates abduction, the scapula begins to rotate laterally as well.

Because of its broad encapsulation of the shoulder, the **deltoid muscle** functions primarily as an abductor of the shoulder, although its posterior muscle fibers also assist in extension and lateral rotation. Its medial fibers assist in flexion and medial rotation at the shoulder. The primary actions of muscles on shoulder movements are summarized at the end of this chapter (see Table 7-19).

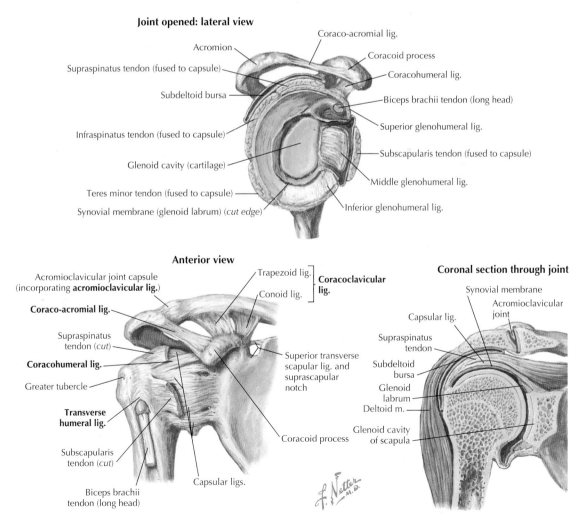

FIGURE 7-4 Shoulder Joint Tendons and Ligaments. (From *Atlas of human anatomy,* ed 6, Plate 408.)

TABLE 7-3 Shoulder Muscles

MUSCLE	PROXIMAL ATTACHMENT (ORIGIN)	DISTAL ATTACHMENT (INSERTION)	INNERVATION	MAIN ACTIONS
Trapezius	Medial third of superior nuchal line; external occipital protuberance, ligamentum nuchae, and spinous processes of C7-T12	Lateral third of clavicle, acromion, and spine of scapula	Spinal root of accessory nerve (cranial nerve XI)	Elevates, retracts, and rotates scapula; superior fibers elevate, middle fibers retract, and inferior fibers depress scapula
Latissimus dorsi	Spinous processes of T7-L5, thoracolumbar fascia, iliac crest, and inferior three or four ribs	Intertubercular sulcus of humerus	Thoracodorsal nerve (C6-C8)	Extends, adducts, and medially rotates humerus at shoulder
Levator scapulae	Transverse processes of C1-C4 vertebrae	Superior part of medial border of scapula	Dorsal scapular and cervical (C3 and C4) nerves	Elevates scapula and tilts its glenoid cavity inferiorly by rotating scapula
Rhomboid minor and major	*Minor:* ligamentum nuchae, spinous processes of C7 and T1 *Major:* spinous processes, T2-T5	Medial border of scapula from level of spine to inferior angle	Dorsal scapular nerve (C4-C5)	Retracts scapula and rotates it to depress glenoid cavity; fixes scapula to thoracic wall
Deltoid	Lateral third of clavicle, acromion, and spine of scapula	Deltoid tuberosity of humerus	Axillary nerve (C5-C6)	*Anterior part:* flexes and medially rotates arm at shoulder *Middle part:* abducts arm at shoulder *Posterior part:* extends and laterally rotates arm at shoulder
Supraspinatus (rotator cuff muscle)	Supraspinous fossa of scapula	Superior facet on greater tubercle of humerus	Suprascapular nerve (C5-C6)	Helps deltoid abduct arm at shoulder and acts with rotator cuff muscles
Infraspinatus (rotator cuff muscle)	Infraspinous fossa of scapula and deep fascia	Middle facet on greater tubercle of humerus	Suprascapular nerve (C5-C6)	Laterally rotates arm at shoulder; helps to hold head in glenoid cavity
Teres minor (rotator cuff muscle)	Lateral border of scapula	Inferior facet on greater tubercle of humerus	Axillary nerve (C5-C6)	Laterally rotates arm at shoulder; helps to hold head in glenoid cavity
Teres major	Dorsal surface of inferior angle of scapula	Medial lip of intertubercular sulcus of humerus	Lower subscapular nerve (C5-C6)	Adducts arm and medially rotates shoulder
Subscapularis (rotator cuff muscle)	Subscapular fossa of scapula	Lesser tubercle of humerus	Upper and lower subscapular nerves (C5-C6)	Medially rotates arm at shoulder and adducts it; helps to hold humeral head in glenoid cavity
Pectoralis major	Medial half of clavicle; sternum; superior six costal cartilages; aponeurosis of external abdominal oblique	Intertubercular sulcus of humerus	Lateral (C5-C7) and medial pectoral (C8-T1) nerves	Flexes, adducts, and medially rotates arm at shoulder
Pectoralis minor	3rd to 5th ribs and deep fascia	Coracoid process of scapula	Medial pectoral nerve (C8-T1)	Depresses and protracts scapula
Serratus anterior	Upper eight ribs	Medial border of scapula	Long thoracic nerve (C5-C7)	Rotates scapula upward and pulls it anterior toward thoracic wall
Subclavius	Junction of 1st rib and costal cartilage	Inferior surface of clavicle	Nerve to subclavius (C5-C6)	Depresses and anchors clavicle

Posterior view

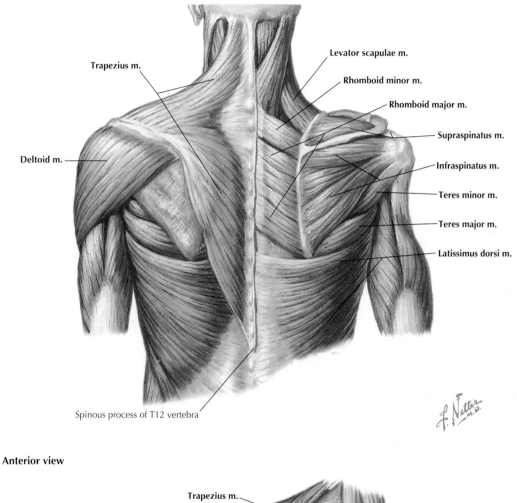

Trapezius m.

Deltoid m.

Spinous process of T12 vertebra

Levator scapulae m.

Rhomboid minor m.

Rhomboid major m.

Supraspinatus m.

Infraspinatus m.

Teres minor m.

Teres major m.

Latissimus dorsi m.

Anterior view

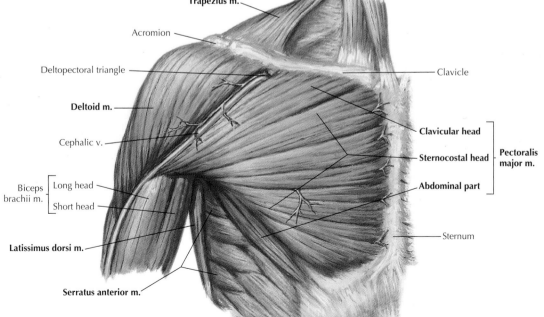

Trapezius m.

Acromion

Deltopectoral triangle

Deltoid m.

Cephalic v.

Biceps brachii m. {
Long head
Short head
}

Latissimus dorsi m.

Serratus anterior m.

Clavicle

Clavicular head

Sternocostal head

Abdominal part

Pectoralis major m.

Sternum

FIGURE 7-5 Muscles Acting on the Shoulder. (From *Atlas of human anatomy,* ed 6, Plate 409.)

Clinical Focus 7-4

Rotator Cuff Injury

The tendons of insertion of the rotator cuff muscles form a musculotendinous cuff about the shoulder joint on its anterior, superior, and posterior aspects. The muscles of the rotator cuff group are as follows:

- Subscapularis
- Infraspinatus
- Supraspinatus
- Teres minor

Repeated abduction and flexion (e.g., a throwing motion) cause wear and tear on the tendons as they rub on the acromion and coraco-acromial ligament, which may lead to cuff tears or rupture. The tendon of the supraspinatus is most vulnerable to injury.

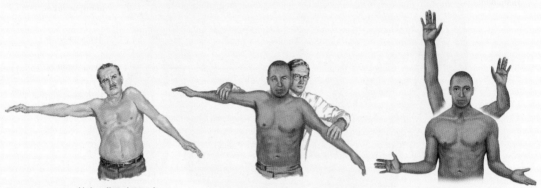

Extensive rupture of left cuff. To bring about abduction, deltoid muscle contracts strongly but only pulls humerus upward toward acromion while scapula rotates and shoulder girdle is elevated. 45° abduction is thus possible.

Test for partial tear of cuff is inability to maintain 90° abduction against mild resistance.

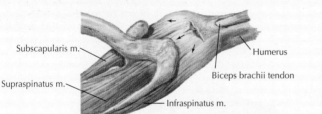

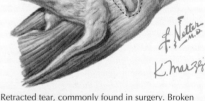

Thickened, edematous biceps brachii tendon

Subscapularis m.

Supraspinatus m.

Humerus

Biceps brachii tendon

Infraspinatus m.

Acute rupture (superior view). Often associated with splitting tear parallel to tendon fibers. Further retraction results in crescentic defect as shown at right.

Retracted tear, commonly found in surgery. Broken line indicates extent of débridement of degenerated tendon for repair.

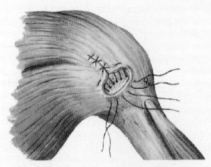

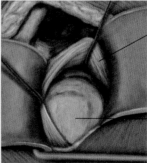

Rotator cuff

Greater tuberosity

Repair. If freshened edges of tear cannot be brought together, notch is created in humerus just beneath articular surface to allow attachment of tendon through drill holes in bone, using strong sutures.

Open surgery for rotator cuff tendon tear. The open rotator cuff repair view demonstrates a large tear of the supraspinatus and infraspinatus tendons.

Shoulder Tendinitis and Bursitis

Movement at the shoulder joint (or almost any joint) can lead to inflammation of the tendons surrounding that joint and secondary inflammation of the bursa that cushions the joint from the overlying muscle or tendon. A painful joint can result, possibly even with calcification within the degenerated tendon. The **supraspinatus muscle tendon** is especially vulnerable because it can become pinched by the greater tubercle of the humerus, the acromion, and the coraco-acromial ligament.

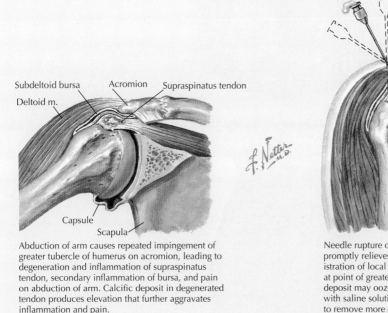
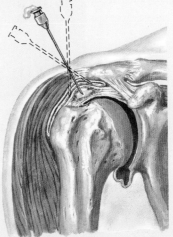

Abduction of arm causes repeated impingement of greater tubercle of humerus on acromion, leading to degeneration and inflammation of supraspinatus tendon, secondary inflammation of bursa, and pain on abduction of arm. Calcific deposit in degenerated tendon produces elevation that further aggravates inflammation and pain.

Needle rupture of deposit in acute tendinitis promptly relieves acute symptoms. After administration of local anesthetic, needle introduced at point of greatest tenderness. Toothpaste-like deposit may ooze from needle. Irrigation of bursa with saline solution using two needles often done to remove more calcific material. Corticosteroid may be injected for additional relief.

4. AXILLA

The axilla (armpit) is a pyramid-shaped region that contains important neurovascular structures that pass through the shoulder region. These neurovascular elements are enclosed in a fascial sleeve called the **axillary sheath**, which is a direct continuation of the prevertebral fascia of the neck. The axilla is a passageway from the neck to the arm and has the following six boundaries (Fig. 7-6):

- **Base (floor):** axillary fascia and skin of armpit.
- **Apex (inlet):** passageway for structures entering or leaving the shoulder and arm; bounded by first rib, clavicle, and superior part of the scapula.
- **Anterior wall:** pectoralis major and minor muscles and clavipectoral fascia.
- **Posterior wall:** subscapularis, teres major, latissimus dorsi, and long head of the triceps muscle.
- **Medial wall:** upper rib cage and intercostal and serratus anterior muscles.
- **Lateral wall:** humerus (intertubercular sulcus).

Important structures in the axilla include the following:

- **Axillary artery:** divided into three parts for descriptive purposes.
- **Axillary vein(s)**
- **Axillary lymph nodes:** five major collections embedded in considerable fat.
- **Brachial plexus of nerves:** ventral rami of C5-T1.
- **Biceps and coracobrachialis muscle:** proximal portions

Anterior view

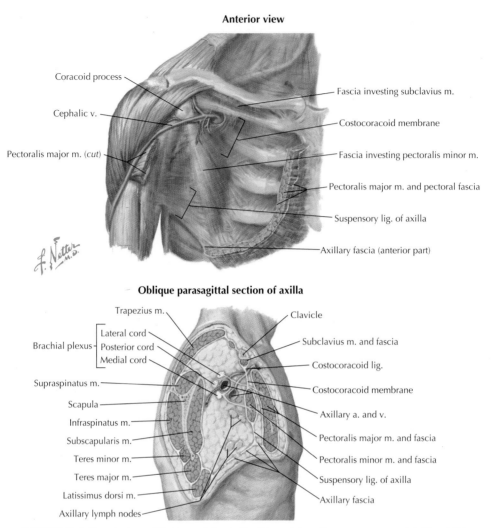

Coracoid process

Cephalic v.

Pectoralis major m. (*cut*)

Fascia investing subclavius m.

Costocoracoid membrane

Fascia investing pectoralis minor m.

Pectoralis major m. and pectoral fascia

Suspensory lig. of axilla

Axillary fascia (anterior part)

Oblique parasagittal section of axilla

Trapezius m.

Brachial plexus
- Lateral cord
- Posterior cord
- Medial cord

Supraspinatus m.

Scapula

Infraspinatus m.

Subscapularis m.

Teres minor m.

Teres major m.

Latissimus dorsi m.

Axillary lymph nodes

Clavicle

Subclavius m. and fascia

Costocoracoid lig.

Costocoracoid membrane

Axillary a. and v.

Pectoralis major m. and fascia

Pectoralis minor m. and fascia

Suspensory lig. of axilla

Axillary fascia

FIGURE 7-6 Boundaries and Features of the Axilla. (From *Atlas of human anatomy,* ed 6, Plate 412.)

- **Axillary tail (of Spence)** of the female breast.

Axillary fasciae include the following:

- **Pectoral fascia:** invests the pectoralis major muscle; attaches to the sternum and clavicle.
- **Clavipectoral fascia:** invests the subclavius and pectoralis minor muscles.
- **Axillary fascia:** forms the base of axilla.
- **Axillary sheath:** invests the axillary neurovascular structures; derivative of the prevertebral fascia of the neck.

Axillary Vessels

The **axillary artery** is the distal continuation of the subclavian artery and begins at the first rib

and is divided into three descriptive parts by the pectoralis minor muscle (Fig. 7-7 and Table 7-4). It continues in the arm as the brachial artery distally at the inferior border of the teres major muscle.

As with most joints, the shoulder joint has a rich vascular **anastomosis.** This anastomosis not only supplies the 16 muscles attaching to the scapula and other shoulder muscles, but also provides collateral circulation to the upper limb should the proximal part of the axillary artery become occluded (proximal to the subscapular branch). This anastomosis includes the following important component arteries (Fig. 7-8):

- **Dorsal scapular (transverse cervical) artery,** a branch of the subclavian (arises from the thyrocervical trunk).

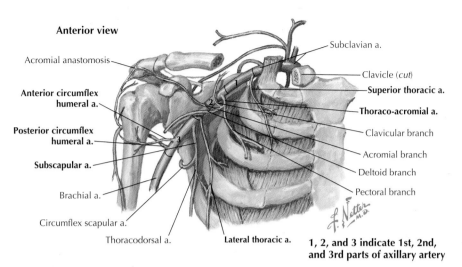

Anterior view

Acromial anastomosis

Anterior circumflex humeral a.

Posterior circumflex humeral a.

Subscapular a.

Brachial a.

Circumflex scapular a.

Thoracodorsal a.

Subclavian a.

Clavicle (*cut*)

Superior thoracic a.

Thoraco-acromial a.

Clavicular branch

Acromial branch

Deltoid branch

Pectoral branch

Lateral thoracic a.

1, 2, and 3 indicate 1st, 2nd, and 3rd parts of axillary artery

FIGURE 7-7 Branches of Axillary Artery. (From *Atlas of human anatomy*, ed 6, Plate 414.)

TABLE 7-4 Branches of Axillary Artery in Its Three Parts

PART	BRANCH	COURSE AND STRUCTURES SUPPLIED	PART	BRANCH	COURSE AND STRUCTURES SUPPLIED
1	Superior thoracic	Supplies first two intercostal spaces	3	Subscapular	Divides into thoracodorsal and circumflex scapular branches
2	Thoraco-acromial	Has clavicular, pectoral, deltoid, and acromial branches		Anterior circumflex humeral	Passes around surgical neck of humerus
	Lateral thoracic	Runs with long thoracic nerve and supplies muscles that it traverses		Posterior circumflex humeral	Runs with axillary nerve through quadrangular space to anastomose with anterior circumflex branch

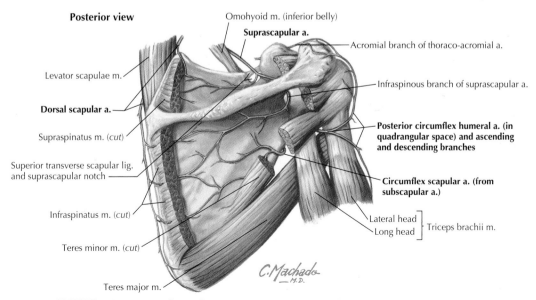

Posterior view

Levator scapulae m.

Dorsal scapular a.

Supraspinatus m. (*cut*)

Superior transverse scapular lig. and suprascapular notch

Infraspinatus m. (*cut*)

Teres minor m. (*cut*)

Teres major m.

Omohyoid m. (inferior belly)

Suprascapular a.

Acromial branch of thoraco-acromial a.

Infraspinous branch of suprascapular a.

Posterior circumflex humeral a. (in quadrangular space) and ascending and descending branches

Circumflex scapular a. (from subscapular a.)

Lateral head

Long head

Triceps brachii m.

FIGURE 7-8 Arteries of Scapular Anastomosis. (From *Atlas of human anatomy*, ed 6, Plate 414.)

Clinical Focus 7-6

Brachial Plexopathy

Damage (trauma, inflammation, tumor, radiation damage, bleeding) to the brachial plexus may present as pain, loss of sensation, and motor weakness. Clinical findings depend on the site of the lesion:

- **Upper plexus lesions:** usually affect the distribution of C5-C6 nerve roots, with the deltoid and biceps muscles affected, and sensory changes that extend below the elbow to the hand.
- **Lower plexus lesions:** usually affect the distribution of C8-T1 nerve roots, with median and ulnar innervated muscles affected; hand weakness and sensory changes involve most of the palmar hand and ulnar aspect of the dorsal hand.

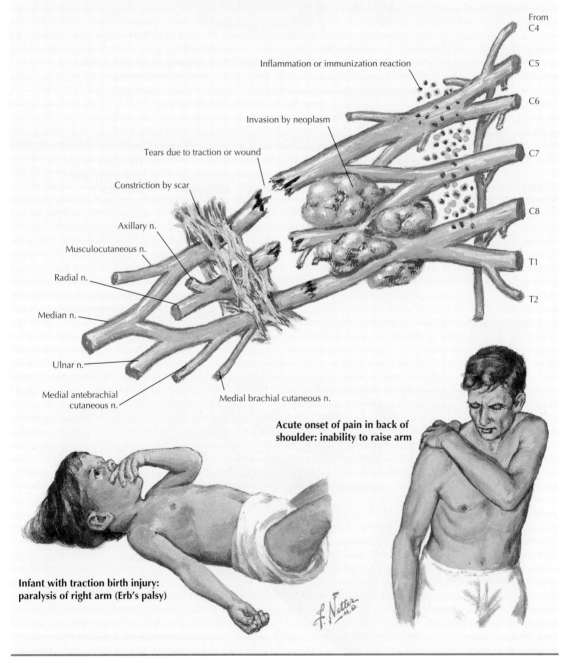

From C4

C5

Inflammation or immunization reaction

C6

Invasion by neoplasm

C7

Tears due to traction or wound

Constriction by scar

C8

Axillary n.

Musculocutaneous n.

T1

Radial n.

T2

Median n.

Ulnar n.

Medial antebrachial cutaneous n.

Medial brachial cutaneous n.

Acute onset of pain in back of shoulder: inability to raise arm

Infant with traction birth injury: paralysis of right arm (Erb's palsy)

- **Suprascapular artery** from the subclavian (thyrocervical trunk) artery.
- **Subscapular artery** and its circumflex scapular and thoracodorsal branches.
- **Posterior and anterior humeral circumflex arteries** passing around the surgical neck of the humerus.
- **Acromial branch of the thoraco-acromial artery** from the second part of the axillary artery.

The **axillary vein** begins at the inferior border of the teres major muscle and is the proximal continuation of the basilic vein (and/or the brachial venae comitantes, which include several small brachial veins that parallel the brachial artery in the arm). When the axillary vein meets the first rib, it becomes the **subclavian vein,** which then drains into the brachiocephalic vein on each side; these two veins then form the **superior vena cava.**

Brachial Plexus

The axillary artery, axillary vein (lies medial to the artery), and cords of the brachial plexus are all bound in the **axillary sheath** (see Fig. 7-6), a continuation of the prevertebral fascia of the neck. In Figure 7-9 the sheath and some parts of the axillary vein have been removed and several muscles reflected for better visualization of the plexus as it invests the axillary artery. Key nerves and branches of the axillary artery also are shown supplying muscles.

Nerves that innervate most of the shoulder muscles and all the muscles of the upper limb arise from the **brachial plexus.** The plexus arises from ventral rami of spinal nerves C5-T1 (Fig. 7-10). The plexus is descriptively divided into five roots (ventral rami), three trunks, six divisions (three anterior, three posterior), three cords (named for their relationship to the axillary artery), and five large terminal branches. Important motor branches of the brachial plexus are described in

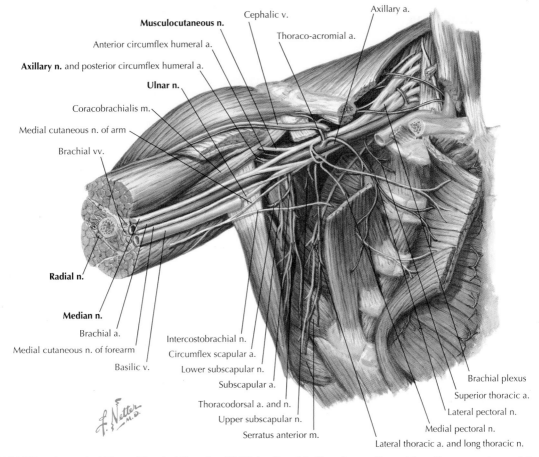

FIGURE 7-9 Brachial Plexus (Terminal Branches Highlighted) and Axillary Artery. (From *Atlas of human anatomy,* ed 6, Plate 415.)

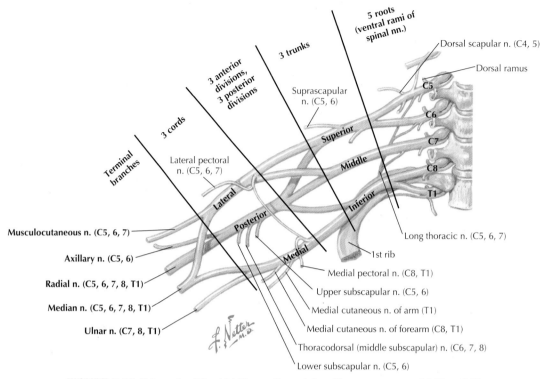

FIGURE 7-10 Schematic of Brachial Plexus. (From *Atlas of human anatomy*, ed 6, Plate 416.)

Table 7-5. The designated ventral root axons contributing to each nerve are generally accurate, although minor variations are normal, as reflected in different textbooks.

Specific nerve lesions related to the brachial plexus (or distal) are fairly common and can occur during obstetric procedures, direct trauma from a cervical rib (extra rib), compression by a neoplasm, radiation injury, bone fractures or joint dislocations, and autoimmune plexopathies.

Despite the complexity of the brachial plexus, its sensory (dermatome) distribution throughout the upper limb is segmental, beginning proximally and lateral over the deltoid muscle and radiating down the lateral arm and forearm to the lateral aspect of the hand. The segmental distribution then courses to the medial side of the hand, back up the medial aspect of the forearm and arm. This distribution is as follows (see also Fig. 7-43):

- **C4:** from the cervical plexus (ventral rami of C1-C4) over the shoulder.
- **C5:** lateral arm over the deltoid and triceps muscles.
- **C6:** lateral forearm over the brachioradialis muscle, thenar eminence, and thumb.

TABLE 7-5 Major Motor Branches of Brachial Plexus

ARISE FROM	NERVE	MUSCLES INNERVATED
Roots	Dorsal scapular	Levator scapulae and rhomboids
	Long thoracic	Serratus anterior
Superior trunk	Suprascapular	Supraspinatus and infraspinatus
	Subclavius	Subclavius
Lateral cord	Lateral pectoral	Pectoralis major
	Musculocutaneous	Anterior compartment muscles of arm
Medial cord	Medial pectoral	Pectoralis minor and major
	Ulnar	Some forearm and most hand muscles
Medial and lateral cords	Median	Most forearm and some hand muscles
Posterior cord	Upper subscapular	Subscapularis
	Thoracodorsal	Latissimus dorsi
	Lower subscapular	Subscapularis and teres major
	Axillary	Deltoid and teres minor
	Radial	Posterior compartment muscles of arm and forearm

Clinical Focus 7-7

Axillary Lipoma

Benign soft tissue tumors occur much more often than malignant tumors. In adults the most common type is the lipoma, composed of mature fat. Presenting as a solitary mass, a lipoma is usually large, soft, and asymptomatic and is more common than all other soft tissue tumors combined. Most lipomas are found in the following locations:

- Axilla
- Shoulders
- Proximal region of the limbs

- Abdomen
- Back

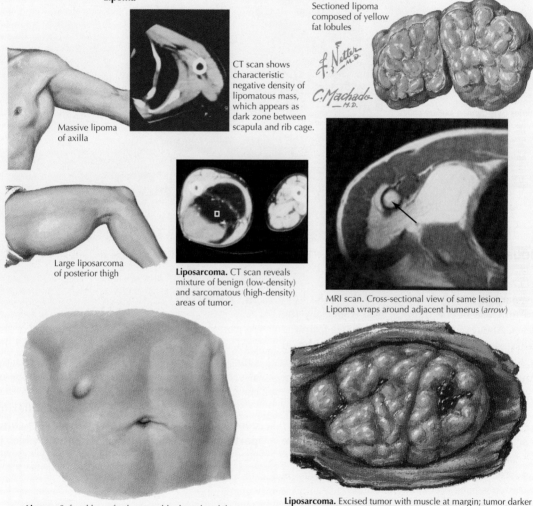

Lipoma

CT scan shows characteristic negative density of lipomatous mass, which appears as dark zone between scapula and rib cage.

Sectioned lipoma composed of yellow fat lobules

Massive lipoma of axilla

Large liposarcoma of posterior thigh

Liposarcoma. CT scan reveals mixture of benign (low-density) and sarcomatous (high-density) areas of tumor.

MRI scan. Cross-sectional view of same lesion. Lipoma wraps around adjacent humerus (*arrow*)

Lipoma. Soft, rubbery, freely moveable dermal nodule

Liposarcoma. Excised tumor with muscle at margin; tumor darker and firmer than benign lipoma

- **C7:** skin of the hand, primarily second through third or fourth digits.
- **C8:** medial two digits (fourth and fifth digits), hypothenar eminence, and medial forearm.
- **T1:** medial arm (some dermatome charts also include anterior forearm).

- **T2:** from the intercostobrachial nerve to the skin of the axilla (not part of the brachial plexus).

Axillary Lymph Nodes

The axillary lymph nodes lie in the fatty connective tissue of the axilla and are the major collection

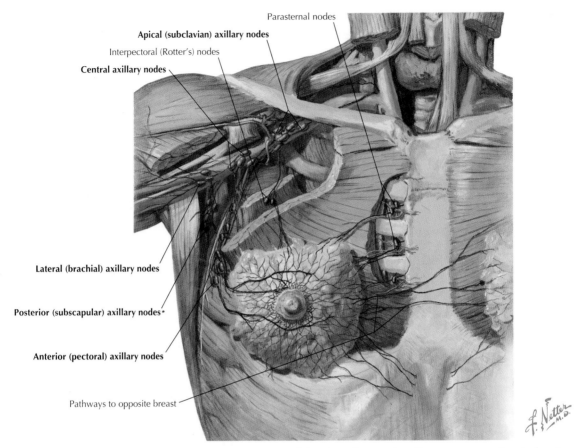

Parasternal nodes

Apical (subclavian) axillary nodes

Interpectoral (Rotter's) nodes

Central axillary nodes

Lateral (brachial) axillary nodes

Posterior (subscapular) axillary nodes

Anterior (pectoral) axillary nodes

Pathways to opposite breast

FIGURE 7-11 Axillary Lymph Nodes and Lymph Drainage of the Breast. (From *Atlas of human anatomy,* ed 6, Plate 181.)

nodes for all lymph draining from the upper limb and portions of the thoracic wall, especially the breast. About 75% of lymphatic drainage from the breast passes through the axillary nodes. The 20 to 30 nodes are divided into the following five groups (Fig. 7-11):

- **Central nodes:** receive lymph from several of the other groups.
- **Lateral (brachial, humeral) nodes:** receive most of the upper limb drainage.
- **Posterior (subscapular) nodes:** drain the upper back, neck, and shoulder.
- **Anterior (pectoral) nodes:** drain the breast and anterior trunk.
- **Apical (subclavian) nodes:** connect with infraclavicular nodes.

Lymph from the breast also can drain superiorly into infraclavicular nodes, into pectoral nodes, medially into parasternal nodes, and inferiorly into abdominal trunk nodes (see also Fig. 3-9 and Clinical Focus 3-3).

5. ARM

As you study the anatomical arrangement of the arm and forearm, organize your study around the functional muscular compartments. We have already discussed the **humerus,** the long bone of the arm (see Fig. 7-3 and Table 7-1).

The arm is divided into an **anterior (flexor) compartment** and a **posterior (extensor) compartment** by an **intermuscular septum,** which is attached medially and laterally to the deep (investing) fascia surrounding the muscles.

Anterior Compartment Arm Muscles, Vessels, and Nerves

Muscles of the anterior compartment exhibit the following features (Fig 7-12 and Table 7-6):

- Are primarily flexors of the forearm at the elbow.
- Are secondarily flexors of the arm at the shoulder (biceps and coracobrachialis).

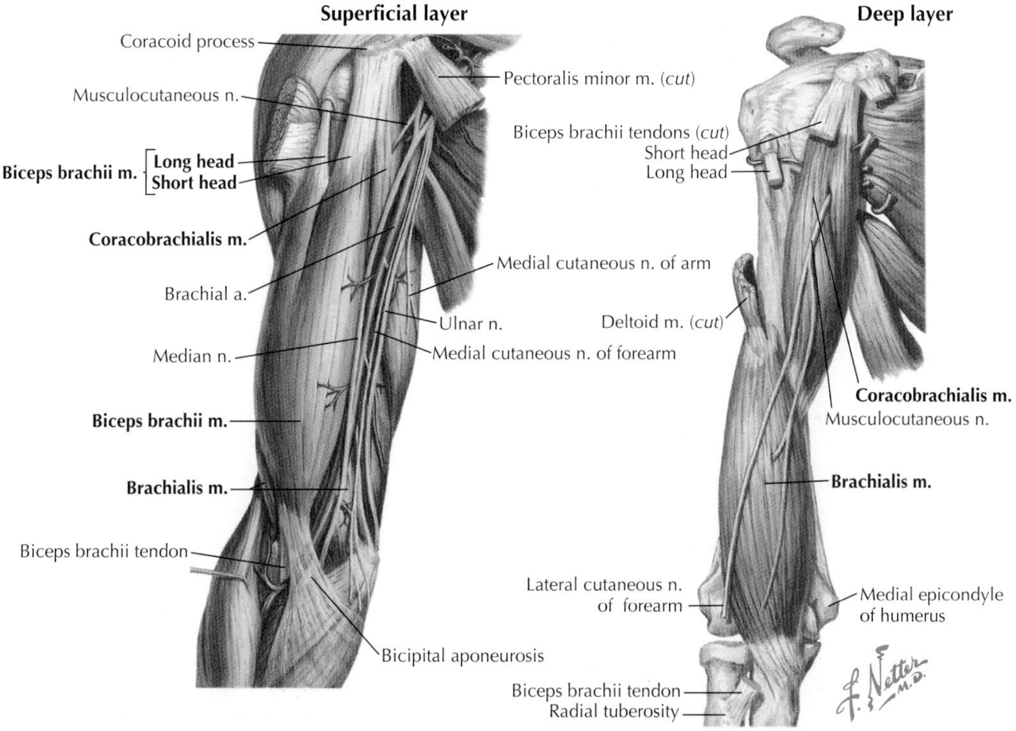

FIGURE 7-12 Anterior Compartment Arm Muscles and Nerves. (From *Atlas of human anatomy,* ed 6, Plate 417.)

TABLE 7-6 Anterior Compartment Arm Muscles

MUSCLE	PROXIMAL ATTACHMENT (ORIGIN)	DISTAL ATTACHMENT (INSERTION)	INNERVATION	MAIN ACTIONS
Biceps brachii	*Short head:* apex of coracoid process of scapula *Long head:* supraglenoid tubercle of scapula	Tuberosity of radius and fascia of forearm via bicipital aponeurosis	Musculocutaneous nerve (C5-C6)	Supinates flexed forearm; flexes forearm at elbow
Brachialis	Distal half of anterior humerus	Coronoid process and tuberosity of ulna	Musculocutaneous nerve (C5-C6), and contribution from radial nerve (C7)	Flexes forearm at elbow in all positions
Coracobrachialis	Tip of coracoid process of scapula	Middle third of medial surface of humerus	Musculocutaneous nerve (C5-C7)	Helps to flex and adduct arm at shoulder

- Can supinate the flexed forearm (biceps only).
- Are innervated by the musculocutaneous nerve.
- Are supplied by the brachial artery and its muscular branches.

Posterior Compartment Arm Muscles, Vessels, and Nerves

Muscles of the posterior compartment exhibit the following features (Fig. 7-13 and Table 7-7):

- Are primarily extensors of the forearm at the elbow.
- Are supplied with blood from the deep artery of the arm (profunda brachii) and its muscular branches.
- Are innervated by the radial nerve.

The artery of the arm is the **brachial artery** and its branches. The brachial artery extends from the inferior border of the teres major muscle to just below the anterior elbow, where it divides into

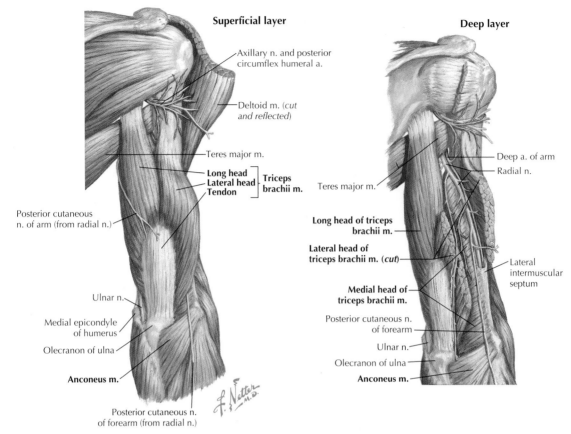

FIGURE 7-13 Posterior Compartment Arm Muscles and Nerves. (From *Atlas of human anatomy,* ed 6, Plate 418.)

TABLE 7-7 Posterior Compartment Arm Muscles

MUSCLE	PROXIMAL ATTACHMENT (ORIGIN)	DISTAL ATTACHMENT (INSERTION)	INNERVATION	MAIN ACTIONS
Triceps brachii	*Long head:* infraglenoid tubercle of scapula *Lateral head:* posterior surface of humerus *Medial head:* posterior surface of humerus, inferior to radial groove	Posterior surface of olecranon of ulna and fascia of forearm	Radial nerve (C6-C8)	Extends forearm at elbow; is chief extensor of elbow; steadies head of abducted humerus (long head)
Anconeus	Lateral epicondyle of humerus	Lateral surface of olecranon and superior part of posterior surface of ulna	Radial nerve (C6-C8)	Assists triceps in extending elbow; abducts ulna during pronation

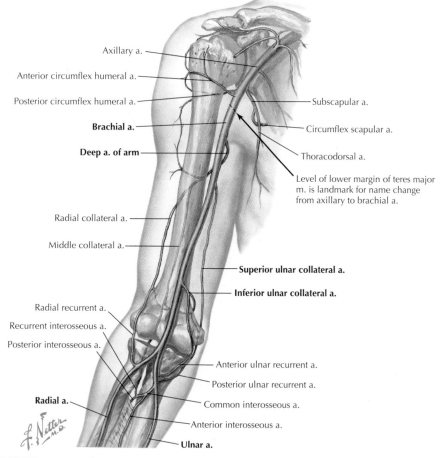

Axillary a.

Anterior circumflex humeral a.

Posterior circumflex humeral a.

Brachial a.

Deep a. of arm

Subscapular a.

Circumflex scapular a.

Thoracodorsal a.

Level of lower margin of teres major
m. is landmark for name change
from axillary to brachial a.

Radial collateral a.

Middle collateral a.

Superior ulnar collateral a.

Inferior ulnar collateral a.

Radial recurrent a.

Recurrent interosseous a.

Posterior interosseous a.

Anterior ulnar recurrent a.

Posterior ulnar recurrent a.

Radial a.

Common interosseous a.

Anterior interosseous a.

Ulnar a.

FIGURE 7-14 Brachial Artery and Its Anastomoses. (From *Atlas of human anatomy,* ed 6, Plate 420.)

TABLE 7-8 Branches of Brachial Artery			
ARTERY	**COURSE**	**ARTERY**	**COURSE**
Brachial	Begins at inferior border of teres major and ends at its bifurcation in cubital fossa	Inferior ulnar collateral	Passes anterior to medial epicondyle of humerus
Deep artery of arm	Runs with radial nerve around humeral shaft	Radial	Is smaller lateral terminal branch of brachial artery
Superior ulnar collateral	Runs with ulnar nerve	Ulnar	Is larger medial terminal branch of brachial artery

the **ulnar** and **radial arteries** (Fig. 7-14 and Table 7-8). A rich anastomosis exists around the elbow joint between branches of the brachial artery and branches of the radial and ulnar arteries. One can feel a brachial pulse by pressing the artery medially at the midarm against the underlying humerus.

As shown in Figure 7-2, the superficial **cephalic** and **basilic veins** course in the subcutaneous tissues of the arm. The **deep brachial veins**

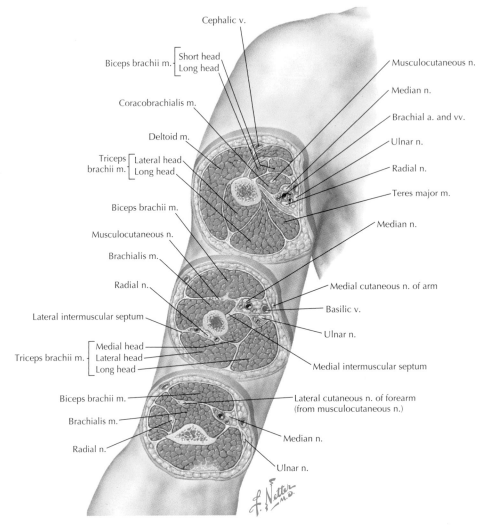

Cephalic v.

Biceps brachii m.
- Short head
- Long head

Coracobrachialis m.

Deltoid m.

Triceps brachii m.
- Lateral head
- Long head

Biceps brachii m.

Musculocutaneous n.

Brachialis m.

Radial n.

Lateral intermuscular septum

Triceps brachii m.
- Medial head
- Lateral head
- Long head

Biceps brachii m.

Brachialis m.

Radial n.

Musculocutaneous n.

Median n.

Brachial a. and vv.

Ulnar n.

Radial n.

Teres major m.

Median n.

Medial cutaneous n. of arm

Basilic v.

Ulnar n.

Medial intermuscular septum

Lateral cutaneous n. of forearm (from musculocutaneous n.)

Median n.

Ulnar n.

FIGURE 7-15 Serial Cross Sections of the Arm. (From *Atlas of human anatomy,* ed 6, Plate 421.)

usually consist of either paired veins or venae comitantes that surround the brachial artery. These veins drain into the basilic and/or axillary vein.

Arm in Cross Section

Cross sections of the arm show the anterior and posterior compartments and their respective flexor and extensor muscles (Fig. 7-15). Note the nerve of each compartment and the medially situated neurovascular bundle containing the brachial artery, median nerve, and ulnar nerve. The median and ulnar nerves do not innervate arm muscles but simply pass through the arm to reach the forearm and hand.

6. FOREARM

Bones and Elbow Joint

The bones of the forearm (defined as elbow to wrist) are the laterally placed **radius** and medial **ulna** (Fig. 7-16 and Table 7-9). The radio-ulnar fibrous (syndesmosis) joint unites both bones by an **interosseous membrane,** which also divides the forearm into anterior and posterior compartments.

The elbow joint is composed of the **humero-ulnar** and **humeroradial joints** for flexion and extension, and the **proximal radio-ulnar joint** for pronation and supination (Figs. 7-17 and 7-18 and Table 7-10).

Deep Tendon Reflexes

A brisk tap to a partially stretched muscle tendon near its point of insertion elicits a deep tendon (muscle stretch) reflex (DTR) dependent on the following:

- Intact afferent (sensory) nerve fibers
- Normal functional synapses in the spinal cord at the appropriate level
- Intact efferent (motor) nerve fibers
- Normal functional neuromuscular junctions on the tapped muscle
- Normal muscle fiber functioning (contraction)

Characteristically, the DTR only involves several spinal cord segments (and their afferent and efferent nerve fibers). If pathology is involved at the level tested, the reflex may be weak or absent, requiring further testing to determine where along the pathway the lesion occurred. For the arm, you should know the following segmental levels for the DTR:

- **Biceps brachii** reflex C5 and C6
- **Triceps brachii** reflex C7 and C8

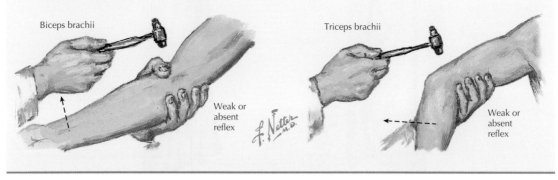

Biceps brachii

Weak or
absent
reflex

Triceps brachii

Weak or
absent
reflex

Fractures of the Humerus

Fractures of the humerus may occur proximally (e.g., surgical neck fractures, which are common in older persons from a fall on an outstretched hand). Humeral fractures also may occur along the midshaft, usually from direct trauma, or distally (uncommon in adults). Proximal fractures mainly occur at the following four sites:

- Humeral head (articular fragment)
- Lesser tuberosity
- Greater tuberosity
- Proximal shaft (surgical neck)

Midshaft fractures usually heal well but may involve entrapment of the radial nerve as it spirals around the shaft to reach the arm's posterior muscle compartment (triceps muscle).

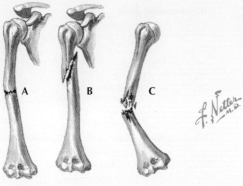

A. Transverse fracture of midshaft
B. Oblique (spiral) fracture
C. Comminuted fracture with marked angulation

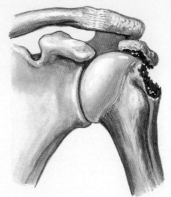

Displaced fracture of greater tuberosity

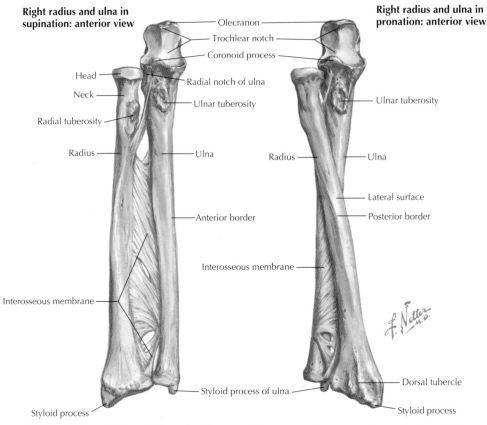

Right radius and ulna in supination: anterior view

- Olecranon
- Trochlear notch
- Coronoid process
- Head
- Neck
- Radial notch of ulna
- Ulnar tuberosity
- Radial tuberosity
- Radius
- Ulna
- Anterior border
- Interosseous membrane
- Interosseous membrane
- Styloid process of ulna
- Styloid process

Right radius and ulna in pronation: anterior view

- Ulnar tuberosity
- Radius
- Ulna
- Lateral surface
- Posterior border
- Interosseous membrane
- Dorsal tubercle
- Styloid process

FIGURE 7-16 Radius and Ulna of the Forearm. (From *Atlas of human anatomy,* ed 6, Plate 425.)

TABLE 7-9 Features of Radius and Ulna

STRUCTURE	DESCRIPTION
Radius	
Long bone	Is shorter than ulna
Proximal head	Articulates with capitulum of humerus and radial notch of ulna
Distal styloid process	Articulates with scaphoid, lunate, and triquetrum carpal bones
Ulna	
Long bone	Is longer than radius
Proximal olecranon	Is attachment point of triceps tendon
Proximal trochlear notch	Articulates with trochlea of humerus
Radial notch	Articulates with head of radius
Distal head	Articulates with disc at distal radio-ulnar joint

TABLE 7-10 Forearm Joints

LIGAMENT	ATTACHMENT	COMMENT
Humero-ulnar (Uniaxial Synovial Hinge [Ginglymus]) Joint		
Capsule	Surrounds joint	Provides flexion and extension
Ulnar (medial) collateral	Medial epicondyle of humerus to coronoid process and olecranon of ulna	Is triangular ligament with anterior, posterior, and oblique bands
Humeroradial Joint		
Capsule	Surrounds joint	Capitulum of humerus to head of radius
Radial (lateral) collateral	Lateral epicondyle of humerus to radial notch of ulna and anular ligament	Is weaker than ulnar collateral ligament but provides posterolateral stability
Proximal Radio-ulnar (Uniaxial Synovial Pivot) Joint		
Anular ligament	Surrounds radial head and radial notch of ulna	Keeps radial head in radial notch; allows pronation and supination

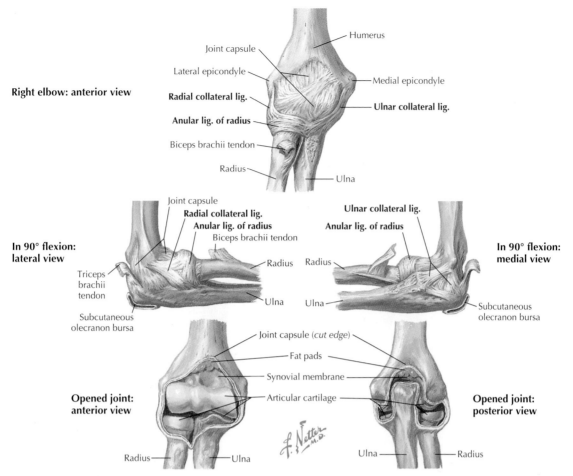

FIGURE 7-17 Elbow Joint and Ligaments. (From *Atlas of human anatomy,* ed 6, Plate 424.)

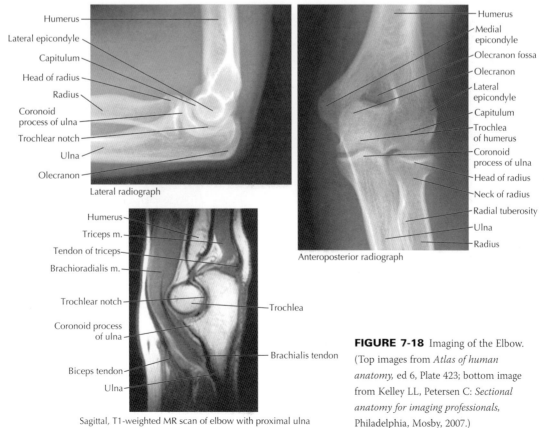

FIGURE 7-18 Imaging of the Elbow. (Top images from *Atlas of human anatomy,* ed 6, Plate 423; bottom image from Kelley LL, Petersen C: *Sectional anatomy for imaging professionals,* Philadelphia, Mosby, 2007.)

Clinical Focus 7-10

Biceps Brachii Rupture

Rupture of the biceps brachii may occur at the tendon (or rarely the muscle belly) and has the highest rate of spontaneous rupture of any tendon in the body. Rupture is seen most often in patients older than 40, in association with rotator cuff injuries (as the tendon begins to undergo degenerative changes), and with repetitive lifting (e.g., weight lifters). Rupture of the long head of the biceps brachii tendon is most common and may occur in the following locations:

- Shoulder joint
- Intertubercular (bicipital) sulcus of the humerus
- Musculotendinous junction

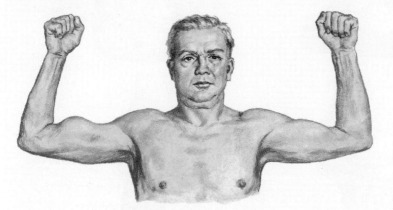

Rupture of tendon of long head of right biceps brachii muscle indicated by active flexion of elbow

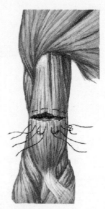

Rupture of belly of biceps brachii muscle; repair with mattress sutures

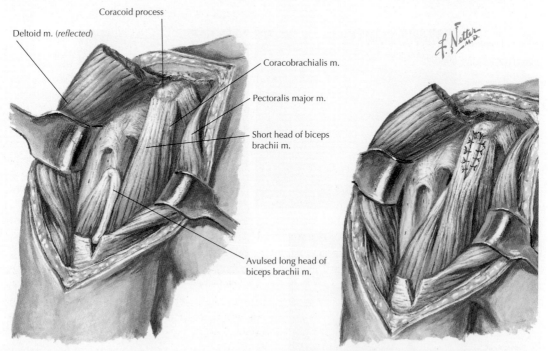

Coracoid process

Deltoid m. (*reflected*)

Coracobrachialis m.

Pectoralis major m.

Short head of biceps brachii m.

Avulsed long head of biceps brachii m.

Exposure shows tendon of long head of biceps brachii muscle avulsed.

For repair, long head tendon brought through slit in short head tendon and sutured to margins and to coracoid process.

Elbow Dislocation

Elbow dislocations occur third in frequency after shoulder and finger dislocations. Dislocation often results from a fall on an outstretched hand and includes the following types:

- Posterior (most common)
- Anterior (rare; may lacerate brachial artery)
- Lateral (uncommon)
- Medial (rare)

Dislocations may be accompanied by fractures of the humeral medial epicondyle, olecranon (ulna), radial head, or coronoid process of the ulna. Injury to the ulnar nerve (most common) or median nerve may accompany these dislocations.

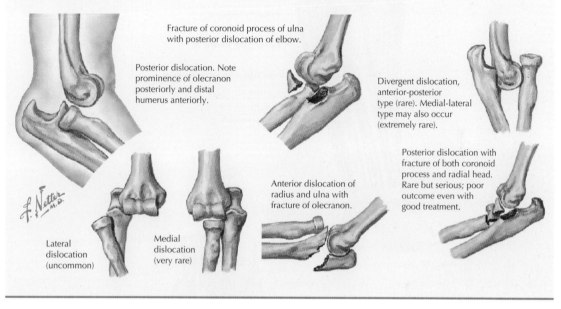

Fracture of coronoid process of ulna with posterior dislocation of elbow.

Posterior dislocation. Note prominence of olecranon posteriorly and distal humerus anteriorly.

Divergent dislocation, anterior-posterior type (rare). Medial-lateral type may also occur (extremely rare).

Posterior dislocation with fracture of both coronoid process and radial head. Rare but serious; poor outcome even with good treatment.

Anterior dislocation of radius and ulna with fracture of olecranon.

Lateral dislocation (uncommon)

Medial dislocation (very rare)

Anterior Compartment Forearm Muscles, Vessels, and Nerves

The muscles of the anterior compartment of the forearm are arranged in two layers, with the muscles of the superficial layer largely arising from the **medial epicondyle** of the humerus (Fig. 7-19 and Table 7-11). The deeper group of anterior forearm muscles arise from the ulna, the radius, and/or the interosseous membrane connecting these two forearm bones. These anterior forearm muscles exhibit the following general features:

- Are primarily flexors of the hand at the wrist and/or finger flexors.
- Two are pronators.
- Secondarily, several can abduct and adduct the hand at the wrist.
- Muscle bellies reside in the forearm, but tendons extend to the wrist or into the hand (except for the pronator muscles).

- Are supplied by the ulnar and radial arteries.
- All except two are innervated by the median nerve (flexor carpi ulnaris and medial half of flexor digitorum profundus innervated by ulnar nerve).

The **cubital fossa** is the region anterior to the elbow and is demarcated by the brachioradialis muscle laterally and the pronator teres muscle medially (Fig. 7-19). The floor of the cubital fossa is formed by the brachialis muscle. The median nerve and brachial artery traverse the cubital fossa and are covered by the bicipital aponeurosis.

Posterior Compartment Forearm Muscles, Vessels, and Nerves

The muscles of the posterior compartment of the forearm also are arranged in a superficial and deep

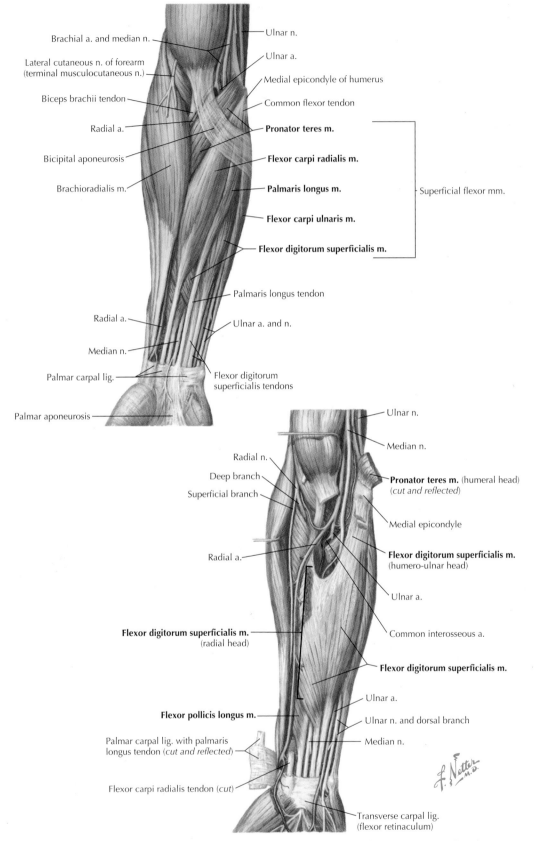

Brachial a. and median n.

Lateral cutaneous n. of forearm
(terminal musculocutaneous n.)

Biceps brachii tendon

Radial a.

Bicipital aponeurosis

Brachioradialis m.

Ulnar n.

Ulnar a.

Medial epicondyle of humerus

Common flexor tendon

Pronator teres m.

Flexor carpi radialis m.

Palmaris longus m.

Flexor carpi ulnaris m.

Flexor digitorum superficialis m.

Superficial flexor mm.

Palmaris longus tendon

Radial a.

Ulnar a. and n.

Median n.

Palmar carpal lig.

Flexor digitorum
superficialis tendons

Palmar aponeurosis

Ulnar n.

Median n.

Radial n.

Deep branch

Superficial branch

Pronator teres m. (humeral head)
(*cut and reflected*)

Medial epicondyle

Radial a.

Flexor digitorum superficialis m.
(humero-ulnar head)

Ulnar a.

Common interosseous a.

Flexor digitorum superficialis m.
(radial head)

Flexor digitorum superficialis m.

Ulnar a.

Flexor pollicis longus m.

Ulnar n. and dorsal branch

Palmar carpal lig. with palmaris
longus tendon (*cut and reflected*)

Median n.

Flexor carpi radialis tendon (*cut*)

Transverse carpal lig.
(flexor retinaculum)

FIGURE 7-19 Anterior Compartment Forearm Muscles and Nerves. (From *Atlas of human anatomy,* ed 6, Plates 432 and 433.)

TABLE 7-11 Anterior Compartment Forearm Muscles

MUSCLE	PROXIMAL ATTACHMENT (ORIGIN)	DISTAL ATTACHMENT (INSERTION)	INNERVATION	MAIN ACTIONS
Pronator teres	Medial epicondyle of humerus and coronoid process of ulna	Middle of lateral surface of radius	Median nerve (C6-C7)	Pronates forearm and flexes elbow
Flexor carpi radialis	Medial epicondyle of humerus	Base of 2nd metacarpal bone	Median nerve (C6-C7)	Flexes hand at wrist and abducts it
Palmaris longus	Medial epicondyle of humerus	Distal half of flexor retinaculum and palmar aponeurosis	Median nerve (C7-C8)	Flexes hand at wrist and tightens palmar aponeurosis
Flexor carpi ulnaris	*Humeral head:* medial epicondyle of humerus *Ulnar head:* olecranon and posterior border of ulna	Pisiform bone, hook of hamate bone, and 5th metacarpal bone	Ulnar nerve (C7-T1)	Flexes hand at wrist and adducts it
Flexor digitorum superficialis	*Humero-ulnar head:* medial epicondyle of humerus, ulnar collateral ligament, and coronoid process of ulna *Radial head:* superior half of anterior radius	Bodies of middle phalanges of medial four digits	Median nerve (C8-T1)	Flexes middle phalanges of medial four digits; also weakly flexes proximal phalanges, forearm, and wrist
Flexor digitorum profundus	Proximal ¾ of medial and anterior surfaces of ulna and interosseous membrane	Palmar bases of distal phalanges of medial four digits	*Medial part:* ulnar nerve *Lateral part:* median nerve	Flexes distal phalanges of medial four digits; assists with flexion of wrist
Flexus pollicis longus	Anterior surface of radius and adjacent interosseous membrane	Base of distal phalanx of thumb	Median nerve (anterior interosseous)	Flexes phalanges of 1st digit (thumb)
Pronator quadratus	Distal ¼ of anterior surface of ulna	Distal ¼ of anterior surface of radius	Median nerve (anterior interosseous) (C7-C8)	Pronates forearm and hand

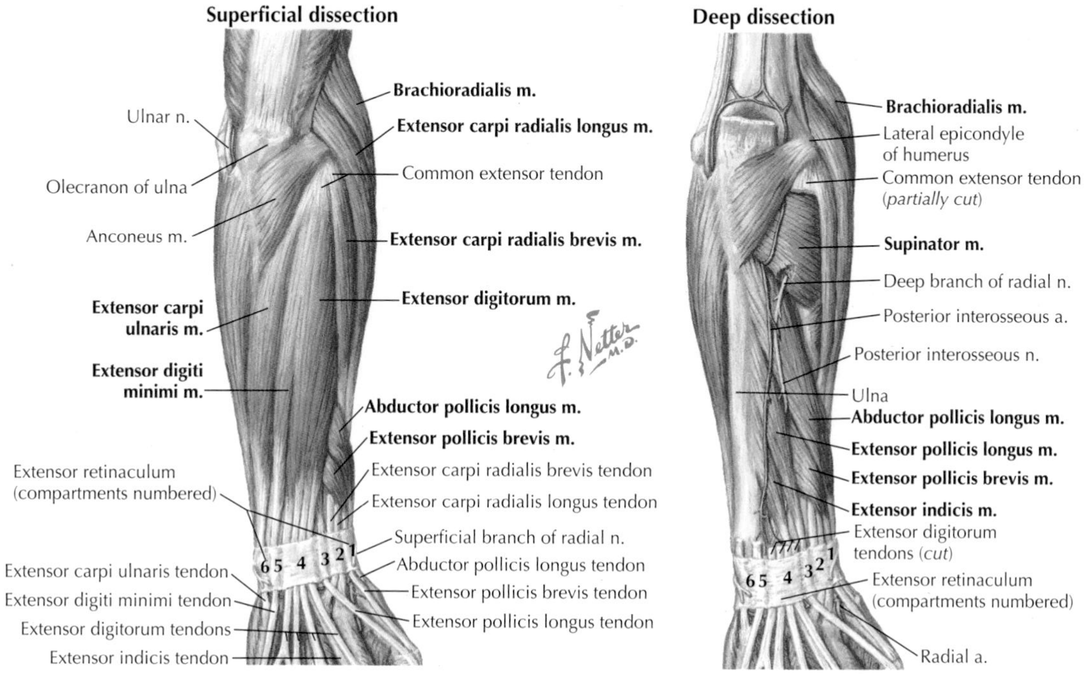

FIGURE 7-20 Posterior Compartment Forearm Muscles and Nerves. (From *Atlas of human anatomy,* ed 6, Plates 430 and 431.)

layer, with the superficial layer of muscles largely arising from the **lateral epicondyle** of the humerus (Fig. 7-20 and Table 7-12). The deeper muscles of the posterior forearm compartment arise from the radius, the ulna, and/or the interosseous membrane connecting these two forearm bones. The posterior forearm muscles exhibit the following general features:

- Are primarily extensors of the hand at the wrist and/or finger extensors; several can adduct or abduct the thumb.
- One is a supinator.
- Secondarily, several can abduct and adduct the hand at the wrist.
- Muscle bellies reside largely in the forearm, but tendons extend to the wrist or into the dorsum of the hand.

- Are supplied by the radial and ulnar arteries (common interosseous branch of the ulnar artery).
- All are innervated by the radial nerve.

The muscles of the forearm are supplied by the **radial** and **ulnar arteries** (see Figs. 7-14, 7-19, and 7-21; Table 7-13). Deeper muscles also receive blood from the **common interosseous** branch of the ulnar artery. **Deep veins** parallel the radial and ulnar arteries and have connections with the superficial veins in the subcutaneous tissue of the forearm.

Forearm in Cross Section

Cross sections of the forearm demonstrate the anterior (flexor-pronator) and posterior (extensor-supinator) compartments and their respective

TABLE 7-12 Posterior Compartment Forearm Muscles and Nerves

MUSCLE	PROXIMAL ATTACHMENT (ORIGIN)	DISTAL ATTACHMENT (INSERTION)	INNERVATION	MAIN ACTIONS
Brachioradialis	Proximal ⅔ of lateral supracondylar ridge of humerus	Lateral surface of distal end of radius	Radial nerve (C5-C6)	Flexes mid-pronated forearm at elbow
Extensor carpi radialis longus	Lateral supracondylar ridge of humerus	Base of 2nd metacarpal bone	Radial nerve (C6-C7)	Extends and abducts hand at wrist
Extensor carpi radialis brevis	Lateral epicondyle of humerus	Base of 3rd metacarpal bone	Radial nerve (deep branch) (C7)	Extends and abducts hand at wrist
Extensor digitorum	Lateral epicondyle of humerus	Extensor expansions of medial four digits	Radial nerve (posterior interosseous) (C7-C8)	Extends medial four digits at MCP joints; extends hand at wrist joint
Extensor digiti minimi	Lateral epicondyle of humerus	Extensor expansion of 5th digit	Radial nerve (posterior interosseous)	Extends 5th digit at MCP and IP joints
Extensor carpi ulnaris	Lateral epicondyle of humerus and posterior border of ulna	Base of 5th metacarpal bone	Radial nerve (posterior interosseous)	Extends and adducts hand at wrist
Supinator	Lateral epicondyle of humerus; radial collateral, and anular ligaments; supinator fossa; and crest of ulna	Lateral, posterior, and anterior surfaces of proximal third of radius	Radial nerve (deep branch) (C6-C7)	Supinates forearm, i.e., rotates radius to turn palm anteriorly
Abductor pollicis longus	Posterior surfaces of ulna, radius, and interosseous membrane	Base of 1st metacarpal bone	Radial nerve (posterior interosseous)	Abducts thumb and extends it at CMC joint
Extensor pollicis brevis	Posterior surfaces of radius and interosseous membrane	Base of proximal phalanx of thumb	Radial nerve (posterior interosseous)	Extends proximal phalanx of thumb at CMC joint
Extensor pollicis longus	Posterior surfaces of middle third of ulna and interosseous membrane	Base of distal phalanx of thumb	Radial nerve (posterior interosseous) (C7-C8)	Extends distal phalanx of thumb at MCP and IP joints
Extensor indicis	Posterior surfaces of ulna and interosseous membrane	Extensor expansion of 2nd digit	Radial nerve (posterior interosseous) (C7-C8)	Extends 2nd digit and helps to extend hand at wrist

CMC, Carpometacarpal *IP*, interphalangeal *MCP*, metacarpophalangeal.

Clinical Focus 7-12

Fracture of the Radial Head and Neck

Fractures to the proximal radius often involve either the head or the neck of the radius. These fractures can result from a fall on an outstretched hand (indirect trauma) or a direct blow to the elbow. Fracture of the radial head is more common in adults, whereas fracture of the neck is more common in children.

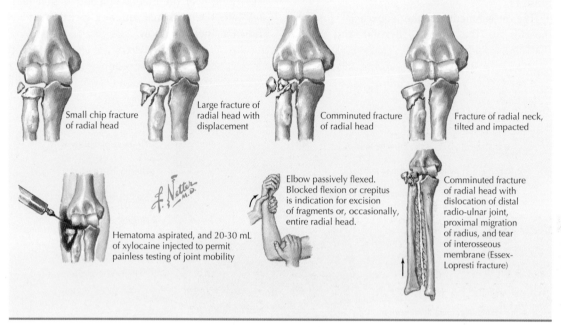

Small chip fracture of radial head

Large fracture of radial head with displacement

Comminuted fracture of radial head

Fracture of radial neck, tilted and impacted

Hematoma aspirated, and 20-30 mL of xylocaine injected to permit painless testing of joint mobility

Elbow passively flexed. Blocked flexion or crepitus is indication for excision of fragments or, occasionally, entire radial head.

Comminuted fracture of radial head with dislocation of distal radio-ulnar joint, proximal migration of radius, and tear of interosseous membrane (Essex-Lopresti fracture)

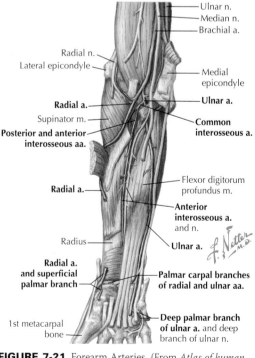

FIGURE 7-21 Forearm Arteries. (From *Atlas of human anatomy*, ed 6, Plate 434.)

TABLE 7-13 Major Branches of the Radial and Ulnar Arteries

ARTERY	COURSE
Radial	Arises from brachial artery in cubital fossa
Radial recurrent branch	Anastomoses with radial collateral artery in arm
Palmar carpal branch	Anastomoses with carpal branch of ulnar artery
Ulnar	Arises from brachial artery in cubital fossa
Anterior ulnar recurrent	Anastomoses with inferior ulnar collateral in arm
Posterior ulnar recurrent	Anastomoses with superior ulnar collateral in arm
Common interosseous	Gives rise to anterior and posterior interosseous arteries
Palmar carpal branch	Anastomoses with carpal branch of radial artery

neurovascular structures (Fig. 7-22). The median nerve innervates all muscles except the flexor carpi ulnaris and the ulnar half of the flexor digitorum profundus (innervated by ulnar nerve) in the anterior compartment. The radial nerve innervates all the posterior compartment muscles.

The attachment of the superficial forearm muscles to the medial (flexors) and lateral (extensors) humeral epicondyles is noteworthy, especially when overused in tennis and golf. Generally, pain from overuse of the forearm extensors is known as "tennis elbow," with the pain felt over the lateral epicondyle and distally into the proximal forearm. Overuse of the forearm flexors may cause pain over the medial epicondyle that radiates into the proximal anterior forearm and is known as "golfer's elbow."

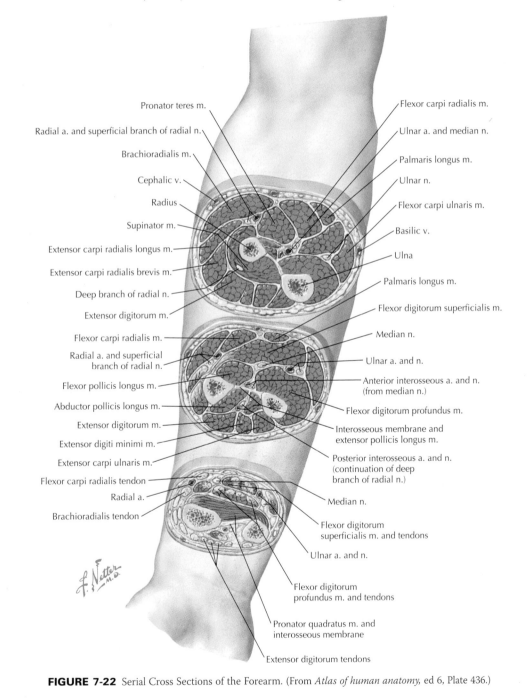

FIGURE 7-22 Serial Cross Sections of the Forearm. (From *Atlas of human anatomy*, ed 6, Plate 436.)

Clinical Focus 7-13

Biomechanics of Forearm Radial Fractures

The ulna is a straight bone with a stable articulation (elbow), but the radius is not uniform in size, proximal to distal. Natural lateral bowing of the radius is essential for optimal pronation and supination. However, when the radius is fractured, the muscles attaching to the bone deform this alignment. Careful reduction of the fracture should attempt to replicate the normal anatomy to maximize pronation and supination, as well as to maintain the integrity of the interosseous membrane.

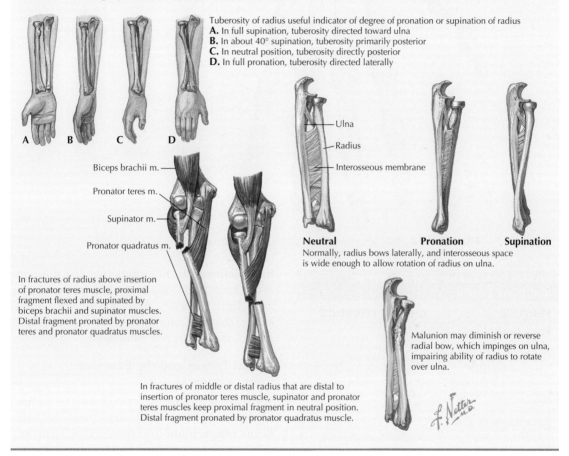

Tuberosity of radius useful indicator of degree of pronation or supination of radius
A. In full supination, tuberosity directed toward ulna
B. In about 40° supination, tuberosity primarily posterior
C. In neutral position, tuberosity directly posterior
D. In full pronation, tuberosity directed laterally

A B C D

Biceps brachii m.

Pronator teres m.

Supinator m.

Pronator quadratus m.

Ulna

Radius

Interosseous membrane

Neutral   **Pronation**   **Supination**
Normally, radius bows laterally, and interosseous space is wide enough to allow rotation of radius on ulna.

In fractures of radius above insertion of pronator teres muscle, proximal fragment flexed and supinated by biceps brachii and supinator muscles. Distal fragment pronated by pronator teres and pronator quadratus muscles.

Malunion may diminish or reverse radial bow, which impinges on ulna, impairing ability of radius to rotate over ulna.

In fractures of middle or distal radius that are distal to insertion of pronator teres muscle, supinator and pronator teres muscles keep proximal fragment in neutral position. Distal fragment pronated by pronator quadratus muscle.

7. WRIST AND HAND

Bones and Joints

The wrist connects the hand to the forearm and is composed of eight **carpal bones** aligned in a proximal and distal row (four carpals in each row). The hand includes the metacarpus (the palm, with five **metacarpal bones**) and five digits with their **phalanges** (Fig. 7-23 and Table 7-14).

The wrist joint is a **radiocarpal synovial joint** between the radius and an articular disc covering the distal ulna, and the proximal articular surfaces of the scaphoid, lunate, and triquetrum (radiocarpal and distal radiocarpal [ulnocarpal in some books] joints), which permits a wide range of movements (Figs. 7-24 and 7-25). Although the **carpal joints** (intercarpal and midcarpal) are within the wrist, they provide for gliding movements and significant wrist extension and flexion.

Carpometacarpal (CMC, carpals to metacarpals), **metacarpophalangeal** (MCP), and **proximal interphalangeal** (PIP) and **distal**

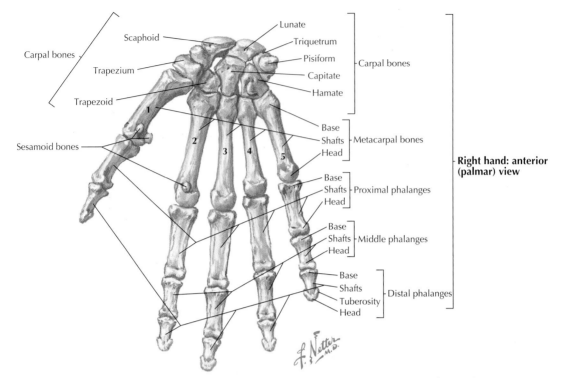

FIGURE 7-23 Wrist and Hand Bones. (From *Atlas of human anatomy*, ed 6, Plate 443.)

TABLE 7-14 Features of the Wrist and Hand Bones

FEATURE	CHARACTERISTICS
Proximal Row of Carpals Scaphoid (boat shaped) Lunate (moon or crescent shaped) Triquetrum (triangular) Pisiform (pea shaped)	Lies beneath anatomical snuffbox; is most commonly fractured carpal All three bones (scaphoid, lunate, triquetrum) articulate with distal radius
Distal Row of Carpals Trapezium (four sided) Trapezoid Capitate (round bone) Hamate (hooked bone)	Distal row articulates with proximal row of carpals and with metacarpals
Metacarpals Numbered 1-5 (thumb to little finger) Two sesamoid bones	Possess a base, shaft, and head Are triangular in cross section Fifth metacarpal most often fractured Are associated with head of first metacarpal
Phalanges Three for each digit except thumb	Possess base, shaft, and head Termed *proximal, middle,* and *distal* Distal phalanx of middle finger often fractured

interphalangeal (DIP) **joints** complete the joints of the hand (Fig. 7-26). Note that the thumb (the first digit) possesses only one interphalangeal joint. Table 7-15 summarizes the movements at each of these wrist and hand joints.

Carpal Tunnel and the Extensor Compartments

The **carpal tunnel** is formed by the arching alignment of the carpal bones and the thick **flexor retinaculum** (transverse carpal ligament), which covers the tunnel on its anterior surface (Fig. 7-27). Structures passing through the carpal tunnel include the following:

- Four flexor digitorum superficialis tendons
- Four flexor digitorum profundus tendons
- One flexor pollicis longus tendon
- Median nerve

The tendon of the flexor carpi radialis lies outside the carpal tunnel but is encased within its own fascial sleeve in the lateral flexor retinaculum. **Synovial sheaths** surround the muscle tendons within the carpal tunnel and permit sliding movements as the muscles contract and relax.

The **extensor tendons** and their synovial sheaths enter the hand by passing on the medial,

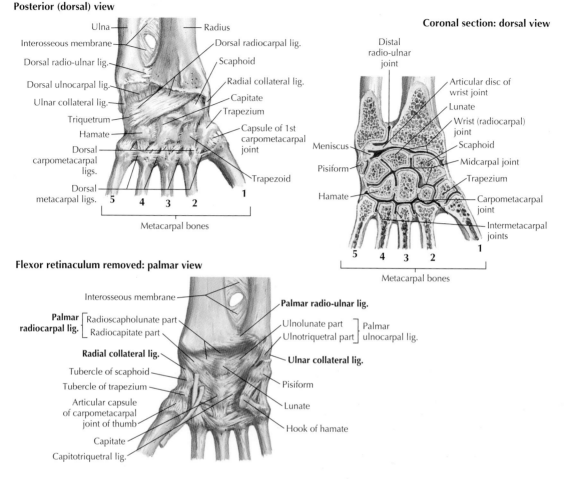

Posterior (dorsal) view

Ulna
Interosseous membrane
Dorsal radio-ulnar lig.
Dorsal ulnocarpal lig.
Ulnar collateral lig.
Triquetrum
Hamate
Dorsal carpometacarpal ligs.
Dorsal metacarpal ligs.

Radius
Dorsal radiocarpal lig.
Scaphoid
Radial collateral lig.
Capitate
Trapezium
Capsule of 1st carpometacarpal joint
Trapezoid

Metacarpal bones   5 4 3 2 1

Coronal section: dorsal view

Distal radio-ulnar joint
Meniscus
Pisiform
Hamate

Articular disc of wrist joint
Lunate
Wrist (radiocarpal) joint
Scaphoid
Midcarpal joint
Trapezium
Carpometacarpal joint
Intermetacarpal joints

Metacarpal bones   5 4 3 2 1

Flexor retinaculum removed: palmar view

Interosseous membrane
Palmar radiocarpal lig. [Radioscapholunate part / Radiocapitate part]
Radial collateral lig.
Tubercle of scaphoid
Tubercle of trapezium
Articular capsule of carpometacarpal joint of thumb
Capitate
Capitotriquetral lig.

Palmar radio-ulnar lig.
Ulnolunate part] Palmar
Ulnotriquetral part] ulnocarpal lig.
Ulnar collateral lig.
Pisiform
Lunate
Hook of hamate

FIGURE 7-24 Wrist Joint Ligaments. (From *Atlas of human anatomy,* ed 6, Plates 441 and 442.)

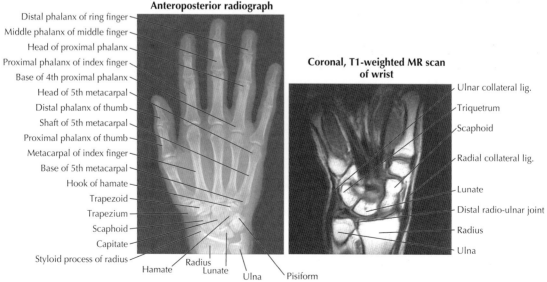

Anteroposterior radiograph

Distal phalanx of ring finger
Middle phalanx of middle finger
Head of proximal phalanx
Proximal phalanx of index finger
Base of 4th proximal phalanx
Head of 5th metacarpal
Distal phalanx of thumb
Shaft of 5th metacarpal
Proximal phalanx of thumb
Metacarpal of index finger
Base of 5th metacarpal
Hook of hamate
Trapezoid
Trapezium
Scaphoid
Capitate
Styloid process of radius
Hamate   Radius
Lunate   Ulna   Pisiform

Coronal, T1-weighted MR scan of wrist

Ulnar collateral lig.
Triquetrum
Scaphoid
Radial collateral lig.
Lunate
Distal radio-ulnar joint
Radius
Ulna

FIGURE 7-25 Radiographic Images of the Wrist and Hand. (Left image from *Atlas of human anatomy,* ed 6, Plate 444; right image from Kelley LL, Petersen C: *Sectional anatomy for imaging professionals,* Philadelphia, Mosby, 2007.)

380   **Chapter 7   Upper Limb**

Metacarpophalangeal and interphalangeal ligaments

Anterior (palmar) view

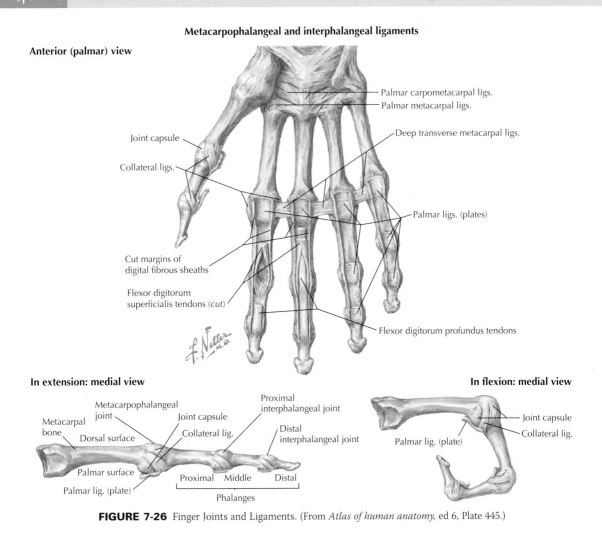

Palmar carpometacarpal ligs.

Palmar metacarpal ligs.

Joint capsule

Deep transverse metacarpal ligs.

Collateral ligs.

Palmar ligs. (plates)

Cut margins of
digital fibrous sheaths

Flexor digitorum
superficialis tendons (cut)

Flexor digitorum profundus tendons

In extension: medial view

In flexion: medial view

Metacarpophalangeal
joint

Proximal
interphalangeal joint

Metacarpal
bone

Joint capsule

Joint capsule

Dorsal surface

Collateral lig.

Collateral lig.

Distal
interphalangeal joint

Palmar lig. (plate)

Palmar surface

Palmar lig. (plate)

Proximal   Middle   Distal

Phalanges

FIGURE 7-26 Finger Joints and Ligaments. (From *Atlas of human anatomy,* ed 6, Plate 445.)

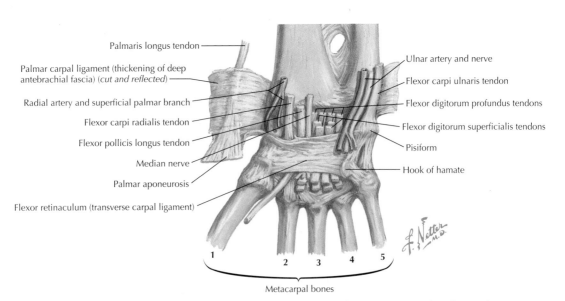

Palmaris longus tendon

Ulnar artery and nerve

Palmar carpal ligament (thickening of deep
antebrachial fascia) (*cut and reflected*)

Flexor carpi ulnaris tendon

Radial artery and superficial palmar branch

Flexor digitorum profundus tendons

Flexor carpi radialis tendon

Flexor digitorum superficialis tendons

Flexor pollicis longus tendon

Pisiform

Median nerve

Hook of hamate

Palmar aponeurosis

Flexor retinaculum (transverse carpal ligament)

1   2   3   4   5

Metacarpal bones

FIGURE 7-27 Palmar View of Carpal Tunnel. (From *Atlas of human anatomy,* ed 6, Plate 441.)

TABLE 7-15 Joints and Ligaments of the Wrist and Hand

LIGAMENT	ATTACHMENT	COMMENT
Radiocarpal (Biaxial Synovial Ellipsoid) Joint		
Capsule and disc	Surrounds joint; radius to scaphoid, lunate, and triquetrum	Provides little support; allows flexion, extension, abduction, adduction, and circumduction
Palmar (volar) radiocarpal ligaments	Radius to scaphoid, lunate, and triquetrum	Are strong and stabilizing
Dorsal radiocarpal	Radius to scaphoid, lunate, and triquetrum	Is weaker ligament
Radial collateral	Radius to scaphoid and triquetrum	Stabilizes proximal row of carpals
Distal Radioulnar (Uniaxial Synovial Pivot) Joint		
Capsule	Surrounds joint; ulnar head to ulnar notch of radius	Is thin superiorly; allows pronation and supination
Palmar and dorsal radio-ulnar	Extends transversely between the two bones	Articular disc binds bones together
Intercarpal (Synovial Plane) Joints		
Proximal row of carpals	Adjacent carpals	Permits gliding and sliding movements
Distal row of carpals	Adjacent carpals	Are united by anterior, posterior, and interosseous ligaments
Midcarpal (Synovial Plane) Joints		
Palmar (volar) intercarpal	Proximal and distal rows of carpals	Is location for ⅓ of wrist extension and ⅔ of flexion; permits gliding and sliding movements
Carpal collaterals	Scaphoid, lunate, and triquetrum to capitate and hamate	Stabilize distal row (ellipsoid synovial joint)
Carpometacarpal (CMC) (Plane Synovial) Joints (except Thumb)		
Capsule	Carpals to metacarpals of digits 2-5	Surrounds joints; allows some gliding movement
Palmar and dorsal CMC	Carpals to metacarpals of digits 2-5	Dorsal ligament strongest
Interosseous CMC	Carpals to metacarpals of digits 2-5	
Thumb (Biaxial Saddle) Joint		
Same ligaments as CMC	Trapezium to 1st metacarpal	Allows flexion, extension, abduction, adduction, and circumduction
		Is common site for arthritis
Metacarpophalangeal (Biaxial Condyloid Synovial) Joint		
Capsule	Metacarpal to proximal phalanx	Surrounds joint; allows flexion, extension, abduction, adduction, and circumduction
Radial and ulnar collaterals	Metacarpal to proximal phalanx	Are tight in flexion and loose in extension
Palmar (volar) plate	Metacarpal to proximal phalanx	If broken digit, cast in flexion or ligament will shorten
Interphalangeal (Uniaxial Synovial Hinge) Joints		
Capsule	Adjacent phalanges	Surrounds joints; allows flexion and extension
Two collaterals	Adjacent phalanges	Are oriented obliquely
Palmar (volar) plate	Adjacent phalanges	Prevents hyperextension

dorsal, and lateral aspects of the wrist beneath the **extensor retinaculum,** which segregates the tendons into six compartments (Fig. 7-28).

Intrinsic Hand Muscles

The intrinsic hand muscles originate and insert in the hand and carry out fine precision movements, whereas the forearm muscles and their tendons that pass into the hand are more important for powerful hand movements such as gripping objects (Fig. 7-29 and Table 7-16). The intrinsic hand muscles of the palm are divided into the thenar eminence or cone of muscles (thumb, first digit), the hypothenar eminence or cone of muscles (little finger, fifth digit), and the interosseous and lumbrical muscles. The **thenar eminence** is

created by the following muscles (all innervated by median nerve):

- Flexor pollicis brevis
- Abductor pollicis brevis
- Opponens pollicis

The **hypothenar eminence** is created by the following muscles (all innervated by ulnar nerve):

- Flexor digiti minimi brevis
- Abductor digiti minimi
- Opponens digiti minimi

Although most intrinsic hand muscles are innervated by the ulnar nerve, the three thenar

Clinical Focus 7-14

Fracture of the Ulna Shaft

Usually, a direct blow to or forced pronation of the forearm is the most common cause of a fracture of the shaft of the ulna. Fracture of the ulna with dislocation of the proximal radio-ulnar joint is termed a **Monteggia fracture.** The radial head usually dislocates anteriorly, but posterior, medial, or lateral dislocation also may occur. Such dislocations may put the posterior interosseous nerve (branch of the radial nerve) at risk.

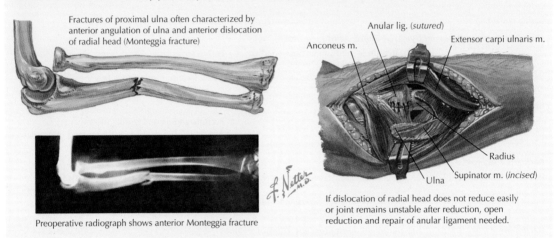

Fractures of proximal ulna often characterized by anterior angulation of ulna and anterior dislocation of radial head (Monteggia fracture)

Anular lig. (*sutured*)

Anconeus m.

Extensor carpi ulnaris m.

Radius

Ulna   Supinator m. (*incised*)

Preoperative radiograph shows anterior Monteggia fracture

If dislocation of radial head does not reduce easily or joint remains unstable after reduction, open reduction and repair of anular ligament needed.

Clinical Focus 7-15

Distal Radial (Colles') Fracture

Fractures of the distal radius account for about 80% of forearm fractures in all age groups and often result from a fall on an outstretched hand. Colles' fracture is an extension-compression fracture of the distal radius that produces a typical "dinner fork" deformity.

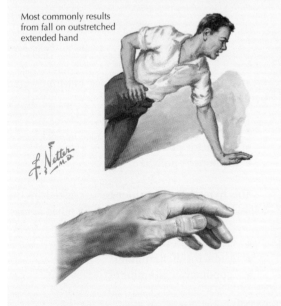

Most commonly results from fall on outstretched extended hand

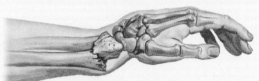

Lateral view of Colles' fracture demonstrates characteristic dinner fork deformity with dorsal and proximal displacement of distal fragment. Note dorsal instead of normal volar slope of articular surface of distal radius.

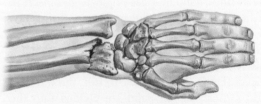

Dorsal view shows radial deviation of hand with ulnar prominence of styloid process of ulna.

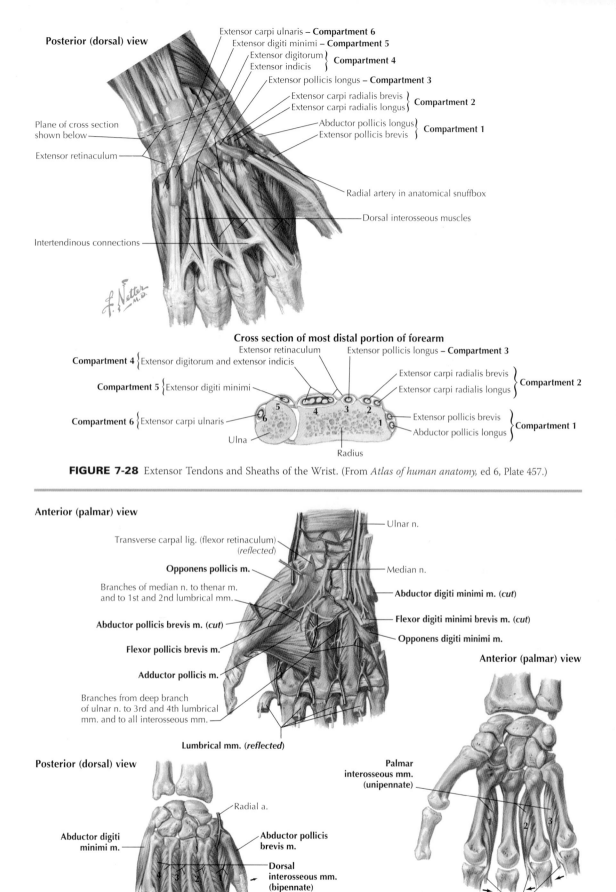

Posterior (dorsal) view

Extensor carpi ulnaris – **Compartment 6**
Extensor digiti minimi – **Compartment 5**
Extensor digitorum }
Extensor indicis } **Compartment 4**
Extensor pollicis longus – **Compartment 3**
Extensor carpi radialis brevis }
Extensor carpi radialis longus } **Compartment 2**
Abductor pollicis longus }
Extensor pollicis brevis } **Compartment 1**

Plane of cross section shown below

Extensor retinaculum

Radial artery in anatomical snuffbox

Dorsal interosseous muscles

Intertendinous connections

f. Netter
M.D.

Cross section of most distal portion of forearm

Extensor retinaculum
Extensor pollicis longus – **Compartment 3**

Compartment 4 {Extensor digitorum and extensor indicis
Compartment 5 {Extensor digiti minimi
Compartment 6 {Extensor carpi ulnaris

Extensor carpi radialis brevis }
Extensor carpi radialis longus } **Compartment 2**

Extensor pollicis brevis }
Abductor pollicis longus } **Compartment 1**

6 5 4 3 2 1

Ulna
Radius

FIGURE 7-28 Extensor Tendons and Sheaths of the Wrist. (From *Atlas of human anatomy,* ed 6, Plate 457.)

Anterior (palmar) view

Ulnar n.

Transverse carpal lig. (flexor retinaculum) (*reflected*)
Opponens pollicis m.
Branches of median n. to thenar m. and to 1st and 2nd lumbrical mm.
Abductor pollicis brevis m. (*cut*)
Flexor pollicis brevis m.
Adductor pollicis m.
Branches from deep branch of ulnar n. to 3rd and 4th lumbrical mm. and to all interosseous mm.

Median n.

Abductor digiti minimi m. (*cut*)
Flexor digiti minimi brevis m. (*cut*)
Opponens digiti minimi m.

Anterior (palmar) view

Lumbrical mm. (*reflected*)

Posterior (dorsal) view

Radial a.

Abductor digiti minimi m.

Abductor pollicis brevis m.

Dorsal interosseous mm. (bipennate)

4 3 2 1

Palmar interosseous mm. (unipennate)

1 2 3

Tendinous slips to extensor expansions (hoods)

C. Machado
M.D.

Note: *Arrows indicate action of muscles.*

FIGURE 7-29 Intrinsic Muscles of the Hand. (From *Atlas of human anatomy,* ed 6, Plate 452.)

TABLE 7-16 Intrinsic Hand Muscles

MUSCLE	PROXIMAL ATTACHMENT (ORIGIN)	DISTAL ATTACHMENT (INSERTION)	INNERVATION	MAIN ACTIONS
Abductor pollicis brevis	Flexor retinaculum and tubercles of scaphoid and trapezium	Lateral side of base of proximal phalanx of thumb	Median nerve (recurrent branch) (C8-T1)	Abducts thumb
Flexor pollicis brevis	Flexor retinaculum and tubercle of trapezium	Lateral side of base of proximal phalanx of thumb	Median nerve (recurrent branch) (C8-T1)	Flexes proximal phalanx of thumb
Opponens pollicis	Flexor retinaculum and tubercle of trapezium	Lateral side of 1st metacarpal bone	Median nerve (recurrent branch) (C8-T1)	Opposes thumb toward center of palm and rotates it medially
Adductor pollicis	*Oblique head:* bases of 2nd and 3rd metacarpals and capitate *Transverse head:* anterior surface of body of 3rd metacarpal	Medial side of base of proximal phalanx of thumb	Ulnar nerve (deep branch) (C8 –T1)	Adducts thumb toward middle digit
Abductor digiti minimi	Pisiform and tendon of flexor carpi ulnaris	Medial side of base of proximal phalanx of 5th digit	Ulnar nerve (deep branch) (C8-T1)	Abducts 5th digit
Flexor digiti minimi brevis	Hook of hamate and flexor retinaculum	Medial side of base of proximal phalanx of 5th digit	Ulnar nerve (deep branch) (C8-T1)	Flexes proximal phalanx of 5th digit
Opponens digiti minimi	Hook of hamate and flexor retinaculum	Palmar surface of 5th metacarpal	Ulnar nerve (deep branch) (C8-T1)	Draws 5th metacarpal anteriorly and rotates it, bringing 5th digit into opposition with thumb
Lumbricals 1 and 2	Lateral two tendons of flexor digitorum profundus	Lateral sides of extensor expansions of 2nd and 3rd digits	Median nerve (C8-T1)	Flex digits at MCP joints and extend IP joints
Lumbricals 3 and 4	Medial three tendons of flexor digitorum profundus	Lateral sides of extensor expansions of 4th and 5th digits	Ulnar nerve (deep branch) (C8-T1)	Flex digits at MCP joints and extend IP joints
Dorsal interossei	Adjacent sides of two metacarpals	Extensor expansions and bases of proximal phalanges of 2nd to 4th digits	Ulnar nerve (deep branch) (C8-T1)	Abduct digits; flex digits at MCP joints and extend IP joints
Palmar interossei	Sides of 2nd, 4th, and 5th metacarpal bones	Extensor expansions of digits and bases of proximal phalanges of 2nd, 4th, and 5th digits	Ulnar nerve (deep branch) (C8-T1)	Adduct digits; flex digits at MCP joints and extend IP joints

IP, Interphalangeal *MCP,* metacarpophalangeal.

muscles and the two lateral lumbricals are innervated by the median nerve.

The blood supply to the hand is by the **radial** and **ulnar arteries,** which anastomose with each other through two **palmar arches** (superficial and deep) (Fig. 7-30 and Table 7-17). Except for the thumb and lateral index finger, the remainder of the hand is supplied largely by the ulnar artery. Corresponding veins drain to the dorsum of the hand and collect in the cephalic (lateral) and basilic (medial) veins (see Fig. 7-2). Deeper veins parallel the arteries and throughout their course in the forearm and arm have connections with the superficial veins. The upper limb veins possess valves to assist in venous return.

Palmar Spaces and Tendon Sheaths

As the long tendons pass through the hand toward the digits, they are surrounded by a **synovial sheath** and, in the digits, a **fibrous digital sheath** that binds them to the phalanges (Figs. 7-30 and 7-31 and Table 7-18). Cross section of the palm

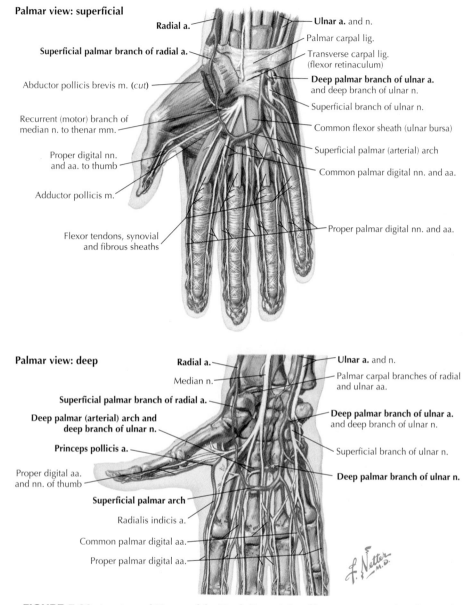

Palmar view: superficial

Radial a.

Superficial palmar branch of radial a.

Abductor pollicis brevis m. (*cut*)

Recurrent (motor) branch of
median n. to thenar mm.

Proper digital nn.
and aa. to thumb

Adductor pollicis m.

Flexor tendons, synovial
and fibrous sheaths

Ulnar a. and n.

Palmar carpal lig.

Transverse carpal lig.
(flexor retinaculum)

Deep palmar branch of ulnar a.
and deep branch of ulnar n.

Superficial branch of ulnar n.

Common flexor sheath (ulnar bursa)

Superficial palmar (arterial) arch

Common palmar digital nn. and aa.

Proper palmar digital nn. and aa.

Palmar view: deep

Radial a.

Median n.

Superficial palmar branch of radial a.

**Deep palmar (arterial) arch and
deep branch of ulnar n.**

Princeps pollicis a.

Proper digital aa.
and nn. of thumb

Superficial palmar arch

Radialis indicis a.

Common palmar digital aa.

Proper palmar digital aa.

Ulnar a. and n.

Palmar carpal branches of radial
and ulnar aa.

Deep palmar branch of ulnar a.
and deep branch of ulnar n.

Superficial branch of ulnar n.

Deep palmar branch of ulnar n.

FIGURE 7-30 Arteries and Nerves of the Hand. (From *Atlas of human anatomy,* ed 6, Plate 453.)

TABLE 7-17 Arteries of the Hand

ARTERY	COURSE	ARTERY	COURSE
Radial		*Ulnar*	
Superficial palmar branch	Forms superficial palmar arch with ulnar artery	Deep palmar branch	Forms deep palmar arch with radial artery
Princeps pollicis	Passes under flexor pollicis longus tendon, and divides into two proper digital arteries to thumb	Superficial palmar arch	Is formed by termination of ulnar artery; gives rise to three common digital arteries, each of which gives rise to two proper digital arteries
Radialis indicis	Passes to index finger on its lateral side		
Deep palmar arch	Is formed by terminal part of radial artery		

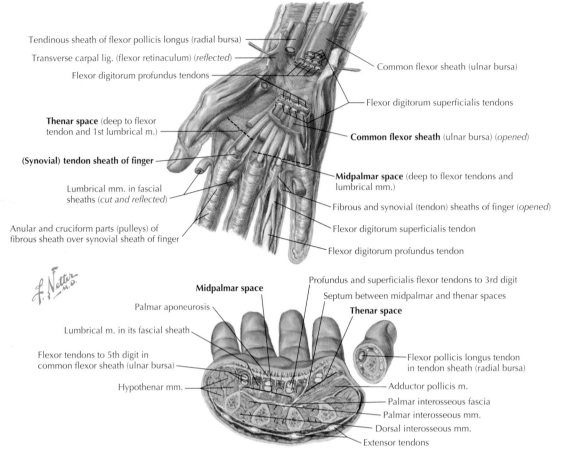

Tendinous sheath of flexor pollicis longus (radial bursa)

Transverse carpal lig. (flexor retinaculum) (reflected)

Flexor digitorum profundus tendons

Thenar space (deep to flexor tendon and 1st lumbrical m.)

(Synovial) tendon sheath of finger

Lumbrical mm. in fascial sheaths (cut and reflected)

Anular and cruciform parts (pulleys) of fibrous sheath over synovial sheath of finger

Common flexor sheath (ulnar bursa)

Flexor digitorum superficialis tendons

Common flexor sheath (ulnar bursa) (opened)

Midpalmar space (deep to flexor tendons and lumbrical mm.)

Fibrous and synovial (tendon) sheaths of finger (opened)

Flexor digitorum superficialis tendon

Flexor digitorum profundus tendon

Profundus and superficialis flexor tendons to 3rd digit

Septum between midpalmar and thenar spaces

Thenar space

Midpalmar space

Palmar aponeurosis

Lumbrical m. in its fascial sheath

Flexor tendons to 5th digit in common flexor sheath (ulnar bursa)

Hypothenar mm.

Flexor pollicis longus tendon in tendon sheath (radial bursa)

Adductor pollicis m.

Palmar interosseous fascia

Palmar interosseous mm.

Dorsal interosseous mm.

Extensor tendons

FIGURE 7-31 Bursae, Spaces, and Tendon Sheaths of the Hand. (From *Atlas of human anatomy*, ed 6, Plate 450.)

TABLE 7-18 Palmar Spaces and Compartments

SPACE	COMMENT
Carpal tunnel	Osseofascial tunnel composed of carpal bones (carpal arch) and overlying flexor retinaculum; contains median nerve and nine tendons
Thenar eminence	Muscle compartment at base of thumb
Thenar space	Potential space just above adductor pollicis muscle
Hypothenar eminence	Muscle compartment at base of little finger
Central compartment	Compartment containing long flexor tendons and lumbrical muscles
Midpalmar space	Potential space deep to central compartment
Adductor compartment	Compartment containing adductor pollicis muscle
Synovial sheaths	Osseofibrous sheaths (tunnels) lined with synovium to facilitate sliding movements

shows that the long flexor tendons segregate out to their respective digits, creating two potential spaces (thenar and midpalmar) of the hand. These spaces can become infected and distended. The long flexor tendons (flexor digitorum superficialis and profundus) course on the palmar side of the digits, with the superficialis tendon splitting to allow the profundus tendon to pass to the distal phalanx (Fig. 7-32). On the dorsum of the digits, the **extensor expansion** (hood) provides for insertion of the long extensor tendons and the insertion of the lumbrical and interosseous muscles. **Lumbricals** and **interossei muscles** flex the MCP joint and extend the PIP and DIP joints (see Table 7-16).

The extensor tendons of the thumb on the dorsum of the hand create the **anatomical snuff-box,** composed of the following tendons visible beneath the raised skin:

Clinical Focus 7-16

Median Nerve Compression and Carpal Tunnel Syndrome

Median nerve compression in the carpal tunnel, the most common compression neuropathy, is often linked to occupational repetitive movements related to wrist flexion and extension, holding the wrist in an awkward position, or strong gripping of objects. Long-term compression often leads to thenar atrophy and weakness of the thumb and index fingers, reflecting the loss of innervation to the muscles distal to the median nerve damage.

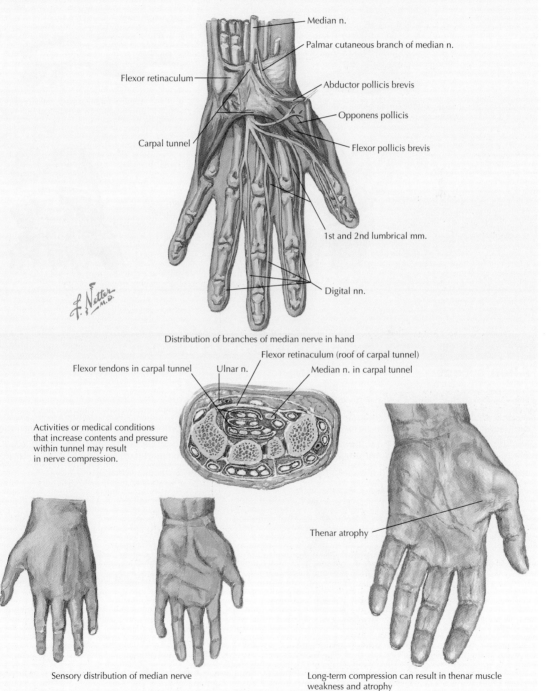

Median n.

Palmar cutaneous branch of median n.

Flexor retinaculum

Abductor pollicis brevis

Opponens pollicis

Carpal tunnel

Flexor pollicis brevis

1st and 2nd lumbrical mm.

Digital nn.

Distribution of branches of median nerve in hand

Flexor retinaculum (roof of carpal tunnel)

Flexor tendons in carpal tunnel   Ulnar n.   Median n. in carpal tunnel

Activities or medical conditions
that increase contents and pressure
within tunnel may result
in nerve compression.

Thenar atrophy

Sensory distribution of median nerve

Long-term compression can result in thenar muscle
weakness and atrophy

Clinical Focus 7-17

Fracture of the Scaphoid

The scaphoid bone is the most frequently fractured carpal bone and may be injured by falling on an extended wrist. Fracture of the middle third (waist) of the bone is most common. Pain and swelling in the "anatomical snuffbox" often occurs, and optimal healing depends on an adequate blood supply from the palmar carpal branch of the radial artery. Loss of the blood supply can lead to nonunion or avascular osteonecrosis.

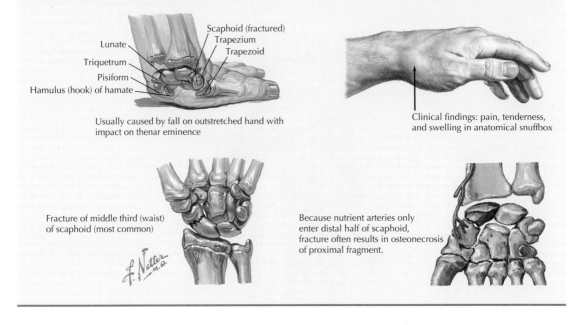

Scaphoid (fractured)
Trapezium
Trapezoid
Lunate
Triquetrum
Pisiform
Hamulus (hook) of hamate

Usually caused by fall on outstretched hand with impact on thenar eminence

Clinical findings: pain, tenderness, and swelling in anatomical snuffbox

Fracture of middle third (waist) of scaphoid (most common)

Because nutrient arteries only enter distal half of scaphoid, fracture often results in osteonecrosis of proximal fragment.

Clinical Focus 7-18

Allen's Test

The Allen's test is used to test the vascular perfusion distal to the wrist. The physician lightly places the thumbs on the patient's ulnar and radial arteries, and the patient makes a tight fist to "blanch" the palmar skin (squeeze the blood into the dorsal venous network). Then, while compressing the radial artery with the thumb, the physician releases the pressure on the ulnar artery and asks the patient to open the clenched fist. Normally the skin will turn pink immediately, indicating normal ulnar artery blood flow through the anastomotic palmar arches. The test is then repeated by occluding the ulnar artery to assess radial artery flow.

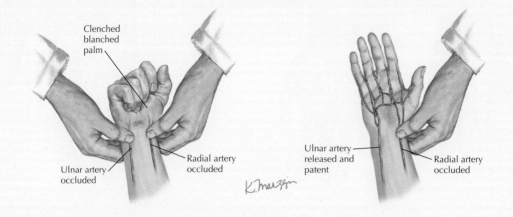

Clenched blanched palm

Ulnar artery occluded

Radial artery occluded

Ulnar artery released and patent

Radial artery occluded

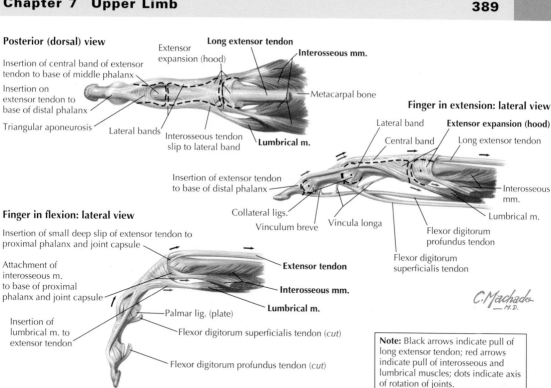

Posterior (dorsal) view

Insertion of central band of extensor tendon to base of middle phalanx

Insertion on extensor tendon to base of distal phalanx

Triangular aponeurosis

Lateral bands

Extensor expansion (hood)

Long extensor tendon

Interosseous mm.

Metacarpal bone

Interosseous tendon slip to lateral band

Lumbrical m.

Finger in extension: lateral view

Lateral band

Central band

Extensor expansion (hood)

Long extensor tendon

Interosseous mm.

Lumbrical m.

Insertion of extensor tendon to base of distal phalanx

Collateral ligs.

Vinculum breve Vincula longa

Flexor digitorum profundus tendon

Flexor digitorum superficialis tendon

Finger in flexion: lateral view

Insertion of small deep slip of extensor tendon to proximal phalanx and joint capsule

Attachment of interosseous m. to base of proximal phalanx and joint capsule

Insertion of lumbrical m. to extensor tendon

Palmar lig. (plate)

Flexor digitorum superficialis tendon (*cut*)

Flexor digitorum profundus tendon (*cut*)

Extensor tendon

Interosseous mm.

Lumbrical m.

Note: Black arrows indicate pull of long extensor tendon; red arrows indicate pull of interosseous and lumbrical muscles; dots indicate axis of rotation of joints.

FIGURE 7-32 Long Tendon Sheaths of the Fingers. (From *Atlas of human anatomy*, ed 6, Plate 451.)

Clinical Focus 7-19

De Quervain Tenosynovitis

In de Quervain tenosynovitis the **tendons of the abductor pollicis longus** and **extensor pollicis brevis** pass through the same tendinous sheath on the dorsum of the wrist (first compartment in the extensor retinaculum). Excessive and repetitive use of the hands in a power grip or twisting-wringing action can cause friction and thickening of the sheath, leading to pain over the styloid process of the radius. This pain is mediated by the **superficial radial nerve** (sensory), and the pain can extend distally into the thumb and radiate up the lateral forearm.

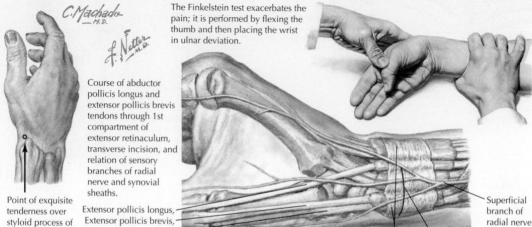

The Finkelstein test exacerbates the pain; it is performed by flexing the thumb and then placing the wrist in ulnar deviation.

Course of abductor pollicis longus and extensor pollicis brevis tendons through 1st compartment of extensor retinaculum, transverse incision, and relation of sensory branches of radial nerve and synovial sheaths.

Point of exquisite tenderness over styloid process of radius and sheath of involved tendons.

Extensor pollicis longus, Extensor pollicis brevis, Abductor pollicis longus tendons

Extensor retinaculum

Skin incision

Superficial branch of radial nerve

- Medially, the tendon of the **extensor pollicis longus**
- Laterally, the tendons of the **abductor pollicis longus** and **extensor pollicis brevis**

The "floor" of the snuffbox contains the **radial artery** (a pulse can be detected here when the artery is pressed against the underlying scaphoid bone) and the terminal end of the **superficial radial nerve,** which passes subcutaneously over this region.

8. UPPER LIMB MUSCLE SUMMARY

Table 7-19 summarizes the actions of major muscles on the joints. The list is not exhaustive and highlights only major muscles responsible for each movement; the separate muscle tables provide more detail. Most joints move because of the action of multiple muscles working on that joint, but this list only focuses on the more important muscles acting on that joint. For example,

---

Clinical Focus 7-20

Proximal Interphalangeal Joint Dislocations

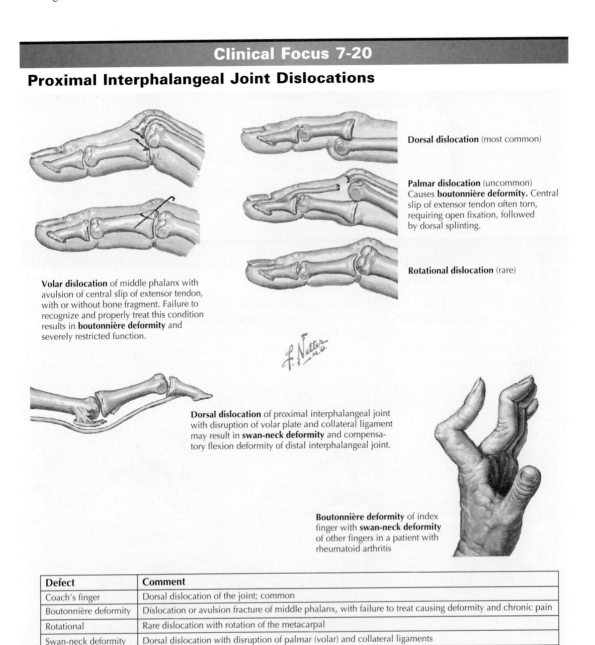

Dorsal dislocation (most common)

Palmar dislocation (uncommon) Causes **boutonnière deformity.** Central slip of extensor tendon often torn, requiring open fixation, followed by dorsal splinting.

Rotational dislocation (rare)

Volar dislocation of middle phalanx with avulsion of central slip of extensor tendon, with or without bone fragment. Failure to recognize and properly treat this condition results in **boutonnière deformity** and severely restricted function.

Dorsal dislocation of proximal interphalangeal joint with disruption of volar plate and collateral ligament may result in **swan-neck deformity** and compensatory flexion deformity of distal interphalangeal joint.

Boutonnière deformity of index finger with **swan-neck deformity** of other fingers in a patient with rheumatoid arthritis

Defect	Comment
Coach's finger	Dorsal dislocation of the joint; common
Boutonnière deformity	Dislocation or avulsion fracture of middle phalanx, with failure to treat causing deformity and chronic pain
Rotational	Rare dislocation with rotation of the metacarpal
Swan-neck deformity	Dorsal dislocation with disruption of palmar (volar) and collateral ligaments

Finger Injuries

Various traumatic finger injuries may occur, causing fractures, disruption of the flexor and extensor tendons, and torn ligaments. Each element must be carefully examined for normal function, including muscle groups, capillary refill (Allen's test), and two-point sensory discrimination.

Mallet finger

Usually caused by direct blow on extended distal phalanx, as in baseball, volleyball

Fracture of metacarpals

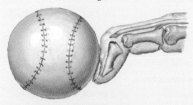

Fractures of metacarpal neck commonly result from end-on blow of fist.

Avulsion of flexor digitorum profundus tendon

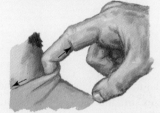

Caused by violent traction on flexed distal phalanx, as in catching on jersey of running football player

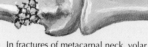

In fractures of metacarpal neck, volar cortex often comminuted, resulting in marked instability after reduction, which often necessitates pinning

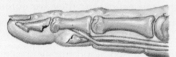

Flexor digitorum profundus tendon may be torn directly from distal phalanx or may avulse small or large bone fragment.

Transverse fractures of metacarpal shaft usually angulated dorsally by pull of interosseous muscles

Thumb injury other than fracture

Stress test for ruptured medial (ulnar) collateral ligament of thumb (gamekeeper thumb)

Adductor pollicis m. and aponeurosis (*cut*)

Torn medial collateral lig.

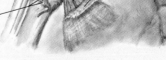

Ruptured medial collateral ligament of metacarpophalangeal joint of thumb

TABLE 7-19 Summary of Actions of Major Upper Limb Muscles*

Scapula

Elevate: levator scapulae, trapezius

Depress: pectoralis minor

Protrude: serratus anterior

Depress glenoid: rhomboids

Elevate glenoid: serratus anterior, trapezius

Retract: rhomboids, trapezius

Shoulder

Flex: pectoralis major, coracobrachialis

Extend: latissimus dorsi, teres major

Abduct: supraspinatus (initiates), deltoid

Adduct: pectoralis major, latissimus dorsi

Rotate medially: subscapularis, teres major, pectoralis major, latissimus dorsi

Rotate laterally: infraspinatus, teres minor

Elbow

Flex: brachialis, biceps

Extend: triceps, anconeus

Radio-ulnar

Pronate: pronators (teres and quadratus)

Supinate: supinator, biceps brachii

Wrist

Flex: flexor carpi radialis, ulnaris

Extend: all extensor carpi muscles

Abduct: flexor/extensor carpi radialis muscles

Adduct: flexor and extensor carpi ulnaris

Circumduct: combination of all movements

Metacarpophalangeal

Flex: interossei and lumbricals

Extend: extensor digitorum

Abduct: dorsal interossei

Adduct: palmar interossei

Circumduct: combination of all movements

Interphalangeal-Proximal

Flex: flexor digitorum superficialis

Extend: interossei and lumbricals

Interphalangeal-Distal

Flex: flexor digitorum profundus

Extend: interossei and lumbricals

*Accessory or secondary actions of muscles are detailed in the muscle tables.

although the brachialis and biceps muscles are the major flexors of the forearm at the elbow, the brachioradialis and many of the forearm muscles originating from the medial epicondyle of the humerus also cross the elbow joint and have a weak flexor action on the elbow.

9. UPPER LIMB ARTERY AND VEIN SUMMARY

Arteries of the Upper Limb

The **left subclavian artery** arises directly from the **aortic arch (1)** while the **right subclavian artery (3)** arises from the **brachiocephalic trunk (2)**. The branches of both subclavian arteries are the same from that point on distally to the hand (Fig. 7-33.). The **brachial artery (5)** bifurcates at the cubital fossa and gives rise to the **ulnar artery (6)** and **radial artery (7)**.

Major anastomoses occur between the subclavian artery and the **axillary artery (4)** around the branches supplying the muscles of the scapula. Likewise, a major anastomosis also occurs around the elbow between collateral arteries from the brachial artery and recurrent branches from the ulnar artery and radial artery. Carpal arteries at the wrist and palmar arches in the hand also participate in anastomoses.

Many of the major arteries also provide small arteries to muscles of the limb (these small branches are not listed) and to nutrient arteries to the adjacent bones (not named). Arteriovenous (AV) anastomoses are direct connections between small arteries and veins and usually are involved in cutaneous thermoregulation. They are numerous in the skin of the fingers, especially nail beds and fingertips.

The joints receive a rich blood supply provided by small articular branches of adjacent arteries. Major pulse points of the upper limb include the following:

- **Brachial pulse:** at the medial aspect of the midarm, where it may be pressed against the humerus.
- **Cubital pulse:** anterior to the elbow in the cubital fossa, where the brachial artery is felt just medial to the biceps brachii muscle tendon.
- **Radial pulse:** at the wrist, just lateral to the flexor carpi radialis muscle tendon; most common site to take a pulse.
- **Ulnar pulse:** at the wrist, just proximolateral to the pisiform carpal bone.

In the outline of arteries, major vessels often dissected in anatomy courses include the

1. **Aortic Arch**
2. **Brachiocephalic Trunk**
3. **Right/Left Subclavian Artery**
   Vertebral artery
   Internal thoracic artery
   Thyrocervical trunk   *+ Dorsal scapular artery*
   Costocervical trunk
4. **Axillary Artery**
   Superior thoracic artery
   Thoraco-acromial artery
   Lateral thoracic artery
   Subscapular artery
   Anterior humeral circumflex artery
   Posterior humeral circumflex artery
5. **Brachial Artery**
   Deep artery of arm
      Radial collateral artery
      Medial collateral artery
   Superior ulnar collateral artery
   Inferior ulnar collateral artery
6. **Ulnar Artery**
   Ulnar recurrent artery
      Anterior ulnar recurrent artery
      Posterior ulnar recurrent artery
   Common interosseous artery
      Anterior interosseous artery
         Median artery
      Posterior interosseous artery
         Perforating branch
         Recurrent interosseous artery
   Dorsal carpal branch
   Palmar carpal branch
   Deep palmar branch
   Superficial palmar arch
   Common palmar digital arteries (3)
      Proper palmar digital arteries
7. **Radial Artery**
   Radial recurrent artery
   Palmar carpal branch
   Superficial palmar branch
   Dorsal carpal branch
      Dorsal carpal arch
      Dorsal metacarpal arteries
      Dorsal digital arteries
   Princeps pollicis artery
   Radialis indicis artery
   Deep palmar arch
      Palmar metacarpal arteries
      Perforating branches

*Direction of blood flow is from top (proximal) to bottom (distal).

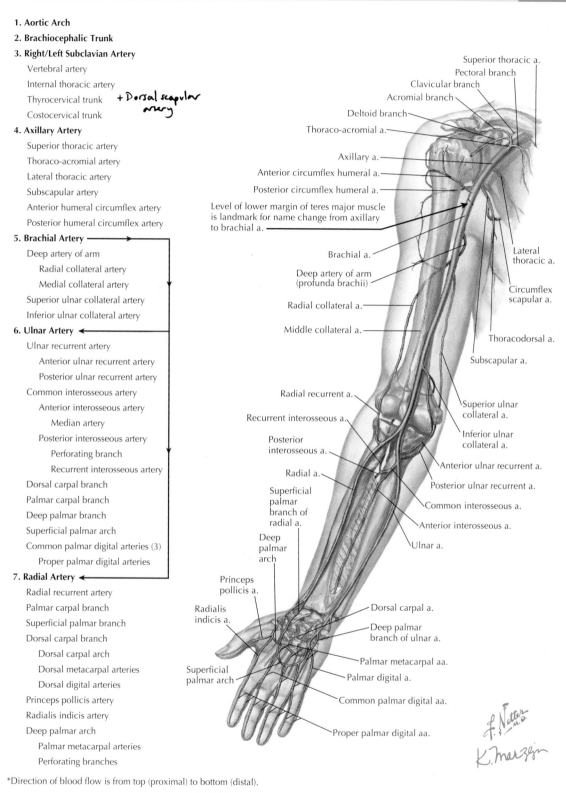

FIGURE 7-33 Arteries of Upper Limb.

Deep Veins

Palmar metacarpal

Deep venous arch

Post. interosseous veins

Ant. interosseous veins

Radial Vein(s)

Ulnar Vein(s)

3. Brachial Vein(s)

Subscapular vein

Circumflex scapular vein

Thoracodorsal vein

Post. circumflex scapular vein

Ant. circumflex scapular vein

Lateral thoracic vein

Thoraco-epigastric veins

Areolar venous plexus (breast)

4. Axillary Vein

5. Subclavian Vein

6. Lt/Rt Brachiocephalic Veins

7. Superior Vena Cava

8. Heart (Right Atrium)

*Direction of blood flow is from distal
(hand) to proximal (heart).

Superficial Veins

Palmar digital veins

Superficial palmar arch

Metacarpal/carpal tributaries

Dorsal venous network of hand

Basilic vein of forearm

Cephalic vein of forearm

Median vein of forearm

Median cubital vein

1. **Basilic Vein**

Thoraco-acromial vein

2. **Cephalic Vein**

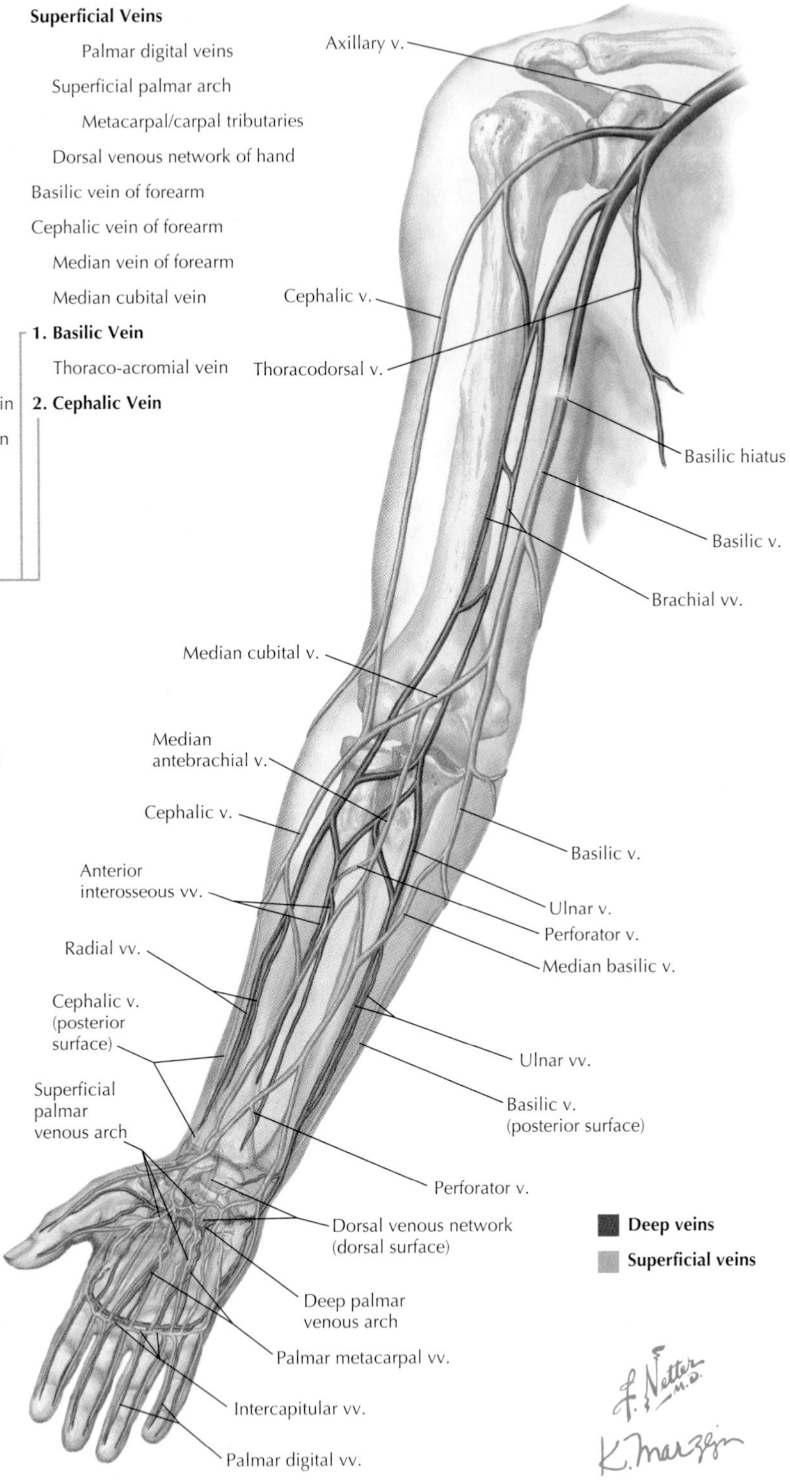

Axillary v.

Cephalic v.

Thoracodorsal v.

Basilic hiatus

Basilic v.

Brachial vv.

Median cubital v.

Median
antebrachial v.

Cephalic v.

Anterior
interosseous vv.

Radial vv.

Cephalic v.
(posterior
surface)

Superficial
palmar
venous arch

Basilic v.

Ulnar v.

Perforator v.

Median basilic v.

Ulnar vv.

Basilic v.
(posterior surface)

Perforator v.

Dorsal venous network
(dorsal surface)

Deep palmar
venous arch

Palmar metacarpal vv.

Intercapitular vv.

Palmar digital vv.

Deep veins

Superficial veins

FIGURE 7-34 Veins of Upper Limb.

first-order arteries (in **bold** and numbered) and their second-order major branches. The third-order and fourth-order arteries are dissected only in more detailed anatomy courses.

Veins of the Upper Limb

The venous drainage begins largely on the dorsum of the hand, with venous blood returning proximally in both a superficial and a deep venous pattern. The **basilic vein (1)** and **cephalic vein (2)** drain into the **axillary vein (4)** in the shoulder. The deep venous drainage via the forearm ulnar and radial veins drains into the **brachial vein (3)**. Often these are multiple veins (venae comitantes) coursing with the single ulnar or radial artery (Fig. 7-34).

The median cubital vein, often coursing between the cephalic and basilic veins in the cubital fossa, is often accessed for venipuncture to withdraw a blood sample. Even the axillary vein usually consists of multiple veins surrounding the single axillary artery. The axillary vein(s) then drains into the **subclavian vein (5)** on each side

(right and left). The subclavian vein(s) then drains into the **left** and **right brachiocephalic veins (6)**, which drain into the **superior vena cava (7)** and then the **heart (right atrium) (8)**.

In the human body the venous system is the *compliance system,* and at rest about 65% of the blood resides in the low-pressure venous system. Veins generally are larger than their corresponding arteries and have thinner walls, and multiple veins often accompany a single artery; the body has many more veins than arteries.

10. UPPER LIMB NERVE SUMMARY

Shoulder Region

Shoulder muscles are largely innervated by the suprascapular (C5, C6), **musculocutaneous** (C5, C6, C7), **long thoracic** (C5, C6, C7), and **axillary** nerves (C5, C6); there may be some variability in spinal segment distribution to these nerves (Fig. 7-35 and Table 7-20).

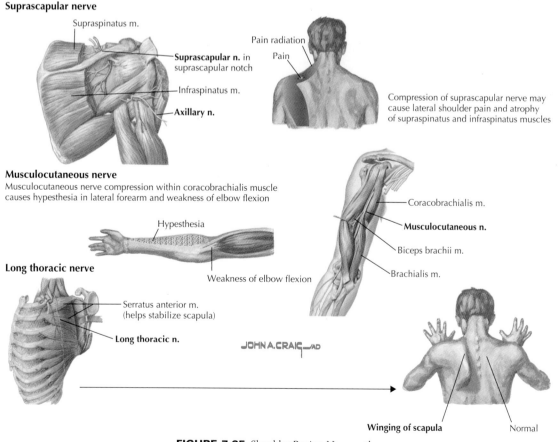

Suprascapular nerve
Supraspinatus m.
Suprascapular n. in suprascapular notch
Pain radiation
Pain
Infraspinatus m.
Axillary n.

Compression of suprascapular nerve may cause lateral shoulder pain and atrophy of supraspinatus and infraspinatus muscles

Musculocutaneous nerve
Musculocutaneous nerve compression within coracobrachialis muscle causes hypesthesia in lateral forearm and weakness of elbow flexion

Hypesthesia
Coracobrachialis m.
Musculocutaneous n.
Biceps brachii m.
Brachialis m.

Long thoracic nerve
Serratus anterior m. (helps stabilize scapula)
Long thoracic n.
Weakness of elbow flexion

JOHN A.CRAIG—AD

Winging of scapula   Normal

FIGURE 7-35 Shoulder Region Neuropathy.

TABLE 7-20 Shoulder Region Neuropathy

INVOLVED NERVE	CONDITION	INVOLVED NERVE	CONDITION
Suprascapular	Posterolateral shoulder pain, which may radiate to arm and neck; weakness in shoulder rotation	Long thoracic	Injury at level of neck caused by stretching during lateral flexion of neck to opposite side; winged scapula
Musculocutaneous	Coracobrachialis compression and weakened flexion at the elbow, with hypesthesia of lateral forearm; weakened supination	Axillary	Rare condition (quadrangular space syndrome) (not shown in illustration); can produce weakness of deltoid muscle and abduction

Radial Nerve in the Arm and Forearm

The **radial nerve** (C5, C6, C7, C8, T1) innervates the muscles that extend the forearm at the elbow (posterior compartment arm muscles) and the skin of the posterior arm, via the inferior lateral and posterior cutaneous nerves of the arm (Fig. 7-36).

The radial nerve innervates the extensor muscles of the wrist and fingers and the supinator muscle (posterior compartment forearm muscles). It also conveys cutaneous sensory information from the posterior forearm and the radial side of the dorsum of the hand. Pure radial nerve sensation (no overlap with other nerves) is tested on the skin overlying the first dorsal interosseous muscle (Fig. 7-37). The radial nerve is vulnerable in fractures of the humeral midshaft or by compression injuries of the arm. It also is vulnerable

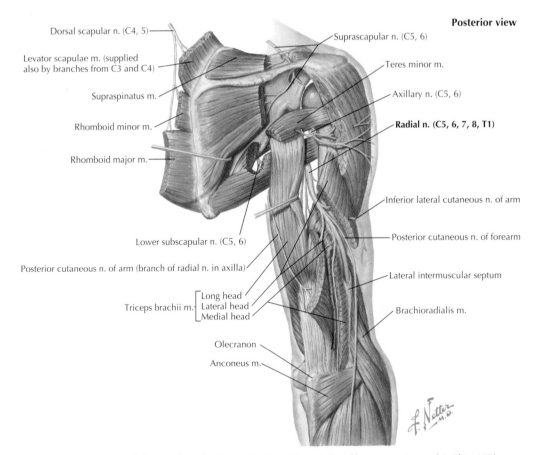

FIGURE 7-36 Radial Nerve Distribution in the Arm. (From *Atlas of human anatomy*, ed 6, Plate 465.)

Clinical Focus 7-22

Radial Nerve Compression

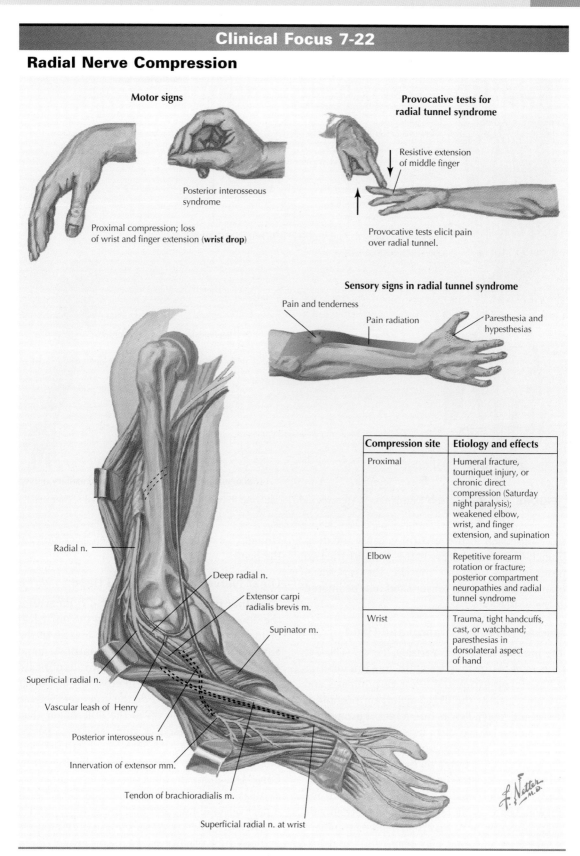

Motor signs

Posterior interosseous syndrome

Proximal compression; loss of wrist and finger extension (**wrist drop**)

Provocative tests for radial tunnel syndrome

Resistive extension of middle finger

Provocative tests elicit pain over radial tunnel.

Sensory signs in radial tunnel syndrome

Pain and tenderness

Pain radiation

Paresthesia and hypesthesias

Radial n.

Deep radial n.

Extensor carpi radialis brevis m.

Supinator m.

Superficial radial n.

Vascular leash of Henry

Posterior interosseous n.

Innervation of extensor mm.

Tendon of brachioradialis m.

Superficial radial n. at wrist

Compression site	Etiology and effects
Proximal	Humeral fracture, tourniquet injury, or chronic direct compression (Saturday night paralysis); weakened elbow, wrist, and finger extension, and supination
Elbow	Repetitive forearm rotation or fracture; posterior compartment neuropathies and radial tunnel syndrome
Wrist	Trauma, tight handcuffs, cast, or watchband; paresthesias in dorsolateral aspect of hand

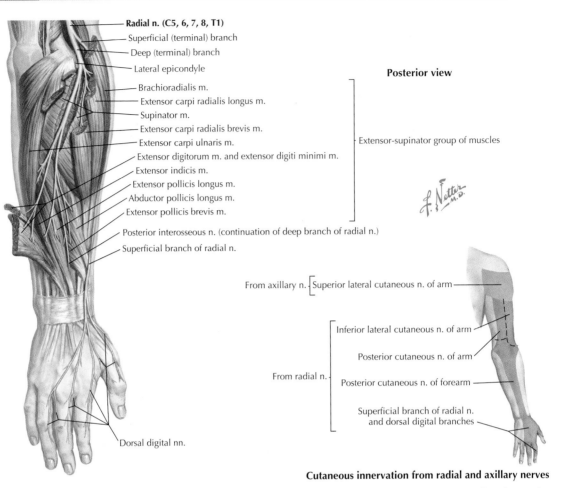

Radial n. (C5, 6, 7, 8, T1)
- Superficial (terminal) branch
- Deep (terminal) branch
- Lateral epicondyle
- Brachioradialis m.
- Extensor carpi radialis longus m.
- Supinator m.
- Extensor carpi radialis brevis m.
- Extensor carpi ulnaris m.
- Extensor digitorum m. and extensor digiti minimi m.
- Extensor indicis m.
- Extensor pollicis longus m.
- Abductor pollicis longus m.
- Extensor pollicis brevis m.
- Posterior interosseous n. (continuation of deep branch of radial n.)
- Superficial branch of radial n.

Extensor-supinator group of muscles

Posterior view

Dorsal digital nn.

From axillary n. { Superior lateral cutaneous n. of arm

From radial n. {
- Inferior lateral cutaneous n. of arm
- Posterior cutaneous n. of arm
- Posterior cutaneous n. of forearm
- Superficial branch of radial n. and dorsal digital branches

Cutaneous innervation from radial and axillary nerves

FIGURE 7-37 Radial Nerve Distribution in Forearm and Dorsal Hand. (From *Atlas of human anatomy,* ed 6, Plate 466.)

to compression in the forearm because the deep branch of the radial nerve passes through the two heads of the supinator muscle. The superficial branch of the nerve is sensory and may be injured at the wrist.

Median Nerve in Forearm and Hand

The **median nerve** (C5 variable, C6, C7, C8, T1) innervates all the muscles of the forearm anterior compartment except the flexor carpi ulnaris and the ulnar half of the flexor digitorum profundus (wrist and finger flexors and forearm pronators). The median nerve also innervates the thenar muscles and first two lumbricals. Pure median nerve sensation is tested on the skin overlying the palmar aspect of the tip of the index finger (Fig. 7-38). Although well protected in the arm, the median nerve is more vulnerable to traumatic injury in the forearm, wrist, and hand. Entrapment at the elbow and wrist may occur, and the recurrent branch of the median nerve on the thenar

eminence may be damaged in deep lacerations of the palm.

Ulnar Nerve in Forearm and Hand

The **ulnar nerve** (C7 variable, C8, T1) innervates the flexor carpi ulnaris muscle and the ulnar half of the flexor digitorum profundus muscle in the anterior forearm and most of the intrinsic hand muscles: hypothenar muscles, two lumbricals, adductor pollicis, and all interossei. Pure ulnar nerve sensation is tested on the skin overlying the palmar aspect of the tip of the little finger (Fig. 7-39). The ulnar nerve is vulnerable as it passes posterior to the medial epicondyle of the humerus; blunt trauma here can elicit the "I hit my funny bone" sensation. The ulnar nerve is also vulnerable as it passes through the cubital tunnel beneath the ulnar collateral ligament and in the ulnar tunnel, where it passes deep to the palmaris brevis muscle and palmar (volar) carpal ligament, just lateral to the pisiform bone.

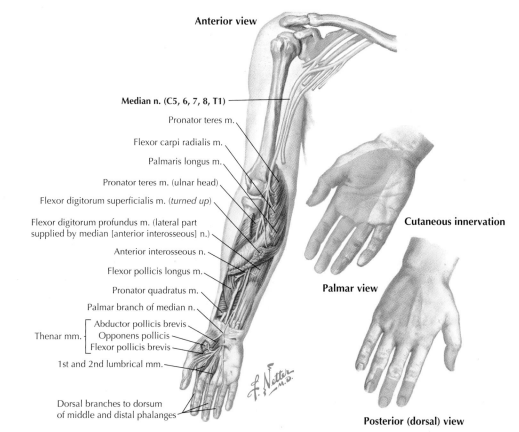

Anterior view

Median n. (C5, 6, 7, 8, T1)

Pronator teres m.

Flexor carpi radialis m.

Palmaris longus m.

Pronator teres m. (ulnar head)

Flexor digitorum superficialis m. (*turned up*)

Flexor digitorum profundus m. (lateral part supplied by median [anterior interosseous] n.)

Anterior interosseous n.

Flexor pollicis longus m.

Pronator quadratus m.

Palmar branch of median n.

Thenar mm. { Abductor pollicis brevis

Opponens pollicis

Flexor pollicis brevis }

1st and 2nd lumbrical mm.

Dorsal branches to dorsum of middle and distal phalanges

Cutaneous innervation

Palmar view

Posterior (dorsal) view

FIGURE 7-38 Median Nerve Distribution in Forearm and Hand. (From *Atlas of human anatomy*, ed 6, Plate 463.)

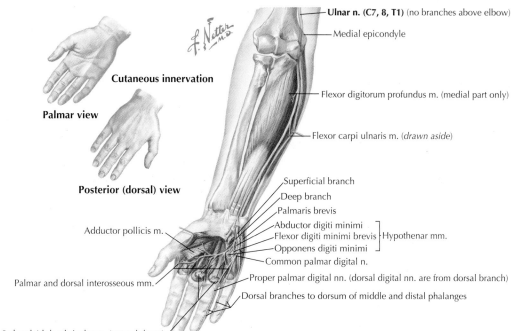

Cutaneous innervation

Palmar view

Posterior (dorsal) view

Adductor pollicis m.

Palmar and dorsal interosseous mm.

3rd and 4th lumbrical mm. (*turned down*)

Ulnar n. (C7, 8, T1) (no branches above elbow)

Medial epicondyle

Flexor digitorum profundus m. (medial part only)

Flexor carpi ulnaris m. (*drawn aside*)

Superficial branch

Deep branch

Palmaris brevis

Abductor digiti minimi

Flexor digiti minimi brevis } Hypothenar mm.

Opponens digiti minimi

Common palmar digital n.

Proper palmar digital nn. (dorsal digital nn. are from dorsal branch)

Dorsal branches to dorsum of middle and distal phalanges

FIGURE 7-39 Ulnar Nerve Distribution in Forearm and Hand. (From *Atlas of human anatomy*, ed 6, Plate 464.)

Proximal Median Nerve Compression

Compression at the elbow is the second most common site of median nerve entrapment after the wrist (carpal tunnel). Repetitive forearm pronation and finger flexion, especially against resistance, can cause muscle hypertrophy and entrap the nerve.

Pronator syndrome

Hypesthesia and activity-induced paresthesias

Pain location

Provocative maneuvers

Compression by flexor digitorum superficialis m.

Flexion of middle finger against resistance

Compression by pronator teres m.

Pronation against resistance

Compression by bicipital aponeurosis

Flexion of wrist against resistance

Median n.

Supracondylar process

Lig. of Struthers

Medial epicondyle

Bicipital aponeurosis

Pronator teres m.
Humeral head

Ulnar head

Flexor digitorum superficialis m. and arch

Flexor pollicis longus m.

Anterior interosseous n.

Anterior interosseous syndrome

Normal   Abnormal

JOHN A.CRAIG—AD

Hand posture in anterior interosseous syndrome due to paresis of flexor digitorum profundis and flexor pollicis longus muscles

Clinical Focus 7-24

Ulnar Tunnel Syndrome

The ulnar tunnel exists at the wrist where the ulnar nerve and artery pass deep to the palmaris brevis muscle and palmar (volar) carpal ligament, just lateral to the pisiform bone. Within the tunnel, the nerve divides into the superficial sensory and deep motor branches. Injury may result from trauma, ulnar artery thrombosis, fractures (hook of the hamate), dislocations (ulnar head, pisiform), arthritis, and repetitive movements. **Claw hand** may be present if the motor components are injured.

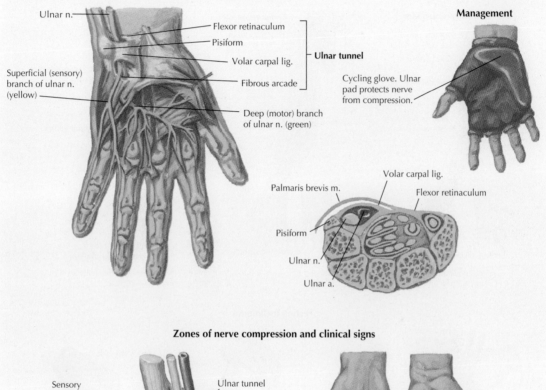

Ulnar n.

Flexor retinaculum

Pisiform

Volar carpal lig.

Fibrous arcade

Superficial (sensory) branch of ulnar n. (yellow)

Deep (motor) branch of ulnar n. (green)

Ulnar tunnel

Management

Cycling glove. Ulnar pad protects nerve from compression.

Palmaris brevis m.

Volar carpal lig.

Flexor retinaculum

Pisiform

Ulnar n.

Ulnar a.

Zones of nerve compression and clinical signs

Sensory

Motor

Ulnar tunnel

Zone I (motor and sensory)

Zone II (motor)

Zone III (sensory)

JOHN A. CRAIG—AD

Sensory findings occur with compression in zones I and III.

Clawing of 4th and 5th fingers

Interosseous atrophy

Motor findings occur with compression in zones I and II (**claw hand**).

Clinical Focus 7-25

Clinical Evaluation of Compression Neuropathy

Compression injury to the radial, median, and ulnar nerves may occur at several sites along each of their courses down the arm and forearm. A review of the applied anatomy and clinical presentation of several common neuropathies is shown in this illustration. Refer to the muscle tables presented in this chapter for a review of the muscle actions and anticipated functional weaknesses.

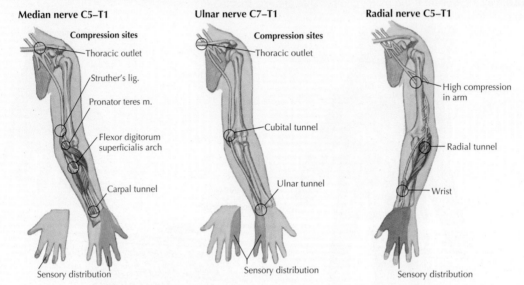

Median nerve C5–T1

Compression sites
Thoracic outlet
Struther's lig.
Pronator teres m.
Flexor digitorum superficialis arch
Carpal tunnel
Sensory distribution

Ulnar nerve C7–T1

Compression sites
Thoracic outlet
Cubital tunnel
Ulnar tunnel
Sensory distribution

Radial nerve C5–T1

High compression in arm
Radial tunnel
Wrist
Sensory distribution

Motor and sensory functions of each nerve assessed individually throughout entire upper extremity to delineate level of compression or entrapment

Testing techniques

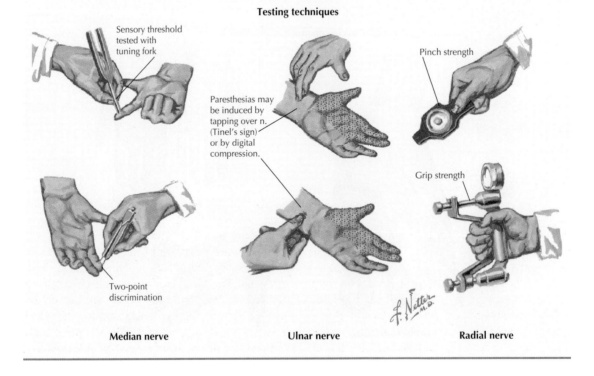

Sensory threshold tested with tuning fork

Paresthesias may be induced by tapping over n. (Tinel's sign) or by digital compression.

Pinch strength

Grip strength

Two-point discrimination

Median nerve   **Ulnar nerve**   **Radial nerve**

Clinical Focus 7-26

Ulnar Nerve Compression in Cubital Tunnel

Cubital tunnel syndrome results from compression of the ulnar nerve as it passes beneath the ulnar collateral ligament and between the two heads of the flexor carpi ulnaris muscle. This syndrome is the second most common compression neuropathy after carpal tunnel syndrome. The tunnel space is significantly reduced with elbow flexion, which compresses and stretches the ulnar nerve. The nerve also may be injured by direct trauma to the subcutaneous portion as it passes around the medial epicondyle.

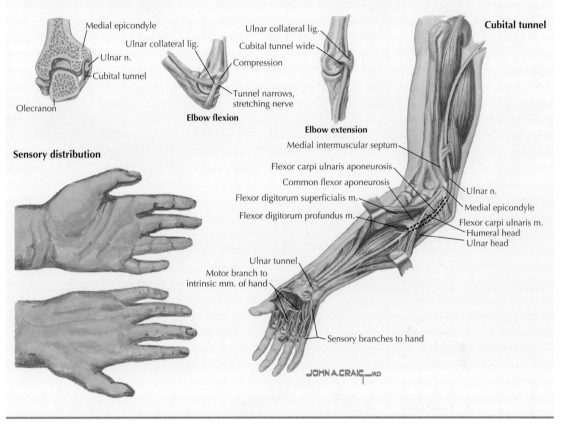

11. EMBRYOLOGY

Appendicular Skeleton

Along the embryonic axis, mesoderm derived from the sclerotome portion of the dermomyotome forms the axial skeleton and gives rise to the skull and spinal column (see Fig. 2-21 for more detailed development). The appendicular skeleton forms from mesenchyme that condenses to form hyaline cartilaginous precursors of limb bones. Upper (and lower) limb bones then develop by **endochondral ossification** from the cartilaginous precursors, except the clavicle, which develops by intramembranous ossification (Fig. 7-40).

Neuromuscular Development

Segmental somites give rise to myotomes that form collections of mesoderm dorsally called **epimeres** (epaxial). These epimeres are innervated by the dorsal rami of the spinal nerves. The epaxial muscles form the intrinsic back muscles. Ventral mesodermal collections form the **hypomeres** (hypaxial), which are innervated by the ventral rami of spinal nerves. Hypaxial muscles in the upper limbs divide into ventral (flexor) and dorsal (extensor) muscles (Fig. 7-41). The terminal branches of the **brachial plexus** (axillary, musculocutaneous, radial, median, and ulnar nerves) then grow into the limb as the

Mesenchymal precartilage primordia of axial and appendicular skeletons at 5 weeks

Precartilage mesenchymal cell condensations of appendicular skeleton at 6th week

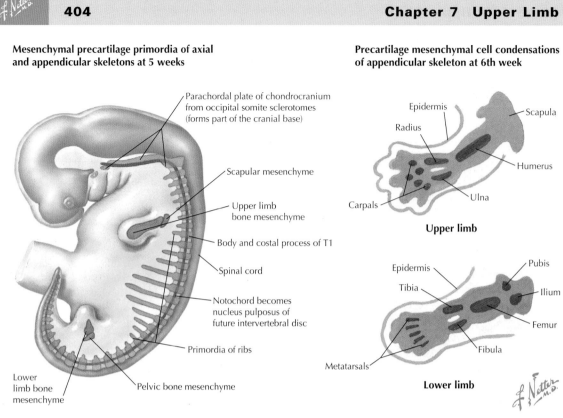

Parachordal plate of chondrocranium from occipital somite sclerotomes (forms part of the cranial base)

Scapular mesenchyme

Upper limb bone mesenchyme

Body and costal process of T1

Spinal cord

Notochord becomes nucleus pulposus of future intervertebral disc

Primordia of ribs

Lower limb bone mesenchyme

Pelvic bone mesenchyme

Epidermis

Radius

Carpals

Scapula

Humerus

Ulna

Upper limb

Epidermis

Tibia

Metatarsals

Pubis

Ilium

Femur

Fibula

Lower limb

FIGURE 7-40 Development of the Appendicular Skeleton.

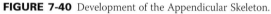

Limbs

Body wall

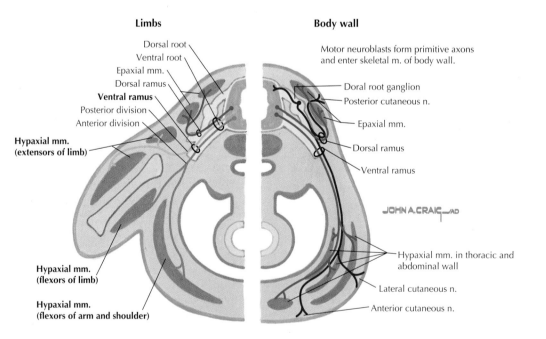

Dorsal root

Ventral root

Epaxial mm.

Dorsal ramus

Ventral ramus

Posterior division

Anterior division

Hypaxial mm. (extensors of limb)

Hypaxial mm. (flexors of limb)

Hypaxial mm. (flexors of arm and shoulder)

Motor neuroblasts form primitive axons and enter skeletal m. of body wall.

Doral root ganglion

Posterior cutaneous n.

Epaxial mm.

Dorsal ramus

Ventral ramus

Hypaxial mm. in thoracic and abdominal wall

Lateral cutaneous n.

Anterior cutaneous n.

Somatic nervous system innervates somatopleure (body wall).

Note: *A schematic cross section showing the body wall and upper limb on the embryo's right side and the embryo body wall only on the left side*

FIGURE 7-41 Neuromuscular Development.

mesoderm develops, supplying the muscles of each compartment.

Limb Bud Rotation and Dermatomes

Initially, as the limb buds grow out from the embryonic trunk, the ventral muscle mass (future flexors) faces medially and the dorsal mass (future extensors) faces laterally (Fig. 7-42). With continued growth and differentiation, the **upper limbs rotate 90 degrees laterally** so that in anatomical position, the ventral flexor muscle compartment faces anteriorly and the dorsal extensor muscle compartment posteriorly. The **lower limbs rotate 90 degrees medially** and are thus 180 degrees out of phase with the upper limbs. (The elbow faces posteriorly, and the knee faces anteriorly.) Thus in the upper limbs the flexors of the shoulder, elbow, and wrist/fingers are positioned anteriorly, and extensor muscles of the same joints are aligned posteriorly.

Although the **dermatome** distribution on the trunk is fairly linear horizontally, on the limbs some spiraling occurs, especially on the lower limb. The upper limb is more uniform, with dermatomes (C4-T2) that closely parallel the myotome innervation from the brachial plexus (C5-T1); a small contributing branch from C4 and T2 to the brachial plexus is normally observed. As noted previously, dermatome maps vary, and overlap of sensory innervation from the dermatome above and below is common (Fig. 7-43).

Changes in position of limbs before birth

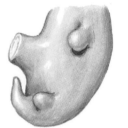 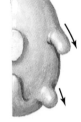

At 5 weeks. Upper and lower limbs have formed as finlike appendages pointing laterally and caudally.

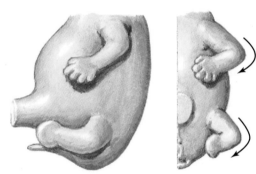

At 6 weeks. Limbs bend anteriorly, so elbows and knees point laterally, palms and soles face trunk.

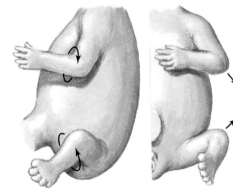

At 7 weeks. Upper and lower limbs have undergone 90° torsion about their long axes, but in opposite directions, so elbows point caudally and posteriorly, and the knees cranially and anteriorly.

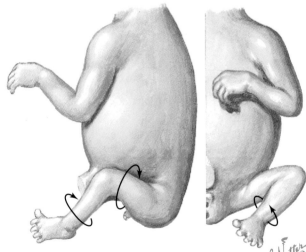

At 8 weeks. Torsion of lower limbs results in twisted or "barber pole" arrangement of their cutaneous innervation.

FIGURE 7-42 Limb Bud Rotation.

Changes in ventral dermatome pattern (cutaneous sensory nerve distribution) during limb development

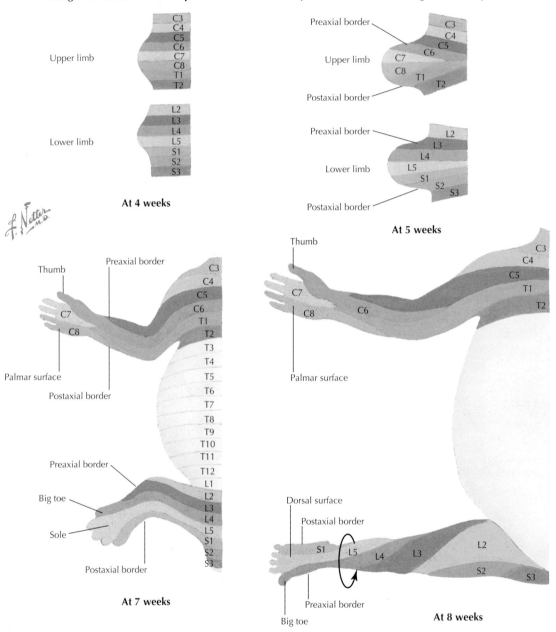

FIGURE 7-43 Limb Bud Rotation and Dermatome Patterns.

Challenge Yourself Questions

1. An elderly woman falls on her outstretched hand and fractures the surgical neck of her humerus. Several weeks later she presents with significant weakness in abduction of her arm and some weakened extension and flexion. Which of the following nerves is most likely injured?

   A. Accessory
   B. Axillary
   C. Radial
   D. Subscapular
   E. Thoracodorsal

2. Cancer spreading via the lymphatics passes into the axillary group of lymph nodes. Which of these axillary groups of nodes is most likely to receive this lymph first?

   A. Anterior (pectoral)
   B. Apical (subclavian)
   C. Central
   D. Lateral (brachial)
   E. Posterior (subscapular)

3. During a routine physical examination, the physician notes an absent biceps tendon reflex. Which spinal cord level is associated with this tendon reflex?

   A. C4-C5
   B. C5-C6
   C. C6-C7
   D. C7-C8
   E. C8-T1

4. A patient with a midshaft compound humeral fracture presents with bleeding and clinical signs of nerve entrapment. Which of the following nerves is most likely injured by the fracture?

   A. Axillary
   B. Median
   C. Musculocutaneous
   D. Radial
   E. Ulnar

5. A baseball pitcher delivers a 97-mph fastball to a batter and suddenly feels a sharp pain in his shoulder on release of the ball. The trainer examines the shoulder and concludes that the pitcher has a rotator cuff injury. Which muscle is most vulnerable and most likely torn by this type of injury?

   A. Infraspinatus
   B. Subscapularis
   C. Supraspinatus
   D. Teres major
   E. Teres minor

6. A fall on an outstretched hand results in swelling and pain on the lateral aspect of the wrist. Radiographic examination confirms a Colles' fracture. Which of the following bones is most likely fractured?

   A. Distal radius
   B. Distal ulna
   C. Lunate
   D. Scaphoid
   E. Trapezium

7. Examining an assembly line worker's complaint of tingling pain in her wrist with muscle weakness and atrophy, her physician diagnoses carpal tunnel syndrome. Which of the following muscles is most likely to be atrophied?

   A. Adductor pollicis
   B. Dorsal interossei
   C. Flexor digitorum superficialis
   D. Lumbricals 3 and 4
   E. Thenar

8. A patient presents with numbness over his medial hand and atrophy of the hypothenar muscles after an injury several days ago over his medial humeral epicondyle. Which of the following nerves most likely was injured?

   A. Anterior interosseous
   B. Musculocutaneous
   C. Recurrent branch of median
   D. Superficial radial
   E. Ulnar

9. During your introductory course to clinical medicine, you are asked to take the radial pulse of your classmate. Which of the following muscle tendons can you use as a guide to locate the radial artery?

    A. Adductor pollicis longus
    B. Brachioradialis
    C. Flexor carpi radialis
    D. Flexor pollicis longus
    E. Palmaris longus

10. A football player has a complete fracture of his radius just proximal to the insertion of the pronator teres muscle. As a result of the actions of the muscles attached to the proximal and distal fragments of the radius, which of the following combinations accurately reflects the orientation of the proximal and distal radial fragments?

    A. Proximal extended, and distal pronated
    B. Proximal extended and pronated, and distal supinated
    C. Proximal flexed, and distal pronated
    D. Proximal flexed, and distal supinated
    E. Proximal flexed and supinated, and distal pronated

11. Intravenous fluid administered into the median cubital vein that enters the basilic vein would then most likely empty into which of the following veins?

    A. Axillary
    B. Brachial
    C. Cephalic
    D. Deep brachial
    E. Subclavian

12. A wrestler comes off the mat holding his right forearm flexed at the elbow and pronated, with his shoulder medially rotated and displaced inferiorly. Which of his bones is most likely broken?

    A. Clavicle
    B. Humerus
    C. Radius
    D. Scapula
    E. Ulna

13. A knife cut results in a horizontal laceration to the thoracic wall extending across the midaxillary and anterior axillary lines just above the level of the T4 dermatome. Which of the following patient presentations will the emergency department physician most likely observe on examining the patient?

    A. Tingling along anterolateral forearm
    B. Supinated forearm
    C. Weakened elbow extension
    D. Weakened elbow flexion
    E. Winged scapula

14. Which of the following tendons is most vulnerable to inflammation and sepsis in the shoulder joint?

    A. Glenoid labrum
    B. Infraspinatus
    C. Long head of biceps
    D. Long head of triceps
    E. Supraspinatus

15. Which of the following muscle-nerve combinations is tested when spreading the fingers against resistance?

    A. Abductor digiti minimi–median
    B. Abductor pollicis brevis–radial
    C. Abductor pollicis longus–median
    D. Dorsal interossei–ulnar
    E. Palmar interossei–ulnar

For each of the descriptions below (16-20), select the nerve from the list (A-K) that is most likely responsible or affected.

(A) Axillary
(B) Dorsal scapular
(C) Long thoracic
(D) Medial cutaneous of arm
(E) Medial cutaneous of forearm
(F) Median
(G) Musculocutaneous
(H) Radial
(I) Suprascapular
(J) Thoracodorsal
(K) Ulnar

_____ 16. A patient presents with a "claw hand" deformity.

_____ 17. When asked to make a fist, the patient is unable to flex the first three fingers into the palm, and the fourth and fifth fingers are partially flexed at the MCP and DIP joints.

_____ 18. Angina pectoris leads to referred pain, which radiates down the arm.

___ 19. Despite injury to the radial nerve in the arm, a patient is still capable of supination of the forearm.

___ 20. Dislocation of the shoulder places this nerve in jeopardy of injury.

Answers to Challenge Yourself Questions

1. B. Fractures of this portion of the humerus can place the axillary nerve in danger of injury. Her muscle weakness confirms that the deltoid muscle especially is weakened, and the deltoid and teres minor are innervated by the axillary nerve.

2. A. 75% of the lymph from the breast passes to the axillary nodes and, of this group of 20-30 nodes, the anterior (pectoral) group of nodes receives the lymph first (the nodes closest to the axillary tail of the upper outer quadrant of the breast).

3. B. The biceps tendon reflex tests the musculocutaneous nerve and especially the C5-C6 contribution. The triceps tendon reflex tests the C7-C8 spinal contributions of the radial nerve.

4. D. The radial nerve spirals around the posterior aspect of the midhumeral shaft and can be stretched or contused by a compound fracture of the humerus. This nerve innervates all the extensor muscles of the upper limb (posterior compartments of the arm and forearm).

5. C. The supraspinatus muscle is most often torn in rotator cuff injuries. Repeated abduction and flexion can cause the tendon to rub on the acromion and coraco-acromial ligament, leading to tears or rupture.

6. A. The Colles' fracture (a fracture of the distal radius) presents with a classic dinner fork deformity with the dorsal and proximal displacement of the distal fragment. This is an extension-compression fracture.

7. E. The thenar muscles are located at the base of the thumb and are innervated by the median nerve (notably, by its recurrent branch), which passes through the carpal tunnel and is prone to injury in excessive repetitive movements at the wrist.

8. E. The ulnar nerve is subcutaneous as it passes around the medial epicondyle of the humerus. In this location, it is vulnerable to compression injury against the bone ("funny bone"), or entrapment in the cubital tunnel (beneath the ulnar collateral ligament).

9. C. The radial pulse can be easily taken at the wrist where the radial artery lies just lateral to the tendon of the flexor carpi radialis muscle.

10. E. The proximal fragment will be flexed and supinated by the biceps brachii and supinator muscles, while the distal fragment will be pronated by the action of the pronator teres and pronator quadratus muscles.

11. A. The median cubital vein may drain into the basilic vein, which then dives deeply and drains into the axillary vein.

12. A. Fractures of the clavicle are relatively common and occur most often in the middle third of the bone. The distal fragment is displaced downward by the weight of the shoulder and drawn medially by the action of the pectoralis major, teres major, and latissimus dorsi muscles.

13. E. This laceration probably severed the long thoracic nerve, which innervates the serratus anterior muscle. During muscle testing, the scapula will "wing" outwardly if this muscle is denervated.

14. C. The long head of the biceps tendon passes through the shoulder joint and attaches to the supraglenoid tubercle of the scapula. An infection in the joint could involve this tendon.

15. D. The dorsal interossei are innervated by the ulnar nerve and abduct the fingers (the little finger and thumb have their own abductors). This action is easily tested in a patient; dorsal interossei abduct the fingers (DAB) and the palmar interossei adduct the fingers (PAD).

16. K. "Claw hand" is a typical deformity of the ulnar nerve. The last two digits may be hyperextended at the MCP joint (unopposed extensor digitorum–radial nerve innervated), flexed at the PIP joint (flexor digitorum superficialis–median nerve innervated) and extended at the DIP joint (loss of flexor digitorum profundus–ulnar nerve, and the action of the unopposed extensor expansion).

17. F. This suggests a lesion to the median nerve. The thenar muscles are affected, as are the long flexors of the digits (flexor digitorum superficialis). Unopposed extension of the first three fingers occurs, and absence of flexion at the PIP joints of fingers 4 and 5 is evident. The position of the hand is that of a "papal" or "benediction" sign.

18. D. Referred pain from myocardial ischemia can be present along the medial aspect of the arm, usually on the left side, and is referred to this area by the medial cutaneous nerve of

the arm (T1). The intercostal brachial nerve (T2) may also contribute.

19. G. While the supinator muscle is denervated (loss of radial nerve), the biceps brachii muscle is innervated by the musculocutaneous nerve and is a powerful supinator when the elbow is flexed.

20. A. The axillary nerve (innervates the deltoid and teres minor muscles) can be injured by shoulder dislocations. This nerve passes through the quadrangular space before innervating its two muscles.

Head and Neck

1. INTRODUCTION

The head and neck area offers a unique challenge for students because of the density of small neurovascular structures; the complexity of its bony features, especially the skull; and the compactness of its anatomy. The head protects the brain, participates in communication and expresses our emotions, and houses the special senses (sight, sound, balance, smell, and taste). The neck connects the head to the thorax and is the conduit for visceral structures passing cranially or caudally within tightly partitioned fascial sleeves.

The anatomy of the head is best understood if you view it as a series of interconnected compartments, which include the following:

- **Cranium:** contains the brain and its meningeal coverings.
- **Orbits:** contain the eye and the muscles that move the eye.
- **Nasal cavities and paranasal sinuses:** form the uppermost part of the respiratory system.
- **Ears:** contain the apparatus for hearing and balance.
- **Oral cavity:** forms the proximal end of the digestive tract.

The anatomy of the neck is composed of a series of concentric-like compartments that provide a conduit for structures passing to the head or thorax, as follows:

- **Musculofascial:** superficial compartment encompassing the outer boundary of the neck.

- **Visceral:** anterocentral compartment that contains the upper respiratory (pharynx, larynx, trachea) and gastrointestinal (GI) tract (pharynx, esophagus), and the thyroid, parathyroid, and thymus glands.
- **Neurovascular:** two anterolateral compartments that contain the common carotid artery, internal jugular vein, and vagus nerve; called the carotid sheath.
- **Prevertebral:** posterocentral compartment that contains the cervical vertebrae and the associated paravertebral muscles.

2. SURFACE ANATOMY

The key surface features of the head and neck and include the following (Fig. 8-1):

- **Glabella:** smooth prominence on the frontal bone above the root of the nose.
- **Zygomatic bone:** the cheekbone, which protrudes below the orbit and is vulnerable to fractures from facial trauma.
- **Ear (auricle or pinna):** skin-covered elastic cartilage with several consistent ridges, including the helix, antihelix, tragus, antitragus, and lobule.
- **Philtrum:** midline infranasal depression of the upper lip.
- **Nasolabial sulcus:** line between the nose and the corner of the lip.
- **Thyroid cartilage:** the laryngeal prominence ("Adam's apple").
- **Jugular (suprasternal) notch:** midline depression between the two sternal heads of the sternocleidomastoid muscle.

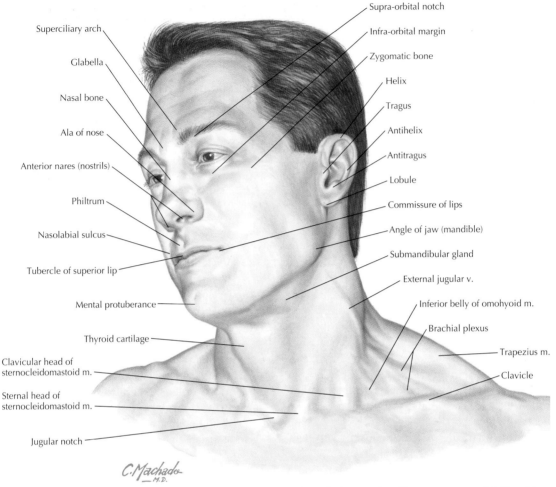

Supra-orbital notch
Superciliary arch
Infra-orbital margin
Glabella
Zygomatic bone
Nasal bone
Helix
Tragus
Ala of nose
Antihelix
Anterior nares (nostrils)
Antitragus
Philtrum
Lobule
Commissure of lips
Nasolabial sulcus
Angle of jaw (mandible)
Tubercle of superior lip
Submandibular gland
External jugular v.
Mental protuberance
Inferior belly of omohyoid m.
Brachial plexus
Thyroid cartilage
Trapezius m.
Clavicular head of sternocleidomastoid m.
Clavicle
Sternal head of sternocleidomastoid m.
Jugular notch

C. Machado
M.D.

FIGURE 8-1 Key Surface Anatomy Landmarks of the Head and Neck. (From *Atlas of human anatomy,* ed 6, Plate 1.)

3. SKULL

The skull is composed of 22 bones (see Chapter 1). Eight of these bones form the cranium (neurocranium, which contains the brain and meninges), and 14 of these form the face (viscerocranium). There are seven associated bones: the auditory ossicles (three in each middle ear) and the unpaired hyoid bone (Fig. 8-2 and Table 8-1). Using your atlas and dry bone specimens, note the complexity of the maxillary, temporal, and sphenoid bones. These bones are in close association with many of the cranial nerves and encase portions of many of our special senses—balance, hearing, smell, sight, and even taste—as the maxillae form a portion of the oral cavity.

Other features of the skull are noted as we review each region of the head. However, general external features include the following (Figs. 8-2 and 8-3):

- **Coronal suture:** region between the frontal and two parietal bones.
- **Sagittal suture:** region between the two parietal bones.
- **Lambdoid suture:** region between the occipital bone and the two parietal bones.
- **Nasion:** point at which the frontal and nasal bones meet.
- **Bregma:** point at which coronal and sagittal sutures meet.
- **Lambda:** point at which sagittal and lambdoid sutures meet.
- **Pterion:** point at which frontal, sphenoid, temporal, and parietal bones meet; the middle meningeal artery lies beneath this region.
- **Asterion:** point at which temporal, parietal, and occipital bones meet.
- **Inion:** the external occipital protuberance.

TABLE 8-1 Bones of the Skull

BONE	DESCRIPTION	BONE	DESCRIPTION
Frontal	Forms forehead, is thicker anteriorly, contains frontal sinuses	Temporal	Paired bones that form the lower portion of the lateral neurocranium and contain the middle and inner ear cavities, and the vestibular system for balance
Nasal	Paired bones that form the root of the nose		
Lacrimal	Small, paired bones that form part of the anteromedial wall of the orbit and contain the lacrimal sac	Sphenoid	Complex bone composed of a central body, and greater and lesser wings
Zygomatic	Paired cheekbones that form the inferolateral rim of the orbit and are frequently fractured by blunt trauma	Occipital	Forms the inferoposterior portion of the neurocranium
		Ethmoid	Forms the ethmoid sinuses, and contributes to the medial, lateral, and superior walls of the nasal cavity
Maxilla	Paired bones that form part of the cheek and contain 16 maxillary teeth		
Mandible	Lower jaw bone that contains 16 mandibular teeth	Inferior concha	Paired bones of the lateral nasal wall that form the inferior nasal concha
Parietal	Forms the superolateral portion of the neurocranium	Vomer	Forms the lower part of the nasal septum
		Palatine	Contributes to the lateral nasal wall, a small part of the nasal septum, and the hard palate

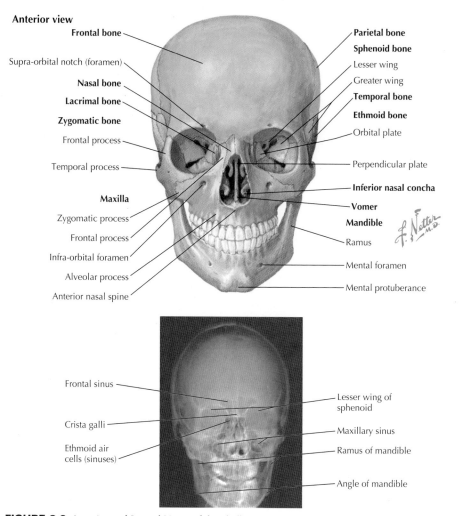

FIGURE 8-2 Anterior and Lateral Views of the Skull. (From *Atlas of human anatomy*, ed 6, Plate 4.)

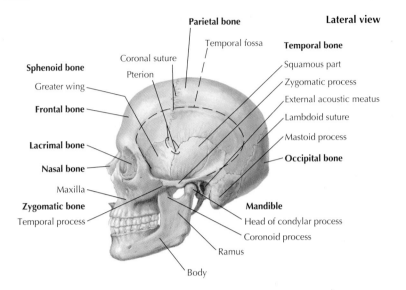

Lateral view

Parietal bone
Temporal fossa
Coronal suture
Pterion
Sphenoid bone
Greater wing
Frontal bone
Lacrimal bone
Nasal bone
Maxilla
Zygomatic bone
Temporal process
Temporal bone
Squamous part
Zygomatic process
External acoustic meatus
Lambdoid suture
Mastoid process
Occipital bone
Mandible
Head of condylar process
Coronoid process
Ramus
Body

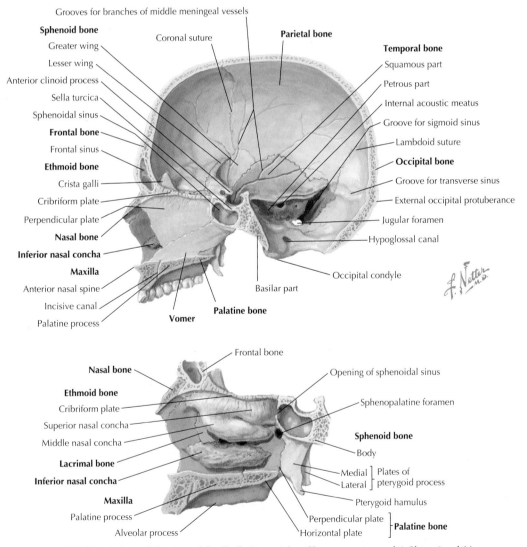

Grooves for branches of middle meningeal vessels
Sphenoid bone
Greater wing
Lesser wing
Anterior clinoid process
Sella turcica
Sphenoidal sinus
Frontal bone
Frontal sinus
Ethmoid bone
Crista galli
Cribriform plate
Perpendicular plate
Nasal bone
Inferior nasal concha
Maxilla
Anterior nasal spine
Incisive canal
Palatine process
Coronal suture
Parietal bone
Temporal bone
Squamous part
Petrous part
Internal acoustic meatus
Groove for sigmoid sinus
Lambdoid suture
Occipital bone
Groove for transverse sinus
External occipital protuberance
Jugular foramen
Hypoglossal canal
Occipital condyle
Basilar part
Vomer
Palatine bone

Frontal bone
Nasal bone
Ethmoid bone
Cribriform plate
Superior nasal concha
Middle nasal concha
Lacrimal bone
Inferior nasal concha
Maxilla
Palatine process
Alveolar process
Opening of sphenoidal sinus
Sphenopalatine foramen
Sphenoid bone
Body
Medial } Plates of
Lateral } pterygoid process
Pterygoid hamulus
Perpendicular plate } **Palatine bone**
Horizontal plate }

FIGURE 8-3 Sagittal Sections of the Skull. (From *Atlas of human anatomy,* ed 6, Plates 6 and 8.)

Clinical Focus 8-1

Skull Fractures

Skull fractures may be classified as follows:

- **Linear:** presents with a distinct fracture line.
- **Comminuted:** presents with multiple fragments (depressed if driven inward; can compress or tear the underlying dura mater).
- **Diastasis:** fracture along a suture line.
- **Basilar:** fracture of the base of the skull.

Any fracture that communicates with a lacerated scalp, a paranasal sinus, or the middle ear is termed a **compound fracture.** Compound depressed fractures must be treated surgically.

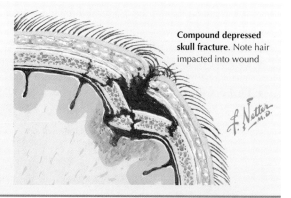

Compound depressed skull fracture. Note hair impacted into wound

Clinical Focus 8-2

Zygomatic Fractures

Trauma to the zygomatic bone (cheekbone) can disrupt the zygomatic complex and its articulations with the frontal, maxillary, temporal, sphenoid, and palatine bones. Often, fractures involve suture lines with the frontal and maxillary bones, resulting in displacement inferiorly, medially, and posteriorly. The typical clinical presentation is illustrated. Ipsilateral ocular and visual changes may include **diplopia** (an upper outer gaze) and **hyphema** (blood in the anterior chamber of the eye), which requires immediate clinical attention.

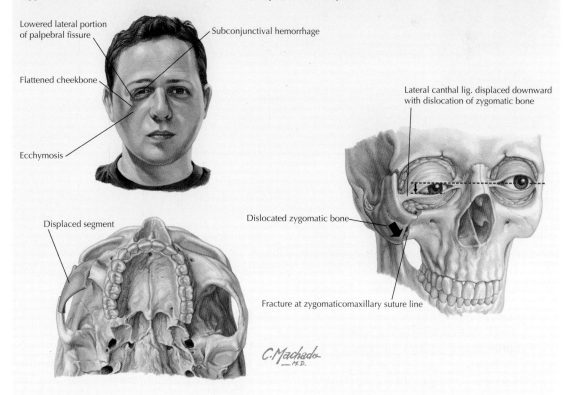

Lowered lateral portion of palpebral fissure

Subconjunctival hemorrhage

Flattened cheekbone

Ecchymosis

Lateral canthal lig. displaced downward with dislocation of zygomatic bone

Displaced segment

Dislocated zygomatic bone

Fracture at zygomaticomaxillary suture line

Midface Fractures

Midface fractures (of the maxilla, naso-orbital complex, and zygomatic bones) were classified by Le Fort as follows:

- **Le Fort I:** horizontal detachment of the maxilla at the level of the nasal floor (ant.-post. views).
- **Le Fort II:** pyramidal fracture that includes both maxillae and nasal bones, medial portions of both maxillary antra, infra-orbital rims, orbits, and orbital floors (ant.-post. views).
- **Le Fort III:** includes Le Fort II and a fracture of both zygomatic bones; may cause airway problems, nasolacrimal apparatus obstruction, and cerebrospinal fluid leakage (ant.-post. views).

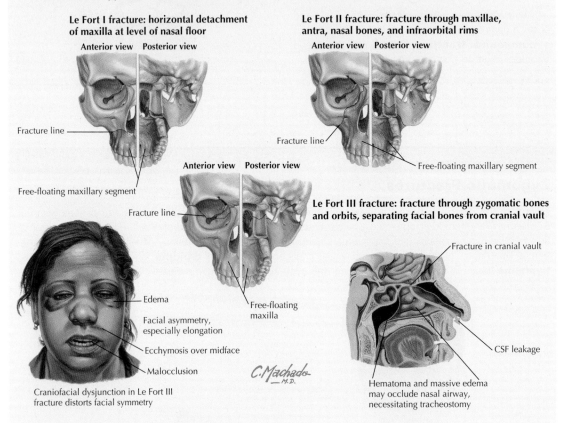

Le Fort I fracture: horizontal detachment of maxilla at level of nasal floor

Anterior view   Posterior view

Fracture line

Free-floating maxillary segment

Anterior view   Posterior view

Fracture line

Edema

Facial asymmetry, especially elongation

Ecchymosis over midface

Malocclusion

Craniofacial dysjunction in Le Fort III fracture distorts facial symmetry

Le Fort II fracture: fracture through maxillae, antra, nasal bones, and infraorbital rims

Anterior view   Posterior view

Fracture line

Free-floating maxillary segment

Free-floating maxilla

Le Fort III fracture: fracture through zygomatic bones and orbits, separating facial bones from cranial vault

Fracture in cranial vault

CSF leakage

Hematoma and massive edema may occlude nasal airway, necessitating tracheostomy

Cranial Fossae

The cranial base is the floor of the neurocranium, which supports the brain, and is divided into the following three **cranial fossae:** (Fig. 8-4):

- **Anterior:** the roof of the orbits; accommodates the frontal lobes of the brain.
- **Middle:** accommodates the temporal lobes of the brain.
- **Posterior:** accommodates the cerebellum, pons, and medulla oblongata of the brain.

Each fossa has numerous foramina (openings) for structures to pass in or out of the neurocranium.

4. BRAIN

Meninges

The brain and spinal cord are surrounded by three membranous connective tissue layers called the *meninges*, which include the following (Fig. 8-5):

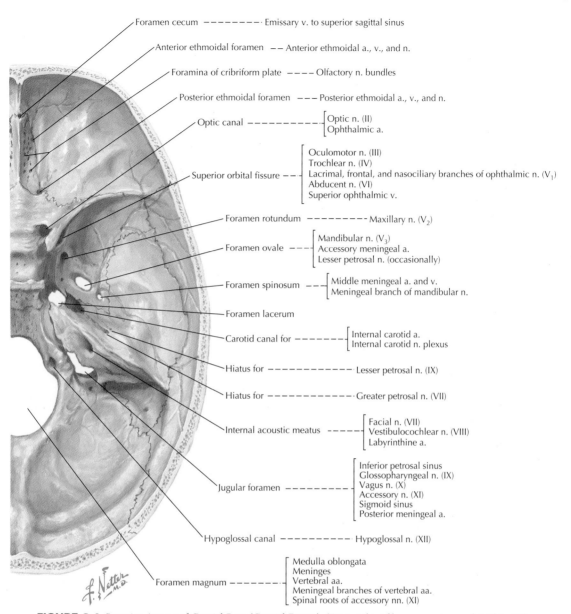

Foramen cecum --------- Emissary v. to superior sagittal sinus

Anterior ethmoidal foramen -- Anterior ethmoidal a., v., and n.

Foramina of cribriform plate ---- Olfactory n. bundles

Posterior ethmoidal foramen --- Posterior ethmoidal a., v., and n.

Optic canal ---------- ⎡Optic n. (II)
                       ⎣Ophthalmic a.

Superior orbital fissure -- ⎡Oculomotor n. (III)
                             │Trochlear n. (IV)
                             ⎨Lacrimal, frontal, and nasociliary branches of ophthalmic n. (V$_1$)
                             │Abducent n. (VI)
                             ⎣Superior ophthalmic v.

Foramen rotundum -------- Maxillary n. (V$_2$)

Foramen ovale --- ⎡Mandibular n. (V$_3$)
                   ⎨Accessory meningeal a.
                   ⎣Lesser petrosal n. (occasionally)

Foramen spinosum --- ⎡Middle meningeal a. and v.
                      ⎣Meningeal branch of mandibular n.

Foramen lacerum

Carotid canal for ------- ⎡Internal carotid a.
                           ⎣Internal carotid n. plexus

Hiatus for ----------- Lesser petrosal n. (IX)

Hiatus for ----------- Greater petrosal n. (VII)

Internal acoustic meatus ----- ⎡Facial n. (VII)
                                ⎨Vestibulocochlear n. (VIII)
                                ⎣Labyrinthine a.

Jugular foramen --------- ⎡Inferior petrosal sinus
                           │Glossopharyngeal n. (IX)
                           │Vagus n. (X)
                           ⎨Accessory n. (XI)
                           │Sigmoid sinus
                           ⎣Posterior meningeal a.

Hypoglossal canal --------- Hypoglossal n. (XII)

Foramen magnum ------- ⎡Medulla oblongata
                        │Meninges
                        ⎨Vertebral aa.
                        │Meningeal branches of vertebral aa.
                        ⎣Spinal roots of accessory nn. (XI)

FIGURE 8-4 Superior Aspect of Cranial Base (Cranial Fossae). (From *Atlas of human anatomy*, ed 6, Plate 13.)

- **Dura mater:** thick outermost meningeal layer that is richly innervated by sensory nerve fibers.
- **Arachnoid mater:** fine, weblike avascular membrane directly beneath the dural surface; the space between the arachnoid and the underlying pia is called the **subarachnoid space** and contains cerebrospinal fluid, which bathes and protects the central nervous system (CNS).
- **Pia mater:** delicate membrane of connective tissue that intimately envelops the brain and spinal cord.

The cranial dura is distinguished from the dura mater covering the spinal cord by its two layers. An outer **periosteal layer** is attached to the inner aspect of the cranium and is supplied by the meningeal arteries, which lie on its surface between it and the bony skull. Imprints of these meningeal artery branches can be seen as depressions on the inner table of bone. This periosteal dura is continuous with the periosteum on the outer surface of the skull at the foramen magnum and where other intracranial foramina open onto the outer skull surface. The inner dural layer is termed the **meningeal layer** and is in close contact with the

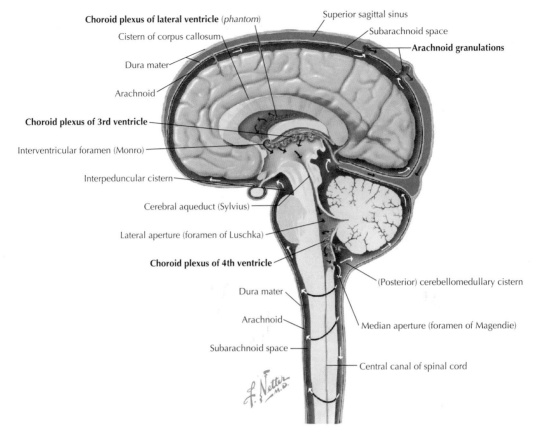

Choroid plexus of lateral ventricle (*phantom*)

Cistern of corpus callosum

Dura mater

Arachnoid

Choroid plexus of 3rd ventricle

Interventricular foramen (Monro)

Interpeduncular cistern

Cerebral aqueduct (Sylvius)

Lateral aperture (foramen of Luschka)

Choroid plexus of 4th ventricle

Dura mater

Arachnoid

Subarachnoid space

Superior sagittal sinus

Subarachnoid space

Arachnoid granulations

(Posterior) cerebellomedullary cistern

Median aperture (foramen of Magendie)

Central canal of spinal cord

FIGURE 8-5 Central Nervous System Meninges, Cerebrospinal Fluid Circulation, and Arachnoid Granulations. (From *Atlas of human anatomy*, ed 6, Plate 110.)

underlying arachnoid mater and is continuous with the spinal dura at the level of the foramen magnum.

The dura mater is richly innervated by meningeal sensory branches of the trigeminal nerve (fifth cranial nerve, CN V); the vagus nerve (CN X), specifically to the posterior cranial fossa; and the upper cervical nerves. A portion of the dura in the posterior cranial fossa also may receive some innervation from the glossopharyngeal nerve (CN IX) and hypoglossal nerve (CN XII). The arachnoid and pia mater lack sensory innervation. The periosteal dura and meningeal dura separate to form thick connective tissue folds or layers that separate various brain regions and lobes (Figs. 8-5, 8-6, and 8-7):

- **Falx cerebri:** double layer of meningeal dura between the cerebral hemispheres.
- **Falx cerebelli:** sickle-shaped layer of meningeal dura that projects between the two cerebellar hemispheres.

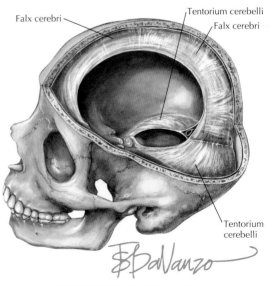

Falx cerebri

Tentorium cerebelli

Falx cerebri

Tentorium cerebelli

FIGURE 8-6 Dural Projections.

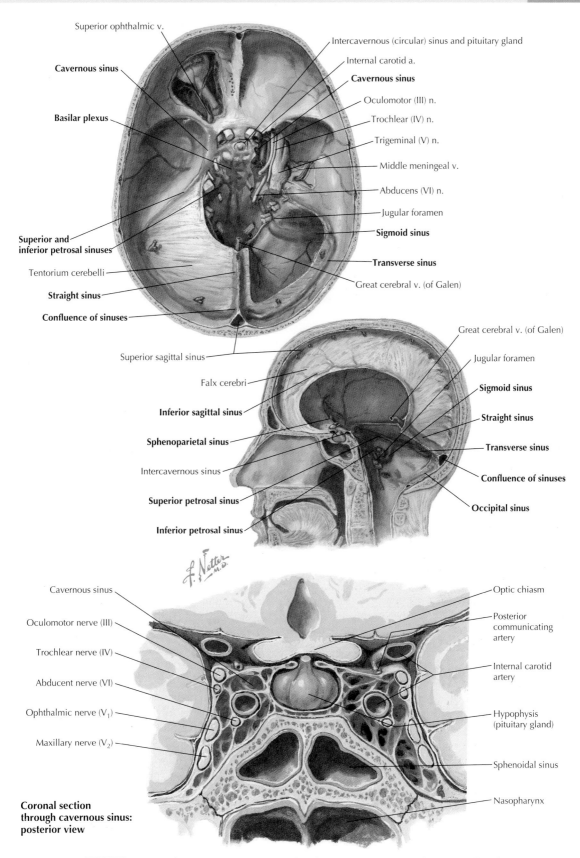

Superior ophthalmic v.

Intercavernous (circular) sinus and pituitary gland

Internal carotid a.

Cavernous sinus

Cavernous sinus

Oculomotor (III) n.

Trochlear (IV) n.

Trigeminal (V) n.

Basilar plexus

Middle meningeal v.

Abducens (VI) n.

Jugular foramen

Sigmoid sinus

Superior and inferior petrosal sinuses

Transverse sinus

Tentorium cerebelli

Great cerebral v. (of Galen)

Straight sinus

Confluence of sinuses

Superior sagittal sinus

Great cerebral v. (of Galen)

Jugular foramen

Falx cerebri

Sigmoid sinus

Inferior sagittal sinus

Straight sinus

Sphenoparietal sinus

Transverse sinus

Intercavernous sinus

Confluence of sinuses

Superior petrosal sinus

Occipital sinus

Inferior petrosal sinus

Cavernous sinus

Optic chiasm

Posterior communicating artery

Oculomotor nerve (III)

Trochlear nerve (IV)

Abducent nerve (VI)

Internal carotid artery

Ophthalmic nerve (V$_1$)

Maxillary nerve (V$_2$)

Hypophysis (pituitary gland)

Sphenoidal sinus

Coronal section through cavernous sinus: posterior view

Nasopharynx

FIGURE 8-7 Dural Venous Sinuses. (From *Atlas of human anatomy,* ed 6, Plates 104 and 105.)

- **Tentorium cerebelli:** fold of meningeal dura that covers the cerebellum and supports the occipital lobes of the cerebral hemispheres.
- **Diaphragma sellae:** horizontal shelf of meningeal dura that forms the roof of the sella turcica covering the pituitary gland; the infundibulum passes through this dural shelf to connect the hypothalamus with the pituitary gland.

Dural Venous Sinuses

The dura also separates to form several large endothelial-lined venous channels between its periosteal and meningeal layers—superior and inferior sagittal, straight, confluence of sinuses, transverse, sigmoid, and cavernous sinuses—and several smaller dural sinuses (Table 8-2 and Fig. 8-7). These **dural venous sinuses** drain blood from the brain, largely posteriorly, then into the internal jugular veins. These sinuses lack valves, however, so the direction of blood flow through the sinuses is pressure dependent. Of particular importance is the **cavernous venous sinus,** which lies on either side of the sella turcica and has an anatomical relationship with the internal carotid artery and several cranial nerves, including III, IV, V_1, V_2, and VI. Injury or inflammation in this region can affect all these important structures. Also, the optic chiasm lies just above this area, so CN II may be involved in any superior expansion of the cavernous sinus (e.g., pituitary tumor).

Subarachnoid Space

The **subarachnoid space** (between the arachnoid and pia mater) contains **cerebrospinal fluid** (CSF), which performs the following functions (Figs. 8-5 and 8-8):

- Supports and cushions the spinal cord and brain.
- Fulfills some functions normally provided by the lymphatic system.
- Occupies a volume of about 150 mL in the subarachnoid space.
- Is produced by **choroid plexuses** in the brain's ventricles.
- Is produced at a rate of about 500 to 700 mL/day.
- Is reabsorbed largely by arachnoid granulations and by small venules along the length of the spinal cord.

The **arachnoid granulations** absorb most of the CSF and deliver it to the dural venous sinuses (see Figs. 8-5 and 8-8). These granulations are composed of convoluted aggregations of arachnoid that extend as "tufts" into the superior sagittal sinus and function as one-way valves for the clearance of CSF; the CSF crosses into the venous sinus, but venous blood cannot enter the subarachnoid space. Small, microscopic arachnoid cell herniations also occur along the spinal cord, where CSF (which circulates at a higher pressure than venous blood) is delivered directly into small spinal cord veins.

TABLE 8-2 Dural Venous Sinuses	
SINUS	**CHARACTERISTICS**
Superior sagittal	Midline sinus along the convex superior border of the falx cerebri
Inferior sagittal	Midline sinus along the inferior free edge of the falx cerebri and joined by the great cerebral vein (of Galen)
Straight	Runs in the attachment of the falx cerebri and the tentorium cerebelli, and is formed by the inferior sagittal sinus and great cerebral vein
Confluence of sinuses	Meeting of superior and inferior sagittal sinuses, the straight sinus, and the occipital sinus
Transverse	Extends from the confluence of sinuses along the lateral edge of the tentorium cerebelli
Sigmoid	Continuation of the transverse sinus that passes inferomedially in an S-shaped pathway to the jugular foramen (becomes internal jugular vein)
Occipital	Runs in the falx cerebelli to the confluence of sinuses
Basilar	Network of venous channels on basilar part of the occipital bone, with connections to the petrosal sinuses; drains into vertebral venous plexus
Cavernous	Lies between dural layers on each side of the sella turcica; connects to the superior ophthalmic veins, pterygoid plexus of veins, sphenoparietal sinuses, petrosal sinuses, and basilar sinus
Sphenoparietal	Runs along the posterior edge of the lesser wing of the sphenoid bone and drains into the cavernous sinus
Emissary veins	Small veins connect the dural sinuses with the diploic veins in the bony skull, which are connected to scalp veins

Scalp, skull, meningeal and cerebral blood vessels

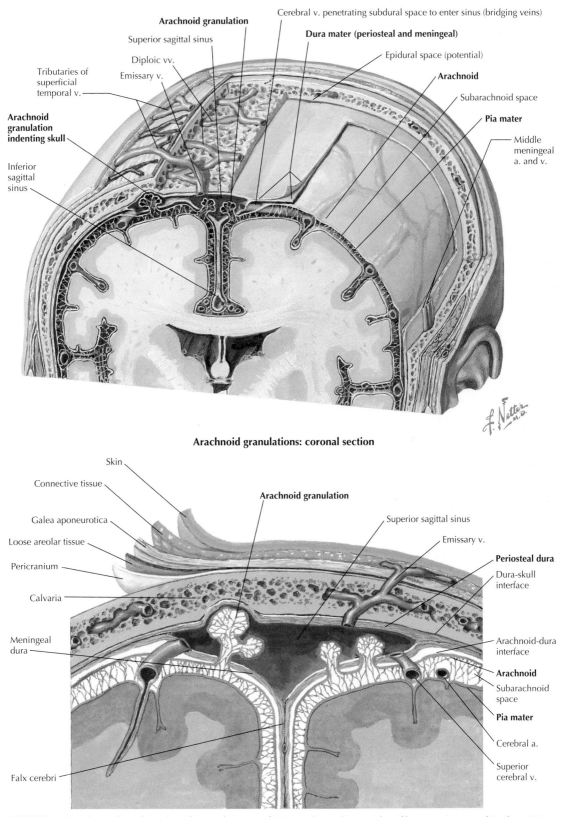

Arachnoid granulation

Superior sagittal sinus

Diploic vv.

Tributaries of superficial temporal v.

Emissary v.

Arachnoid granulation indenting skull

Inferior sagittal sinus

Cerebral v. penetrating subdural space to enter sinus (bridging veins)

Dura mater (periosteal and meningeal)

Epidural space (potential)

Arachnoid

Subarachnoid space

Pia mater

Middle meningeal a. and v.

Arachnoid granulations: coronal section

Skin

Connective tissue

Galea aponeurotica

Loose areolar tissue

Pericranium

Calvaria

Meningeal dura

Falx cerebri

Arachnoid granulation

Superior sagittal sinus

Emissary v.

Periosteal dura

Dura-skull interface

Arachnoid-dura interface

Arachnoid

Subarachnoid space

Pia mater

Cerebral a.

Superior cerebral v.

FIGURE 8-8 Relationship of Arachnoid Granulations and Venous Sinus. (From *Atlas of human anatomy*, ed 6, Plates 101 and 103.)

Hydrocephalus

Hydrocephalus is the accumulation of excess CSF within the brain's ventricular system. It is caused by over-production or decreased absorption of CSF or by blockage of one of the passageways for CSF flow in the subarachnoid space.

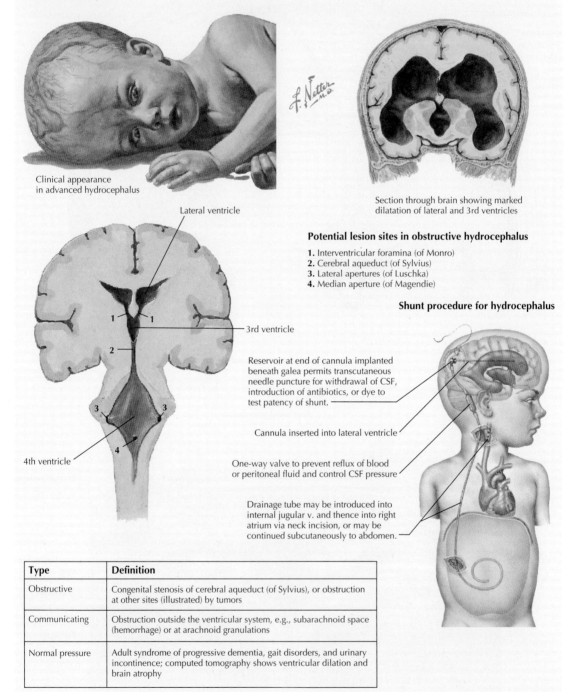

Clinical appearance
in advanced hydrocephalus

Section through brain showing marked
dilatation of lateral and 3rd ventricles

Lateral ventricle

Potential lesion sites in obstructive hydrocephalus

1. Interventricular foramina (of Monro)
2. Cerebral aqueduct (of Sylvius)
3. Lateral apertures (of Luschka)
4. Median aperture (of Magendie)

Shunt procedure for hydrocephalus

3rd ventricle

Reservoir at end of cannula implanted
beneath galea permits transcutaneous
needle puncture for withdrawal of CSF,
introduction of antibiotics, or dye to
test patency of shunt.

Cannula inserted into lateral ventricle

4th ventricle

One-way valve to prevent reflux of blood
or peritoneal fluid and control CSF pressure

Drainage tube may be introduced into
internal jugular v. and thence into right
atrium via neck incision, or may be
continued subcutaneously to abdomen.

Type	Definition
Obstructive	Congenital stenosis of cerebral aqueduct (of Sylvius), or obstruction at other sites (illustrated) by tumors
Communicating	Obstruction outside the ventricular system, e.g., subarachnoid space (hemorrhage) or at arachnoid granulations
Normal pressure	Adult syndrome of progressive dementia, gait disorders, and urinary incontinence; computed tomography shows ventricular dilation and brain atrophy

Meningitis

Meningitis is a serious condition defined as an inflammation of the arachnoid and pia mater. It results most often from bacterial or aseptic causes. Aseptic causes include viral infections, drug reactions, and systemic diseases. Patients with meningitis usually present with the following symptoms:

- Headache
- Fever

- Seizures
- Painful stiff neck

Diagnosis is made by performing a lumbar puncture and examining the CSF.

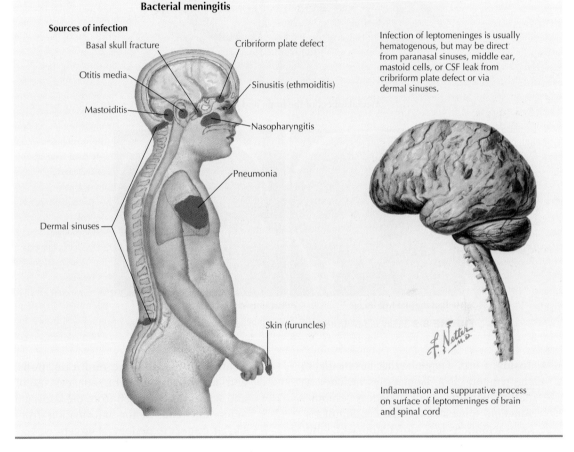

Bacterial meningitis

Sources of infection

Basal skull fracture

Cribriform plate defect

Otitis media

Sinusitis (ethmoiditis)

Mastoiditis

Nasopharyngitis

Pneumonia

Dermal sinuses

Skin (furuncles)

Infection of leptomeninges is usually hematogenous, but may be direct from paranasal sinuses, middle ear, mastoid cells, or CSF leak from cribriform plate defect or via dermal sinuses.

Inflammation and suppurative process on surface of leptomeninges of brain and spinal cord

Gross Anatomy of the Brain

The most notable feature of the human brain is its large cerebral hemispheres (Fig. 8-9). Several circumscribed regions of the cerebral cortex are associated with specific functions, and key surface landmarks of the typical human cerebrum are used to divide the brain into lobes: four or five, depending on classification, with the fifth either the insula or the limbic lobe. The lobes and their functions are as follows:

- **Frontal:** mediates precise voluntary motor control, learned motor skills, planned

movement, eye movement, expressive speech, personality, working memory, complex problem solving, emotions, judgment, socialization, olfaction, and drive.
- **Parietal:** affects sensory input, spatial discrimination, sensory representation and integration, taste, and receptive speech.
- **Occipital:** affects visual input and processing.
- **Temporal:** mediates auditory input and auditory memory integration, spoken language (dominant side), and body language (nondominant side).

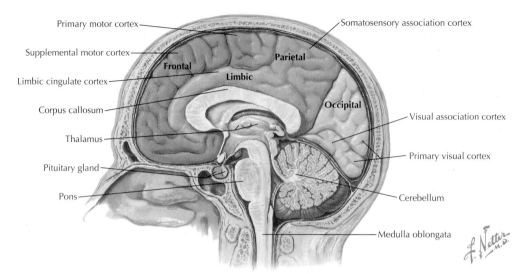

Primary motor cortex

Supplemental motor cortex

Limbic cingulate cortex

Corpus callosum

Thalamus

Pituitary gland

Pons

Somatosensory association cortex

Parietal

Frontal

Limbic

Occipital

Visual association cortex

Primary visual cortex

Cerebellum

Medulla oblongata

Medial aspect of the brain and brainstem

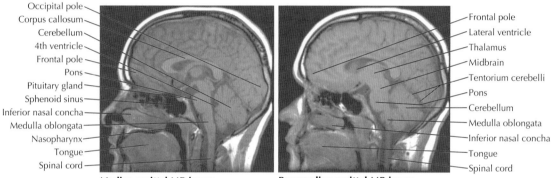

Occipital pole
Corpus callosum
Cerebellum
4th ventricle
Frontal pole
Pons
Pituitary gland
Sphenoid sinus
Inferior nasal concha
Medulla oblongata
Nasopharynx
Tongue
Spinal cord

Frontal pole
Lateral ventricle
Thalamus
Midbrain
Tentorium cerebelli
Pons
Cerebellum
Medulla oblongata
Inferior nasal concha
Tongue
Spinal cord

Median sagittal MR image   **Paramedian sagittal MR image**

FIGURE 8-9 Brain and Brainstem. (From *Atlas of human anatomy,* ed 6, Plate 107.)

- **Insula:** a fifth deep lobe that lies medial to the temporal lobe (sometimes included as part of temporal lobe); influences vestibular function, some language, perception of visceral sensations (e.g., upset stomach), emotions, and limbic functions.
- **Limbic:** also sometimes considered a fifth medial lobe (cingulate cortex); influences emotions and some autonomic functions.

Other key areas of the brain include the following components (Fig. 8-9):

- **Thalamus:** gateway to the cortex; simplistically functions as an "executive secretary" to the cortex (relay center between cortical and subcortical areas).
- **Cerebellum:** coordinates smooth motor activities, and processes muscle position; possible role in behavior and cognition.

- **Brainstem:** includes the **midbrain, pons, and medulla oblongata;** conveys motor and sensory information from the body and autonomic and motor information from higher centers to peripheral targets.

Internally, the brain contains **four ventricles,** two lateral ventricles, and a central third and fourth ventricle (Fig. 8-10). Cerebrospinal fluid, produced by the choroid plexus (see Fig. 8-5), circulates through these ventricles and then enters the subarachnoid space through **two lateral apertures** (foramina of Luschka) or a **median aperture** (foramen of Magendie) in the fourth ventricle.

Blood Supply to the Brain

Arteries supplying the brain arise largely from the following two pairs of arteries (Fig. 8-11 and Table 8-3):

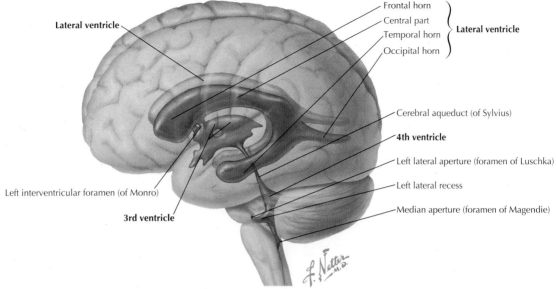

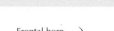

FIGURE 8-10 Ventricular System of the Brain. (From *Atlas of human anatomy,* ed 6, Plate 109.)

Clinical Focus 8-6

Subarachnoid Hemorrhage

Subarachnoid hemorrhage usually occurs from an arterial source and results in the collection of blood between the arachnoid and pia mater. The most common cause of subarachnoid hemorrhage is the rupture of a saccular, or berry, aneurysm.

Distribution of cerebral aneurysms

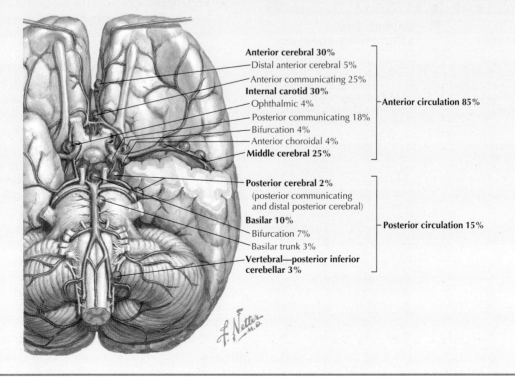

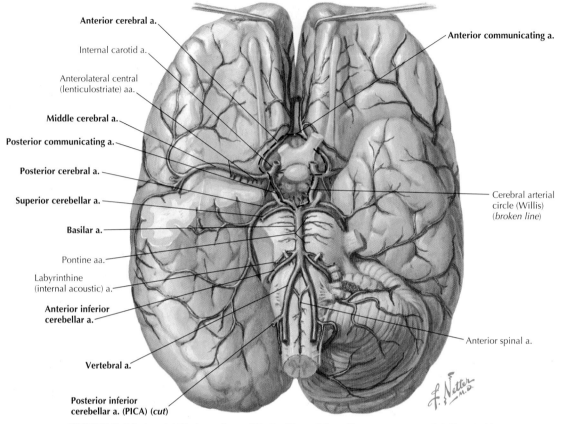

Anterior cerebral a.

Internal carotid a.

Anterolateral central
(lenticulostriate) aa.

Middle cerebral a.

Posterior communicating a.

Posterior cerebral a.

Superior cerebellar a.

Basilar a.

Pontine aa.

Labyrinthine
(internal acoustic) a.

**Anterior inferior
cerebellar a.**

Vertebral a.

**Posterior inferior
cerebellar a. (PICA)** (*cut*)

Anterior communicating a.

Cerebral arterial
circle (Willis)
(*broken line*)

Anterior spinal a.

FIGURE 8-11 Arterial Circle on Base of Brain. (From *Atlas of human anatomy,* ed 6, Plate 140.)

TABLE 8-3 Blood Supply to the Brain

ARTERY	COURSE AND STRUCTURES SUPPLIED
Vertebral	From subclavian artery; supplies cerebellum
Posterior inferior cerebellar	From vertebral artery; supplies the posteroinferior cerebellum
Basilar	From both vertebrals; supplies brainstem, cerebellum, and cerebrum
Anterior inferior cerebellar	From basilar; supplies inferior cerebellum
Superior cerebellar	From basilar; supplies superior cerebellum
Posterior cerebral	From basilar; supplies inferior cerebrum and occipital lobe
Posterior communicating	Cerebral arterial circle (of Willis)
Internal carotid (IC)	From common carotid; supplies cerebral lobes and eye
Middle cerebral	From IC; supplies lateral aspect of cerebral hemispheres
Anterior communicating	Cerebral arterial circle (of Willis)
Anterior cerebral	From IC; supplies cerebral hemispheres (except occipital lobe)

- **Vertebrals:** arise from the subclavian artery, ascend through the transverse foramina of the C1-C6 vertebrae, and enter the foramen magnum of the skull.
- **Internal carotids:** arise from the common carotid in the neck, ascend in the neck, enter the carotid canal, and traverse the foramen lacerum to terminate as the middle and anterior cerebral arteries, which anastomose with the **arterial circle of Willis.**

The **vertebral arteries** give rise to the anterior and posterior spinal arteries (a portion of the supply to the spinal cord) and the posterior inferior cerebellar arteries, and then join at about the level of the junction between the medulla and pons to form the **basilar artery** (Fig. 8-11). The **internal carotid arteries** each give rise to an ophthalmic artery, a posterior communicating artery, a middle cerebral artery, and an anterior cerebral artery. Table 8-3 summarizes the brain regions supplied by these vessels and their major branches.

Text continued on p. 433.

Epidural Hematomas

Epidural hematomas result most often from motor vehicle crashes, falls, and sports injuries. The blood collects between the periosteal dura and bony cranium. The source of the bleeding is usually arterial (85%); common locations include the frontal, temporal (middle meningeal artery is very susceptible, especially where it lies deep to the pterion), and occipital regions.

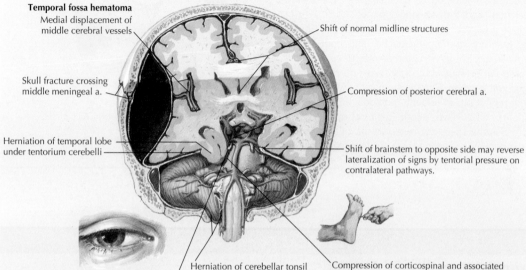

Temporal fossa hematoma
Medial displacement of middle cerebral vessels

Shift of normal midline structures

Skull fracture crossing middle meningeal a.

Compression of posterior cerebral a.

Herniation of temporal lobe under tentorium cerebelli

Shift of brainstem to opposite side may reverse lateralization of signs by tentorial pressure on contralateral pathways.

Herniation of cerebellar tonsil

Compression of corticospinal and associated pathways, resulting in contralateral hemiparesis, deep tendon hyperreflexia, and Babinski's sign

Compression of oculomotor (III) n. leading to ipsilateral pupil dilatation and 3rd cranial n. muscle palsy

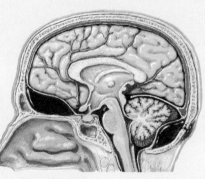

Posterior fossa hematoma
Occipital trauma and/or fracture: headache, meningismus, cerebellar and cranial n. signs, Cushing's triad

Subfrontal hematoma
Frontal trauma: headache, poor cerebration, intermittent disorientation, anisocoria

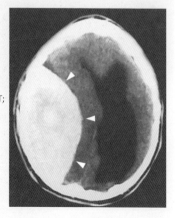

Epidural hematoma (*arrowheads*) as seen in an axial CT; note the mass effect of the hematoma and the midline shift of the brain with dilated ventricles. *(From Major NM: A practical approach to radiology, Philadelphia, Saunders, 2006.)*

Clinical Focus 8-8

Subdural Hematomas

Subdural hematomas are usually caused by an acute venous hemorrhage of the cortical bridging veins draining cortical blood into the superior sagittal sinus. Half are associated with skull fractures. In a subdural hematoma the blood collects between the meningeal dura and the arachnoid mater. Clinical signs include a decreasing level of consciousness, ipsilateral pupillary dilation, headache, and contralateral hemiparesis. These hematomas may develop within 1 week after injury but often present with clinical signs within hours. Chronic subdural hematomas are most common in elderly persons and alcoholic patients who have some brain atrophy, which increases the space traversed by the bridging veins and renders the stretched vein susceptible to tearing.

Burst

Section showing acute subdural hematoma on right side and subdural hematoma associated with temporal lobe intracerebral hematoma ("burst" temporal lobe) on left

Clinical Focus 8-9

Transient Ischemic Attack

A transient ischemic attack is a temporary interruption of focal brain circulation that results in a neurologic deficit that lasts less than 24 hours, usually 15 minutes to 1 hour. The most common cause of TIA is embolic disease from the heart, carotid, or cerebral vessels, which may temporarily block a vessel. The onset of the deficit is abrupt, and recovery is gradual. The most common deficits include the following:

- Hemiparesis
- Hemisensory loss
- Aphasia
- Confusion
- Hemianopia
- Ataxia
- Vertigo

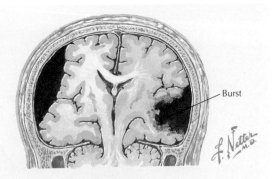

Atheroma with or without clot at bifurcation of internal carotid artery into anterior and middle cerebral arteries

At siphon within cavernous sinus

Dissection of internal carotid artery

Atheroma with or without clot at bifurcation of common carotid artery (most common)

At origin of common carotid artery (uncommon)

Potential sites for emboli in TIA

Clinical Focus 8-10

Stroke

Cerebrovascular accident (CVA) or stroke is a localized brain injury caused by a vascular episode that lasts more than 24 hours, whereas a transient ischemic attack (TIA) is a focal ischemic episode lasting less than 24 hours. Stroke is classified into the following two types:

- **Ischemic** (80%): infarction; thrombotic or embolic, resulting from atherosclerosis of the extracranial (usually carotid) and intracranial arteries or from underlying heart disease.
- **Hemorrhagic:** occurs when a cerebral vessel weakens and ruptures (subarachnoid or intracerebral hemorrhage), which causes intracranial bleeding, usually affecting a larger brain area.

Ischemic Stroke

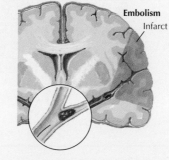

Embolism
Infarct

Clot fragment carried from heart
or more proximal a.

Thrombosis
Infarct

Clot in carotid a. extends directly to
middle cerebral a.

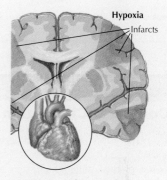

Hypoxia
Infarcts

Hypotension and poor cerebral
perfusion: border zone infarcts, no
vascular occlusion

Hemorrhagic Stroke

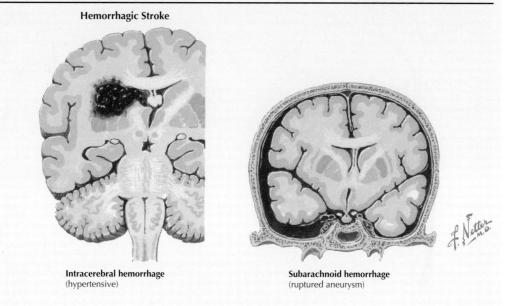

Intracerebral hemorrhage
(hypertensive)

Subarachnoid hemorrhage
(ruptured aneurysm)

Carotid–Cavernous Sinus Fistula

More common than symptomatic intracavernous sinus aneurysms but less common than subarachnoid saccular (berry) aneurysms, carotid–cavernous sinus fistulas often result from trauma and are more common in men. These high-pressure (arterial) low-flow lesions are characterized by an orbital bruit, exophthalmos, chemosis, and extra-ocular muscle palsy involving CN III, IV, and VI. Blood collecting in the cavernous sinus drains by several venous pathways because the sinus has connections with other dural venous sinuses as well as with the ophthalmic veins and pterygoid plexus of veins in the infratemporal region.

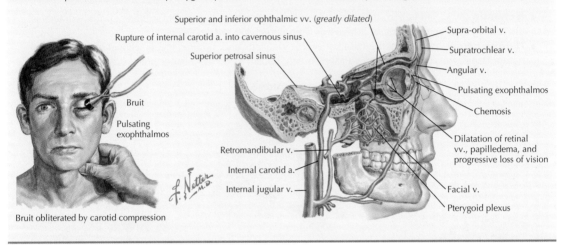

Collateral Circulation after Internal Carotid Artery Occlusion

If a major artery such as the internal carotid becomes occluded, extracranial and intracranial (circle of Willis) anastomoses may provide collateral routes of circulation. These routes are more likely to develop when occlusion is gradual, as in atherosclerosis, rather than acute, as in embolic obstruction.

Reversal of flow through ophthalmic artery

Via circle of Willis

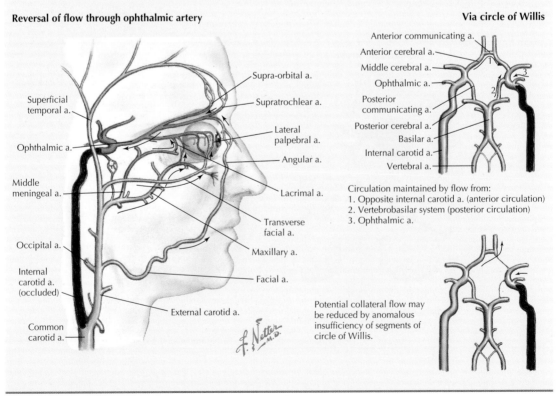

Clinical Focus 8-13

Vascular (Multi-infarct) Dementia

Dementia is an acquired neurologic syndrome that presents with multiple cognitive deficits. By definition, dementia includes short-term memory impairment, behavioral disturbance, and/or difficulties with daily functioning and independence. Dementia can be classified as degenerative, vascular, alcoholic, or human immunodeficiency virus (HIV) related. Vascular dementias are caused by anoxic damage from small infarcts and account for about 15% to 20% of dementia cases. Multi-infarct dementia is associated with heart disease, diabetes mellitus, hypertension, and inflammatory diseases.

Clinical characteristics

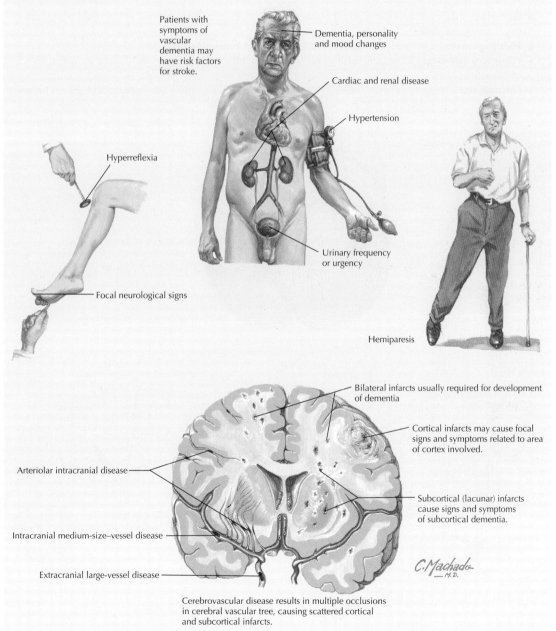

Patients with symptoms of vascular dementia may have risk factors for stroke.

Dementia, personality and mood changes

Cardiac and renal disease

Hypertension

Hyperreflexia

Urinary frequency or urgency

Focal neurological signs

Hemiparesis

Bilateral infarcts usually required for development of dementia

Cortical infarcts may cause focal signs and symptoms related to area of cortex involved.

Arteriolar intracranial disease

Subcortical (lacunar) infarcts cause signs and symptoms of subcortical dementia.

Intracranial medium-size–vessel disease

Extracranial large-vessel disease

Cerebrovascular disease results in multiple occlusions in cerebral vascular tree, causing scattered cortical and subcortical infarcts.

Clinical Focus 8-14

Brain Tumors

Clinical signs and symptoms of brain tumors depend on the location and the degree to which intracranial pressure (ICP) is elevated. Slow-growing tumors in relatively silent areas (e.g., frontal lobes) may go undetected and can become quite large before symptoms occur. Small tumors in key brain areas can lead to seizures, hemiparesis, or aphasia. Increased ICP can initiate broader damage by compressing critical brain structures. Early symptoms of increased ICP include malaise, headache, nausea, papilledema, and less often abducent nerve palsy and Parinaud's syndrome. Classic signs of hydrocephalus are loss of upward gaze, downward ocular deviation ("setting sun" syndrome), lid retraction, and light-near dissociation of pupils. Primary tumors include the following:

- **Gliomas:** arise from astrocytes or oligodendrocytes; glioblastoma multiforme is the most malignant form (astrocytic series).
- **Meningiomas:** arise from the arachnoid mater and can extend into the brain.
- **Pituitary tumors:** can expand in the sella turcica and affect CN II, III, IV, V_1, V_2, and VI; about 15% of primary tumors.
- **Neuromas:** acoustic neuroma, a benign tumor of CN VIII, is a common example; about 7% of primary tumors.

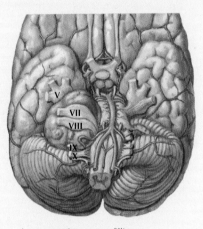

Large acoustic neuroma filling
cerebellopontine angle, distorting
brainstem and cranial nerves
V, VII, VIII, IX, X

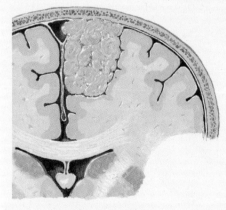

Meningioma invading superior sagittal sinus

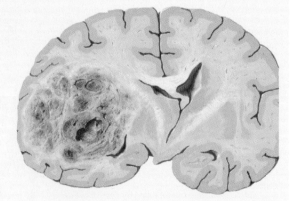

Large, hemispheric glioblastoma multiforme
with central areas of necrosis. Brain distorted
to opposite side.

Clinical Focus 8-15

Metastatic Brain Tumors

Metastatic brain tumors are more common than primary brain tumors. Most spread via the bloodstream, with cells seeded between the white matter (fiber tract pathways) and gray matter (cortical neurons). Some tumors metastasize directly from head and neck cancers or through Batson's vertebral venous plexus. Presentation often includes headache (50%), seizures (25%), and elevated intracranial pressure.

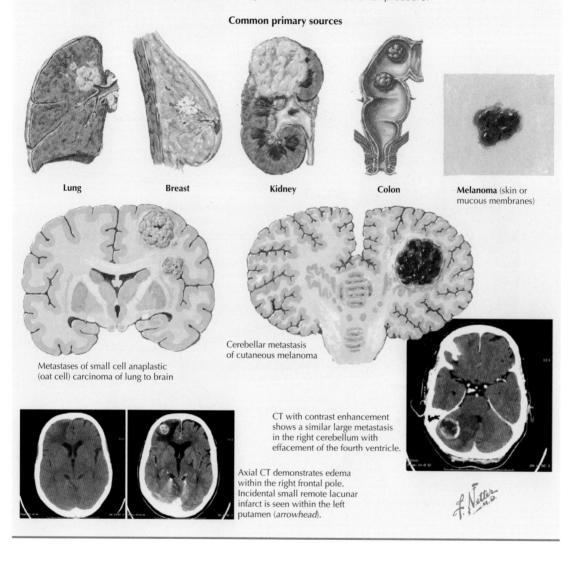

Common primary sources

Lung   Breast   Kidney   Colon   Melanoma (skin or
                                                                                                    mucous membranes)

Metastases of small cell anaplastic
(oat cell) carcinoma of lung to brain

Cerebellar metastasis
of cutaneous melanoma

CT with contrast enhancement
shows a similar large metastasis
in the right cerebellum with
effacement of the fourth ventricle.

Axial CT demonstrates edema
within the right frontal pole.
Incidental small remote lacunar
infarct is seen within the left
putamen (*arrowhead*).

Cranial Nerves

See Chapter 1 for an overview of the general organization of the nervous system.

In addition to the 31 pairs of spinal nerves, 12 pairs of cranial nerves arise from the brain. As with the spinal nerves, cranial nerves are part of the peripheral nervous system and are identified both by name and by Roman numerals I to XII (Fig. 8-12). Cranial nerves are somewhat unique and may contain the following multiple functional components:

- **General (G):** same general functions as spinal nerves.

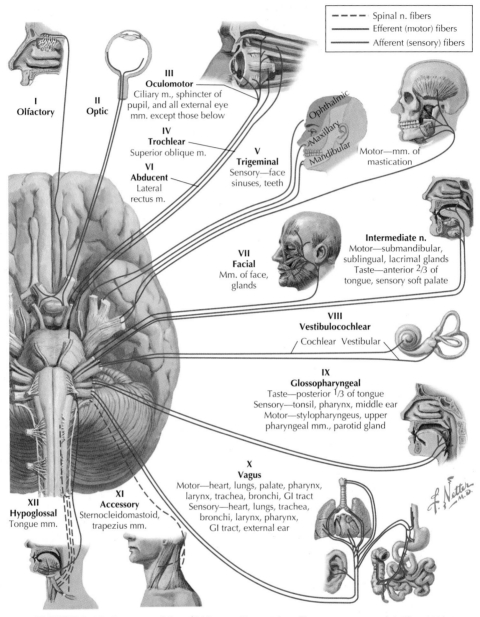

-----	Spinal n. fibers
———	Efferent (motor) fibers
———	Afferent (sensory) fibers

I Olfactory

II Optic

III Oculomotor
Ciliary m., sphincter of pupil, and all external eye mm. except those below

IV Trochlear
Superior oblique m.

VI Abducent
Lateral rectus m.

V Trigeminal
Sensory—face sinuses, teeth

Ophthalmic
Maxillary
Mandibular

Motor—mm. of mastication

Intermediate n.
Motor—submandibular, sublingual, lacrimal glands
Taste—anterior 2/3 of tongue, sensory soft palate

VII Facial
Mm. of face, glands

VIII Vestibulocochlear
Cochlear   Vestibular

IX Glossopharyngeal
Taste—posterior 1/3 of tongue
Sensory—tonsil, pharynx, middle ear
Motor—stylopharyngeus, upper pharyngeal mm., parotid gland

X Vagus
Motor—heart, lungs, palate, pharynx, larynx, trachea, bronchi, GI tract
Sensory—heart, lungs, trachea, bronchi, larynx, pharynx, GI tract, external ear

XII Hypoglossal
Tongue mm.

XI Accessory
Sternocleidomastoid, trapezius mm.

FIGURE 8-12 Overview of Cranial Nerves. (From *Atlas of human anatomy,* ed 6, Plate 119.)

- **Special (S):** functions found only in cranial nerves (special senses).
- **Afferent (A)** or **efferent (E):** sensory or motor functions, respectively.
- **Somatic (S)** or **visceral (V):** related to skin and skeletal muscle innervation (**somatic**), or to smooth muscle, cardiac muscle, and glands (**visceral**).

By convention, each cranial nerve is classified as either general (G) or special (S), and then somatic (S) or visceral (V), and finally as afferent (A) or efferent (E). For example, a cranial nerve that is classified GVE (general visceral efferent) means it contains motor fibers to visceral structures, such as a parasympathetic or sympathetic fiber from the spinal cord.

In general, cranial nerves are described as follows (Table 8-4):

- **CN I** and **II:** arise from the forebrain; are really *tracts* of the brain for the special senses of smell and sight; they are brain extensions surrounded by all three meningeal

TABLE 8-4 Functional Components of the Cranial Nerves

CRANIAL NERVE	FUNCTIONAL COMPONENT
I Olfactory nerve	SSA (Special sense of smell)
II Optic nerve	SSA (Special sense of sight)
III Oculomotor nerve	GSE (Motor to extra-ocular muscles)
	GVE (Parasympathetic to smooth muscle in eye)
IV Trochlear nerve	GSE (Motor to one extra-ocular muscle)
V Trigeminal nerve	GSA (Sensory to face, orbit, nose, and anterior tongue)
	SVE (Motor to skeletal muscles)
VI Abducent nerve	GSE (Motor to one extra-ocular muscle)
VII Facial nerve	GSA (Sensory to skin of ear)
	SVA (Special sense of taste to anterior tongue)
	GVE (Motor to salivary, nasal, and lacrimal glands)
	SVE (Motor to facial muscles)
VIII Vestibulocochlear nerve	SSA (Special sense of hearing and balance)
IX Glossopharyngeal nerve	GSA (Sensory to posterior tongue)
	SVA (Special sense of taste—posterior tongue)
	GVA (Sensory from middle ear, pharynx, carotid body, and sinus)
	GVE (Motor to parotid gland)
	SVE (Motor to one muscle of pharynx)
X Vagus nerve	GSA (Sensory external ear)
	SVA (Special sense of taste—epiglottis)
	GVA (Sensory from pharynx, larynx, and thoracic and abdominal organs)
	GVE (Motor to thoracic and abdominal organs)
	SVE (Motor to muscles of pharynx/larynx)
XI Accessory nerve	GSE (Motor to two muscles)
XII Hypoglossal nerve	GSE (Motor to tongue muscles)

coverings, with CSF in the subarachnoid space—but still are classified as cranial nerves.

- **CN III, IV,** and **VI:** move the extra-ocular skeletal muscles of the eyeball.
- **CN V:** has three divisions; V_1 and V_2 are sensory, and V_3 is both motor and sensory.
- **CN VII, IX,** and **X:** are both motor and sensory.
- **CN VIII:** is the special sense of hearing and balance, but unlike CN I and II, is not a brain tract.

- **CN XI** and **XII:** are motor to skeletal muscle.
- **CN III, VII, IX,** and **X:** also contain parasympathetic (visceral) fibers of origin, although many of these autonomic fibers "jump" onto branches of CN V to reach their targets, because the branches of CN V pass almost everywhere in the head.

Rather than describe each cranial nerve and all its branches in detail at this time, we will review each nerve anatomically and clinically as we encounter it in the various regions of the head and neck. It may be helpful to refer back to this section each time you are introduced to a new region and its cranial nerve innervation. Autonomic components of the cranial nerves and their autonomic ganglia are summarized in Figure 1-25; the more complex cranial nerves also are summarized at the end of this chapter.

5. SCALP AND FACE

Layers of the Scalp

The layers of the **SCALP** include the following:

- **S**kin
- **C**onnective tissue that contains the blood vessels of the scalp
- **A**poneurosis (galea aponeurotica) of the epicranial muscles (frontalis and occipitalis)
- **L**oose connective tissue deep to the aponeurosis, which contains emissary veins that communicate with the cranial diploë and dural sinuses within the cranium
- **P**eriosteum (pericranium) on the surface of the bony skull

The loose connective tissue layer allows the skin to move over the skull when one rubs the head and also allows infections to spread through this layer. Small emissary veins communicate with this layer and can pass infections intracranially.

Muscles of Facial Expression

The muscles of facial expression are skeletal muscles that lie in the subcutaneous tissue of the face. They are all innervated by the terminal motor branches of the facial nerve (CN VII), and most originate from the underlying facial skeleton but insert into the skin or facial cartilages (Fig. 8-13). Table 8-5 summarizes several of the major facial muscles, which are derived from the second branchial arch (see Embryology).

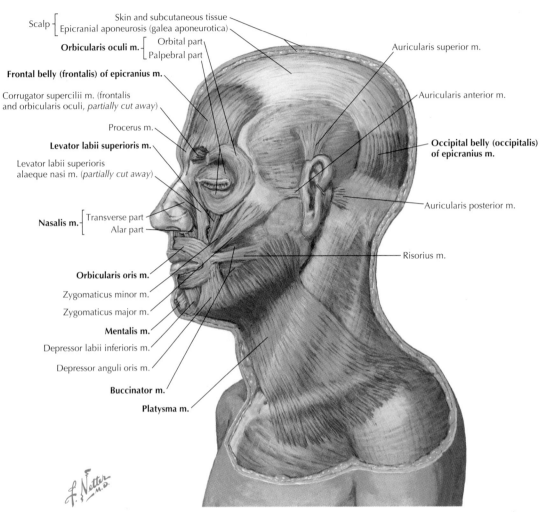

Scalp [Skin and subcutaneous tissue
Epicranial aponeurosis (galea aponeurotica)

Orbicularis oculi m. [Orbital part
Palpebral part

Frontal belly (frontalis) of epicranius m.

Corrugator supercilii m. (frontalis and orbicularis oculi, *partially cut away*)

Procerus m.

Levator labii superioris m.

Levator labii superioris alaeque nasi m. (*partially cut away*)

Nasalis m. [Transverse part
Alar part

Orbicularis oris m.

Zygomaticus minor m.

Zygomaticus major m.

Mentalis m.

Depressor labii inferioris m.

Depressor anguli oris m.

Buccinator m.

Platysma m.

Auricularis superior m.

Auricularis anterior m.

Occipital belly (occipitalis) of epicranius m.

Auricularis posterior m.

Risorius m.

FIGURE 8-13 Muscles of Facial Expression. (From *Atlas of human anatomy,* ed 6, Plate 25.)

TABLE 8-5 Summary of Major Facial Muscles

MUSCLE	ORIGIN	INSERTION	MAIN ACTIONS
Frontalis	Skin of forehead	Epicranial aponeurosis	Elevates eyebrows and forehead; wrinkles forehead
Orbicularis oculi	Medial orbital margin, medial palpebral ligament, and lacrimal bone	Skin around margin of orbit; tarsal plate	Closes eyelids; orbital part forcefully and palpebral part for blinking
Nasalis	Superior part of canine ridge of maxilla	Nasal cartilages	Draws ala of nose toward septum to compress opening
Orbicularis oris	Median plane of maxilla superiorly and mandible inferiorly; other fibers from deep surface of skin	Mucous membrane of lips	Closes and protrudes lips (e.g., purses them during whistling)
Levator labii superioris	Frontal process of maxilla and infra-orbital region	Skin of upper lip and alar cartilage	Elevates lip, dilates nostril, raises angle of mouth
Platysma	Superficial fascia of deltoid and pectoral regions	Mandible, skin of cheek, angle of mouth, and orbicularis oris	Depresses mandible and tenses skin of lower face and neck
Mentalis	Incisive fossa of mandible	Skin of chin	Elevates and protrudes lower lip and wrinkles chin
Buccinator	Mandible, pterygomandibular raphe, and alveolar processes of maxilla and mandible	Angle of mouth	Presses cheek against molar teeth, thereby aiding chewing

Innervation of the facial muscles is by the five terminal branches of CN VII. The facial nerve enters the internal acoustic meatus, passes through the facial canal in the petrous portion of the temporal bone, and then descends to emerge from the stylomastoid foramen. CN VII then passes through the parotid salivary gland and distributes over the face and neck (Fig. 8-14). The five terminal motor (branchial motor) branches are as follows:

- **Temporal**
- **Zygomatic**
- **Buccal**
- **Marginal mandibular**
- **Cervical**

The sensory innervation of the face is by the **three divisions of the trigeminal nerve** (CN V), with some contributions by the cervical plexus. Figure 8-15 lists the specific nerves for each

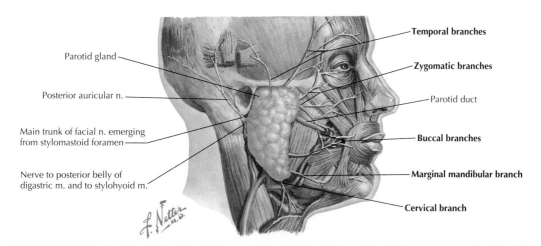

FIGURE 8-14 Terminal Branches of Facial Nerve and Parotid Gland. (From *Atlas of human anatomy*, ed 6, Plate 24.)

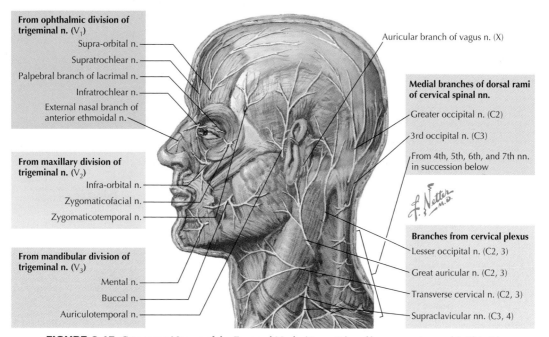

FIGURE 8-15 Cutaneous Nerves of the Face and Neck. (From *Atlas of human anatomy*, ed 6, Plate 2.)

Clinical Focus 8-16

Trigeminal Neuralgia

Trigeminal neuralgia (or tic douloureux) is a neurologic condition characterized by episodes of brief, intense facial pain over one of the three areas of distribution of CN V. The pain is so intense that the patient winces, which produces a facial muscle tic.

Zones of skin innervation of trigeminal nerve divisions, where pain may occur in trigeminal neuralgia

Ophthalmic n. zone

Maxillary n. zone

Common trigger points

Mandibular n. zone

Characteristic	Description
Etiology	Uncertain; possibly vascular compression of trigeminal sensory ganglion by superior cerebellar artery
Presentation	Recurrent, lancinating, burning pain, usually affecting V_2 or V_3 unilaterally (<6% involve V_1), usually in a person older than 50 years
Triggers	Touch; draft of cool air

Clinical Focus 8-17

Herpes Zoster (Shingles)

Herpes zoster, or shingles, is the most common infection of the peripheral nervous system (PNS). It is an acute neuralgia confined to the dermatome distribution of a specific spinal or cranial sensory nerve root.

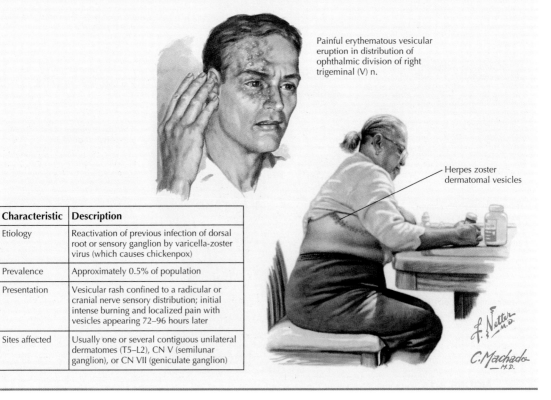

Painful erythematous vesicular eruption in distribution of ophthalmic division of right trigeminal (V) n.

Herpes zoster dermatomal vesicles

Characteristic	Description
Etiology	Reactivation of previous infection of dorsal root or sensory ganglion by varicella-zoster virus (which causes chickenpox)
Prevalence	Approximately 0.5% of population
Presentation	Vesicular rash confined to a radicular or cranial nerve sensory distribution; initial intense burning and localized pain with vesicles appearing 72–96 hours later
Sites affected	Usually one or several contiguous unilateral dermatomes (T5–L2), CN V (semilunar ganglion), or CN VII (geniculate ganglion)

Clinical Focus 8-18

Facial Nerve (Bell's) Palsy

Acute, unilateral idiopathic facial palsy is the most common cause of facial muscle weakness and cranial neuropathy. Facial nerve palsy also may be caused by herpes simplex virus (HSV) infection. Manifestations associated with lesions at various points along the path of CN VII are illustrated.

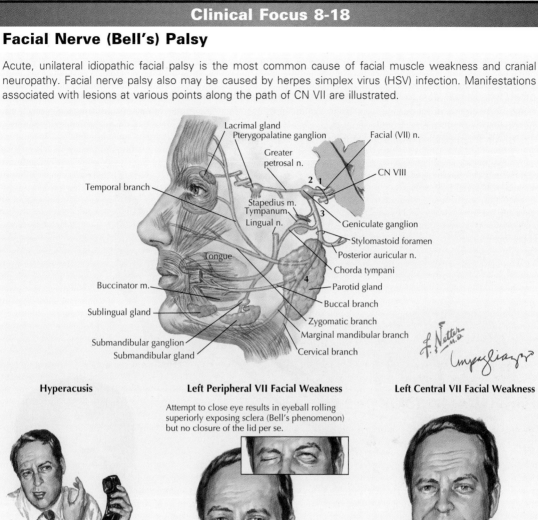

Hyperacusis

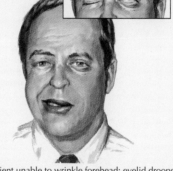

This may be early or initial symptom of a peripheral VII nerve palsy: patient holds phone away from ear because of painful sensitivity to sound. Loss of taste also may occur on affected side.

Left Peripheral VII Facial Weakness

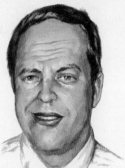

Attempt to close eye results in eyeball rolling superiorly exposing sclera (Bell's phenomenon) but no closure of the lid per se.

Patient unable to wrinkle forehead; eyelid droops very slightly; cannot show teeth at all on affected side in attempt to smile; and lower lip droops slightly.

Left Central VII Facial Weakness

Incomplete smile with very subtle flattening of affected nasolabial fold; relative preservation of brow and forehead movement.

Sites of lesions and their manifestations (sites numbered in top image)

1. Intracranial and/or internal auditory meatus
All symptoms of 2, 3, and 4, plus deafness due to involvement of eighth cranial nerve.

2. Geniculate ganglion
All symptoms of 3 and 4, plus pain behind ear. Herpes of tympanum and of external auditory meatus may occur.

3. Facial canal
All symptoms of 4, plus loss of taste in anterior tongue and decreased salivation on affected side due to chorda tympani involvement. Hyperacusis due to effect on nerve branch to stapedius muscle.

4. Below stylomastoid foramen (parotid gland tumor, trauma)
Facial paralysis (mouth draws to opposite side; on affected side, patient unable to close eye or wrinkle forehead; food collects between teeth and cheek due to paralysis of buccinator muscle).

Tetanus

The PNS motor unit is vulnerable to three bacteria-produced toxins: tetanospasmin (motor neuron), diphtheria toxin (peripheral nerve), and botulin (neuromuscular junction). The hearty spore of *Clostridium tetani* is commonly found in soil, dust, and feces and can enter the body through wounds, blisters, burns, skin ulcers, insect bites, and surgical procedures. Symptoms include restlessness, low-grade fever, and stiffness or soreness. Eventually, nuchal rigidity, trismus (lockjaw), dysphagia, laryngospasm, and acute, massive muscle spasms can occur. Prophylaxis (immunization) is the best management.

Organisms enter through large, small, or even unrecognized wound. Deep, infected punctures are most susceptible, because organisms thrive best anaerobically.

Toxin produced locally passes via bloodstream or along nerves to CNS.

Spasm of jaw, facial, and neck muscles (trismus [lockjaw], risus sardonicus) and dysphagia are often early symptoms.

Motor neurons of spinal cord (anterior horn) and of brainstem become hyperactive because toxin specifically attacks inhibitory (Renshaw) cells.

Complete tetanic spasm in advanced disease. Patient rigid in moderate opisthotonos, with arms extended, abdomen boardlike. Respiratory arrest may occur.

division. All the sensory neurons in CN V reside in the **trigeminal (semilunar, gasserian) ganglion.** The trigeminal nerve is divided as follows:

- **Ophthalmic (V₁) division:** exits the skull via the superior orbital fissure.
- **Maxillary (V₂) division:** exits the skull via the foramen rotundum.
- **Mandibular (V₃) division:** exits the skull via the foramen ovale.

The blood supply to the face includes the following vessels (Fig. 8-16):

- **Facial artery:** arises from the external carotid artery.
- **Superficial temporal artery:** one of the terminal branches of the external carotid artery.
- **Ophthalmic artery**: arises from the internal carotid artery and distributes over the forehead.
- **Facial vein:** drains into the internal jugular vein, directly or as a common facial vein.

- **Retromandibular vein:** formed by the union of the maxillary and superficial temporal veins; ultimately drains into the external and/or the internal jugular vein.
- **Ophthalmic veins:** tributaries from the forehead drain into superior and inferior ophthalmic veins in the orbit (and also anastomose with the facial vein) and then posteriorly into the cavernous dural sinus and/or the pterygoid plexus of veins in the infratemporal region (see Fig. 8-28).

6. ORBIT AND EYE

Bony Orbit

The bones contributing to the orbit include the following (Fig. 8-17):

- **Frontal** (orbital surface)
- **Maxilla** (orbital surface)
- **Zygomatic** (orbital surface)
- **Sphenoid**

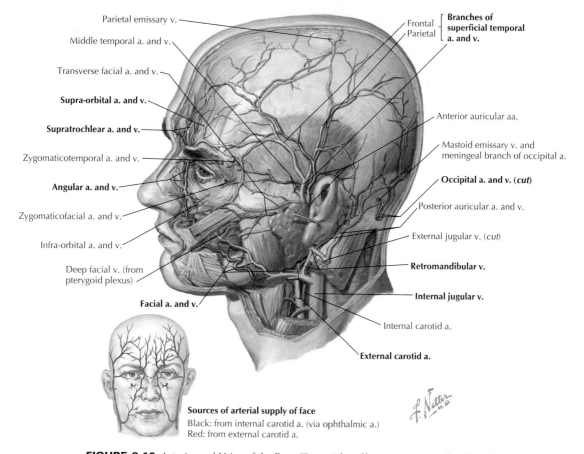

FIGURE 8-16 Arteries and Veins of the Face. (From *Atlas of human anatomy*, ed 6, Plate 3.)

Parietal emissary v.
Middle temporal a. and v.
Transverse facial a. and v.
Supra-orbital a. and v.
Supratrochlear a. and v.
Zygomaticotemporal a. and v.
Angular a. and v.
Zygomaticofacial a. and v.
Infra-orbital a. and v.
Deep facial v. (from pterygoid plexus)
Facial a. and v.

Frontal
Parietal — Branches of superficial temporal a. and v.
Anterior auricular aa.
Mastoid emissary v. and meningeal branch of occipital a.
Occipital a. and v. (*cut*)
Posterior auricular a. and v.
External jugular v. (*cut*)
Retromandibular v.
Internal jugular v.
Internal carotid a.
External carotid a.

Sources of arterial supply of face
Black: from internal carotid a. (via ophthalmic a.)
Red: from external carotid a.

Right orbit: frontal and slightly lateral view

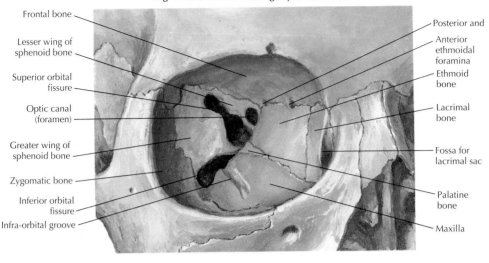

Frontal bone

Lesser wing of
sphenoid bone

Superior orbital
fissure

Optic canal
(foramen)

Greater wing of
sphenoid bone

Zygomatic bone

Inferior orbital
fissure

Infra-orbital groove

Posterior and

Anterior
ethmoidal
foramina

Ethmoid
bone

Lacrimal
bone

Fossa for
lacrimal sac

Palatine
bone

Maxilla

Muscle attachments and nerves and vessels entering right orbit

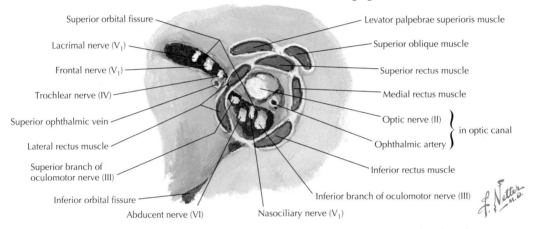

Superior orbital fissure

Lacrimal nerve (V₁)

Frontal nerve (V₁)

Trochlear nerve (IV)

Superior ophthalmic vein

Lateral rectus muscle

Superior branch of
oculomotor nerve (III)

Inferior orbital fissure

Abducent nerve (VI)

Nasociliary nerve (V₁)

Levator palpebrae superioris muscle

Superior oblique muscle

Superior rectus muscle

Medial rectus muscle

Optic nerve (II)

Ophthalmic artery

Inferior rectus muscle

Inferior branch of oculomotor nerve (III)

in optic canal

FIGURE 8-17 Bony Orbit and Its Openings. (From *Atlas of human anatomy*, ed 6, Plate 4.)

- **Palatine** (orbital plate)
- **Ethmoid** (orbital plate)
- **Lacrimal**

The back of the orbit has three large openings that include the following:

- **Superior orbital fissure:** CN III, IV, VI, and V₁ (frontal, lacrimal, and nasociliary nerves) pass through the fissure along with the ophthalmic vein.
- **Inferior orbital fissure:** CN V₂ and infra-orbital vessels pass through this fissure.
- **Optic canal:** CN II and the ophthalmic artery pass through this canal.

The periosteum of the orbital bones is a distinct layer of connective tissue called the **periorbita.** It is continuous with the pericranium (periosteum) covering the skull and, where the orbit communicates with the cranial cavity (e.g., superior orbital fissure), the periorbita is continuous with the periosteal layer of the dura mater.

Eyelids and Lacrimal Apparatus

The eyelids protect the eyeballs and keep the corneas moist. Each eyelid contains a **tarsal plate** of dense connective tissue; **tarsal glands** that secrete an oily mixture into the tears; modified **sebaceous glands** associated with each eyelash; **apocrine glands** (modified sweat glands); **accessory lacrimal glands** along the inner surface of the upper eyelid; and in the superior eyelid only, a small slip of **smooth muscle (superior tarsal**

Clinical Focus 8-20

Orbital Blow-out Fracture

A massive zygomaticomaxillary complex fracture or a direct blow to the front of the orbit (e.g., by baseball or fist) may cause a rapid increase in intraorbital pressure resulting in a blow-out fracture of the thin orbital floor. In severe comminuted fractures of the orbital floor, the orbital soft tissues may herniate into the underlying maxillary paranasal sinus. Clinical signs include diplopia, infra-orbital nerve paresthesia, enophthalmos, edema, and ecchymosis.

Clinical findings

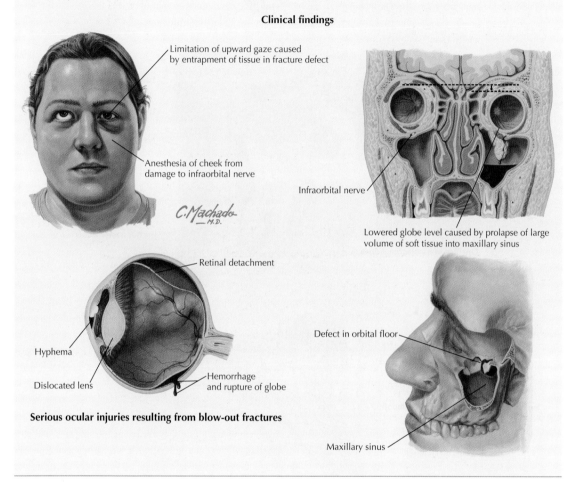

Limitation of upward gaze caused by entrapment of tissue in fracture defect

Anesthesia of cheek from damage to infraorbital nerve

C. Machado —M.D.

Infraorbital nerve

Lowered globe level caused by prolapse of large volume of soft tissue into maxillary sinus

Retinal detachment

Hyphema

Dislocated lens

Hemorrhage and rupture of globe

Defect in orbital floor

Maxillary sinus

Serious ocular injuries resulting from blow-out fractures

[Müller's] muscle), which attaches to the tarsal plate along with the levator palpebrae superioris muscle (Fig. 8-18). The tears contain albumins, lactoferrin, lysozyme, lipids, metabolites, and electrolytes. The lacrimal glands secrete continuously, and as one blinks, the tears are evenly spread across the conjunctiva and cornea. Tears not only keep the eye surface moist but also possess antimicrobial properties. The lacrimal apparatus includes the following:

- **Lacrimal glands:** secrete tears; innervated by the facial nerve parasympathetics

- **Lacrimal ducts:** excretory ducts of the glands
- **Lacrimal canaliculi:** collect tears into openings on the medial aspect of each lid called the puncta, and convey them to the lacrimal sacs
- **Lacrimal sacs:** collect tears and release them into the nasolacrimal duct when one blinks (contraction of the orbicularis oculi muscle)
- **Nasolacrimal ducts:** convey tears from lacrimal sacs to the inferior meatus of the nasal cavity

Superior palpebral conjunctiva:
tarsal (meibomian) glands shining through

Corneoscleral junction (corneal limbus)

Bulbar conjunctiva over sclera

Inferior conjunctival fornix

Inferior palpebral conjunctiva:
tarsal glands shining through

Superior lacrimal papilla and punctum

Plica semilunaris

Lacrimal caruncle in lacrimal lake

Inferior lacrimal papilla and punctum

Frontal bone (*cut away*)

Lacrimal gland

Palpebral part of lacrimal gland

Excretory ducts of lacrimal gland

Plica semilunaris and lacrimal lake

Lacrimal caruncle

Opening of nasolacrimal duct

Lacrimal canaliculi

Lacrimal sac

Nasolacrimal duct

Middle nasal concha

Nasal cavity

Inferior nasal meatus

Inferior nasal concha (*cut*)

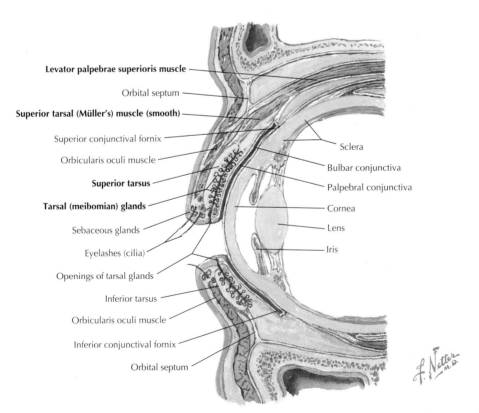

Levator palpebrae superioris muscle

Orbital septum

Superior tarsal (Müller's) muscle (smooth)

Superior conjunctival fornix

Orbicularis oculi muscle

Superior tarsus

Tarsal (meibomian) glands

Sebaceous glands

Eyelashes (cilia)

Openings of tarsal glands

Inferior tarsus

Orbicularis oculi muscle

Inferior conjunctival fornix

Orbital septum

Sclera

Bulbar conjunctiva

Palpebral conjunctiva

Cornea

Lens

Iris

FIGURE 8-18 Eyelids and Lacrimal Apparatus. (From *Atlas of human anatomy,* ed 6, Plates 83 and 84.)

Clinical Focus 8-21

Clinical Testing of the Extra-ocular Muscles

Because extra-ocular muscles act as synergists and antagonists and may be responsible for multiple movements, it is difficult to test each muscle individually. However, the generalist physician can check extra-ocular muscle (or nerve) impairment by assessing the ability of individual muscles to elevate or depress the globe with the eye abducted or adducted, thereby aligning the globe with the *pull* (line of contraction) of the muscle. Generally, intorsion and extorsion are too difficult to assess in a routine eye examination. The examiner can use an H pattern to assess how each eye tracks movement of an object (the tester's finger). For example, when the finger is held up and to the right of the patient's eyes, the patient must primarily use the superior rectus (SR) muscle of the right eye and the inferior oblique (IO) muscle of the left eye to focus on the finger. Pure abduction is done by the lateral rectus, and pure adduction is done by the medial rectus. In all other cases, two muscles elevate the eye (SR and IO, with minimal intorsion or extorsion) and two muscles depress the eye (inferior rectus and superior oblique, with minimal intorsion or extorsion) in abduction and adduction, respectively. At the end of this test, the examiner can bring the finger directly to the midline to test convergence (medial rectus muscles). If an eye movement disorder is detected by this method, a clinical specialist may be consulted for further evaluation.

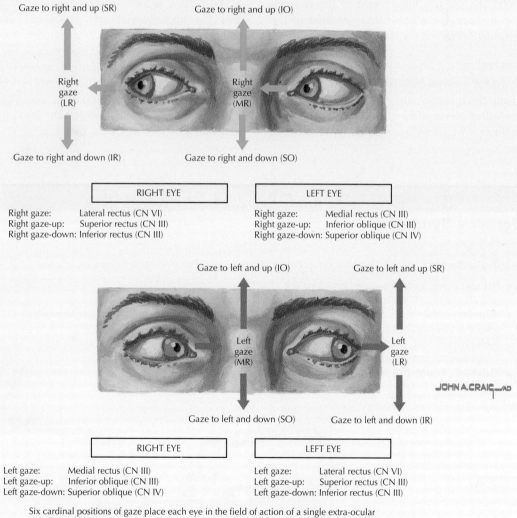

Gaze to right and up (SR) Gaze to right and up (IO)

Right gaze (LR) Right gaze (MR)

Gaze to right and down (IR) Gaze to right and down (SO)

RIGHT EYE

LEFT EYE

Right gaze: Lateral rectus (CN VI)
Right gaze-up: Superior rectus (CN III)
Right gaze-down: Inferior rectus (CN III)

Right gaze: Medial rectus (CN III)
Right gaze-up: Inferior oblique (CN III)
Right gaze-down: Superior oblique (CN IV)

Gaze to left and up (IO) Gaze to left and up (SR)

Left gaze (MR) Left gaze (LR)

Gaze to left and down (SO) Gaze to left and down (IR)

JOHN A.CRAIG—AD

RIGHT EYE

LEFT EYE

Left gaze: Medial rectus (CN III)
Left gaze-up: Inferior oblique (CN III)
Left gaze-down: Superior oblique (CN IV)

Left gaze: Lateral rectus (CN VI)
Left gaze-up: Superior rectus (CN III)
Left gaze-down: Inferior rectus (CN III)

Six cardinal positions of gaze place each eye in the field of action of a single extra-ocular muscle, and allow testing of the action of each muscle and its innervation.

The lacrimal glands receive secretomotor parasympathetic fibers from the facial nerve (CN VII) that originate in the **superior salivatory nucleus.** These preganglionic parasympathetic fibers travel in the greater petrosal nerve and in the nerve of the pterygoid canal (vidian nerve), and the fibers then synapse in the **pterygopalatine ganglion.** Postganglionic parasympathetic fibers travel through the maxillary nerve (V_2), zygomatic nerve, and lacrimal nerve (V_1) to the lacrimal gland (see Fig. 8-70). Postganglionic sympathetic nerves from the superior cervical ganglion (SCG) jump from the internal carotid plexus in the form of the deep petrosal nerve, join the greater petrosal nerve, and form the nerve of the pterygoid canal. These postganglionic sympathetic fibers then follow the same course up to the lacrimal glands. The sensory innervation of the lacrimal gland is through the ophthalmic division of the trigeminal nerve (via the lacrimal branch).

Muscles

The orbital muscles include six extra-ocular skeletal muscles that move the eyeball and one skeletal muscle that elevates the upper eyelid (Fig. 8-19 and Table 8-6). In addition to the movements of elevation, depression, abduction, and adduction, the superior rectus and superior oblique muscles medially rotate (intorsion) the eyeball, and the inferior rectus and inferior oblique muscles laterally rotate (extorsion) the eyeball. The actions of the extra-ocular muscles detailed in Table 8-6 reflect their "anatomical" actions; because of how the muscles insert into the globe, any single action of the eye often involves multiple muscles contracting at the same time. For example, two muscles elevate the eyeball (superior rectus, inferior oblique), and three muscles abduct the eyeball (lateral rectus, superior oblique, inferior oblique). Clinically, one needs to "isolate" the multiple actions of the muscles so that an individual muscle's action can be assessed (e.g., elevation or depression; see Clinical Focus 8-21).

The levator palpebrae superioris muscle elevates the upper eyelid and, from its inferior surface, has a small amount of smooth muscle **(superior tarsal muscle)** connecting it to the tarsal plate. This smooth muscle is innervated by postganglionic sympathetic fibers from the superior cervical ganglion. The interruption of this sympathetic pathway can lead to a moderate ptosis, or drooping, of the upper eyelid.

Clinical Focus 8-22

Horner's Syndrome

Horner's syndrome occurs when there is a lesion somewhere along the pathway of the sympathetic fibers traveling to the head, usually from the sympathetic trunk distally. The cardinal signs are as follows:

- **Ptosis:** drooping of the upper eyelid on the affected side caused by paralysis of the superior tarsal smooth muscle in the free edge of the levator palpebrae superioris muscle.
- **Miosis:** pupillary constriction on the affected side caused by the paralysis of the pupillary dilator smooth muscle in the iris.
- **Anhidrosis:** loss of sweating on the affected side of the head caused by loss of sweat gland innervation by the sympathetic fibers.
- **Flushed, warm dry skin:** vasodilation of the subcutaneous arteries on the affected side caused by a lack of sympathetic vasoconstriction tone and sweat gland innervation.

Interruption of the sympathetic fibers outside the brain causes ipsilateral ptosis, anhidrosis, and miosis without abnormal ocular mobility.

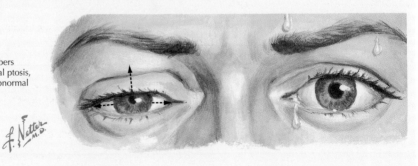

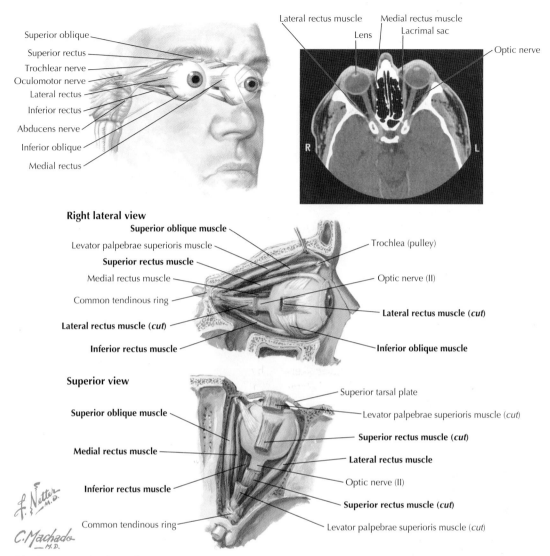

FIGURE 8-19 Orbital Muscles. (From *Atlas of human anatomy,* ed 6, Plate 86; CT image from Kelley LL, Petersen C: *Sectional anatomy for imaging professionals,* Philadelphia, Mosby, 2007.)

TABLE 8-6 Summary of Orbital Muscles

MUSCLE	ORIGIN	INSERTION	INNERVATION	MAIN ACTIONS
Levator palpebrae superioris	Lesser wing of sphenoid bone, anterosuperior optic canal	Tarsal plate and skin of upper eyelid	Oculomotor nerve	Elevates upper eyelid
Superior rectus	Common tendinous ring	Sclera just posterior to cornea	Oculomotor nerve	Elevates, adducts, and rotates eyeball medially
Inferior rectus	Common tendinous ring	Anterior sclera	Oculomotor nerve	Depresses, adducts, and rotates eyeball laterally
Medial rectus	Common tendinous ring	Anterior sclera	Oculomotor nerve	Adducts eyeball
Lateral rectus	Common tendinous ring	Anterior sclera	Abducent nerve	Abducts eyeball
Superior oblique	Body of sphenoid bone	Passes through trochlea and inserts into sclera	Trochlear nerve	Medially rotates, depresses, and abducts eyeball
Inferior oblique	Floor of orbit	Sclera deep to lateral rectus muscle	Oculomotor nerve	Laterally rotates and elevates and abducts eyeball

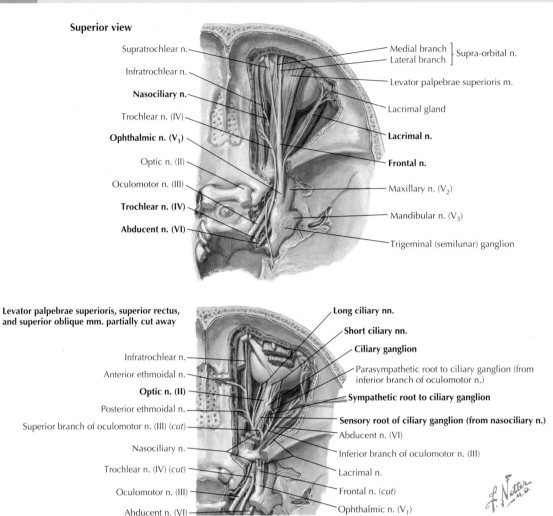

Superior view

Supratrochlear n.

Infratrochlear n.

Nasociliary n.

Trochlear n. (IV)

Ophthalmic n. (V₁)

Optic n. (II)

Oculomotor n. (III)

Trochlear n. (IV)

Abducent n. (VI)

Medial branch ⎫
Lateral branch ⎬ Supra-orbital n.

Levator palpebrae superioris m.

Lacrimal gland

Lacrimal n.

Frontal n.

Maxillary n. (V₂)

Mandibular n. (V₃)

Trigeminal (semilunar) ganglion

Levator palpebrae superioris, superior rectus, and superior oblique mm. partially cut away

Infratrochlear n.

Anterior ethmoidal n.

Optic n. (II)

Posterior ethmoidal n.

Superior branch of oculomotor n. (III) (cut)

Nasociliary n.

Trochlear n. (IV) (cut)

Oculomotor n. (III)

Abducent n. (VI)

Long ciliary nn.

Short ciliary nn.

Ciliary ganglion

Parasympathetic root to ciliary ganglion (from inferior branch of oculomotor n.)

Sympathetic root to ciliary ganglion

Sensory root of ciliary ganglion (from nasociliary n.)

Abducent n. (VI)

Inferior branch of oculomotor n. (III)

Lacrimal n.

Frontal n. (cut)

Ophthalmic n. (V₁)

FIGURE 8-20 Nerves of the Orbit. (From *Atlas of human anatomy,* ed 6, Plate 88.)

TABLE 8-7 Features of the Eyeball

STRUCTURE	DEFINITION	STRUCTURE	DEFINITION
Sclera	Outer fibrous layer of eyeball	Refractive media	Light rays focused by the cornea, aqueous humor, lens, and vitreous humor
Cornea	Transparent part of outer layer; very sensitive to pain		
Choroid	Vascular middle layer of eyeball	Retina	Optically receptive part of optic nerve (optic retina); contains rods (dim light vision) and cones (color vision)
Conjunctiva	Thin membrane that lines the inner aspect of the eyelids and reflects onto the sclera, ending at the scleral-corneal junction		
		Macula lutea	Yellowish region of retina lateral to the optic disc that contains the fovea centralis
Ciliary body	Vascular and muscular extension of choroid anteriorly	Fovea centralis	Area of macula with the most acute vision; contains only cones and is the center of the visual axis (ideal focus point)
Ciliary process	Radiating pigmented ridge on ciliary body; secretes aqueous humor that fills posterior and anterior chambers		
Iris	Contractile diaphragm with central aperture (pupil)	Optic disc	Nonreceptive area (blind spot) where retinal ganglion cell nerve axons leave the retina in the optic nerve and pass to the brain
Lens	Transparent lens supported in capsule by zonular fibers		

Interruption of the innervation of the levator palpebrae superioris from CN III can lead to a significant ptosis.

Nerves in the Orbit

Three cranial nerves innervate the extra-ocular skeletal muscles (Table 8-6), one cranial nerve mediates the special sense of sight (CN II), and one cranial nerve conveys general sensory information from the orbit and eye (CN V_1) (Fig. 8-20). The major branches of the **ophthalmic nerve** (CN V_1) include the following:

- **Frontal:** runs on the superior aspect of the levator palpebrae superioris muscle and ends as the supratrochlear and supra-orbital nerves; sensory to forehead, scalp, frontal sinus, and upper eyelid.
- **Lacrimal:** courses laterally on the superior aspect of the lateral rectus muscle to the lacrimal gland; sensory to conjunctiva and skin of the upper eyelid, and the lacrimal gland.
- **Nasociliary:** gives rise to short and long ciliary nerves, posterior and anterior ethmoidal nerves, and infratrochlear nerve; sensory to iris and cornea, sphenoid and ethmoid sinuses, lower eyelid, lacrimal sac, and skin of the anterior nose.

The **optic nerve** (CN II) is actually a brain tract that conveys sensory information from the retina, via the ganglion cell axons, to the brain (see Fig. 8-12). The optic nerve is covered by the same three dural layers as the rest of the CNS, and the retina is really our "window" into the brain (see Clinical Focus 8-25).

In addition to supplying four of the seven skeletal muscles in the orbit (see Table 8-6), the **oculomotor nerve** (CN III) also provides **parasympathetic** fibers, which exhibit the following features (see Fig. 8-68):

- Parasympathetic fibers arise centrally from the **nucleus of Edinger-Westphal** (preganglionic fibers) and course along CN III and its inferior division to synapse in the **ciliary ganglion** on postganglionic parasympathetic neurons.
- Postganglionic parasympathetic fibers then course via **short ciliary nerves** to the eyeball.
- These postganglionic fibers innervate the **sphincter muscle of the pupil** (sphincter

pupillae) and the **ciliary muscle** for accommodation.

Sympathetic innervation to the eyeball is arranged as follows (see Figs. 8-67 and 8-68):

- Sympathetic innervation arises from the **upper thoracic intermediolateral cell column** of the spinal cord (T1-T2) and sends preganglionic fibers into the sympathetic trunk, where these fibers ascend to synapse in the **superior cervical ganglion** (SCG).
- Postganglionic sympathetic fibers course along the internal carotid artery, enter the orbit on the ophthalmic artery and ophthalmic nerve, and pass through the ciliary ganglion or along the **long and short ciliary nerves** to the eyeball.
- These postganglionic fibers innervate the **dilator muscle of the pupil** (dilator pupillae) and the **superior tarsal muscle** of the upper eyelid.

Eyeball (Globe)

The human eyeball measures about 25 mm in diameter, is tethered in the bony orbit by six extra-ocular muscles that move the globe, and is cushioned by fat that surrounds the posterior two thirds of the globe (Fig. 8-21). The outer fibrous white coat of the eyeball is the **sclera** and is continuous anteriorly with the transparent cornea. A middle vascular layer called the **choroid** is continuous anteriorly with the ciliary body, ciliary process, and iris. The inner layer is the optically receptive **retina** posteriorly and an anterior nonvisual retinal extension that lines the internal surface of the ciliary body and iris (Table 8-7).

The large chamber behind the lens is the **vitreous chamber** (body) and is filled with a gel-like substance called the **vitreous humor,** which helps cushion and protect the fragile retina during rapid eye movements (see Fig. 8-21).

The chamber between the cornea and the iris is the **anterior chamber;** the space between the iris and lens is the **posterior chamber.** Both chambers are filled with **aqueous humor,** which is produced by the ciliary body and circulates from the posterior chamber, through the pupil, and into the anterior chamber, where it is absorbed by the trabecular meshwork into the **scleral venous sinus** (canal of Schlemm) at the angle of the cornea and iris.

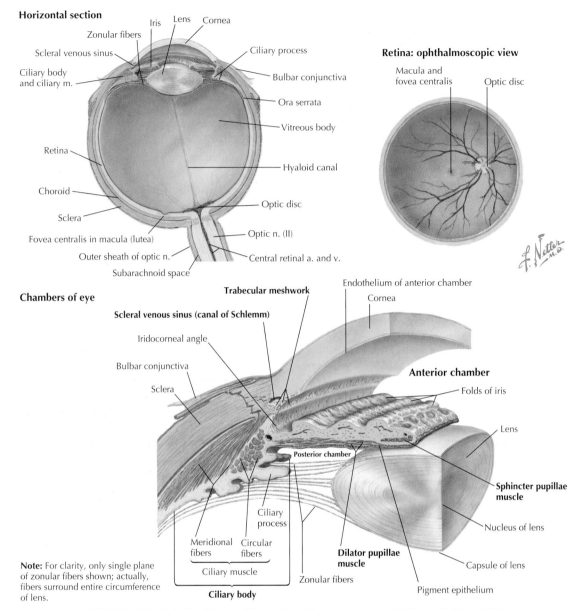

Horizontal section

Iris   Lens   Cornea
Zonular fibers
Scleral venous sinus
Ciliary body
and ciliary m.
Retina
Choroid
Sclera
Fovea centralis in macula (lutea)
Outer sheath of optic n.
Subarachnoid space

Ciliary process
Bulbar conjunctiva
Ora serrata
Vitreous body
Hyaloid canal
Optic disc
Optic n. (II)
Central retinal a. and v.

Retina: ophthalmoscopic view

Macula and
fovea centralis   Optic disc

Chambers of eye

Trabecular meshwork
Scleral venous sinus (canal of Schlemm)
Iridocorneal angle
Bulbar conjunctiva
Sclera

Endothelium of anterior chamber
Cornea

Anterior chamber
Folds of iris
Lens
**Sphincter pupillae
muscle**
Nucleus of lens
Capsule of lens
Pigment epithelium

Posterior chamber

Ciliary
process
Meridional   Circular
fibers   fibers
Ciliary muscle
**Dilator pupillae
muscle**
Zonular fibers

Ciliary body

Note: For clarity, only single plane
of zonular fibers shown; actually,
fibers surround entire circumference
of lens.

FIGURE 8-21 Eyeball and Retina. (From *Atlas of human anatomy,* ed 6, Plates 89, 90, and 92.)

Retina

The retina consists of the optic or **neural retina,** which is sensitive to light, and the **nonvisual retina,** which lines the internal surface of the ciliary body and iris. The junction separating the neural from the nonvisual retina is called the ora serrata (see Fig. 8-21).

The neural retina is composed of an outer **retinal pigmented epithelium** lying adjacent to the vascular choroid and a photosensitive region consisting of photoreceptive cells: **rods** are more sensitive to light and the receptors for low-light conditions (gray tones); **cones** are less sensitive to low light but very sensitive to red, green, and blue regions of the visual spectrum. Interspersed layers of conducting and association neurons and supporting cells lie more internally in the retina, closer to the vitreous body.

The axons of ganglion cells ultimately convey the photosensory information to the **optic disc,** where the cells course in the optic nerve and are relayed centrally. The optic disc is our "blind spot" because no cones or rods are present in this region of the retina.

Clinical Focus 8-23

Eyelid Infections and Conjunctival Disorders

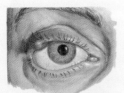

Acute meibomianitis

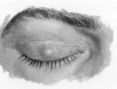

Chalazion

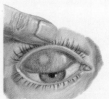

Chalazion; lid everted

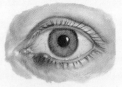

Hordeolum (sty) of lower lid

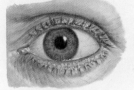

Blepharitis

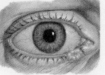

Carcinoma of lower lid

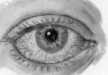

Conjunctivitis

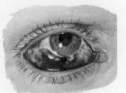

Subconjunctival hemorrhage

Condition	Description
Meibomianitis	Inflammation of meibomian (tarsal) glands
Chalazion	Cyst formation in meibomian gland
Hordeolum (sty)	Infection of sebaceous gland at base of eyelash follicle
Blepharitis	Inflammation of eyelash margin (scaly or ulcerated)
Conjunctival hyperemia (bloodshot eye)	Dilated, congested conjunctival vessels caused by local irritants (e.g., dust, smoke) (not illustrated)
Conjunctivitis (pink eye)	Common inflammation; result of injection of conjunctival vessels caused by allergy, infection, or external irritant
Subconjunctival hemorrhage	Painless, homogeneous red area; result of rupture of subconjunctival capillaries

Clinical Focus 8-24

Papilledema

The optic nerve is a tract of the brain and is therefore surrounded by the three meningeal layers that cover the CNS. The subarachnoid space extends along the nerve to the point where it attaches to the posterior aspect of the eyeball. If ICP is increased, this pressure also compresses the optic nerve and its venous return through the retinal veins. This results in edema of the optic disc, which can be detected by ophthalmoscopic examination (see Fig. 8-21).

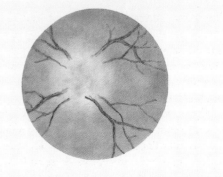

Clinical Focus 8-25

Diabetic Retinopathy

Diabetic retinopathy develops in almost all patients with type 1 diabetes mellitus (DM) and in 50% to 80% of patients with type 2 DM of 20 years' duration or more. Retinopathy can progress rapidly in pregnant women with type 1 DM. Diabetic retinopathy is the number-one cause of blindness in middle-aged individuals and the fourth leading cause of blindness overall in the United States.

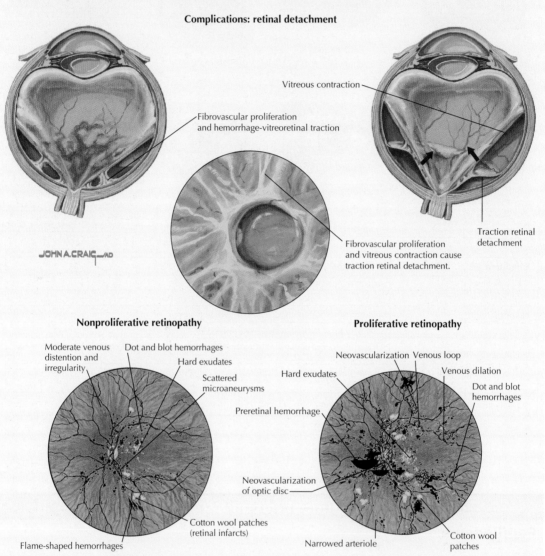

Complications: retinal detachment

Vitreous contraction

Fibrovascular proliferation and hemorrhage-vitreoretinal traction

Fibrovascular proliferation and vitreous contraction cause traction retinal detachment.

Traction retinal detachment

JOHN A.CRAIG—AD

Nonproliferative retinopathy

Moderate venous distention and irregularity

Dot and blot hemorrhages

Hard exudates

Scattered microaneurysms

Preretinal hemorrhage

Neovascularization of optic disc

Cotton wool patches (retinal infarcts)

Flame-shaped hemorrhages

Proliferative retinopathy

Neovascularization　Venous loop

Hard exudates

Venous dilation

Dot and blot hemorrhages

Narrowed arteriole

Cotton wool patches

Characteristic	Description
Etiology	Hyperglycemia through an interaction of hemodynamic, biochemical, and hormonal mechanisms leading to capillary endothelial cell damage (retinal hemorrhages, venous distention, microaneurysms, edema, and microangiopathy)
Types	Nonproliferative and proliferative (abnormal neovascularization and fibrosis)
Complications	Vitreous hemorrhage, retinal edema, retinal detachment

Clinical Focus 8-26

Glaucoma

Glaucoma is an optic neuropathy that can lead to visual field deficits and is often associated with elevated intraocular pressure (IOP).

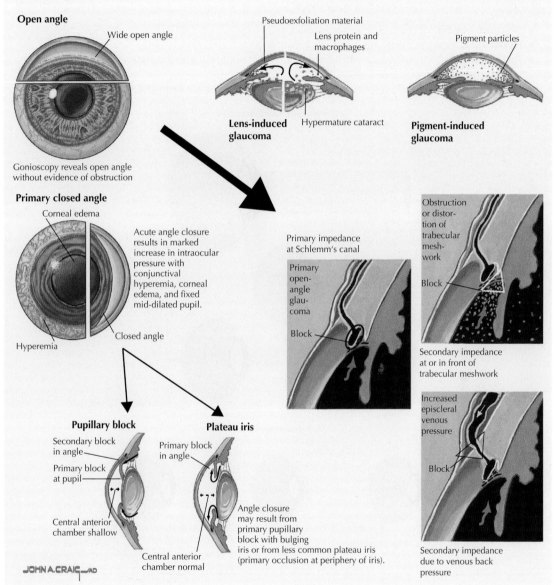

Open angle

Wide open angle

Gonioscopy reveals open angle without evidence of obstruction

Pseudoexfoliation material

Lens protein and macrophages

Lens-induced glaucoma

Hypermature cataract

Pigment particles

Pigment-induced glaucoma

Primary closed angle

Corneal edema

Acute angle closure results in marked increase in intraocular pressure with conjunctival hyperemia, corneal edema, and fixed mid-dilated pupil.

Hyperemia

Closed angle

Primary impedance at Schlemm's canal

Primary open-angle glaucoma

Block

Obstruction or distortion of trabecular meshwork

Block

Secondary impedance at or in front of trabecular meshwork

Pupillary block

Secondary block in angle

Primary block at pupil

Central anterior chamber shallow

Plateau iris

Primary block in angle

Central anterior chamber normal

Angle closure may result from primary pupillary block with bulging iris or from less common plateau iris (primary occlusion at periphery of iris).

Increased episcleral venous pressure

Block

Secondary impedance due to venous back pressure

JOHN A.CRAIG—AD

Characteristic	Description
Etiology	Usually increased resistance to outflow of aqueous humor, which leads to increased IOP (reference range, 10–21 mm Hg)
Types	Primary open-angle glaucoma (POAG) most common; closed angle (iris blocks trabecular meshwork)
Risk factors	African-American, family history, age, increased IOP
POAG pathogenesis	Blocked canal of Schlemm (angle is normal) or from obstruction or malfunction of anterior segment angle
Closed-angle pathogenesis	Age-related anatomical changes that block angle or secondary to diseases that pull iris over angle

Clinical Focus 8-27

Ocular Refractive Disorders

Ametropias are the aberrant focusing of light rays on a site other than the optimal site on the retina (macula). Optically, the cornea, lens, and axial length of the eyeball must be in precise balance to achieve sharp focus on the macula. Common disorders include the following:

- **Myopia:** nearsightedness; 80% of ametropias
- **Hyperopia:** farsightedness; age-related occurrence
- **Astigmatism:** nonspherical cornea causes focusing at multiple locations instead of at a single point; affects 25% to 40% of the U.S. population.
- **Presbyopia:** age-related progressive loss of accommodative ability (lens is less flexible).

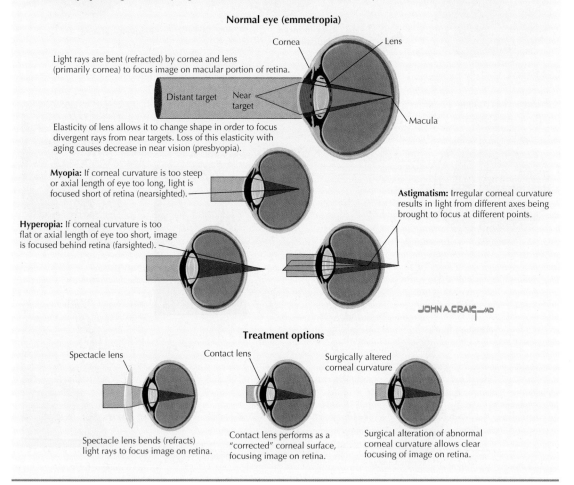

Normal eye (emmetropia)

Light rays are bent (refracted) by cornea and lens (primarily cornea) to focus image on macular portion of retina.

Cornea   Lens

Distant target   Near target

Macula

Elasticity of lens allows it to change shape in order to focus divergent rays from near targets. Loss of this elasticity with aging causes decrease in near vision (presbyopia).

Myopia: If corneal curvature is too steep or axial length of eye too long, light is focused short of retina (nearsighted).

Astigmatism: Irregular corneal curvature results in light from different axes being brought to focus at different points.

Hyperopia: If corneal curvature is too flat or axial length of eye too short, image is focused behind retina (farsighted).

JOHN A.CRAIG—AD

Treatment options

Spectacle lens

Contact lens

Surgically altered corneal curvature

Spectacle lens bends (refracts) light rays to focus image on retina.

Contact lens performs as a "corrected" corneal surface, focusing image on retina.

Surgical alteration of abnormal corneal curvature allows clear focusing of image on retina.

The **fovea centralis** is the central focusing area and most sensitive portion of the retina. This region is thin because most of the other layers of the retina are absent. Here the photoreceptor layer consists only of cones, specialized for color vision and acute discrimination.

Accommodation of the Lens

The **ciliary body** contains smooth muscle arranged in a circular fashion like a sphincter (see Fig. 8-21). When relaxed, it pulls a set of zonular fibers attached to the elastic lens taut and flattens the lens for viewing objects at some distance from the eye. When focusing on near objects, the sphincter-like ciliary muscle (parasympathetically innervated by CN III) contracts and constricts closer to the lens, relaxing the zonular fibers and allowing the elastic lens to round up for accommodation (near vision).

Cataract

A cataract is an opacity, or cloudy area, in the crystalline lens. Risk factors for cataracts include age, smoking, alcohol use, sun exposure, low educational status, diabetes, and systemic steroid use. Treatment is most often surgical, involving lens removal (patient becomes extremely farsighted); vision is corrected with glasses, contact lenses, or implanted plastic lens (intraocular lens).

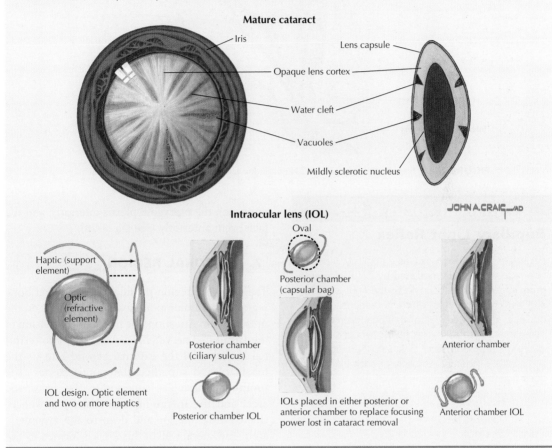

Mature cataract

Iris
Lens capsule
Opaque lens cortex
Water cleft
Vacuoles
Mildly sclerotic nucleus

JOHN A.CRAIG—AD

Intraocular lens (IOL)

Oval
Haptic (support element)
Optic (refractive element)
Posterior chamber (capsular bag)
Posterior chamber (ciliary sulcus)
Anterior chamber
IOL design. Optic element and two or more haptics
Posterior chamber IOL
IOLs placed in either posterior or anterior chamber to replace focusing power lost in cataract removal
Anterior chamber IOL

Blood Supply to the Orbit and Eye

The **ophthalmic artery** arises from the internal carotid artery just as it exits the cavernous sinus, and it supplies the orbit and eye by the following branches (Fig. 8-22):

- **Central artery of the retina:** travels in the optic nerve; occlusion leads to blindness.
- **Short and long posterior ciliary arteries**: pierce the sclera and supply the ciliary body, iris, and choroid.
- **Lacrimal arteries:** supply the gland, conjunctiva, and eyelids.
- **Ethmoidal arteries:** supply the ethmoid and frontal sinuses, nasal cavity, and external anterior nose.

- **Medial palpebrae arteries:** supply the eyelids.
- **Muscular arteries**: supply skeletal muscles of the orbit and smooth muscles of the eyeball.
- **Dorsal nasal arteries:** supply the lateral nose and lacrimal sac.
- **Supra-orbital artery:** passes through supra-orbital notch and supplies the forehead and scalp.
- **Supratrochlear artery:** supplies the forehead and scalp.

The venous drainage is by the **superior and inferior ophthalmic veins,** with connections to the cavernous sinus posteriorly (principal

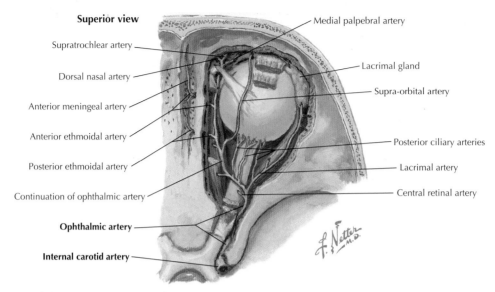

Superior view

Supratrochlear artery

Dorsal nasal artery

Anterior meningeal artery

Anterior ethmoidal artery

Posterior ethmoidal artery

Continuation of ophthalmic artery

Ophthalmic artery

Internal carotid artery

Medial palpebral artery

Lacrimal gland

Supra-orbital artery

Posterior ciliary arteries

Lacrimal artery

Central retinal artery

FIGURE 8-22 Branches of Ophthalmic Artery. (From *Atlas of human anatomy*, ed 6, Plate 87.)

Clinical Focus 8-29

Pupillary Light Reflex

Bright light stimulation causes a pupillary constriction response that is mediated by CN II afferents (from the retina) responding to the light stimulus and evoking a bilateral efferent response in the nucleus of Edinger-Westphal preganglionic parasympathetic fibers. These fibers synapse in the ciliary ganglion and send postganglionic fibers to the pupillary constrictor muscle of each iris, which constricts the pupils symmetrically and bilaterally, limiting the light's effect on the retina.

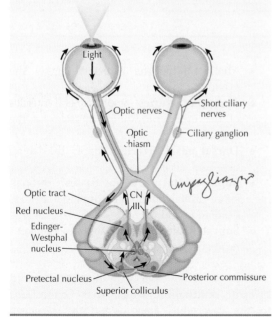

Light

Optic nerves

Short ciliary nerves

Optic chiasm

Ciliary ganglion

Optic tract

CN III

Red nucleus

Edinger-Westphal nucleus

Pretectal nucleus

Posterior commissure

Superior colliculus

drainage), the pterygoid plexus inferiorly, and the facial vein anteriorly (see Fig. 8-28).

7. TEMPORAL REGION

The temporal region includes the temporal bone region and infratemporal fossa, and focuses on the muscles of mastication, the mandibular division of the trigeminal nerve (CN V_3), and the two terminal branches of the external carotid artery—the maxillary and superficial temporal arteries. The **temporal fossa** lies superior to the zygomatic arch, and the **infratemporal fossa** is a wedge-shaped area inferior and deep to the zygomatic arch. The lateral wall of this fossa is formed by the mandibular ramus.

Muscles of Mastication

The muscles of mastication provide a coordinated set of movements that facilitate biting and chewing (grinding action of lower jaw). These muscles participate in movements of elevation, retrusion (retraction), and protrusion of the mandible. Embryologically, the muscles are derived from the first branchial arch, and all are innervated by CN V_3 (Fig. 8-23 and Table 8-8).

The **temporomandibular joint** (TMJ) is the articulation between the condylar process of the mandible and the squamous portion of the temporal bone (mandibular fossa) (Figs. 8-24 and 8-25 and Table 8-9). The TMJ is a modified hinge-type synovial joint. Unlike most synovial joints, the TMJ surfaces are covered with fibrous cartilage

Clinical Focus 8-30

Mandibular Dislocation

Temporomandibular joint dislocation (subluxation) occurs when the mandibular condyle moves anterior to the articular eminence and the mouth has the appearance of being wide open. TMJ dislocation can be quite painful and can occur from a variety of actions, including a large yawn. Once the ligaments are stretched, subsequent dislocations may occur more frequently.

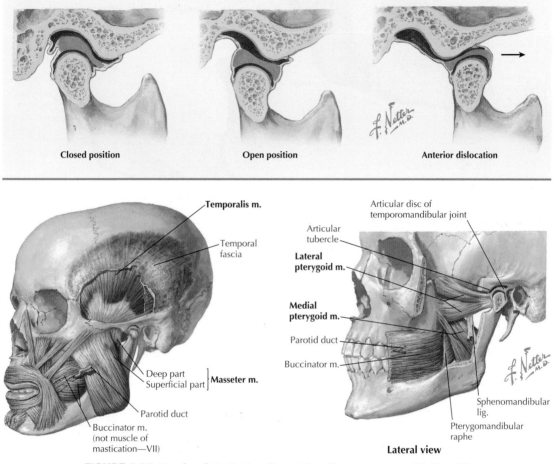

Closed position   Open position   Anterior dislocation

FIGURE 8-23 Muscles of Mastication. (From *Atlas of human anatomy*, ed 6, Plate 48.)

TABLE 8-8 Summary of the Muscles of Mastication

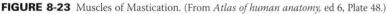

MUSCLE	ORIGIN	INSERTION	MAIN ACTIONS
Temporalis*	Floor of temporal fossa and deep temporal fascia	Ramus of mandible and coronoid process	Elevates mandible; posterior fibers retrude mandible
Masseter	Zygomatic arch	Ramus of mandible and coronoid process	Elevates and protrudes mandible; deep fibers retrude mandible
Lateral pterygoid	*Superior head*: infratemporal surface of greater wing of sphenoid *Inferior head*: lateral pterygoid plate	Pterygoid fovea, capsule of TMJ, articular disc	Acting together, protrude mandible; acting alone and alternately, produces side-to-side movements
Medial pterygoid	*Deep head*: medial surface of lateral pterygoid plate and palatine bone *Superficial head*: tuberosity of maxilla	Ramus of medial mandible, inferior to mandibular foramen	Elevates mandible; acting together, protrude mandible; acting alone, protrudes side of jaw; acting alternately, produces grinding motion

*All innervated by CN V_3.

Mandible of adult: anterolateral superior view

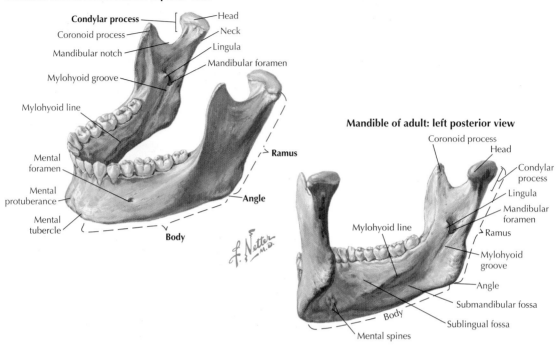

Mandible of adult: left posterior view

FIGURE 8-24 Mandible. (From *Atlas of human anatomy,* ed 6, Plate 17.)

Lateral view

Jaws closed

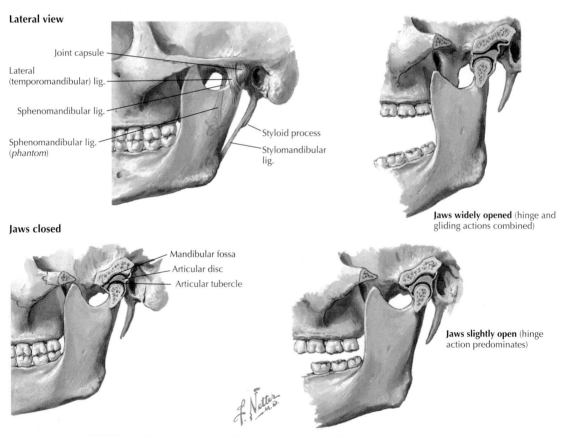

Jaws widely opened (hinge and gliding actions combined)

Jaws slightly open (hinge action predominates)

FIGURE 8-25 Temporomandibular Joint. (From *Atlas of human anatomy,* ed 6, Plate 18.)

TABLE 8-9 Features of the TMJ

LIGAMENT	ATTACHMENT	COMMENT
Capsule	Temporal fossa and tubercle to mandibular head	Permits side-to-side motion, protrusion, and retrusion
Lateral (TMJ)	Temporal to mandible	Thickened fibrous band of capsule
Articular disc	Between temporal bone and mandible	Divides joint into two synovial compartments
Stylomandibular	Styloid process to posterior ramus and angle of jaw	Limits anterior protrusion of mandible
Sphenomandibular	Spine of sphenoid to lingula of mandible	May act as a pivot by providing tension during opening and closing

Clinical Focus 8-31

Mandibular Fractures

Because of its vulnerable location, the mandible is the second most fractured facial bone, after the nasal bone. The mandible's U shape renders it liable to multiple fractures (more than 50%). The most common sites are the cuspid (canine tooth) area and the third molar area. Oozing blood from the mandible collects in loose tissues of the mouth floor (ecchymosis) and is virtually pathognomonic of a fracture.

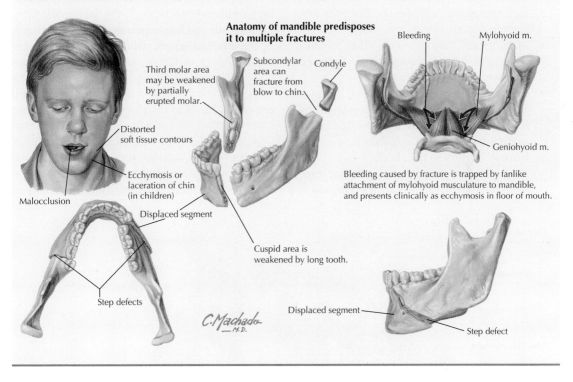

Parotid Gland

The parotid gland is the largest of the three pairs of salivary glands and occupies the retromandibular space between the mandibular ramus and mastoid process (see Figs. 8-14 and 8-16). It is encased within the parotid sheath, a tough extension of the deep cervical fascia. The **parotid duct** courses medially across the medial border of the masseter muscle and then dives deeply into the buccal fat pad, piercing the buccinator muscle of the cheek and opening in the mouth just lateral to the second maxillary (upper) molar. As noted previously, the terminal portion of the facial nerve to the face exits the stylomastoid foramen and passes through the parotid gland to distribute to

rather than hyaline cartilage and the joint cavity is divided by a fibrocartilaginous articular disc.

the muscles of facial expression (Fig. 8-14). The parotid gland is innervated by secretomotor parasympathetic fibers from the glossopharyngeal nerve (CN IX), which we will review in the next section (see Fig. 8-71).

Infratemporal Fossa

The wedge-shaped infratemporal fossa is the space inferior to the zygomatic arch, medial to the mandibular ramus and posterior to the maxilla. CN V_3, the largest division of CN V, exits the **foramen ovale,** which is located in the roof of the fossa, and its branches in this region include the following (Fig. 8-26):

- **Muscular:** small motor nerves to the four muscles of mastication, and to the tensor veli palatini, mylohyoid, anterior belly of the digastric, and tensor tympani (in middle ear); embryologically, derived from the first branchial arch.
- **Meningeal:** accompanies the middle meningeal artery through the **foramen spinosum;** sensory to the dura.
- **Auriculotemporal:** conveys CN IX postganglionic parasympathetic secretory fibers from the **otic ganglion** to the parotid gland; sensory to the auricle and temple.
- **Buccal:** sensory to the cheek.
- **Lingual:** conveys CN VII preganglionic parasympathetics of the **chorda tympani** to

the **submandibular ganglion,** and taste fibers from the tongue to the geniculate ganglion of CN VII; sensory to the tongue. These sensory fibers have their cell bodies in the trigeminal ganglion of CN V.
- **Inferior alveolar:** passes into the mandibular canal and is sensory to the mandibular teeth and gums via inferior dental and gingival branches and to the chin via the mental branch from the inferior alveolar nerve. The **mylohyoid branch** that leaves the inferior alveolar nerve before it enters the mandibular canal courses in the mylohyoid groove of the medial mandible and innervates the mylohyoid and anterior belly of the digastric muscles.

Parasympathetic preganglionic fibers from the glossopharyngeal nerve (CN IX) **(inferior salivatory nucleus)** run through the middle ear tympanic plexus and **lesser petrosal nerve** to synapse in the **otic ganglion,** which is located on the medial aspect of CN V_3 as it exits the foramen ovale (see Figs. 8-69 and 8-71). Secretomotor postganglionic fibers join the **auriculotemporal nerve** and travel to the parotid gland, which they innervate.

Additionally, parasympathetic preganglionic fibers from CN VII **(superior salivatory nucleus)** pass through the middle ear and exit through a small fissure (petrotympanic) in the temporal

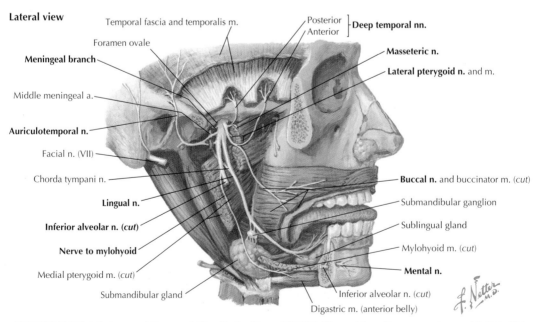

Lateral view

Temporal fascia and temporalis m.

Foramen ovale

Meningeal branch

Middle meningeal a.

Auriculotemporal n.

Facial n. (VII)

Chorda tympani n.

Lingual n.

Inferior alveolar n. (cut)

Nerve to mylohyoid

Medial pterygoid m. (cut)

Submandibular gland

Posterior / Anterior ⎤ **Deep temporal nn.**

Masseteric n.

Lateral pterygoid n. and m.

Buccal n. and buccinator m. (cut)

Submandibular ganglion

Sublingual gland

Mylohyoid m. (cut)

Mental n.

Inferior alveolar n. (cut)

Digastric m. (anterior belly)

FIGURE 8-26 Infratemporal Fossa and Mandibular Nerve (CN V_3). (From *Atlas of human anatomy*, ed 6, Plate 50.)

Clinical Focus 8-32

Rhinosinusitis

Rhinosinusitis is an inflammation of the paranasal sinuses (usually the ethmoid and maxillary sinuses) and the nasal cavity. Physical examination of the paranasal sinuses is usually sufficient to make the diagnosis, although a CT of the sinus may help in difficult cases.

Characteristic	Description
Etiology	Respiratory viral infection or bacterial infection (often secondary); deviation of nasal septum
Pathogenesis	Obstruction of discharge of normal sinus secretions compromises normal sterility of sinuses
Signs and symptoms	Nasal congestion, facial pain and/or pressure, purulent discharge, fever, headache, painful maxillary teeth, halitosis

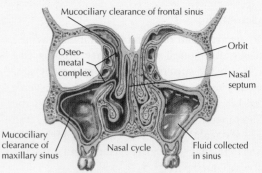

Mucociliary clearance of frontal sinus

Orbit

Osteo-meatal complex

Nasal septum

Mucociliary clearance of maxillary sinus

Nasal cycle

Fluid collected in sinus

Cilia drain sinuses by propelling mucus toward natural ostia (mucociliary clearance)

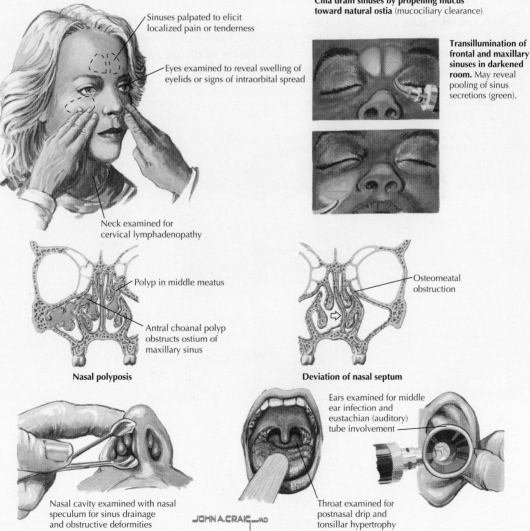

Sinuses palpated to elicit localized pain or tenderness

Eyes examined to reveal swelling of eyelids or signs of intraorbital spread

Neck examined for cervical lymphadenopathy

Transillumination of frontal and maxillary sinuses in darkened room. May reveal pooling of sinus secretions (green).

Polyp in middle meatus

Antral choanal polyp obstructs ostium of maxillary sinus

Nasal polyposis

Osteomeatal obstruction

Deviation of nasal septum

Nasal cavity examined with nasal speculum for sinus drainage and obstructive deformities

Ears examined for middle ear infection and eustachian (auditory) tube involvement

Throat examined for postnasal drip and tonsillar hypertrophy

JOHN A. CRAIG—AD

bone as the **chorda tympani nerve,** to join the lingual branch of CN V_3 and pass to the **submandibular ganglion,** where the fibers synapse (see Fig. 8-70). Secretomotor postganglionic fibers then innervate the submandibular and sublingual salivary glands.

Vascular Supply

The external carotid artery terminates as the superficial temporal and maxillary arteries (see Fig. 8-16). The **superficial temporal artery** supplies the scalp and upper face via its transverse facial branch. The **maxillary artery** supplies the infratemporal region, nasal cavities, palate, and maxillary teeth (Fig. 8-27). For descriptive purposes, the maxillary artery is divided into the following three parts:

- **Retromandibular:** arteries enter foramina and supply dura, mandibular teeth and gums, ear, and chin.

- **Pterygoid:** branches supply muscles of mastication and buccinator.
- **Pterygopalatine:** branches enter foramina and supply maxillary teeth and gums, orbital floor, nose, paranasal sinuses, palate, auditory tube, and superior pharynx.

Major branches of the maxillary artery include the inferior alveolar and middle meningeal branches from the first (retromandibular) part, branches to the muscles of mastication from the second (pterygoid) part, and the superior alveolar, infra-orbital, greater palatine, and sphenopalatine branches from the third (pterygopalatine) part (Fig. 8-27). The terminal portion of the maxillary artery passes into the **pterygopalatine fossa** (see Fig. 8-27) to gain access to the nasal cavity and nasopharynx. Here it is joined by the maxillary nerve (CN V_2) and its branches.

The infratemporal fossa is largely drained by **veins of the pterygoid plexus** (Fig. 8-28), which

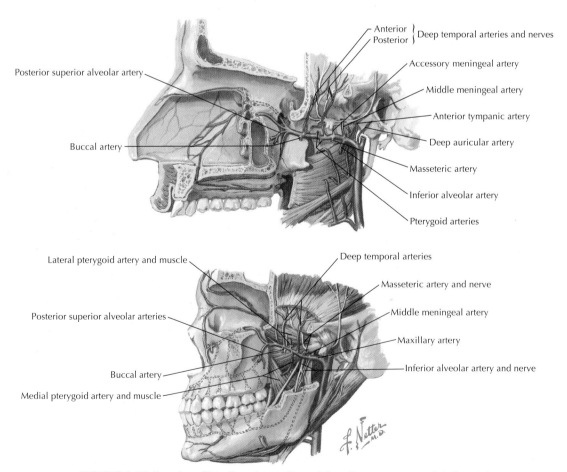

FIGURE 8-27 Branches of Maxillary Artery. (From *Atlas of human anatomy,* ed 6, Plate 51.)

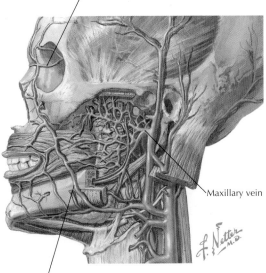

Ophthalmic v.

Maxillary vein

Facial v.

FIGURE 8-28 Pterygoid Plexus of Veins. (From *Atlas of human anatomy,* ed 6, Plate 73.)

have extensive anastomoses with dural, ophthalmic, and facial veins. Tributaries from each of the areas supplied by the branches of the maxillary artery ultimately drain into the pterygoid venous plexus and/or its principal anastomotic veins. These veins are valveless, so flow can go in either direction based on gravity and pressure.

8. PARANASAL SINUSES AND NASAL CAVITY

Paranasal Sinuses

The four paired paranasal sinuses are the frontal, ethmoid, maxillary, and sphenoid sinuses, named for the bones in which they reside (Fig. 8-29). The paranasal sinuses surround the nose and orbits and are lined with respiratory epithelium (pseudostratified columnar with cilia). The sinuses lighten the weight of the facial skeleton, assist in warming and humidifying inspired air, add

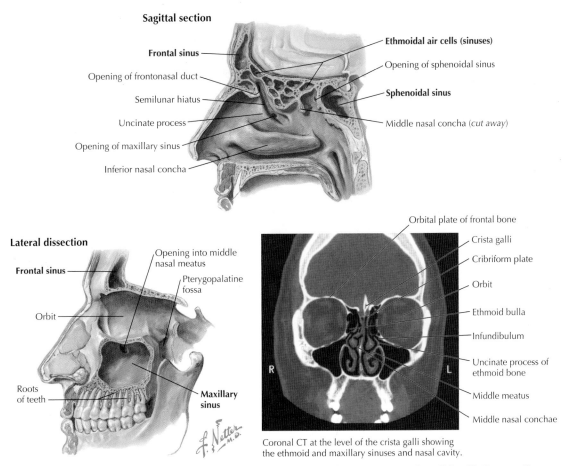

Sagittal section

Frontal sinus

Opening of frontonasal duct

Semilunar hiatus

Uncinate process

Opening of maxillary sinus

Inferior nasal concha

Ethmoidal air cells (sinuses)

Opening of sphenoidal sinus

Sphenoidal sinus

Middle nasal concha (*cut away*)

Lateral dissection

Frontal sinus

Orbit

Roots of teeth

Opening into middle nasal meatus

Pterygopalatine fossa

Maxillary sinus

Orbital plate of frontal bone

Crista galli

Cribriform plate

Orbit

Ethmoid bulla

Infundibulum

Uncinate process of ethmoid bone

Middle meatus

Middle nasal conchae

R   L

Coronal CT at the level of the crista galli showing the ethmoid and maxillary sinuses and nasal cavity.

FIGURE 8-29 Paranasal Sinuses. (From *Atlas of human anatomy,* ed 6, Plate 44; CT image from Kelley LL, Petersen C: *Sectional anatomy for imaging professionals,* Philadelphia, Mosby, 2007.)

resonance to the voice, and drain mucus secretions into the nasal cavities. Sneezing and blowing the nose, as well as gravity, help to drain the paranasal sinuses of mucus.

The innervation, blood supply, and drainage of the paranasal sinuses include the following (see Figs. 8-27 to 8-29, 8-31, 8-33, and 8-34):

- **Frontal sinus:** sensory fibers from V_1 (supra-orbital); anterior ethmoidal arteries (from ophthalmic); the frontal sinus drains via the frontonasal duct into the **semilunaris hiatus** (middle meatus).
- **Ethmoid sinus:** sensory fibers from V_1 (nasociliary nerve's ethmoidal branches) and V_2 (orbital branches); blood from ethmoidal arteries (from ophthalmic); the anterior ethmoid sinus drains into the **semilunaris hiatus** (middle meatus); the middle ethmoid sinus drains into the **ethmoid bulla** (middle meatus); and the posterior ethmoid sinus drains into the **superior meatus.**
- **Sphenoid sinus:** sensory fibers from V_2 (orbital branches); pharyngeal arteries (from maxillary); the sphenoid sinus drains into the **spheno-ethmoidal recess** above the superior concha.
- **Maxillary sinus:** sensory fibers from V_2 (infra-orbital and alveolar branches); infra-orbital and alveolar arteries (from maxillary); the maxillary sinus drains into the **semilunar hiatus** (middle meatus).

Note also that the **nasolacrimal duct** drains tears into the **inferior meatus;** thus your nose "runs" when you cry.

External Nose

The upper portion of the external nose is continuous with the forehead (frontal bone) through the nasal bones and laterally by the maxillae. The inferior two thirds of the external nose is cartilaginous and formed by the lateral processes of the septal cartilage, a midline septal cartilage, a major alar cartilage (tip of the nose), and several small, minor alar cartilages (Fig 8-30).

Nasal Cavities

Air entering the nose passes through the following areas (Fig. 8-31):

Anterolateral view

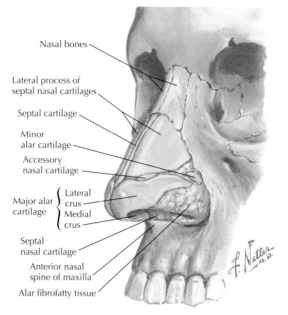

Nasal bones

Lateral process of septal nasal cartilages

Septal cartilage

Minor alar cartilage

Accessory nasal cartilage

Major alar cartilage { Lateral crus / Medial crus }

Septal nasal cartilage

Anterior nasal spine of maxilla

Alar fibrofatty tissue

FIGURE 8-30 Structure of External Nose. (From *Atlas of human anatomy*, ed 6, Plate 35.)

- **Nares:** anterior apertures or nostrils.
- **Vestibule:** dilated portion of the nose inside each aperture; highly vascular epithelium with hair.
- **Respiratory region:** nasal cavity proper, lined with highly vascular respiratory epithelium and three conchae, which increase the surface area for filtering, warming, and humidifying inspired air; conchae covered by respiratory epithelium are called **turbinates.**
- **Olfactory region:** small, apical region of nasal cavity where the olfactory receptors reside.
- **Choanae:** posterior apertures where the nasal cavity communicates with the nasopharynx.

Bones of the nasal cavity include the following (Fig. 8-32):

- **Ethmoid:** unpaired bone that contains the ethmoid air cells (sinuses); contributes to the roof and the lateral and medial walls of the nasal cavity.
- **Sphenoid:** unpaired bone that contains the sphenoid sinus; forms the posterior part of the cavity.

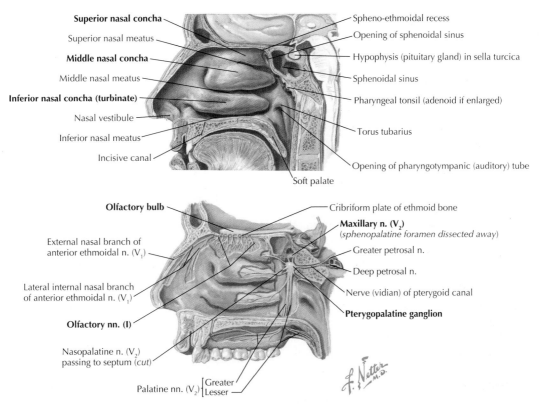

Superior nasal concha
Superior nasal meatus
Middle nasal concha
Middle nasal meatus
Inferior nasal concha (turbinate)
Nasal vestibule
Inferior nasal meatus
Incisive canal
Soft palate

Spheno-ethmoidal recess
Opening of sphenoidal sinus
Hypophysis (pituitary gland) in sella turcica
Sphenoidal sinus
Pharyngeal tonsil (adenoid if enlarged)
Torus tubarius
Opening of pharyngotympanic (auditory) tube

Olfactory bulb
External nasal branch of anterior ethmoidal n. (V₁)
Lateral internal nasal branch of anterior ethmoidal n. (V₁)
Olfactory nn. (I)
Nasopalatine n. (V₂) passing to septum (cut)
Palatine nn. (V₂) [Greater Lesser]

Cribriform plate of ethmoid bone
Maxillary n. (V₂) (sphenopalatine foramen dissected away)
Greater petrosal n.
Deep petrosal n.
Nerve (vidian) of pterygoid canal
Pterygopalatine ganglion

FIGURE 8-31 Lateral Wall of Nasal Cavity. (From *Atlas of human anatomy,* ed 6, Plates 36 and 39.)

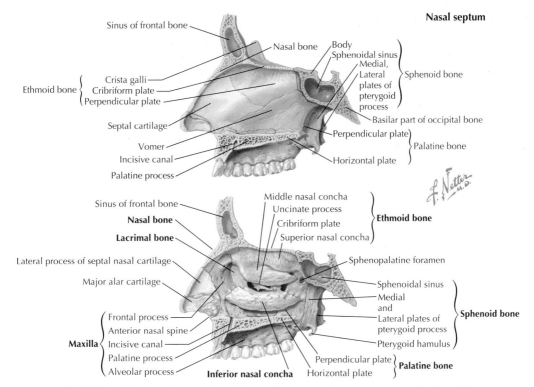

Sinus of frontal bone
Nasal bone
Ethmoid bone {
Crista galli
Cribriform plate
Perpendicular plate }
Septal cartilage
Vomer
Incisive canal
Palatine process

Nasal septum
Body
Sphenoidal sinus
Medial, Lateral plates of pterygoid process } Sphenoid bone
Basilar part of occipital bone
Perpendicular plate } Palatine bone
Horizontal plate

Sinus of frontal bone
Nasal bone
Lacrimal bone
Lateral process of septal nasal cartilage
Major alar cartilage
Maxilla {
Frontal process
Anterior nasal spine
Incisive canal
Palatine process
Alveolar process }

Middle nasal concha
Uncinate process
Cribriform plate
Superior nasal concha } Ethmoid bone
Sphenopalatine foramen
Sphenoidal sinus
Medial and Lateral plates of pterygoid process } Sphenoid bone
Pterygoid hamulus
Perpendicular plate } Palatine bone
Horizontal plate
Inferior nasal concha

FIGURE 8-32 Bones Forming Nasal Cavity. (From *Atlas of human anatomy,* ed 6, Plate 37.)

Clinical Focus 8-33

Nosebleed

A nosebleed, or **epistaxis,** is a common occurrence and often involves the richly vascularized region of the vestibule and the anteroinferior aspect of the nasal septum (Kiesselbach's area). Nosebleeds usually result from trauma to the septal branch of the superior labial artery from the facial artery.

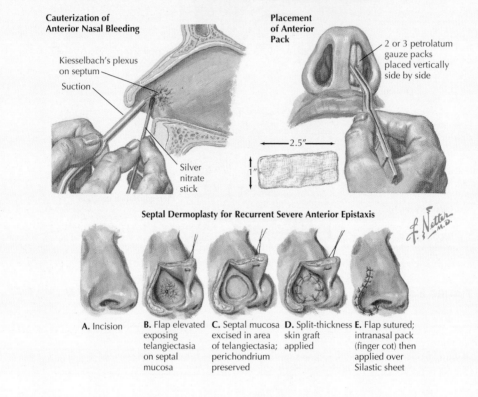

Cauterization of Anterior Nasal Bleeding

Kiesselbach's plexus on septum

Suction

Silver nitrate stick

Placement of Anterior Pack

2 or 3 petrolatum gauze packs placed vertically side by side

2.5"

1"

Septal Dermoplasty for Recurrent Severe Anterior Epistaxis

A. Incision

B. Flap elevated exposing telangiectasia on septal mucosa

C. Septal mucosa excised in area of telangiectasia; perichondrium preserved

D. Split-thickness skin graft applied

E. Flap sutured; intranasal pack (finger cot) then applied over Silastic sheet

- **Frontal:** unpaired bone that contains the frontal sinus; forms part of the roof and septum of the cavity.
- **Vomer:** unpaired bone that contributes to the septum.
- **Nasal:** paired bones that form part of the anterior roof and lateral wall.
- **Maxilla:** paired bones that form the floor, septum, and lateral walls of the cavity.
- **Palatine:** paired bones that form the floor, septum, and lateral walls of the cavity.
- **Lacrimal:** bone that forms part of the lateral wall of the nasal cavity.
- **Inferior nasal concha:** paired bones that form part of the lateral wall.

Blood Supply and Innervation

Blood supply to the nasal cavities originates from the following major arteries (Fig. 8-33):

- **Ophthalmic:** anterior and posterior ethmoidal arteries
- **Maxillary:** sphenopalatine (terminal branch of the maxillary) and its septal branches, and the greater palatine arteries
- **Facial:** lateral nasal, septal branches, and superior labial artery

Corresponding veins drain the floor, lateral walls, and nasal septum, with most of the venous return passing into the **pterygoid plexus of veins** (Fig. 8-33). Some venous drainage also passes into the facial vein anteriorly and into the inferior ophthalmic veins superiorly.

The innervation of the nasal cavity includes the following (Fig. 8-34; see also Fig. 8-70):

- **Olfactory:** CN I olfactory receptors (special sense of smell) in the olfactory epithelium convey axons that pass from the upper part

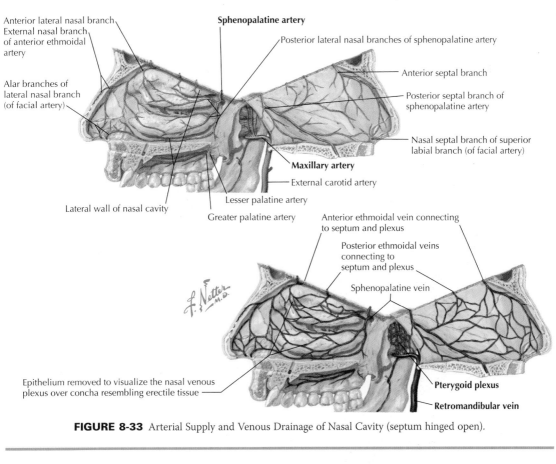

Anterior lateral nasal branch
External nasal branch
of anterior ethmoidal
artery

Alar branches of
lateral nasal branch
(of facial artery)

Sphenopalatine artery

Posterior lateral nasal branches of sphenopalatine artery

Anterior septal branch

Posterior septal branch of
sphenopalatine artery

Nasal septal branch of superior
labial branch (of facial artery)

Maxillary artery

External carotid artery

Lateral wall of nasal cavity

Lesser palatine artery

Greater palatine artery

Anterior ethmoidal vein connecting
to septum and plexus

Posterior ethmoidal veins
connecting to
septum and plexus

Sphenopalatine vein

Epithelium removed to visualize the nasal venous
plexus over concha resembling erectile tissue

Pterygoid plexus

Retromandibular vein

FIGURE 8-33 Arterial Supply and Venous Drainage of Nasal Cavity (septum hinged open).

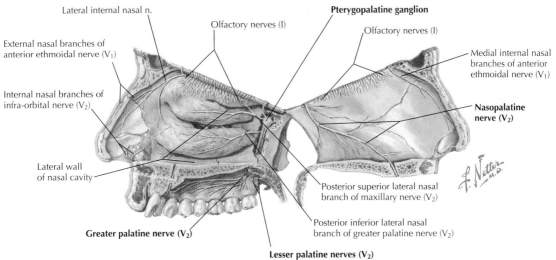

Lateral internal nasal n.

Olfactory nerves (I)

Pterygopalatine ganglion

Olfactory nerves (I)

External nasal branches of
anterior ethmoidal nerve (V_1)

Internal nasal branches of
infra-orbital nerve (V_2)

Medial internal nasal
branches of anterior
ethmoidal nerve (V_1)

Nasopalatine
nerve (V_2)

Lateral wall
of nasal cavity

Posterior superior lateral nasal
branch of maxillary nerve (V_2)

Greater palatine nerve (V_2)

Posterior inferior lateral nasal
branch of greater palatine nerve (V_2)

Lesser palatine nerves (V_2)

FIGURE 8-34 Nerve Supply of the Nose (septum hinged open).

of the nasal cavity, through the cribriform plate, and synapse in the olfactory bulbs, which are actually brain tracts surrounded by the three meningeal layers, not unlike CN II.

- **Ophthalmic:** CN V_1 general afferents are conveyed by the anterior and posterior ethmoidal nerves of the nasociliary nerve in the orbit to the trigeminal (sensory) ganglion.

- **Maxillary:** CN V_2 general afferents are conveyed to the trigeminal (sensory) ganglion via small nasal branches and by the nasopalatine nerve on the septum.

- **Sympathetics:** comprised largely of post-ganglionic sympathetic vasomotor fibers from the SCG that reach the nose by traveling on blood vessels and existing nerves (mostly V_2); other fibers also may course via the **deep petrosal nerve** to the nerve of the pterygoid canal and distribute with branches of CN V_2.
- **Parasympathetics:** preganglionic secreto-motor fibers to the mucosal glands of the nose and paranasal sinuses come from the **superior salivatory nucleus** of CN VII and travel via the greater petrosal nerve and the nerve of the pterygoid canal; the fibers synapse in the **pterygopalatine ganglion;** postganglionic parasympathetic fibers then distribute on existing nerves of CN V_2.

9. EAR

The human ear consists of the following three parts (Fig. 8-35):

- **External:** the auricle (pinna), external acoustic meatus, and tympanic membrane (eardrum)
- **Middle:** the air-filled tympanic cavity between the eardrum and labyrinthine wall, which contains the three middle ear ossicles—**malleus, incus,** and **stapes**—and the stapedius and tensor tympani muscles; communicates posteriorly with the mastoid antrum and anteriorly with the auditory (pharyngotympanic, eustachian) tube
- **Internal (inner):** acoustic apparatus (cochlea) and vestibular apparatus (vestibule with the utricle and saccule, and semicircular canals)

External Ear

The **auricle** is composed of skin and elastic cartilage and helps funnel sound waves into the external acoustic meatus. It is innervated by auricular branches from CN V_3, VII, and X and by the lesser occipital (C2) and greater auricular (C2-3) nerves. The **external acoustic meatus** is about 2.5 cm long and is composed of cartilage (lateral third) and bone. Its lining of skin contains hairs and modified sweat glands (ceruminous glands) that secrete earwax that protects the skin. It is innervated mostly by CN V_3 and X, with minor contributions from CN VII and IX. The **tympanic**

membrane lies at an oblique angle (Fig. 8-35), sloping medially from posterosuperior to antero-inferior, and is attached on its medial side to the handle of the malleus, which creates a depression in its middle called the *umbo.* Because of its oblique position and the umbo, the tympanic membrane gives off a reflection of light when viewed with an otoscope (the cone of light). Its external surface is innervated by CN V_3, VII, and X and its internal surface by CN IX.

Middle Ear

The middle ear cavity resembles a box with six sides and is air filled and lined with a mucous membrane. Its boundaries include the following (Fig. 8-36):

- *Roof:* **tegmen tympani,** a layer of bone that is part of the petrous portion of the temporal bone.
- *Floor:* **jugular fossa,** a thin layer of bone separating the middle ear from the internal jugular vein.
- *Posterior wall:* an incomplete wall with a small aperture (aditus ad antrum) leading to the **mastoid air cells.**
- *Anterior wall:* an incomplete wall with a thin, bony lower portion separating the cavity from the internal carotid artery (in the carotid canal) and superiorly an opening for the **auditory** (pharyngotympanic; eustachian) **tube** and tensor tympani muscle.
- *Lateral wall:* the **tympanic membrane** and **epitympanic recess** above the eardrum; the chorda tympani branch of CN VII passes through the cavity.
- *Medial wall:* the **labyrinthine wall** exhibiting superiorly a prominence of the lateral semicircular canal and a second prominence for the CN VII; the **oval** (fenestra vestibuli) **window** for the base of the stapes; a promontory (basal turn of the cochlea), with the tympanic nerve plexus (CN IX) ·on its surface; and most inferiorly the **round** (fenestra cochlea) **window** covered with a membrane.

Vibrations of the eardrum cause the three middle ear ossicles to vibrate, which causes the base of the stapes to vibrate against the oval window and thus initiates a wave action within the fluid-filled **scala vestibuli** (filled with **perilymph**) and **scala tympani** of the cochlea (described in

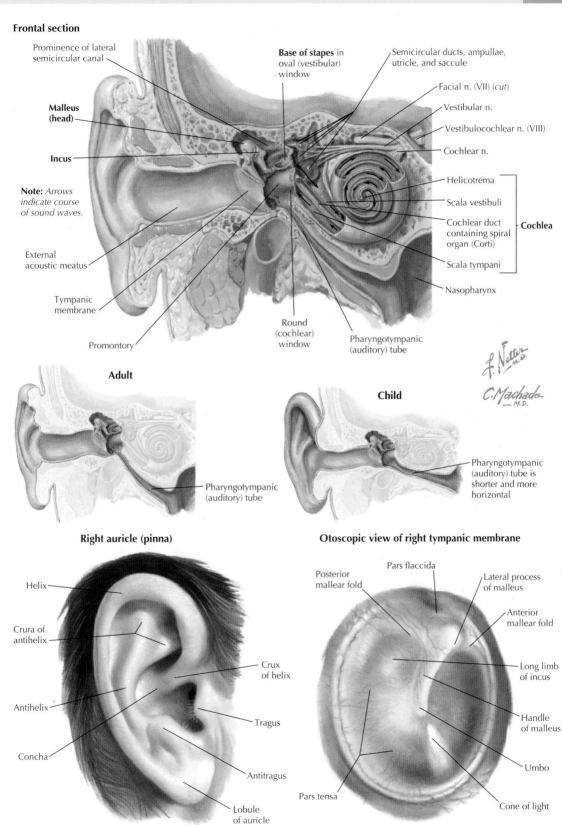

Frontal section

Prominence of lateral semicircular canal

Malleus (head)

Incus

Note: *Arrows indicate course of sound waves.*

External acoustic meatus

Tympanic membrane

Promontory

Base of stapes in oval (vestibular) window

Round (cochlear) window

Pharyngotympanic (auditory) tube

Semicircular ducts, ampullae, utricle, and saccule

Facial n. (VII) *(cut)*

Vestibular n.

Vestibulocochlear n. (VIII)

Cochlear n.

Helicotrema

Scala vestibuli

Cochlear duct containing spiral organ (Corti)

Scala tympani

Nasopharynx

Cochlea

Adult

Child

Pharyngotympanic (auditory) tube

Pharyngotympanic (auditory) tube is shorter and more horizontal

Right auricle (pinna)

Helix

Crura of antihelix

Antihelix

Concha

Crux of helix

Tragus

Antitragus

Lobule of auricle

Otoscopic view of right tympanic membrane

Pars flaccida

Posterior mallear fold

Lateral process of malleus

Anterior mallear fold

Long limb of incus

Handle of malleus

Umbo

Cone of light

Pars tensa

FIGURE 8-35 General Anatomy of Right Ear. (From *Atlas of human anatomy*, ed 6, Plates 94 and 95.)

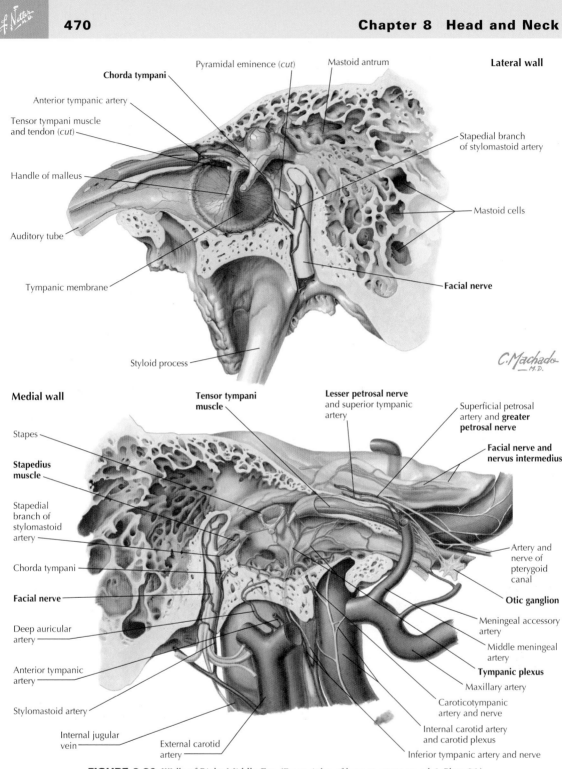

Chorda tympani

Pyramidal eminence (*cut*)

Mastoid antrum

Lateral wall

Anterior tympanic artery

Tensor tympani muscle and tendon (*cut*)

Stapedial branch of stylomastoid artery

Handle of malleus

Auditory tube

Mastoid cells

Tympanic membrane

Facial nerve

Styloid process

Medial wall

Tensor tympani muscle

Lesser petrosal nerve and superior tympanic artery

Superficial petrosal artery and **greater petrosal nerve**

Stapes

Facial nerve and nervus intermedius

Stapedius muscle

Stapedial branch of stylomastoid artery

Chorda tympani

Artery and nerve of pterygoid canal

Facial nerve

Otic ganglion

Deep auricular artery

Meningeal accessory artery

Middle meningeal artery

Anterior tympanic artery

Tympanic plexus

Maxillary artery

Stylomastoid artery

Caroticotympanic artery and nerve

Internal jugular vein

External carotid artery

Internal carotid artery and carotid plexus

Inferior tympanic artery and nerve

FIGURE 8-36 Walls of Right Middle Ear. (From *Atlas of human anatomy*, ed 6, Plate 96.)

the next section). The **stapedius** (smallest skeletal muscle in the body) and **tensor tympani muscles** dampen excessive vibrations in the stapes (stapedius) and eardrum (tensor) in response to loud noises.

The innervation of the middle ear is via the tympanic branch of CN IX to the **tympanic plexus** lying beneath the mucosa of the promontory on the medial wall of the middle ear. The **lesser petrosal preganglionic parasympathetic nerve** arises from this plexus, passes through the petrous portion of the temporal bone, runs in a hiatus just inferior to the greater petrosal nerve, and courses to the foramen ovale, where it

Clinical Focus 8-34

Acute Otitis Externa and Otitis Media

Acute otitis externa (swimmer's ear) involves inflammation or bacterial infection of the external acoustic meatus, usually because the protective earwax has been washed from the ear. **Otitis media** is an inflammation of the middle ear and is common in children younger than 15 years because the auditory tube is short and relatively horizontal at this age, which limits drainage by gravity and provides a route for infection from the nasopharynx. When viewed with an otoscope, the normal translucent appearance of the tympanic membrane is gone, the eardrum is erythematous and bulging, and the cone of light is absent.

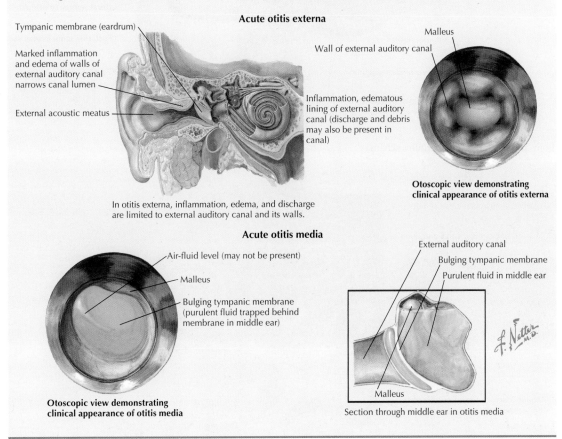

Acute otitis externa

Tympanic membrane (eardrum)

Marked inflammation and edema of walls of external auditory canal narrows canal lumen

External acoustic meatus

Malleus

Wall of external auditory canal

Inflammation, edematous lining of external auditory canal (discharge and debris may also be present in canal)

Otoscopic view demonstrating clinical appearance of otitis externa

In otitis externa, inflammation, edema, and discharge are limited to external auditory canal and its walls.

Acute otitis media

Air-fluid level (may not be present)

Malleus

Bulging tympanic membrane (purulent fluid trapped behind membrane in middle ear)

External auditory canal

Bulging tympanic membrane

Purulent fluid in middle ear

Malleus

Otoscopic view demonstrating clinical appearance of otitis media

Section through middle ear in otitis media

synapses in the **otic ganglion.** The postganglionic parasympathetic fibers of the otic ganglion innervate the parotid salivary gland through the auriculotemporal branch of CN V₃.

Internal Ear

The internal ear houses the special senses of hearing and balance and comprises the following two elements (Fig. 8-37):

- **Bony labyrinth:** includes the vestibule, the three semicircular canals, and the cochlea,

which are all housed within the temporal bone and filled with **perilymph.**

- **Membranous labyrinth:** is suspended within the perilymph of the bony labyrinth and is filled with **endolymph**; consists of the **cochlear duct** (the organ of hearing) and the **utricle, saccule,** and **semicircular ducts** (the organs of balance).

Vibrations of the middle ear ossicles and the base plate of the stapes on the oval window initiate a wave action within the perilymph-filled scala vestibuli and scala tympani of the cochlea (see

Right membranous labyrinth with nerves: posteromedial view

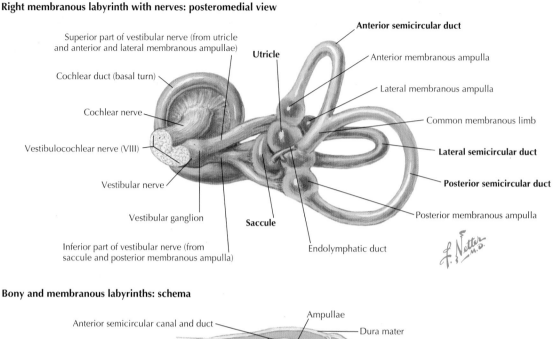

Superior part of vestibular nerve (from utricle and anterior and lateral membranous ampullae)

Cochlear duct (basal turn)

Cochlear nerve

Vestibulocochlear nerve (VIII)

Vestibular nerve

Vestibular ganglion

Inferior part of vestibular nerve (from saccule and posterior membranous ampulla)

Anterior semicircular duct

Utricle

Anterior membranous ampulla

Lateral membranous ampulla

Common membranous limb

Lateral semicircular duct

Posterior semicircular duct

Posterior membranous ampulla

Saccule

Endolymphatic duct

Bony and membranous labyrinths: schema

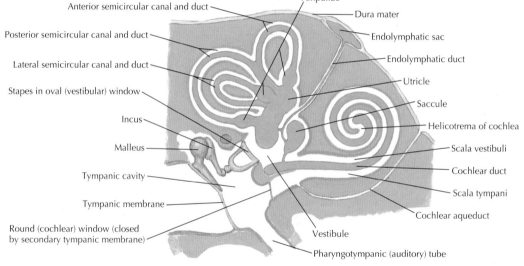

Anterior semicircular canal and duct

Posterior semicircular canal and duct

Lateral semicircular canal and duct

Stapes in oval (vestibular) window

Incus

Malleus

Tympanic cavity

Tympanic membrane

Round (cochlear) window (closed by secondary tympanic membrane)

Ampullae

Dura mater

Endolymphatic sac

Endolymphatic duct

Utricle

Saccule

Helicotrema of cochlea

Scala vestibuli

Cochlear duct

Scala tympani

Cochlear aqueduct

Vestibule

Pharyngotympanic (auditory) tube

FIGURE 8-37 Structures of Right Internal Ear. (From *Atlas of human anatomy,* ed 6, Plates 97 and 98.)

Fig. 8-35, *top* image). This wave action causes the deflection and depolarization of tiny hair cells within the **organ of Corti** (membranous labyrinth). This stimulates action potentials in the afferent axons of the spiral ganglion cells that are conveyed centrally to the brain through the vestibulocochlear nerve (CN VIII), with final processing in the auditory cortex of the temporal lobe.

A similar mechanism of depolarization also occurs in the endolymph of the vestibular system (hair cells and a single kinocilium), where the receptors for equilibrium involve the following two functional components:

- **Static:** a special receptor called the **macula** resides in each **utricle** and **saccule;** participate in positioning of the head and linear acceleration, as well as gravity and low-frequency vibrations (saccule only).
- **Dynamic:** special receptors called the **crista ampullaris** reside in the ampulla of each semicircular canal (anterior, lateral, and posterior canals) and participate in angular (rotational) movements of the head.

Vestibular afferents passing back to the CNS provide input to help modulate and coordinate

Weber and Rinne Tests

Sensorineural hearing loss suggests a disorder of the internal ear or the cochlear division of CN VIII. **Conductive** hearing loss suggests a disorder of the external or middle ear (eardrum, ear ossicles, or both). The Weber and Rinne tests offer an easy way to differentiate between sensorineural and conductive hearing loss.

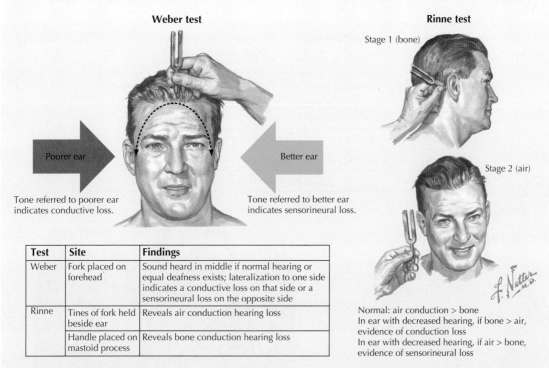

Weber test

Poorer ear

Better ear

Tone referred to poorer ear indicates conductive loss.

Tone referred to better ear indicates sensorineural loss.

Rinne test

Stage 1 (bone)

Stage 2 (air)

Test	Site	Findings
Weber	Fork placed on forehead	Sound heard in middle if normal hearing or equal deafness exists; lateralization to one side indicates a conductive loss on that side or a sensorineural loss on the opposite side
Rinne	Tines of fork held beside ear	Reveals air conduction hearing loss
	Handle placed on mastoid process	Reveals bone conduction hearing loss

Normal: air conduction > bone
In ear with decreased hearing, if bone > air, evidence of conduction loss
In ear with decreased hearing, if air > bone, evidence of sensorineural loss

Cochlear Implant

Two million Americans have profound bilateral deafness. A cochlear implant consists of a speech processor and implanted electrodes. An external microphone detects sound, which is converted by the processor into electrical signals transmitted to the cochlear implant and vestibulocochlear nerve.

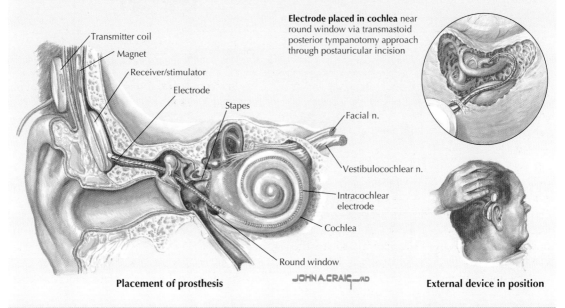

Transmitter coil

Magnet

Receiver/stimulator

Electrode

Stapes

Electrode placed in cochlea near round window via transmastoid posterior tympanotomy approach through postauricular incision

Facial n.

Vestibulocochlear n.

Intracochlear electrode

Cochlea

Round window

Placement of prosthesis

JOHN A. CRAIG—AD

External device in position

Vertigo

Vertigo involves the peripheral vestibular system or its CNS connections and is characterized by the illusion or perception of motion. Central types of vertigo may be caused by multiple sclerosis, migraine, vascular disease associated with the vestibulobasilar region, or brainstem tumors, especially at the cerebellopontine angle.

Peripheral type	Cause
Acute vestibulopathy	Viral infection
Endolymphatic hydrops (Ménière's disease)	Excess endolymph secondary to impaired resorption
Benign paroxysmal positional vertigo	Accumulation of otoconial debris in semicircular canals
Vestibular schwannoma (acoustic neuroma)	Benign tumor of vestibulocochlear nerve
Chronic otitis media	Infection or cholesteatoma

Causes of vertigo

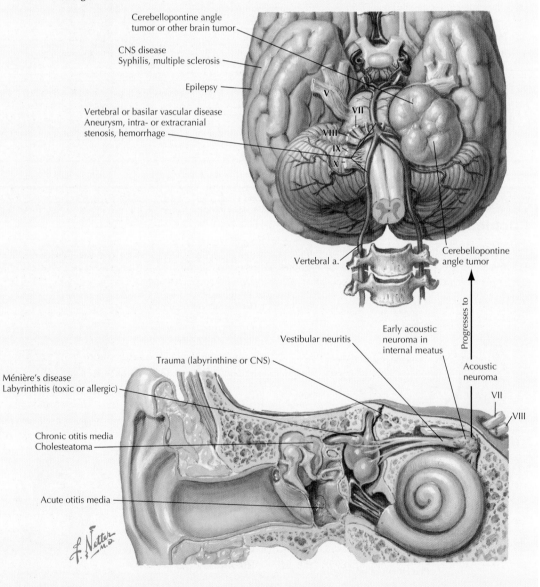

Clinical Focus 8-38

Clinical Focus 8-38

Removal of an Acoustic Neuroma

The translabyrinthine approach to acoustic neuroma removal takes advantage of the anatomy of CN VIII. The tumor often is encapsulated within the vestibular division of CN VIII in the internal acoustic meatus. The approach is via the mastoid air cells, with removal of the semicircular canals and resection of the tumor. Early treatment can spare the cochlear division of CN VIII, and thus hearing, and also spare the facial nerve from involvement.

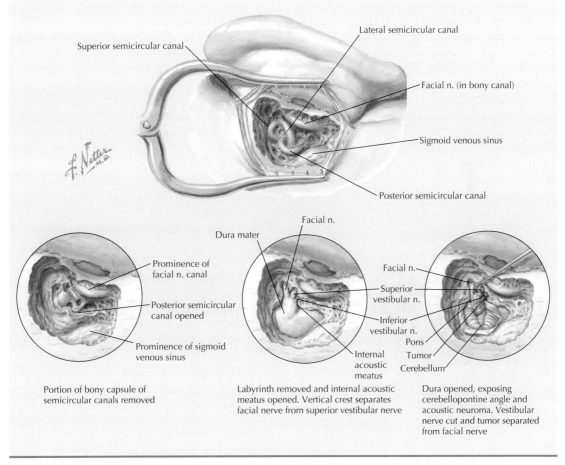

Superior semicircular canal

Lateral semicircular canal

Facial n. (in bony canal)

Sigmoid venous sinus

Posterior semicircular canal

Facial n.

Dura mater

Prominence of facial n. canal

Posterior semicircular canal opened

Prominence of sigmoid venous sinus

Portion of bony capsule of semicircular canals removed

Facial n.

Superior vestibular n.

Inferior vestibular n.

Internal acoustic meatus

Labyrinth removed and internal acoustic meatus opened. Vertical crest separates facial nerve from superior vestibular nerve

Facial n.

Pons

Tumor

Cerebellum

Dura opened, exposing cerebellopontine angle and acoustic neuroma. Vestibular nerve cut and tumor separated from facial nerve

muscle movement, tone, and posture, as well as regulate head and neck movements and coordinate eye movements.

10. ORAL CAVITY

The mouth consists of an **oral vestibule,** the space between the teeth and lips or cheeks, and the **oral cavity proper,** internal to the teeth and gums. Features of the oral cavity proper include the palate (hard and soft), teeth, gums (gingivae), tongue, and salivary glands (see Figs. 8-41 and 8-42). The mucosa of the hard palate, cheeks,

tongue, and lips contain numerous minor salivary glands that secrete directly into the oral cavity. Paired collections of lymphoid tissue called the **palatine tonsils** lie between the palatoglossal and palatopharyngeal folds (contain small skeletal muscles of the same name) and "guard" the entrance into the oropharynx.

Muscles

The tongue is a strong muscular organ (gram for gram, one of the strongest muscles in the body) consisting of **intrinsic** skeletal muscle arranged in four different planes, all innervated by the hypoglossal nerve, CN XII:

- Superior longitudinal
- Inferior longitudinal
- Transverse
- Vertical

Additionally, three extrinsic skeletal muscles originate outside the tongue and insert into it (Fig. 8-38 and Table 8-10). The **genioglossus muscle** depresses and protrudes the tongue. The **hypoglossus** and **styloglossus muscles** retract the tongue during swallowing, pushing the bolus of food up against the palate as it is pushed posteriorly into the oropharynx (see Fig. 8-56). The **palatoglossus muscle** can be considered both a muscle of the tongue and a muscle of the palate. Because it is innervated by the vagus nerve rather than the hypoglossal nerve, the palatoglossus may be grouped with the palate muscles.

The surface of the tongue is characterized by small lingual papillae, divided into four types (Fig. 8-39):

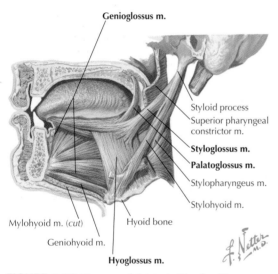

FIGURE 8-38 Tongue and Extrinsic Muscles. (From *Atlas of human anatomy,* ed 6, Plate 59.)

- **Filiform:** numerous slender projections that lack taste buds; give the tongue its rough feel.
- **Fungiform:** larger mushroom-shaped papillae (may appear as red caps) scattered on the dorsum of the tongue's surface; possess taste buds.
- **Circumvallate:** larger papillae that lie in a row just anterior to the sulcus terminalis; possess taste buds.
- **Foliate:** lie along the sides of the tongue and are rudimentary in humans; possess taste buds.

The tongue receives its blood supply largely by the **lingual artery** (from the external carotid artery) and is innervated by the following five cranial nerves (Fig. 8-40):

- **Mandibular:** via lingual nerve; for general sensation to the anterior two thirds of the tongue.
- **Facial:** via **chorda tympani nerve**, which joins the lingual nerve; for taste on the anterior two thirds of the tongue.
- **Glossopharyngeal:** general sensation and taste to the posterior third of the tongue.
- **Vagus:** via the internal branch of the superior laryngeal nerve, for general sensation and taste on the base of the tongue at the epiglottic region.
- **Hypoglossal:** motor to the intrinsic and extrinsic tongue muscles, except palatoglossus.

Salivary Glands

Whereas there are thousands of microscopic minor salivary glands in the oral and lingual mucosa, there also are three pairs of larger salivary glands (Fig. 8-41 and Table 8-11). Saliva contains water, mucins, α-amylase for initial digestion of

TABLE 8-10 Extrinsic Tongue Muscles				
MUSCLE	**ORIGIN**	**INSERTION**	**INNERVATION**	**MAIN ACTIONS**
Genioglossus	Mental spine of mandible	Dorsum of tongue and hyoid bone	Hypoglossal nerve	Depresses and protrudes tongue
Hyoglossus	Body and greater horn of hyoid bone	Lateral and inferior aspect of tongue	Hypoglossal nerve	Depresses and retracts tongue
Styloglossus	Styloid process and stylohyoid ligament	Lateral and inferior aspect of tongue	Hypoglossal nerve	Retracts tongue and draws it up for swallowing
Palatoglossus	Palatine aponeurosis of soft palate	Lateral aspect of tongue	Vagus nerve and pharyngeal plexus	Elevates posterior tongue

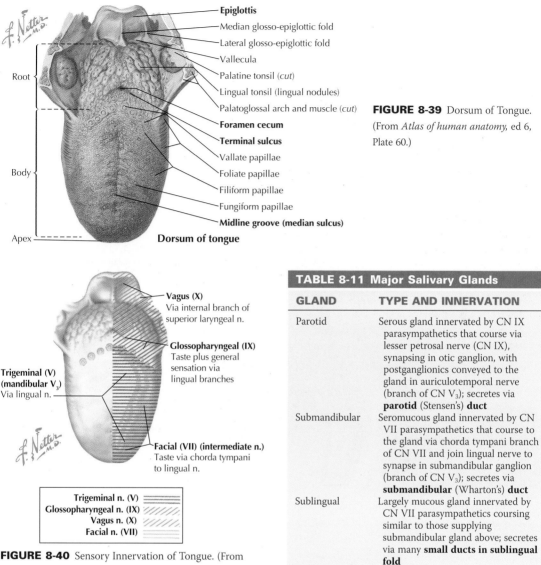

Epiglottis
Median glosso-epiglottic fold
Lateral glosso-epiglottic fold
Vallecula
Palatine tonsil (*cut*)
Lingual tonsil (lingual nodules)
Palatoglossal arch and muscle (*cut*)
Foramen cecum
Terminal sulcus
Vallate papillae
Foliate papillae
Filiform papillae
Fungiform papillae
Midline groove (median sulcus)

Root
Body
Apex

Dorsum of tongue

FIGURE 8-39 Dorsum of Tongue. (From *Atlas of human anatomy*, ed 6, Plate 60.)

Vagus (X)
Via internal branch of superior laryngeal n.

Glossopharyngeal (IX)
Taste plus general sensation via lingual branches

Trigeminal (V)
(mandibular V₃)
Via lingual n.

Facial (VII) (intermediate n.)
Taste via chorda tympani to lingual n.

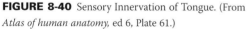

Trigeminal n. (V)
Glossopharyngeal n. (IX)
Vagus n. (X)
Facial n. (VII)

FIGURE 8-40 Sensory Innervation of Tongue. (From *Atlas of human anatomy*, ed 6, Plate 61.)

TABLE 8-11 Major Salivary Glands	
GLAND	**TYPE AND INNERVATION**
Parotid	Serous gland innervated by CN IX parasympathetics that course via lesser petrosal nerve (CN IX), synapsing in otic ganglion, with postganglionics conveyed to the gland in auriculotemporal nerve (branch of CN V₃); secretes via **parotid** (Stensen's) **duct**
Submandibular	Seromucous gland innervated by CN VII parasympathetics that course to the gland via chorda tympani branch of CN VII and join lingual nerve to synapse in submandibular ganglion (branch of CN V₃); secretes via **submandibular** (Wharton's) **duct**
Sublingual	Largely mucous gland innervated by CN VII parasympathetics coursing similar to those supplying submandibular gland above; secretes via many **small ducts in sublingual fold**

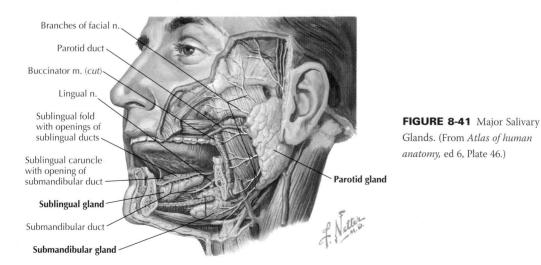

Branches of facial n.
Parotid duct
Buccinator m. (*cut*)
Lingual n.
Sublingual fold with openings of sublingual ducts
Sublingual caruncle with opening of submandibular duct
Sublingual gland
Submandibular duct
Submandibular gland
Parotid gland

FIGURE 8-41 Major Salivary Glands. (From *Atlas of human anatomy*, ed 6, Plate 46.)

carbohydrates, lysozyme to control bacterial flora, bicarbonate ions for buffering, antibodies, and the calcium and phosphate essential for healthy teeth. We produce about 1.2 L of saliva each day. As summarized in Table 8-11, the three pairs of salivary glands are innervated by parasympathetic nerve fibers from CN VII (submandibular and sublingual glands) and CN IX (parotid gland).

Palate

The palate forms the floor of the nasal cavity and the roof of the oral cavity. The palate is divided as follows (Figs. 8-42 and 8-43):

- **Hard palate:** bony anterior two thirds of the palate; formed by the palatal process of the maxilla and horizontal process of the

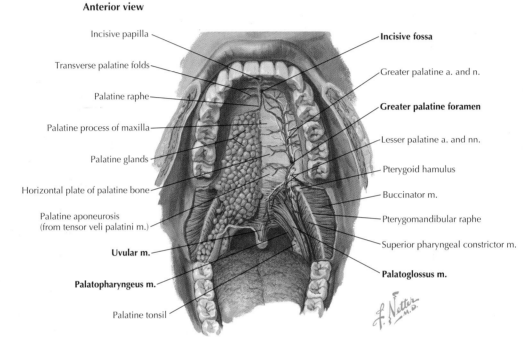

Anterior view

Incisive papilla

Transverse palatine folds

Palatine raphe

Palatine process of maxilla

Palatine glands

Horizontal plate of palatine bone

Palatine aponeurosis (from tensor veli palatini m.)

Uvular m.

Palatopharyngeus m.

Palatine tonsil

Incisive fossa

Greater palatine a. and n.

Greater palatine foramen

Lesser palatine a. and nn.

Pterygoid hamulus

Buccinator m.

Pterygomandibular raphe

Superior pharyngeal constrictor m.

Palatoglossus m.

FIGURE 8-42 Oral Cavity with Partial Dissection of Palate. (From *Atlas of human anatomy,* ed 6, Plate 57.)

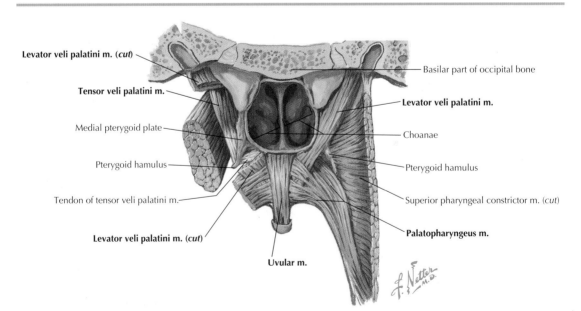

Levator veli palatini m. (*cut*)

Tensor veli palatini m.

Medial pterygoid plate

Pterygoid hamulus

Tendon of tensor veli palatini m.

Levator veli palatini m. (*cut*)

Uvular m.

Basilar part of occipital bone

Levator veli palatini m.

Choanae

Pterygoid hamulus

Superior pharyngeal constrictor m. (*cut*)

Palatopharyngeus m.

FIGURE 8-43 Posterior View of Soft Palate Muscles. (From *Atlas of human anatomy,* ed 6, Plate 57.)

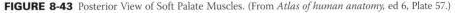

palatine bone; covered by a thick mucosa that overlies numerous mucus-secreting palatal glands.

- **Soft palate:** posterior third of the palate; composed of a mucosa and mucus-secreting palatal glands, with five muscles that contribute to the soft palate and its movements; closes off the nasopharynx during swallowing.

Sensory innervation of the hard palate is largely via the **nasopalatine** and **greater palatine nerves** (CN V$_2$), whereas sensory innervation of the soft palate is largely through the **lesser palatine nerves** (CN V$_2$) (Fig. 8-42). The muscles of the soft palate are summarized in Table 8-12.

Teeth and Gums (Gingivae)

The **maxillary teeth** (upper jaw) number 16 in adults: 4 incisors, 2 canines, 4 premolars (bicuspids), and 6 molars (tricuspids). The **mandibular teeth** (lower jaw) also have 16 teeth of the same, for a total of 32 adult teeth (Fig. 8-44). The third set of molars are the last to erupt and are commonly referred to as the "wisdom teeth." Children possess 20 deciduous teeth (4 incisors, 2 canines,

TABLE 8-12 Muscles of the Soft Palate

MUSCLE	SUPERIOR ATTACHMENT (ORIGIN)	INFERIOR ATTACHMENT (INSERTION)	INNERVATION	MAIN ACTIONS
Levator veli palatini	Auditory tube and temporal bone	Palatine aponeurosis	Vagus nerve via pharyngeal plexus	Elevates soft palate during swallowing
Tensor veli palatini	Scaphoid fossa of medial pterygoid plate, spine of sphenoid, and auditory tube	Palatine aponeurosis	Mandibular nerve	Tenses soft palate and opens auditory tube during swallowing and yawning
Palatoglossus	Palatine aponeurosis of soft palate	Side of tongue	Vagus nerve via pharyngeal plexus	Elevates posterior tongue
Palatopharyngeus	Hard palate and palatine aponeurosis	Lateral wall of pharynx	Vagus nerve via pharyngeal plexus	Tenses soft palate; pulls walls of pharynx superiorly, anteriorly, and medially during swallowing
Musculus uvulae	Nasal spine and palatine aponeurosis	Mucosa of uvula	Vagus nerve via pharyngeal plexus	Shortens, elevates, and retracts uvula

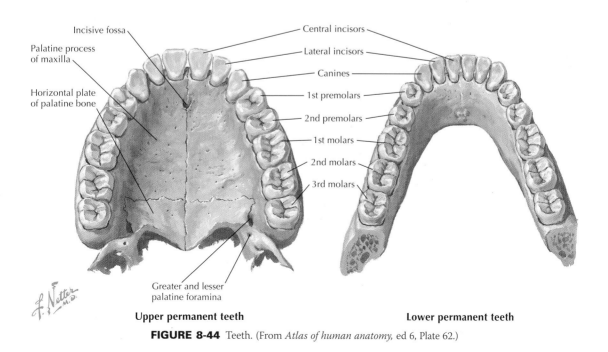

Incisive fossa

Palatine process of maxilla

Horizontal plate of palatine bone

Central incisors

Lateral incisors

Canines

1st premolars

2nd premolars

1st molars

2nd molars

3rd molars

Greater and lesser palatine foramina

Upper permanent teeth   **Lower permanent teeth**

FIGURE 8-44 Teeth. (From *Atlas of human anatomy,* ed 6, Plate 62.)

Common Oral Lesions

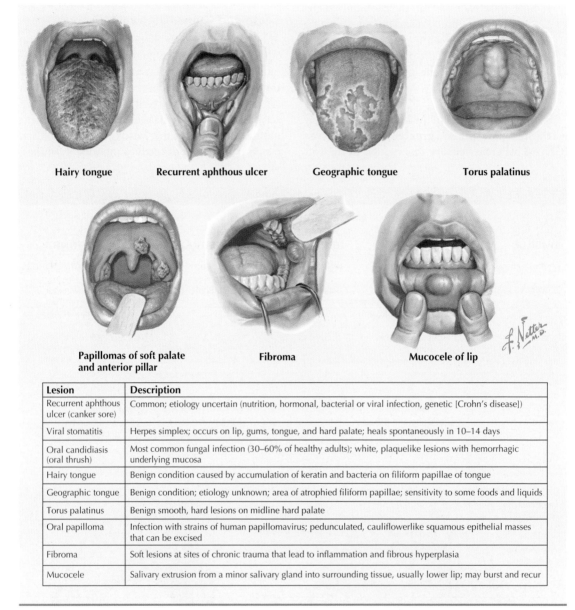

Hairy tongue   Recurrent aphthous ulcer   Geographic tongue   Torus palatinus

Papillomas of soft palate   Fibroma   Mucocele of lip
and anterior pillar

Lesion	Description
Recurrent aphthous ulcer (canker sore)	Common; etiology uncertain (nutrition, hormonal, bacterial or viral infection, genetic [Crohn's disease])
Viral stomatitis	Herpes simplex; occurs on lip, gums, tongue, and hard palate; heals spontaneously in 10–14 days
Oral candidiasis (oral thrush)	Most common fungal infection (30–60% of healthy adults); white, plaquelike lesions with hemorrhagic underlying mucosa
Hairy tongue	Benign condition caused by accumulation of keratin and bacteria on filiform papillae of tongue
Geographic tongue	Benign condition; etiology unknown; area of atrophied filiform papillae; sensitivity to some foods and liquids
Torus palatinus	Benign smooth, hard lesions on midline hard palate
Oral papilloma	Infection with strains of human papillomavirus; pedunculated, cauliflowerlike squamous epithelial masses that can be excised
Fibroma	Soft lesions at sites of chronic trauma that lead to inflammation and fibrous hyperplasia
Mucocele	Salivary extrusion from a minor salivary gland into surrounding tissue, usually lower lip; may burst and recur

and 4 molars in each jaw), which usually have erupted by the third year of life. The central mandibular incisors usually are the first deciduous teeth to erupt at about the sixth or seventh month of age.

The maxillary teeth receive sensory innervation by the anterior, middle, and posterior superior alveolar nerves from CN V_2 and the mandibular teeth by the inferior alveolar nerve (CN V_3).

The maxillary buccal (side facing the cheek) gingivae receive sensory innervation by the same nerves from CN V_2 as the maxillary teeth, but the lingual (side facing the tongue) gingivae are innervated by the greater palatine and nasopalatine nerves of CN V_2. The mandibular buccal gingivae receive sensory innervation by the buccal and mental nerves from CN V_3, and the lingual gingivae from the lingual nerve (CN V_3).

Clinical Focus 8-40

Cancer of the Oral Cavity

Squamous cell carcinoma (SCC) accounts for more than 90% of cancers in this region, so the information here focuses on SCC. All these lesions may present with palpable submental, submandibular, and upper cervical lymph nodes.

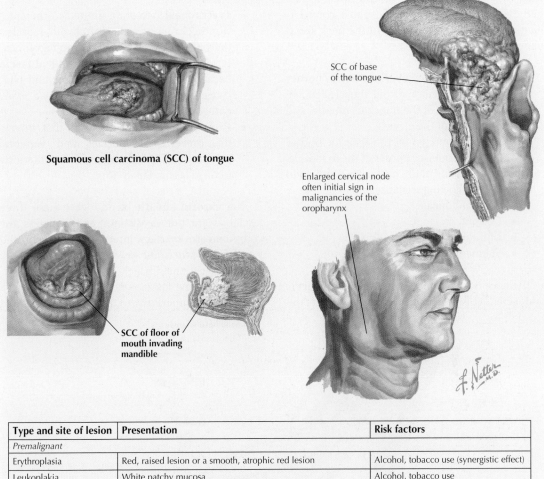

SCC of base of the tongue

Squamous cell carcinoma (SCC) of tongue

Enlarged cervical node often initial sign in malignancies of the oropharynx

SCC of floor of mouth invading mandible

Type and site of lesion	Presentation	Risk factors
Premalignant		
Erythroplasia	Red, raised lesion or a smooth, atrophic red lesion	Alcohol, tobacco use (synergistic effect)
Leukoplakia	White patchy mucosa	Alcohol, tobacco use
Malignant		
Lip SCC (90% lower lip)	Nonhealing, crusting ulcerative lesion or scaly, hyperkeratotic lesion at vermilion border of lip	Ultraviolet (sun) exposure
Tongue SCC	Anterolateral tongue; nonhealing ulcer; exophytic lesion	Alcohol, tobacco use
Floor of mouth	Anterior tongue; may infiltrate mandible; trismus if muscles of mastication involved	Alcohol, tobacco use
Oropharynx SCC	Ulcerative or infiltrating mucosal lesions; pain; dysphagia	Alcohol, tobacco use

The blood to the maxillary teeth comes from the anterior (a branch of the infra-orbital branch of the maxillary artery) and posterior (a branch of the maxillary artery) superior alveolar arteries. The blood supply to the mandibular teeth comes from the inferior alveolar artery (branch of the maxillary artery). The venous drainage is from corresponding veins, most of which drain into the pterygoid plexus of veins in the infratemporal fossa.

11. NECK

The neck is divided descriptively into two major triangles. Each triangle contains key structures used as landmarks by anatomists and physicians operating in this area. The neck is a vertical conduit for structures entering or leaving the head. It is tightly bound in several fascial layers that divide the neck into descriptive compartments. The two major triangles of the neck are as follows (Fig. 8-45):

- **Posterior:** bounded by the posterior border of the sternocleidomastoid muscle (SCM), anterior border of the trapezius muscle, and middle third of the clavicle.
- **Anterior:** bounded by the anterior border of the SCM, inferior border of the mandible, and the midline of the neck; also subdivided into the following triangles:
  - Submandibular
  - Carotid
  - Muscular
  - Submental

The neck is surrounded by a **superficial cervical fascia** that lies deep to the skin and invests the platysma muscle (a muscle of facial expression). A second **deep cervical fascia** tightly invests the neck structures and is divided into the following three layers (Fig. 8-46):

- **Investing:** surrounds the neck and invests the trapezius and SCM muscles (*red* fascia, Fig. 8-46).
- **Pretracheal** (visceral): limited to the anterior neck; invests the infrahyoid muscles, thyroid gland, trachea, and esophagus; posteriorly called the **buccopharyngeal fascia** because it covers the buccinator and pharyngeal constrictor muscles (*purple, blue,* and *green* fasciae, Fig. 8-46).
- **Prevertebral:** tubular sheath that invests the prevertebral muscles and vertebral column; includes the **alar fascia** anteriorly (*orange* fascia, Fig. 8-46).

The **carotid sheath** blends with these three fascial layers but is distinct and contains the common carotid artery, internal jugular vein, and vagus nerve (*dark blue* fascial sheath in Fig. 8-46, *top* cross-sectional image).

The investing fascia is not limited to the neck but extends superiorly to the hyoid bone and

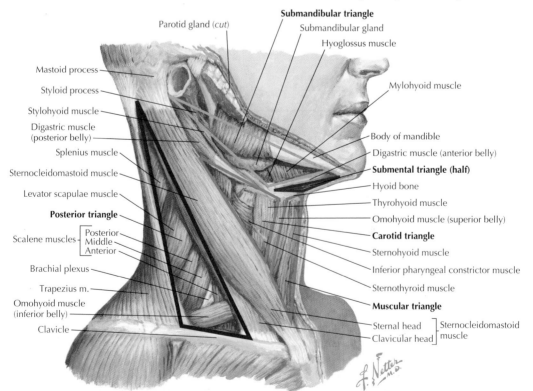

FIGURE 8-45 Triangles of the Neck.

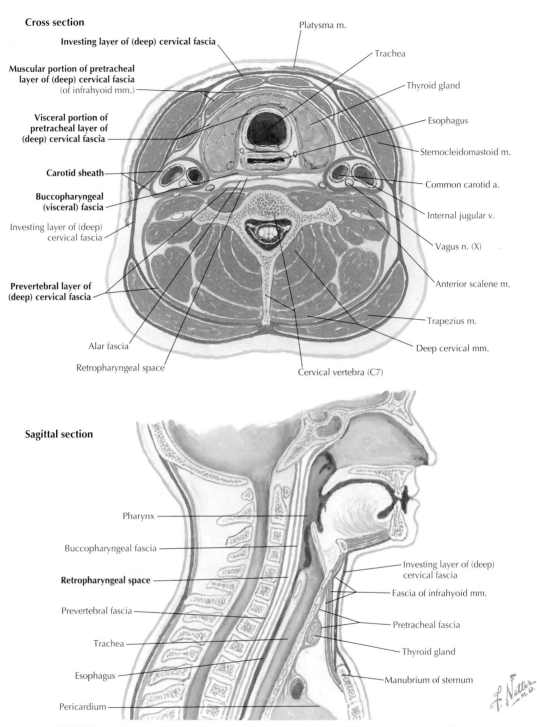

Cross section

Investing layer of (deep) cervical fascia

Muscular portion of pretracheal layer of (deep) cervical fascia (of infrahyoid mm.)

Visceral portion of pretracheal layer of (deep) cervical fascia

Carotid sheath

Buccopharyngeal (visceral) fascia

Investing layer of (deep) cervical fascia

Prevertebral layer of (deep) cervical fascia

Alar fascia

Retropharyngeal space

Platysma m.

Trachea

Thyroid gland

Esophagus

Sternocleidomastoid m.

Common carotid a.

Internal jugular v.

Vagus n. (X)

Anterior scalene m.

Trapezius m.

Deep cervical mm.

Cervical vertebra (C7)

Sagittal section

Pharynx

Buccopharyngeal fascia

Retropharyngeal space

Prevertebral fascia

Trachea

Esophagus

Pericardium

Investing layer of (deep) cervical fascia

Fascia of infrahyoid mm.

Pretracheal fascia

Thyroid gland

Manubrium of sternum

FIGURE 8-46 Cervical Fascial Layers and Spaces. (From *Atlas of human anatomy*, ed 6, Plate 26.)

envelops the submandibular salivary gland. As it courses along the inferior margin of the mandible, the investing fascia also envelops the parotid salivary gland and then extends to the mastoid process and zygomatic arch.

Muscles

The muscles of the anterior and posterior triangles are summarized in Figure 8-47 and Table 8-13. The **suprahyoid muscles** raise the hyoid bone toward a stabilized mandible during swallowing.

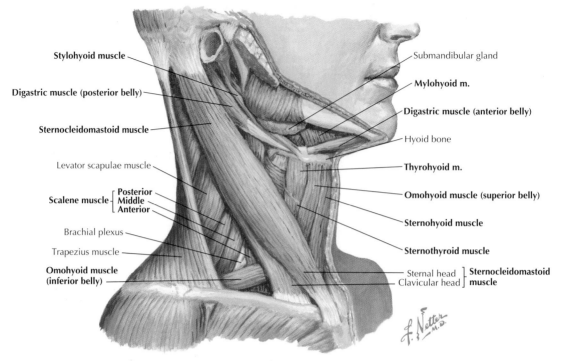

FIGURE 8-47 Muscles of the Neck. (From *Atlas of human anatomy,* ed 6, Plate 29.)

TABLE 8-13 Muscles of the Neck

MUSCLE	ORIGIN	INSERTION	INNERVATION	MAIN ACTIONS
Sternocleidomastoid	*Sternal head:* manubrium *Clavicular head:* medial third of clavicle	Mastoid process and lateral half of superior nuchal line	Spinal root of cranial nerve CN XI and C2-C3	Tilts head to one side, i.e., laterally flexes and rotates head so face is turned superiorly toward opposite side; acting together, muscles flex neck
Posterior scalene	Posterior tubercles of transverse processes of C4-C6	2nd rib	C6-C8	Flexes neck laterally; elevates 2nd rib
Middle scalene	Posterior tubercles of transverse processes of C2-C7	1st rib	C3-C8	Flexes neck laterally; elevates 1st rib
Anterior scalene	Anterior tubercles of transverse processes of C3-C6	1st rib	C5-C7	Flexes neck laterally; elevates 1st rib
Digastric	*Anterior belly:* digastric fossa of mandible *Posterior belly:* mastoid notch	Intermediate tendon to hyoid bone	*Anterior belly:* mylohyoid nerve, a branch of inferior alveolar nerve *Posterior belly:* facial nerve	Depresses mandible; raises hyoid bone and steadies it during swallowing and speaking
Sternohyoid	Manubrium of sternum and medial end of clavicle	Body of hyoid bone	C1-C3 from ansa cervicalis	Depresses hyoid bone after swallowing
Sternothyroid	Posterior surface of manubrium	Oblique line of thyroid lamina	C2 and C3 from ansa cervicalis	Depresses larynx after swallowing
Thyrohyoid	Oblique line of thyroid cartilage	Body and greater horn of hyoid bone	C1 via hypoglossal nerve	Depresses hyoid bone and elevates larynx when hyoid bone is fixed
Omohyoid	Superior border of scapula near suprascapular notch	Inferior border of hyoid bone	C1-C3 from ansa cervicalis	Depresses, retracts, and fixes hyoid bone
Mylohyoid	Mylohyoid line of mandible	Raphe and body of hyoid bone	Mylohyoid nerve, a branch of inferior alveolar nerve of V_3	Elevates hyoid bone, floor of mouth, and tongue during swallowing and speaking
Stylohyoid	Styloid process	Body of hyoid bone	Facial nerve	Elevates and retracts hyoid bone

The **infrahyoid muscles** depress the hyoid bone and larynx during swallowing and vocalization.

Cervical Plexus

The (spinal) accessory nerve (CN XI) exits the jugular foramen and crosses the posterior triangle, innervating the SCM and trapezius muscles (Fig. 8-48). However, the **cervical plexus**, composed of the **ventral rami of C1-C4,** innervates most of the neck muscles and provides sensory innervation to the anterior and lateral neck (Table 8-14). Additional innervation includes:

- The mylohyoid nerve (CN V₃) innervates the mylohyoid muscle and anterior belly of the digastric muscle beneath the chin.

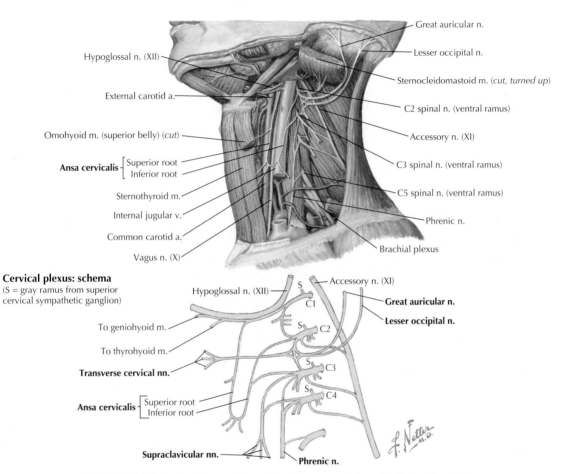

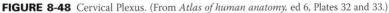

FIGURE 8-48 Cervical Plexus. (From *Atlas of human anatomy*, ed 6, Plates 32 and 33.)

TABLE 8-14 Cervical Plexus			
NERVE	**INNERVATION**	**NERVE**	**INNERVATION**
C1	Travels with cranial nerve CN XII to innervate geniohyoid and thyrohyoid muscles	Supraclavicular	From C3 to C4, are anterior, middle, and posterior sensory branches to skin over clavicle and shoulder region
Ansa cervicalis	Is C1-C3 loop that sends motor branches to infrahyoid muscles	Phrenic	From C3 to C5, is motor and sensory nerve to diaphragm
Lesser occipital	From C2, is sensory to neck and scalp posterior to ear	Motor branches	Are small twigs that supply scalene muscles, levator scapulae, and prevertebral muscles
Great auricular	From C2 to C3, is sensory over parotid gland and posterior ear		
Transverse cervical	From C2 to C3, is sensory to anterior triangle of neck		

- The facial nerve (CN VII) innervates the platysma muscle through its cervical branch.
- The glossopharyngeal nerve (CN IX) supplies the carotid body and sinus (visceral sensory).
- The vagus nerve (CN X) supplies the larynx through its superior and recurrent (inferior) laryngeal nerves.
- The hypoglossal nerve (CN XII) loops through the neck to innervate the tongue.

Blood Supply

The arterial supply to the neck is by the **subclavian artery** (Fig. 8-49 and Table 8-15) and some of the branches of the **external carotid artery,** a branch of the common carotid artery (Fig. 8-50 and Table 8-16). The subclavian artery is divided for descriptive purposes into three parts: part 1 lies medial, part 2 lies posterior, and part 3 lies lateral to the anterior scalene muscle. Of the

TABLE 8-15 Branches of the Subclavian Artery

BRANCH	COURSE
Part 1	
Vertebral	Ascends through C6 to C1 transverse foramina and enters foramen magnum
Internal thoracic	Descends parasternally to anastomose with superior epigastric artery
Thyrocervical trunk	Gives rise to inferior thyroid, transverse cervical, and suprascapular arteries
Part 2	
Costocervical trunk	Gives rise to deep cervical and superior intercostal arteries
Part 3	
Dorsal scapular	Is inconstant; may also arise from transverse cervical artery

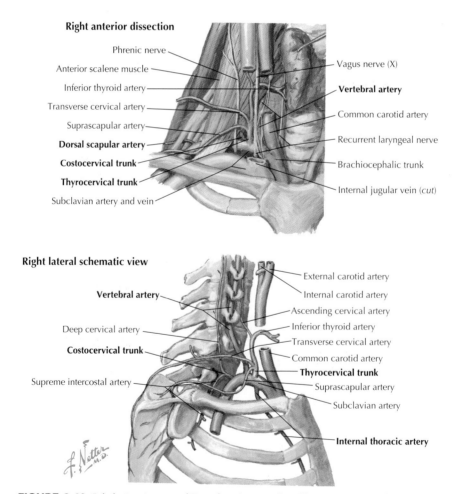

Right anterior dissection

Phrenic nerve
Anterior scalene muscle
Inferior thyroid artery
Transverse cervical artery
Suprascapular artery
Dorsal scapular artery
Costocervical trunk
Thyrocervical trunk
Subclavian artery and vein

Vagus nerve (X)
Vertebral artery
Common carotid artery
Recurrent laryngeal nerve
Brachiocephalic trunk
Internal jugular vein (cut)

Right lateral schematic view

Vertebral artery
Deep cervical artery
Costocervical trunk
Supreme intercostal artery

External carotid artery
Internal carotid artery
Ascending cervical artery
Inferior thyroid artery
Transverse cervical artery
Common carotid artery
Thyrocervical trunk
Suprascapular artery
Subclavian artery
Internal thoracic artery

FIGURE 8-49 Subclavian Artery and Branches. (From *Atlas of human anatomy,* ed 6, Plate 33.)

TABLE 8-16 Branches of the External Carotid Artery

BRANCH	COURSE AND STRUCTURES SUPPLIED
Superior thyroid	Supplies thyroid gland, larynx, and infrahyoid muscles
Ascending pharyngeal	Supplies pharyngeal region, middle ear, meninges, and prevertebral muscles
Lingual	Passes deep to hyoglossus muscle to supply the tongue
Facial	Courses over the mandible and supplies the face
Occipital	Supplies SCM and anastomoses with costocervical trunk
Posterior auricular	Supplies region posterior to ear
Maxillary	Passes into infratemporal fossa (described later)
Superficial temporal	Supplies face, temporalis muscle, and lateral scalp

branches of the subclavian artery listed in Table 8-15, the vertebral artery and the thyrocervical trunk and its branches are the primary blood supply to the neck. Of the branches of the external carotid artery listed in Table 8-16, the superior thyroid, the ascending pharyngeal, and the lingual also contribute to the blood supply of the neck.

The venous drainage of the neck is highly variable, but most of the blood ultimately drains into **tributaries of the external and internal jugular veins** (Fig. 8-51). The external jugular vein is formed by the posterior auricular and posterior branches of the retromandibular veins, while the internal jugular vein begins at the jugular foramen as a continuation of the sigmoid dural sinus (the small inferior petrosal sinus also ends at this point).

The **thoracic lymphatic duct** ascends through the thorax just anterior to the vertebral bodies, enters the root of the neck by passing posterior to the left carotid sheath, and loops inferiorly

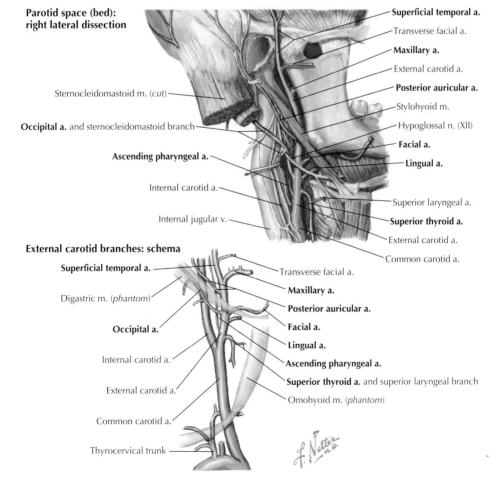

FIGURE 8-50 External Carotid Artery and Branches. (From *Atlas of human anatomy*, ed 6, Plate 34.)

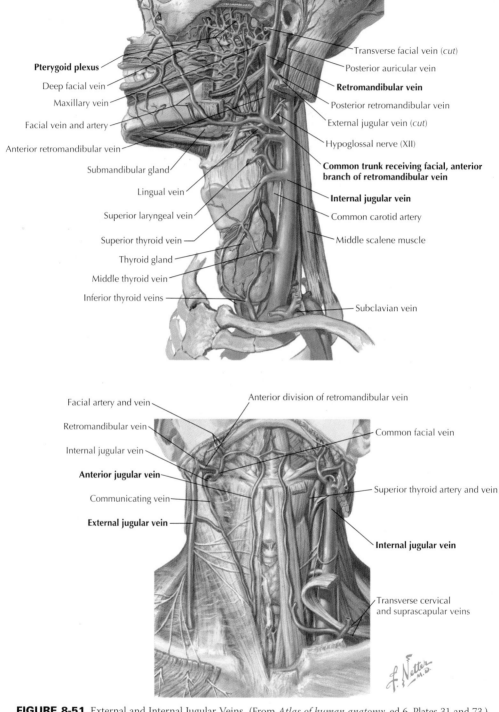

Pterygoid plexus

Deep facial vein

Maxillary vein

Facial vein and artery

Anterior retromandibular vein

Submandibular gland

Lingual vein

Superior laryngeal vein

Superior thyroid vein

Thyroid gland

Middle thyroid vein

Inferior thyroid veins

Transverse facial vein (*cut*)

Posterior auricular vein

Retromandibular vein

Posterior retromandibular vein

External jugular vein (*cut*)

Hypoglossal nerve (XII)

Common trunk receiving facial, anterior branch of retromandibular vein

Internal jugular vein

Common carotid artery

Middle scalene muscle

Subclavian vein

Facial artery and vein

Retromandibular vein

Internal jugular vein

Anterior jugular vein

Communicating vein

External jugular vein

Anterior division of retromandibular vein

Common facial vein

Superior thyroid artery and vein

Internal jugular vein

Transverse cervical and suprascapular veins

FIGURE 8-51 External and Internal Jugular Veins. (From *Atlas of human anatomy*, ed 6, Plates 31 and 73.)

to empty into the junction between the left subclavian vein and left internal jugular vein (see Figs. 3-12 and 3-26). The smaller **right lymphatic duct** collects lymph from the right side of the head, neck, thorax, and right upper limb and drains it into the corresponding junction of

the right subclavian vein and right internal jugular vein.

Thyroid and Parathyroid Glands

The **thyroid gland** lies at the C5-T1 vertebral level, anterior to the trachea, and is a ductless endocrine gland that weighs about 20 grams (Fig. 8-52 and Table 8-17). The thyroid gland has two lateral lobes connected by an isthmus that lies anterior to the second to fourth tracheal cartilaginous rings. It is enveloped in the visceral layer of the pretracheal fascia (*blue* fascia in Fig. 8-46). In about 50% of cases, a pyramidal lobe may extend superiorly from the isthmus, demarcating the embryonic migratory pathway of the thyroid from the base of the tongue (see Clinical Focus 8-49). The thyroid gland secretes thyroxine (T_4), triiodothyronine (T_3), and calcitonin and performs the following functions:

- Increases the metabolic rate of tissues.
- Increases the consumption of oxygen.
- Increases heart rate, ventilation, and renal function.
- Is required for growth hormone production and is important in CNS growth.
- Increases the deposition of calcium and phosphate in bones (calcitonin).

TABLE 8-17 Features of the Thyroid Gland

STRUCTURE	CHARACTERISTICS
Lobes	Right and left, with a thin isthmus joining them
Blood supply	Superior and inferior thyroid arteries
Venous drainage	Superior, middle, and inferior thyroid veins
Pyramidal lobe	Variable (50% of time) superior extension of thyroid tissue

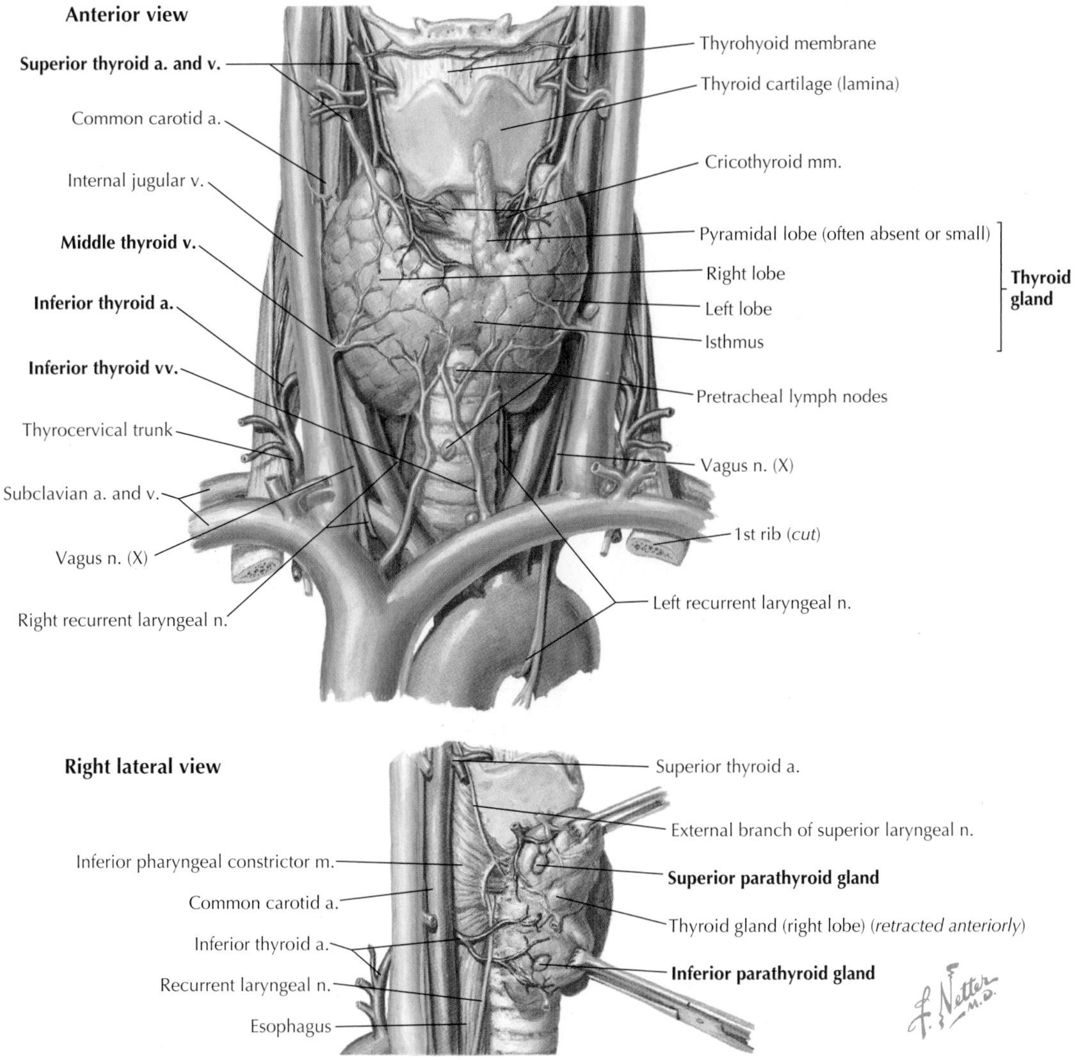

FIGURE 8-52 Thyroid and Parathyroid Glands and Blood Supply. (From *Atlas of human anatomy*, ed 6, Plates 76 and 78.)

Clinical Focus 8-41

Hyperthyroidism with Diffuse Goiter (Graves' Disease)

Graves' disease is the most common cause of hyperthyroidism in patients younger than 40. Excess synthesis and release of thyroid hormone (T_3 and T_4) result in thyrotoxicosis, which upregulates tissue metabolism and leads to symptoms, indicating increased metabolism. Besides Graves' disease, hyperthyroidism can be caused by benign growth of the thyroid gland, benign growth of the anterior pituitary gland, thyroiditis, the ingestion of excessive amounts of thyroid hormones and iodine, and tumors of the ovaries.

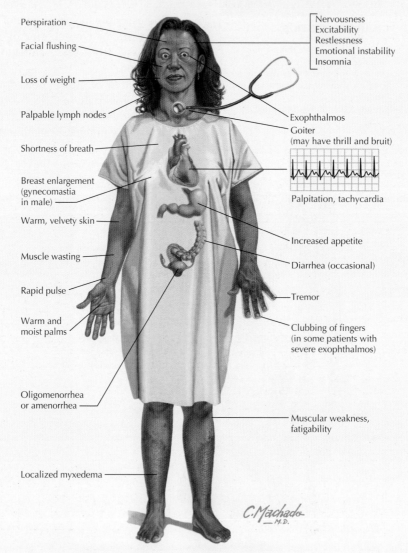

Perspiration

Facial flushing

Loss of weight

Palpable lymph nodes

Shortness of breath

Breast enlargement
(gynecomastia
in male)

Warm, velvety skin

Muscle wasting

Rapid pulse

Warm and
moist palms

Oligomenorrhea
or amenorrhea

Localized myxedema

Nervousness
Excitability
Restlessness
Emotional instability
Insomnia

Exophthalmos
Goiter
(may have thrill and bruit)

Palpitation, tachycardia

Increased appetite

Diarrhea (occasional)

Tremor

Clubbing of fingers
(in some patients with
severe exophthalmos)

Muscular weakness,
fatigability

C. Machado
_M.D.

Characteristic	Description
Etiology	Autoimmune disease with antibodies directed against thyroid-stimulating hormone (TSH) receptor, stimulating release of hormone or increasing thyroid epithelial cell activity; familial predisposition
Prevalence	Seven times more common in women than in men; peak incidence between 20 and 40 years of age
Signs	Thyrotoxicosis (hyperfunctional state), lid lag, exophthalmos (infiltrative increase in retrobulbar connective tissue and extra-ocular muscles), pretibial myxedema (thickened skin on leg); most common cause of endogenous hyperthyroidism

Primary Hypothyroidism

Primary hypothyroidism is a disease in which the thyroid gland produces inadequate amounts of thyroid hormone to meet the body's needs. Thyroid-stimulating hormone (TSH) levels are elevated. In addition to the autoimmune form of the disease, hypothyroidism also may occur from thyroidectomy and radiation-related damage.

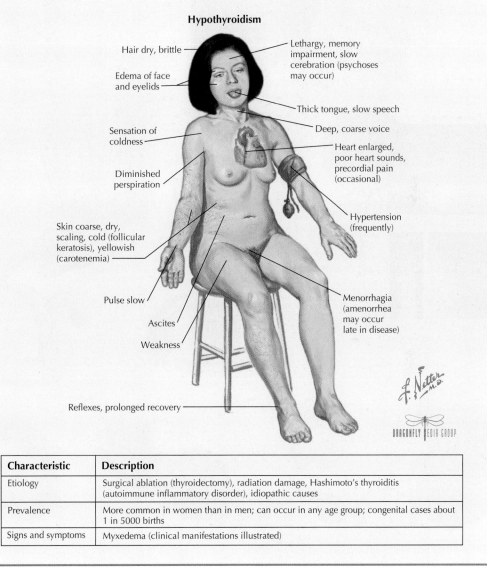

Hypothyroidism

Characteristic	Description
Etiology	Surgical ablation (thyroidectomy), radiation damage, Hashimoto's thyroiditis (autoimmune inflammatory disorder), idiopathic causes
Prevalence	More common in women than in men; can occur in any age group; congenital cases about 1 in 5000 births
Signs and symptoms	Myxedema (clinical manifestations illustrated)

The **parathyroid glands** are paired superior and inferior glands (number and location can vary significantly) located on the posterior aspect of the thyroid gland (see Fig. 8-52). The parathyroid glands secrete parathyroid hormone (PTH) in response to low calcium levels in the bloodstream and perform the following functions:

- Cause the resorption and release of calcium from bone; 99% of the body's calcium is stored in bone.
- Cause the resorption of calcium by the kidney.
- Alter vitamin D metabolism, critical for calcium absorption from the GI tract.

Clinical Focus 8-43

Manifestations of Primary Hyperparathyroidism

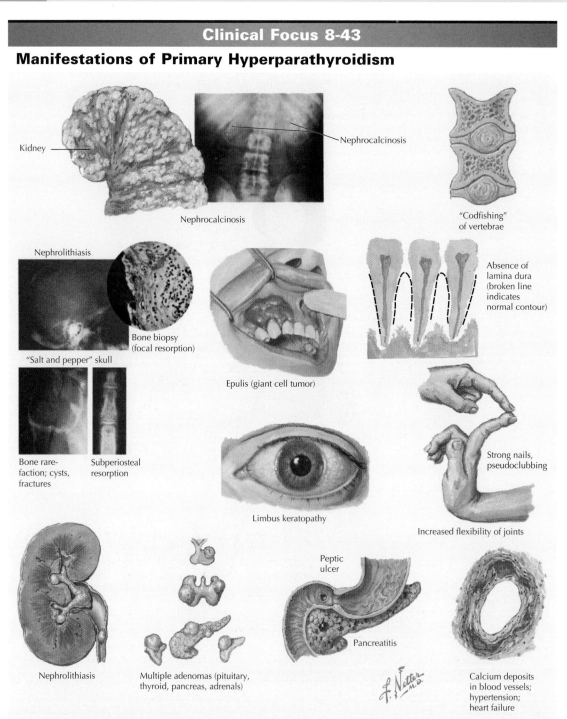

Kidney

Nephrocalcinosis

Nephrocalcinosis

"Codfishing" of vertebrae

Nephrolithiasis

Bone biopsy (focal resorption)

Absence of lamina dura (broken line indicates normal contour)

"Salt and pepper" skull

Epulis (giant cell tumor)

Bone rare-faction; cysts, fractures

Subperiosteal resorption

Strong nails, pseudoclubbing

Limbus keratopathy

Increased flexibility of joints

Peptic ulcer

Pancreatitis

Nephrolithiasis

Multiple adenomas (pituitary, thyroid, pancreas, adrenals)

Calcium deposits in blood vessels; hypertension; heart failure

Characteristic	Description
Etiology	Hypertrophy of parathyroid glands (>85% are solitary benign adenomas), which leads to secretion of excess parathyroid hormone that causes increased calcium levels
Presentation	Mild or nonspecific symptoms including fatigue, constipation, polyuria, polydipsia, depression, skeletal pain, and nausea
Prevalence	Approximately 100,000 new cases/year in the United States; 2:1 prevalence in women, which increases with age
Management	Surgical removal of parathyroid glands

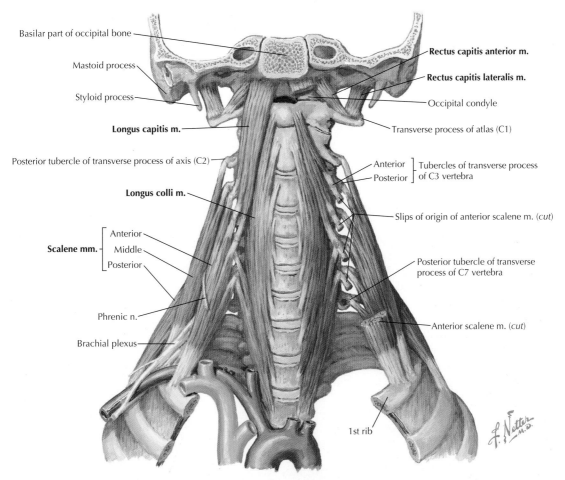

Basilar part of occipital bone

Mastoid process

Styloid process

Longus capitis m.

Posterior tubercle of transverse process of axis (C2)

Longus colli m.

Scalene mm. — Anterior / Middle / Posterior

Phrenic n.

Brachial plexus

Rectus capitis anterior m.

Rectus capitis lateralis m.

Occipital condyle

Transverse process of atlas (C1)

Anterior / Posterior — Tubercles of transverse process of C3 vertebra

Slips of origin of anterior scalene m. (*cut*)

Posterior tubercle of transverse process of C7 vertebra

Anterior scalene m. (*cut*)

1st rib

FIGURE 8-53 Prevertebral Muscles. (From *Atlas of human anatomy,* ed 6, Plate 30.)

TABLE 8-18 Prevertebral Muscles

MUSCLE	INFERIOR ATTACHMENT	SUPERIOR ATTACHMENT	INNERVATION	MAIN ACTIONS
Longus colli	Body of T1-T3 with attachments to bodies of C4-C7 and transverse processes of C3-C6	Anterior tubercle of C1 (atlas), transverse processes of C4-C6, and bodies of C2-C6	C2-C6 spinal nerves	Flexes cervical vertebrae; allows slight rotation
Longus capitis	Anterior tubercles of C3-C6 transverse processes	Basilar part of occipital bone	C2-C3 spinal nerves	Flexes head
Rectus capitis anterior	Lateral mass of C1 (atlas)	Base of occipital bone, anterior to occipital condyle	C1-C2 spinal nerves	Flexes head
Rectus capitis lateralis	Transverse process of C1 (atlas)	Jugular process of occipital bone	C1-C2 spinal nerves	Flexes and helps stabilize head

Prevertebral Muscles

A group of deep neck flexor muscles called the prevertebral muscles lie surrounded by the prevertebral fascia adjacent to the bodies of the cervical and upper thoracic vertebrae (Fig. 8-53 and Table 8-18). Generally, these muscles stabilize the cervical vertebrae and flex the neck. Additionally, the **scalene muscles** (posterior, middle and anterior) help elevate the rib cage and laterally flex the neck (see Table 8-13). The ventral rami of the nerves forming the cervical plexus (C1-C4) and brachial plexus (C5-T1) pass laterally between the anterior and middle scalene muscles. The **phrenic nerve** (ventral rami of C3-C5), which innervates the diaphragm, emerges from between the middle and anterior scalene muscles and can usually be found lying on the anterior surface of the anterior scalene as it descends to enter the thoracic cavity (see Figs. 8-48, 8-49, and 8-53).

12. PHARYNX

The **pharynx** (throat), a fibromuscular tube, connects the nasal and oral cavities of the head with the larynx and esophagus in the neck (Fig. 8-54). It extends from the base of the skull to the cricoid cartilage, where it is continuous with the esophagus. The pharynx is subdivided as follows:

- **Nasopharynx:** lies posterior to the nasal cavity above the soft palate.
- **Oropharynx:** extends from the soft palate to the superior tip of the epiglottis; lies posterior to the oral cavity.

- **Laryngopharynx:** extends from the tip of the epiglottis to the inferior aspect of the cricoid cartilage; also known clinically as the *hypopharynx*.

The muscles of the pharynx participate in swallowing (deglutition) and contract serially from superior to inferior to move a bolus of food from the oropharynx and laryngopharynx into the proximal esophagus (Fig. 8-55 and Table 8-19).

The blood supply to the pharynx is via branches of the **thyrocervical trunk** (subclavian), especially the ascending cervical artery (see Figs. 8-49 and Table 8-15) and the **external carotid artery** (principally its superior thyroid, facial, ascending pharyngeal, and maxillary branches) (see Fig. 8-50 and Table 8-16). Venous drainage is via the pharyngeal venous plexus, the pterygoid plexus of veins, and the facial, lingual, and superior thyroid veins, all of which drain primarily into the internal jugular vein (see Fig. 8-51).

The sensory innervation of the nasopharynx is by the pharyngeal branch of V_2; sensory innervation to the oropharynx is by CN IX; and sensory

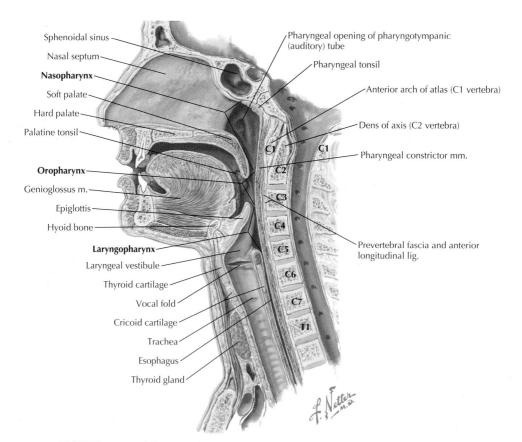

FIGURE 8-54 Subdivisions of the Pharynx. (From *Atlas of human anatomy,* ed 6, Plate 64.)

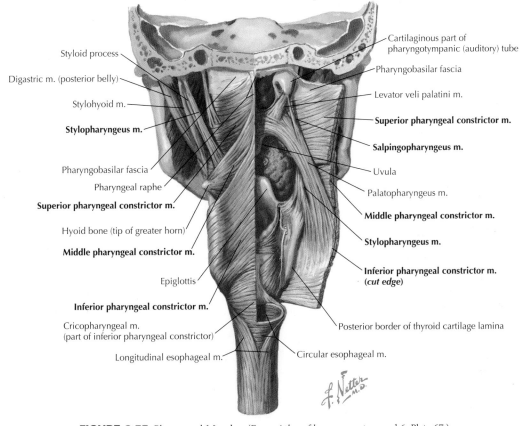

FIGURE 8-55 Pharyngeal Muscles. (From *Atlas of human anatomy,* ed 6, Plate 67.)

TABLE 8-19 Pharyngeal Muscles

MUSCLE	ORIGIN	INSERTION	INNERVATION	MAIN ACTIONS
Superior pharyngeal constrictor	Hamulus, pterygomandibular raphe, mylohyoid line of mandible	Median raphe of pharynx	Vagus via pharyngeal plexus	Constricts wall of pharynx during swallowing
Middle pharyngeal constrictor	Stylohyoid ligament and horns of hyoid bone	Median raphe of pharynx	Vagus via pharyngeal plexus	Constricts wall of pharynx during swallowing
Inferior pharyngeal constrictor	Oblique line of thyroid cartilage, and cricoid cartilage	Median raphe of pharynx	Vagus via pharyngeal plexus	Constricts wall of pharynx during swallowing
Salpingopharyngeus	Auditory (pharyngotympanic) tube	Side of pharynx wall	Vagus via pharyngeal plexus	Elevates pharynx and larynx during swallowing and speaking
Stylopharyngeus	Medial aspect of styloid process	Posterior and superior borders of thyroid cartilage	Glossopharyngeal nerve	Elevates pharynx and larynx during swallowing and speaking

innervation of the laryngopharynx is by CN X. The motor innervation is by CN X and its pharyngeal plexus, except the stylopharyngeus muscle, which is innervated by CN IX.

Swallowing, or **deglutition,** includes the following sequence of events (Fig. 8-56):

- The tongue pushes the bolus of food up against the hard palate.
- The soft palate elevates to close off the nasopharynx.
- The tongue pushes the bolus back into the oropharynx.

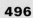

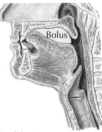 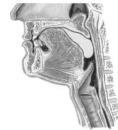 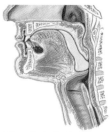

A. The tip of the tongue contacts the anterior part of palate while the bolus is pushed posteriorly in a groove between tongue and palate. The soft palate is drawn upward as a bulge forms in the upper part of posterior pharyngeal wall (Passavant's ridge) and approaches the rising soft palate.

B. As tongue gradually presses more of its dorsal surface against the hard palate, the bolus is pushed posteriorly into the oropharynx. The soft palate is drawn superiorly to contact Passavant's ridge and closes off the nasopharynx. A receptive space is created in the oropharynx as the root of the tongue moves slightly anterior. The stylopharyngeus and upper pharyngeal constrictor mm. contract to raise the pharyngeal wall over the bolus.

C. When the bolus has reached the vallecula, the hyoid and larynx move superior and anterior while the epiglottis is tipped inferiorly. A "stripping wave" on the posterior pharyngeal wall moves inferiorly.

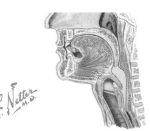 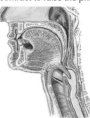 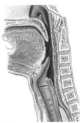

D. The soft palate is pulled inferiorly and approximated to the root of tongue by contraction of the palatopharyngeus and pressure of the descending "stripping wave." The oropharyngeal cavity is closed by contraction of upper pharyngeal constrictors. Relaxation of the cricopharyngeus permits entry of the bolus into the esophagus. A trickle of food may enter the laryngeal aditus.

E. "Stripping wave" reaches vallecula and presses out the last of the bolus. The cricopharyngeus remains relaxed and the bolus has largely passed into the esophagus.

F. "Stripping wave" passes the pharynx and the epiglottis begins to turn superiorly as the hyoid and larynx descend. Communication with the nasopharynx is re-established.

G. All structures of the pharynx return to their resting position as the "stripping wave" passes into the esophagus, pushing the bolus before it.

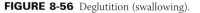

FIGURE 8-56 Deglutition (swallowing).

- As the bolus reaches the epiglottis, the larynx elevates and the tip of the epiglottis tips downward over the laryngeal opening (aditus).
- Contractions of the pharyngeal constrictors squeeze the bolus into two streams that pass on either side of the epiglottis and down along the piriform recesses and into the upper esophagus.
- The soft palate pulls downward to assist in moving the bolus around the epiglottis.
- The laryngeal vestibule and rima glottidis (space between the vocal folds) close to protect the larynx.
- Once the bolus is in the esophagus, all structures return to their starting positions.

The superior openings into the pharynx (nasal and oral cavities) are "guarded" by a ring of lymphoid tissue in the mucosa that composes **Waldeyer's tonsillar ring** and includes the following (Fig. 8-57):

- **Tubal tonsils:** lymphoid tissue adjacent to the opening of the auditory tube; may be continuous with the pharyngeal tonsils.
- **Pharyngeal tonsils:** lie in the posterior wall and roof of the nasopharynx; called **adenoids** when enlarged.
- **Palatine tonsils:** guard the oropharynx and lie between the palatoglossal and palatopharyngeal folds; receive a rich blood supply from branches of facial, lingual, ascending pharyngeal, and maxillary arteries of the external carotid.
- **Lingual tonsils:** collection of lymphoid nodules on the posterior third of the tongue.

13. LARYNX

The **larynx** (voice box) is a musculoligamentous and cartilaginous structure that lies at the C3-C6 vertebral level, just superior to the trachea. It functions both as a sphincter to close off the

Medial view
Median (sagittal) section

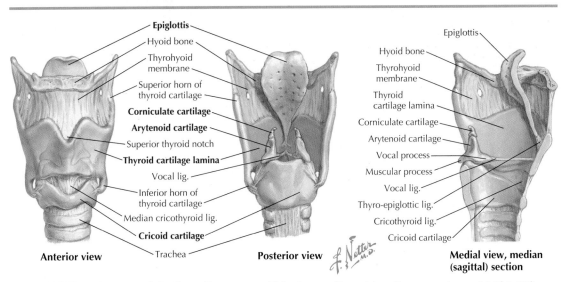

Sphenoidal sinus
Pharyngeal tonsil
Torus tubarius
Opening of auditory tube
Salpingopharyngeal fold
Palatine glands
Uvula
Palatine tonsil
Palatopharyngeal arch
Palatoglossal arch
Tongue (*drawn forward*)
Lingual tonsil
Epiglottis
Vallecula

FIGURE 8-57 Tonsils. (From *Atlas of human anatomy,* ed 6, Plate 68.)

Anterior view

Epiglottis
Hyoid bone
Thyrohyoid membrane
Superior horn of thyroid cartilage
Corniculate cartilage
Arytenoid cartilage
Superior thyroid notch
Thyroid cartilage lamina
Vocal lig.
Inferior horn of thyroid cartilage
Median cricothyroid lig.
Cricoid cartilage
Trachea

Posterior view

Medial view, median (sagittal) section

Epiglottis
Hyoid bone
Thyrohyoid membrane
Thyroid cartilage lamina
Corniculate cartilage
Arytenoid cartilage
Vocal process
Muscular process
Vocal lig.
Thyro-epiglottic lig.
Cricothyroid lig.
Cricoid cartilage

FIGURE 8-58 Laryngeal Cartilages, Ligaments, and Membranes. (From *Atlas of human anatomy,* ed 6, Plate 79.)

airway and as a "reed instrument" to produce sound. Its framework consists of nine cartilages joined by ligaments and membranes (Fig. 8-58 and Table 8-20).

The intrinsic skeletal muscles of the larynx attach to the laryngeal cartilages and act largely to adjust the tension on the vocal folds (ligaments, cords); to open or close the **rima glottidis** (space between the vocal folds); and to open or close the **rima vestibuli,** which is the space above the vestibular folds (false folds) (Fig. 8-59). The opening or closing of the rima vestibuli is important during swallowing, preventing aspiration into the trachea,

TABLE 8-20 Laryngeal Cartilages	
CARTILAGE	**DESCRIPTION**
Thyroid	Two hyaline laminae and laryngeal prominence (Adam's apple)
Cricoid	Signet ring–shaped hyaline cartilage just inferior to thyroid
Epiglottis	Spoon-shaped elastic plate attached to thyroid cartilage
Arytenoid	Paired pyramidal cartilages that rotate on cricoid cartilage
Corniculate	Paired cartilages that lie on apex of arytenoid cartilages
Cuneiform	Paired cartilages in ary-epiglottic folds that have no articulations

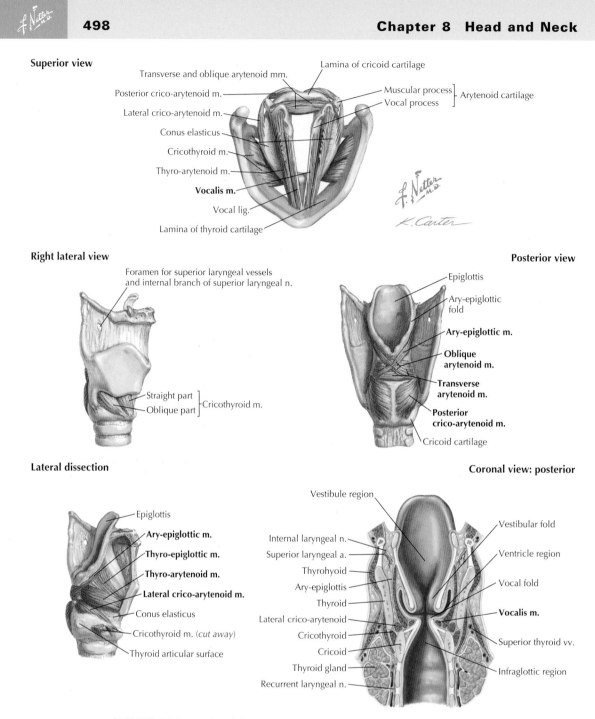

Superior view

Transverse and oblique arytenoid mm.
Posterior crico-arytenoid m.
Lateral crico-arytenoid m.
Conus elasticus
Cricothyroid m.
Thyro-arytenoid m.
Vocalis m.
Vocal lig.
Lamina of thyroid cartilage

Lamina of cricoid cartilage
Muscular process
Vocal process
Arytenoid cartilage

Right lateral view

Foramen for superior laryngeal vessels
and internal branch of superior laryngeal n.

Straight part
Oblique part
Cricothyroid m.

Posterior view

Epiglottis
Ary-epiglottic fold
Ary-epiglottic m.
Oblique arytenoid m.
Transverse arytenoid m.
Posterior crico-arytenoid m.
Cricoid cartilage

Lateral dissection

Epiglottis
Ary-epiglottic m.
Thyro-epiglottic m.
Thyro-arytenoid m.
Lateral crico-arytenoid m.
Conus elasticus
Cricothyroid m. (*cut away*)
Thyroid articular surface

Coronal view: posterior

Vestibule region
Internal laryngeal n.
Superior laryngeal a.
Thyrohyoid
Ary-epiglottis
Thyroid
Lateral crico-arytenoid
Cricothyroid
Cricoid
Thyroid gland
Recurrent laryngeal n.

Vestibular fold
Ventricle region
Vocal fold
Vocalis m.
Superior thyroid vv.
Infraglottic region

FIGURE 8-59 Muscles of the Larynx. (From *Atlas of human anatomy,* ed 6, Plate 80.)

but also adjusts the size of the vestibule during phonation, which enhances the quality of the sound. All these muscles are innervated by the **recurrent branch of CN X,** except the cricothyroid muscle, which is innervated by the external branch of the **superior laryngeal nerve (CN X).** Sensation above the vocal folds is conveyed by the superior laryngeal nerve and by the recurrent laryngeal nerve below the vocal folds.

The vocal folds (vocal ligaments covered with mucosa) control phonation similar to a reed instrument. Vibrations of the folds produce sounds as air passes through the rima glottidis. The **posterior crico-arytenoid muscles** are important because they are the *only* laryngeal muscles that abduct the vocal folds and maintain the opening of the rima glottidis. The vestibular folds are protective in function.

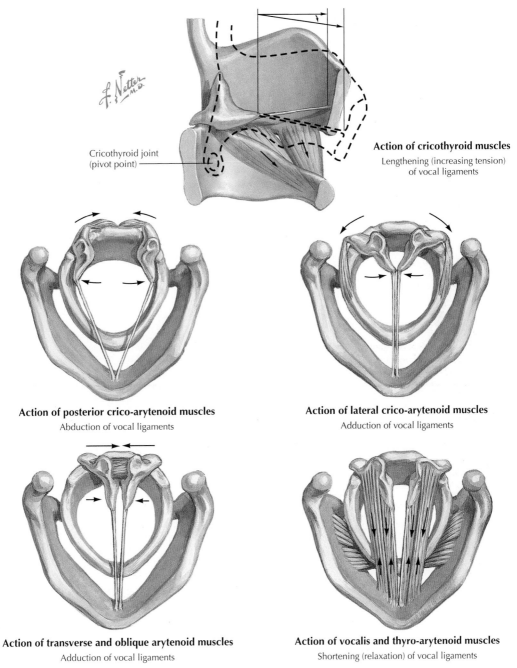

Action of cricothyroid muscles
Lengthening (increasing tension)
of vocal ligaments

Cricothyroid joint
(pivot point)

Action of posterior crico-arytenoid muscles
Abduction of vocal ligaments

Action of lateral crico-arytenoid muscles
Adduction of vocal ligaments

Action of transverse and oblique arytenoid muscles
Adduction of vocal ligaments

Action of vocalis and thyro-arytenoid muscles
Shortening (relaxation) of vocal ligaments

FIGURE 8-60 Action of Intrinsic Muscles of Larynx. (From *Atlas of human anatomy*, ed 6, Plate 81.)

Rotation of the arytenoid cartilages moves the vocal folds medially (adduction) by the action of the lateral crico-arytenoid muscle and the transverse and oblique arytenoid muscles. This action narrows the space between the vocal folds (rima glottidis), and the air rushing through the rima glottidis vibrates the vocal folds and their mucosal lining (higher tones) (Fig. 8-60). Lateral (abduction) movement of the arytenoid cartilages widens the rima glottidis, producing lower tones. The vocal folds also can be lengthened (increased tension on the vocal ligaments), producing a higher pitch, or shortened (relaxation of the ligaments), producing a lower pitch, by the cricothyroid joint, a synovial joint that allows the thyroid cartilage to be tilted anteriorly. The **cricothyroid muscles** tilt it anteriorly, increasing the tension, and the **thyro-arytenoid muscles** tilt the thyroid

Emergency Airway: Cricothyrotomy

When all other methods of establishing an airway have been exhausted or determined to be unsuitable, an incision can be made through the skin and the underlying cricothyroid membrane to gain access to the trachea. The site of the incision can be judged by locating the thyroid notch and sliding your finger inferiorly until the space between the thyroid and cricoid cartilages is palpated (about one fingerbreadth inferior to the thyroid notch). If the patient has a midline pyramidal lobe arising from the thyroid gland, this procedure may lacerate that tissue and cause significant bleeding.

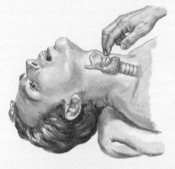

Thyroid cartilage
Cricoid cartilage
Thyroid gland

Cricothyroid membrane identified by palpating for transverse indentation between thyroid cartilage and cricoid cartilage

Cricothyroid membrane opened with scalpel, knife, or other sharp instrument that may be at hand. Opening may be enlarged by twisting instrument and patency preserved by inserting rubber tubing or any other suitable object available

Manifestations of Hoarseness

Hoarseness can be caused by any condition that results in improper vibration or coaptation of the vocal folds.

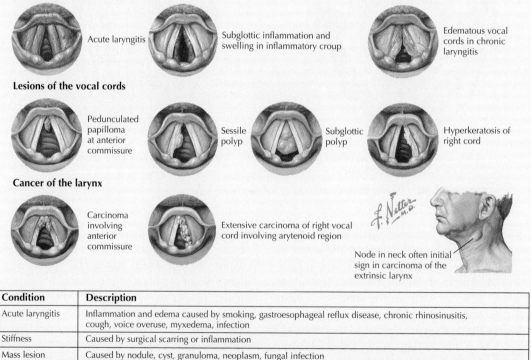

Inflammation of the larynx

Acute laryngitis

Subglottic inflammation and swelling in inflammatory croup

Edematous vocal cords in chronic laryngitis

Lesions of the vocal cords

Pedunculated papilloma at anterior commissure

Sessile polyp

Subglottic polyp

Hyperkeratosis of right cord

Cancer of the larynx

Carcinoma involving anterior commissure

Extensive carcinoma of right vocal cord involving arytenoid region

Node in neck often initial sign in carcinoma of the extrinsic larynx

Condition	Description
Acute laryngitis	Inflammation and edema caused by smoking, gastroesophageal reflux disease, chronic rhinosinusitis, cough, voice overuse, myxedema, infection
Stiffness	Caused by surgical scarring or inflammation
Mass lesion	Caused by nodule, cyst, granuloma, neoplasm, fungal infection
Paralysis or paresis	Occurs after viral infection, recurrent laryngeal nerve lesion, or stroke; can have congenital causes or be iatrogenic

cartilage back into position to relax the vocal ligaments. As males reach puberty, the thyroid cartilage enlarges and the vocal ligaments become longer and thicker, leading to a deeper sound in their voice. The quality of everyone's voice also is influenced by the shape of the oral and pharyngeal spaces, nose and paranasal sinuses, tongue and lips, and soft palate.

The arterial supply to the larynx is by the **superior laryngeal artery,** a branch of the superior thyroid artery off the external carotid artery, and by the **inferior laryngeal artery,** a branch of the inferior thyroid artery off the thyrocervical trunk of the subclavian artery (Figs. 8-49 and 8-50). The venous drainage is by laryngeal veins that drain into the superior and inferior thyroid veins (Figs. 8-51 and 8-52).

14. HEAD AND NECK VASCULAR AND LYMPHATIC SUMMARY

Arteries of the head and neck largely include branches derived from the following major vessels (Fig. 8-61):

- **Subclavian artery:** supplies the lower neck (thyrocervical and costocervical trunks), thyroid gland, thoracic wall, shoulder, upper back, and brain (vertebral branches).

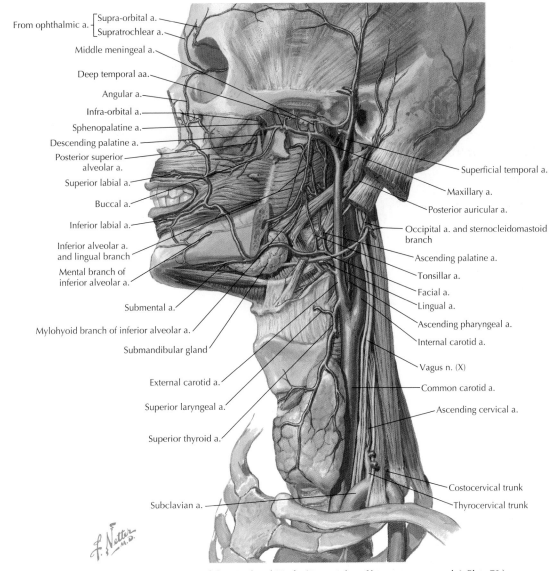

FIGURE 8-61 Major Arteries of the Head and Neck. (From *Atlas of human anatomy*, ed 6, Plate 72.)

- **External carotid artery:** supplies the thyroid gland, larynx, pharynx, neck, oral cavity, face, nasal cavity, meninges, and temporal and infratemporal regions via its eight primary branches.
- **Internal carotid artery:** supplies the brain, orbit, eyeball, lacrimal glands, forehead, and ethmoid sinuses.

The venous drainage of the head and neck ultimately collects in the following major veins (numerous variations and anastomoses exist between these veins) (Fig. 8-62):

- **Retromandibular vein:** receives tributaries from the temporal and infratemporal regions (pterygoid plexus), orbit, nasal cavity, pharynx, and oral cavity.
- **Internal jugular vein:** drains the brain (dural venous sinuses), face, thyroid gland, and neck.
- **External jugular vein:** drains the superficial neck, lower neck and shoulder, and upper back (often communicates with the retromandibular vein) (see Fig. 8-51).

Lymph nodes and vessels of the head and neck tend to follow the venous drainage, with most of

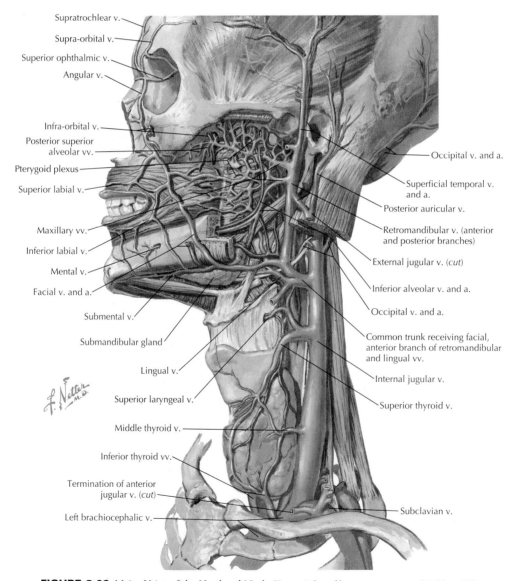

FIGURE 8-62 Major Veins of the Head and Neck. (From *Atlas of human anatomy,* ed 6, Plate 73.)

the lymph ultimately collecting in the **deep cervical lymphatic chain** (jugulodigastric and juguloomohyoid nodes), which courses along the internal jugular veins (Fig. 8-63). Superficial cervical nodes drain the superficial structures of the neck along lymphatic vessels that parallel the external jugular vein. The right side drains into the right lymphatic duct, and the left side drains into the thoracic duct (see Fig. 1-15).

15. HEAD AND NECK ARTERIOVENOUS SUMMARY

Arteries of the Head and Neck
(see Fig. 8-64)

After the **ascending aorta (1)** gives rise to the two coronary arteries, it forms the **aortic arch (2)**, which gives rise to three branches: the **brachiocephalic artery (3)**, the **left common carotid artery,** and the **left subclavian artery** (Fig. 8-64). The brachiocephalic artery is short and gives rise to the **right common carotid artery (4)** and the **right subclavian artery (7)**.

The common carotid artery, both right and left sides, ascends in the neck and divides into the **internal carotid artery (5),** which passes superiorly to become intracranial (giving off only several very small branches), and the **external carotid artery (6).**

The external carotid artery gives rise to eight major branches to the neck, face, and occipital region and terminates as the **superficial temporal artery** on the lateral aspect of the head and as the **maxillary artery**. The **maxillary**

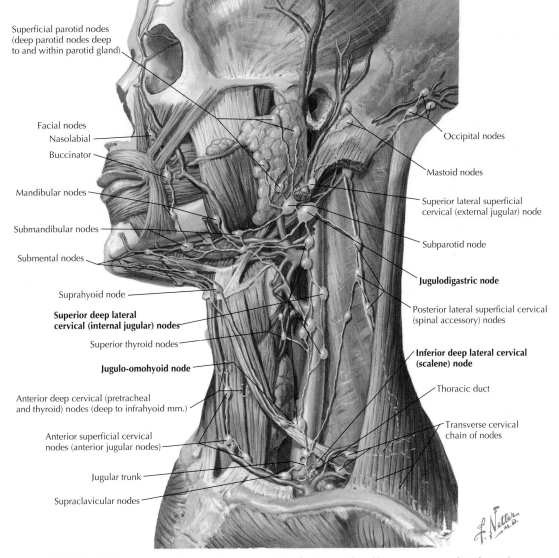

Superficial parotid nodes
(deep parotid nodes deep
to and within parotid gland)

Facial nodes
Nasolabial

Buccinator

Mandibular nodes

Submandibular nodes

Submental nodes

Suprahyoid node

**Superior deep lateral
cervical (internal jugular) nodes**

Superior thyroid nodes

Jugulo-omohyoid node

Anterior deep cervical (pretracheal
and thyroid) nodes (deep to infrahyoid mm.)

Anterior superficial cervical
nodes (anterior jugular nodes)

Jugular trunk

Supraclavicular nodes

Occipital nodes

Mastoid nodes

Superior lateral superficial
cervical (external jugular) node

Subparotid node

Jugulodigastric node

Posterior lateral superficial cervical
(spinal accessory) nodes

**Inferior deep lateral cervical
(scalene) node**

Thoracic duct

Transverse cervical
chain of nodes

FIGURE 8-63 Major Lymphatics of the Head and Neck. (From *Atlas of human anatomy*, ed 6, Plate 74.)

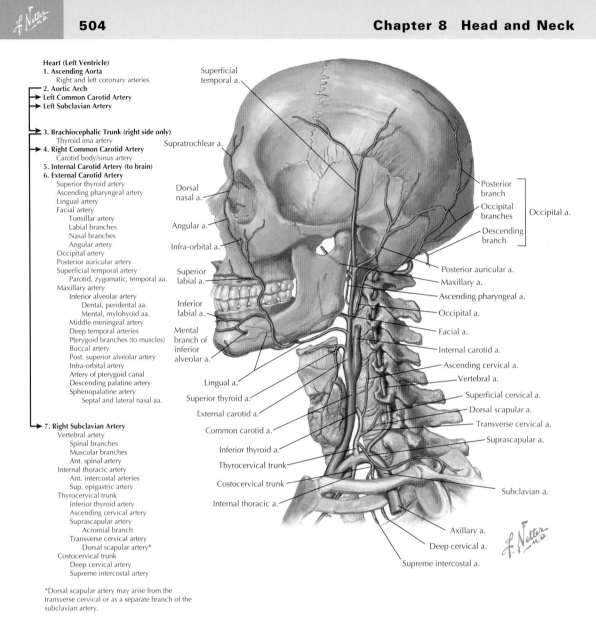

Heart (Left Ventricle)
1. Ascending Aorta
    Right and left coronary arteries
2. Aortic Arch
   Left Common Carotid Artery
   Left Subclavian Artery

3. Brachiocephalic Trunk (right side only)
    Thyroid ima artery
4. Right Common Carotid Artery
    Carotid body/sinus artery
5. Internal Carotid Artery (to brain)
6. External Carotid Artery
    Superior thyroid artery
    Ascending pharyngeal artery
    Lingual artery
    Facial artery
        Tonsillar artery
        Labial branches
        Nasal branches
        Angular artery
    Occipital artery
    Posterior auricular artery
    Superficial temporal artery
        Parotid, zygomatic, temporal aa.
    Maxillary artery
        Inferior alveolar artery
            Dental, peridental aa.
            Mental, mylohyoid aa.
        Middle meningeal artery
        Deep temporal arteries
        Pterygoid branches (to muscles)
        Buccal artery
        Post. superior alveolar artery
        Infra-orbital artery
        Artery of pterygoid canal
        Descending palatine artery
        Sphenopalatine artery
            Septal and lateral nasal aa.

7. Right Subclavian Artery
    Vertebral artery
        Spinal branches
        Muscular branches
        Ant. spinal artery
    Internal thoracic artery
        Ant. intercostal arteries
        Sup. epigastric artery
    Thyrocervical trunk
        Inferior thyroid artery
        Ascending cervical artery
        Suprascapular artery
            Acromial branch
        Transverse cervical artery
            Dorsal scapular artery*
    Costocervical trunk
        Deep cervical artery
        Supreme intercostal artery

*Dorsal scapular artery may arise from the
transverse cervical or as a separate branch of the
subclavian artery.

Superficial temporal a.
Supratrochlear a.
Dorsal nasal a.
Angular a.
Infra-orbital a.
Superior labial a.
Inferior labial a.
Mental branch of inferior alveolar a.
Lingual a.
Superior thyroid a.
External carotid a.
Common carotid a.
Inferior thyroid a.
Thyrocervical trunk
Costocervical trunk
Internal thoracic a.

Posterior branch
Occipital branches
Descending branch
Occipital a.
Posterior auricular a.
Maxillary a.
Ascending pharyngeal a.
Occipital a.
Facial a.
Internal carotid a.
Ascending cervical a.
Vertebral a.
Superficial cervical a.
Dorsal scapular a.
Transverse cervical a.
Suprascapular a.
Subclavian a.
Axillary a.
Deep cervical a.
Supreme intercostal a.

FIGURE 8-64 Arteries of the Head and Neck.

artery itself gives off about 15 additional branches to the infratemporal region and its muscles, the meninges, mandible, maxilla, orbit, palate, and nasal cavities.

The **subclavian artery (7)** (both sides) gives off four major branches: one to the posterior brain and cervical spinal cord (vertebral artery), an artery to the thorax (internal thoracic artery), and branches to the neck and shoulder region, via its thyrocervical and costocervical trunks.

The subclavian artery then becomes the axillary artery after crossing the first rib.

A rich vascular supply is given to the brain by the two vertebral and two internal carotid arteries. The infratemporal fossa, jaws, and nasal cavity receive a rich blood supply by the maxillary artery, as does the neck, especially the thyroid and parathyroid endocrine glands (superior and inferior thyroid arteries). A rich vascular anastomosis also exists around the shoulder joint and scapula by the branches of the subclavian and axillary arteries (see Figs. 7-7 and 7-8).

Veins of the Head and Neck

The veins of the head and neck have numerous interconnections (Fig. 8-65). The dural venous sinuses converge at the sigmoid dural sinus to form the **superior bulb of the jugular vein (1)** at

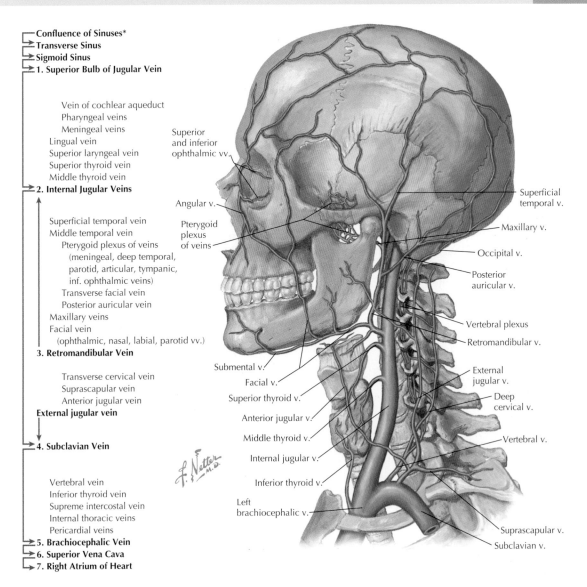

Confluence of Sinuses*
Transverse Sinus
Sigmoid Sinus
1. Superior Bulb of Jugular Vein

Vein of cochlear aqueduct
Pharyngeal veins
Meningeal veins
Lingual vein
Superior laryngeal vein
Superior thyroid vein
Middle thyroid vein
2. Internal Jugular Veins

Superficial temporal vein
Middle temporal vein
Pterygoid plexus of veins
(meningeal, deep temporal,
parotid, articular, tympanic,
inf. ophthalmic veins)
Transverse facial vein
Posterior auricular vein
Maxillary veins
Facial vein
(ophthalmic, nasal, labial, parotid vv.)
3. Retromandibular Vein

Transverse cervical vein
Suprascapular vein
Anterior jugular vein
External jugular vein

4. Subclavian Vein

Vertebral vein
Inferior thyroid vein
Supreme intercostal vein
Internal thoracic veins
Pericardial veins
5. Brachiocephalic Vein
6. Superior Vena Cava
7. Right Atrium of Heart

*Distal (dural sinuses) to Heart (right atrium)

FIGURE 8-65 Veins of the Head and Neck.

the jugular foramen (CN IX, X, and XI also exit the skull here). The veins outlined are bilateral (right and left veins) and can often communicate across the midline of the face and neck. The **internal jugular vein (2)** then descends within the carotid sheath and receives numerous tributaries from the head and face; one major tributary is the **retromandibular vein (3),** which itself receives tributaries from the head and facial regions (listed separately in the outline). The retromandibular vein communicates directly not only with the internal jugular vein but also with the anterior jugular vein and external jugular vein(s), which are in the superficial fascia. Both the internal jugular vein and the tributaries of the retromandibular

vein and external jugular vein drain inferiorly to join the with the **subclavian vein (4).** The subclavian vein and internal jugular vein then form the **brachiocephalic vein (5)** on the right and left side. The brachiocephalic vein receives small tributaries from the superior mediastinum, including the inferior thyroid, vertebral, intercostal, pericardial, laryngeal, esophageal and bronchial veins. The left and right brachiocephalic veins then join to form the **superior vena cava (6)** on the right aspect of the superior mediastinum, and the SVC then drains into the **right atrium of the heart (7).**

Variations and interconnections are common, especially with the smaller veins. The ophthalmic veins of the orbit drain into the facial veins and into the infratemporal fossa and the pterygoid plexus of veins. Ultimately, these veins and their tributaries drain into the retromandibular vein and internal jugular vein. A rich venous anastomosis also exits in the neck as three pairs of veins drain the thyroid/parathyroid endocrine glands (superior, middle, and inferior thyroid veins).

16. CRANIAL NERVE SUMMARY

Autonomic Innervation

The autonomic distribution to the head involves preganglionic axons that arise from neurons in the CNS and synapse in peripheral ganglia (Fig. 8-66). Postganglionic axons then arise from neurons in these peripheral ganglia and course to their respective targets (smooth muscle and glands). Except for the parasympathetic fibers to the eye (constrictor of the pupil and ciliary muscle for accommodation) and parotid salivary gland, *all* the other parasympathetics arise from the superior salivatory nucleus of the facial nerve (CN VII) via the intermediate portion (nervus intermedius) of the facial nerve. These preganglionic fibers then course either in the **greater petrosal nerve** to the pterygopalatine ganglion or via the **chorda tympani nerve** to the submandibular ganglion. The vagus nerve (not shown) provides parasympathetic innervation to the neck, thorax, and upper two thirds of the abdominal viscera, but none to the head region.

Preganglionic sympathetic fibers from the upper thoracic spinal cord levels (T1-T2) ascend via the sympathetic trunk and synapse in the **SCG.**

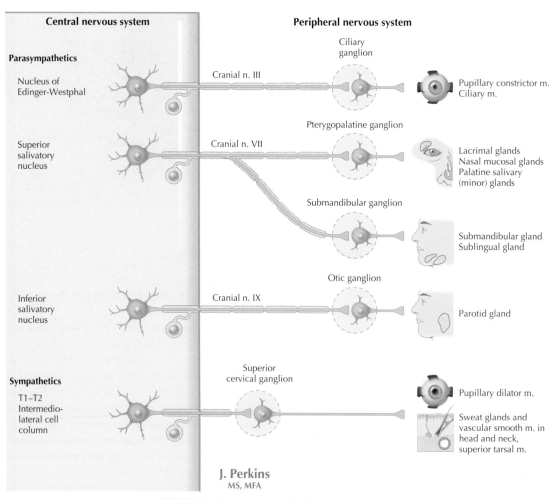

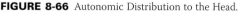

FIGURE 8-66 Autonomic Distribution to the Head.

Postganglionic axons from the SCG then course along blood vessels or existing nerves to reach their targets, mainly vasomotor, sweat glands, and some smooth muscle (Fig. 8-67).

Cranial Nerves

We reviewed the general components of the cranial nerves earlier in this chapter (see Table 8-4), so we will focus this summary selectively on the more complex cranial nerves.

Oculomotor, Trochlear, and Abducent Nerves

The oculomotor nerve (CN III) innervates five muscles in the orbit (general somatic efferents; see Table 8-6) and conveys parasympathetic preganglionic fibers from the **Edinger-Westphal nucleus** to the **ciliary ganglion.** (Postganglionic fibers mediate pupillary constriction and accommodation.) The trochlear nerve (CN IV) innervates the superior oblique muscle, and the abducent nerve (CN VI) innervates the lateral rectus muscle (Fig. 8-68).

Trigeminal Nerve

The trigeminal nerve (CN V), the **major sensory nerve of the head**, conveys general somatic afferents centrally to the **trigeminal sensory ganglion** via its ophthalmic (V_1), maxillary (V_2), and mandibular (V_3) divisions. Its mandibular division also innervates skeletal muscles derived from the **first embryonic branchial arch.** Because of the

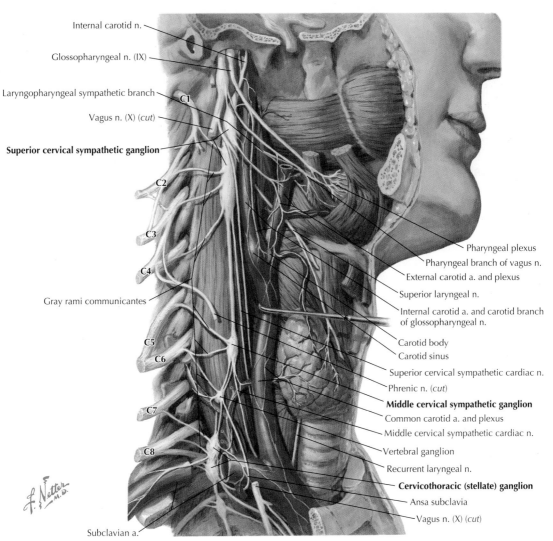

FIGURE 8-67 Sympathetic Ganglia and Nerves to the Head. (From *Atlas of human anatomy*, ed 6, Plate 131.)

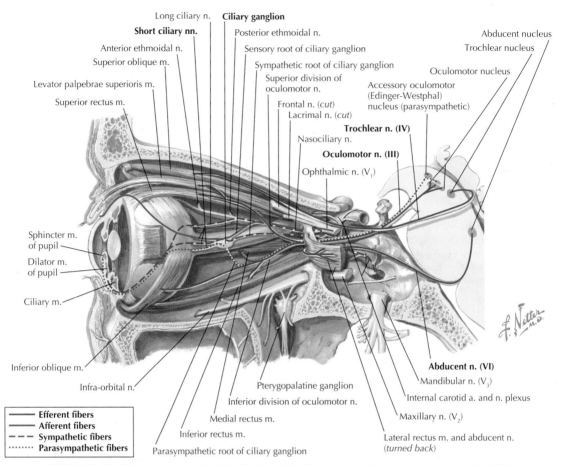

FIGURE 8-68 Pathway Summary for CN III, IV, and VI. (From *Atlas of human anatomy*, ed 6, Plate 122.)

extensive distribution of CN V, most of the parasympathetic fibers from CN III, VII, and IX course with branches of CN V to reach their targets: smooth muscle and glands (Fig. 8-69).

Facial Nerve

The facial nerve (CN VII), the **major motor nerve of the head,** conveys general somatic efferents to skeletal muscles derived from the **second embryonic branchial arch.** Additionally, CN VII sends preganglionic parasympathetic fibers from the **superior salivatory nucleus** via the intermediate nerve to the **pterygopalatine ganglia** via the greater petrosal nerve and the nerve of the pterygoid canal, and to the **submandibular ganglia** via chorda tympani and lingual nerves. The facial nerve also conveys special visceral afferents from taste receptors on the anterior two thirds of the tongue along the chorda tympani to the **geniculate sensory ganglion** of CN VII (Fig. 8-70).

Glossopharyngeal Nerve

The glossopharyngeal nerve (CN IX) innervates the stylopharyngeus muscle (derived from the **third embryonic branchial arch**), sends preganglionic parasympathetics from the **inferior salivatory nucleus** via the lesser petrosal nerve to the **otic ganglion** (innervates the parotid gland), and conveys special visceral afferents from taste receptors on the posterior third of the tongue to the sensory ganglia of CN IX. General visceral afferents also return from the carotid sinus (baroreceptors) and carotid body (chemoreceptors), and general somatic afferents return from the posterior tongue, palatine tonsils, pharynx, and middle ear (Fig. 8-71).

Vagus Nerve

The vagus nerve (CN X) innervates the pharyngeal and laryngeal muscles of the **fourth embryonic branchial arch** via its superior laryngeal

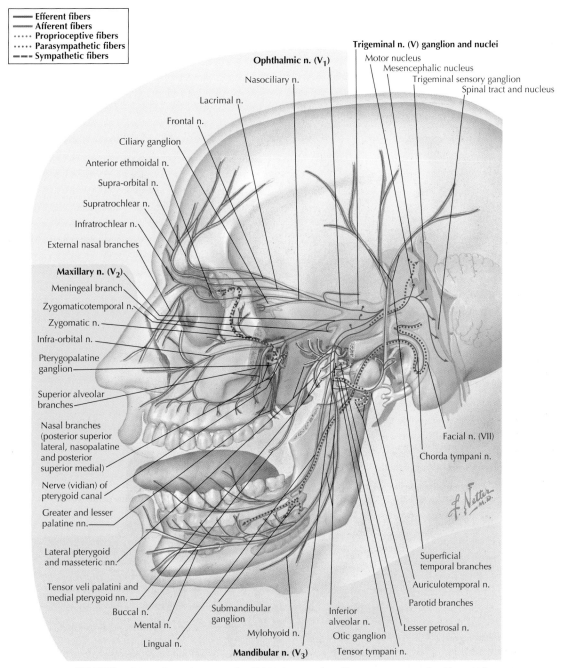

Efferent fibers
Afferent fibers
Proprioceptive fibers
Parasympathetic fibers
Sympathetic fibers

Trigeminal n. (V) ganglion and nuclei
Motor nucleus
Mesencephalic nucleus
Trigeminal sensory ganglion
Spinal tract and nucleus

Ophthalmic n. (V₁)
Nasociliary n.
Lacrimal n.
Frontal n.
Ciliary ganglion
Anterior ethmoidal n.
Supra-orbital n.
Supratrochlear n.
Infratrochlear n.
External nasal branches

Maxillary n. (V₂)
Meningeal branch
Zygomaticotemporal n.
Zygomatic n.
Infra-orbital n.
Pterygopalatine ganglion
Superior alveolar branches
Nasal branches (posterior superior lateral, nasopalatine and posterior superior medial)
Nerve (vidian) of pterygoid canal
Greater and lesser palatine nn.
Lateral pterygoid and masseteric nn.
Tensor veli palatini and medial pterygoid nn.
Buccal n.
Mental n.
Lingual n.

Submandibular ganglion
Mylohyoid n.

Mandibular n. (V₃)

Inferior alveolar n.
Otic ganglion
Tensor tympani n.

Facial n. (VII)
Chorda tympani n.

Superficial temporal branches
Auriculotemporal n.
Parotid branches
Lesser petrosal n.

FIGURE 8-69 Pathway Summary for CN V. (From *Atlas of human anatomy,* ed 6, Plate 123.)

nerve and the **sixth embryonic branchial arch** via the recurrent laryngeal nerve. CN X also sends preganglionic parasympathetic fibers from its **dorsal nucleus** to smooth muscle and glands of the neck, thorax (including cardiac muscle of the heart), and proximal two thirds of the abdominal GI tract, with its fibers synapsing in **terminal ganglia** in or near the structures innervated. Afferents arise from visceral structures of the same thoracic and GI regions and from aortic baroreceptors and chemoreceptors. Special sensory fibers from taste buds on the epiglottis and general somatic afferents arising from skin around the ear, larynx, external acoustic meatus,

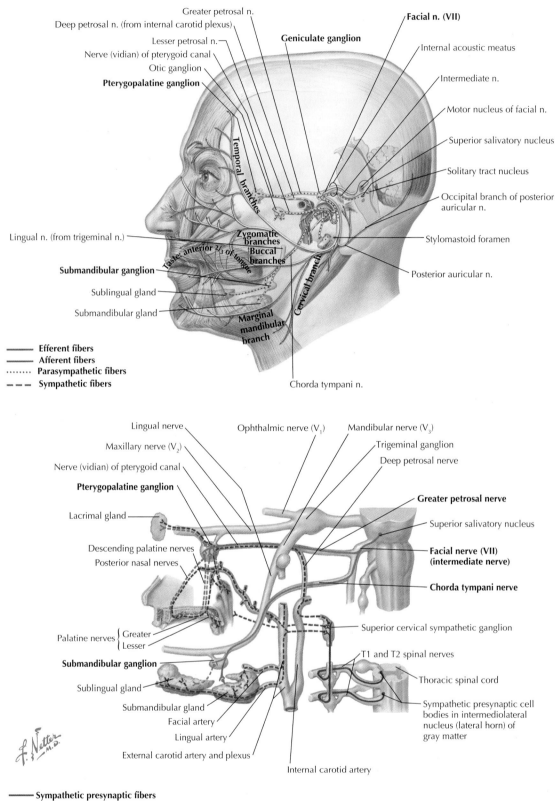

Greater petrosal n.

Deep petrosal n. (from internal carotid plexus)

Geniculate ganglion

Facial n. (VII)

Lesser petrosal n.

Nerve (vidian) of pterygoid canal

Internal acoustic meatus

Otic ganglion

Intermediate n.

Pterygopalatine ganglion

Motor nucleus of facial n.

Superior salivatory nucleus

Solitary tract nucleus

Temporal branches

Occipital branch of posterior auricular n.

Lingual n. (from trigeminal n.)

Zygomatic branches

Buccal branches

Stylomastoid foramen

Taste: anterior ⅔ of tongue

Submandibular ganglion

Cervical branch

Posterior auricular n.

Sublingual gland

Submandibular gland

Marginal mandibular branch

_____ Efferent fibers
_____ Afferent fibers
········· Parasympathetic fibers
– – – Sympathetic fibers

Chorda tympani n.

Lingual nerve

Ophthalmic nerve (V₁)

Mandibular nerve (V₃)

Maxillary nerve (V₂)

Trigeminal ganglion

Nerve (vidian) of pterygoid canal

Deep petrosal nerve

Pterygopalatine ganglion

Greater petrosal nerve

Lacrimal gland

Superior salivatory nucleus

Descending palatine nerves

**Facial nerve (VII)
(intermediate nerve)**

Posterior nasal nerves

Chorda tympani nerve

Palatine nerves { Greater / Lesser

Superior cervical sympathetic ganglion

Submandibular ganglion

T1 and T2 spinal nerves

Sublingual gland

Thoracic spinal cord

Submandibular gland

Facial artery

Sympathetic presynaptic cell bodies in intermediolateral nucleus (lateral horn) of gray matter

Lingual artery

External carotid artery and plexus

Internal carotid artery

_____ Sympathetic presynaptic fibers
– – – Sympathetic postsynaptic fibers
_____ Parasympathetic presynaptic fibers
– – – Parasympathetic postsynaptic fibers

FIGURE 8-70 Pathway Summary for CN VII. (From *Atlas of human anatomy,* ed 6, Plates 124 and 134.)

Clinical Focus 8-46

Nerve Lesions

A lesion of the **vagus nerve** is easily detected by asking the patient to say "ah." If the nerve is intact, the soft palate and uvula will elevate symmetrically. If the vagus nerve has a lesion on one side, the elevation will be asymmetrical, with the palate and uvula deviating away from the lesioned side.

Lesion of the **hypoglossal nerve** peripherally (lower motor neuron) will cause the tongue to deviate toward the side of the lesioned nerve when the patient is asked to stick out the tongue. The ipsilateral tongue will also show evidence of muscle atrophy.

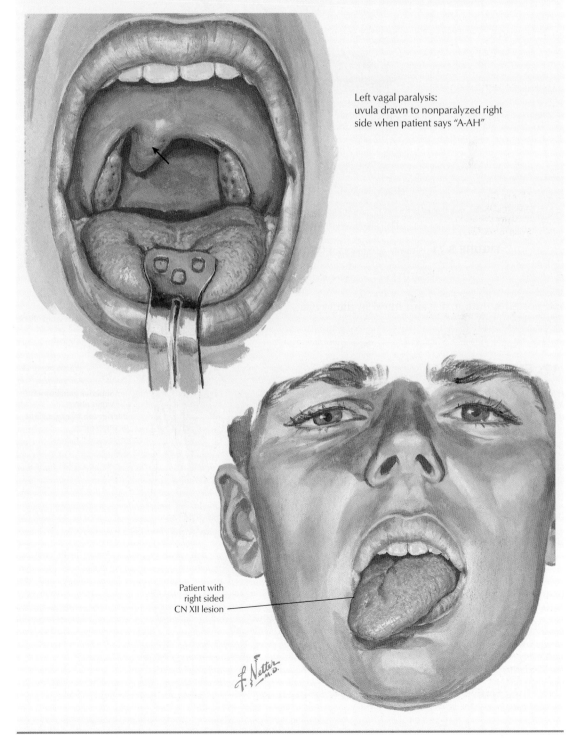

Left vagal paralysis: uvula drawn to nonparalyzed right side when patient says "A-AH"

Patient with right sided CN XII lesion

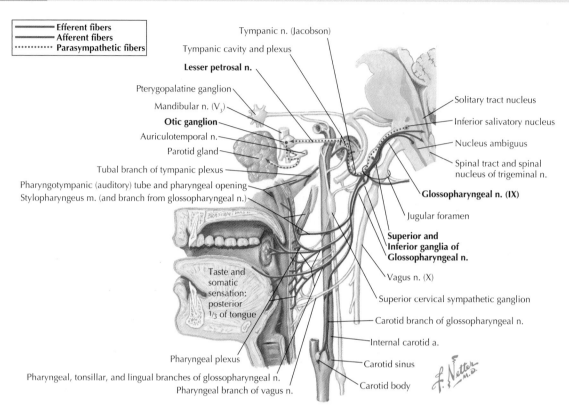

Efferent fibers
Afferent fibers
Parasympathetic fibers

Tympanic n. (Jacobson)
Tympanic cavity and plexus
Lesser petrosal n.
Pterygopalatine ganglion
Mandibular n. (V₃)
Otic ganglion
Auriculotemporal n.
Parotid gland
Tubal branch of tympanic plexus
Pharyngotympanic (auditory) tube and pharyngeal opening
Stylopharyngeus m. (and branch from glossopharyngeal n.)
Taste and somatic sensation: posterior ⅓ of tongue
Pharyngeal plexus
Pharyngeal, tonsillar, and lingual branches of glossopharyngeal n.
Pharyngeal branch of vagus n.

Solitary tract nucleus
Inferior salivatory nucleus
Nucleus ambiguus
Spinal tract and spinal nucleus of trigeminal n.
Glossopharyngeal n. (IX)
Jugular foramen
Superior and Inferior ganglia of Glossopharyngeal n.
Vagus n. (X)
Superior cervical sympathetic ganglion
Carotid branch of glossopharyngeal n.
Internal carotid a.
Carotid sinus
Carotid body

FIGURE 8-71 Pathway Summary for CN IX. (From *Atlas of human anatomy*, ed 6, Plate 126.)

and posterior dura mater also travel in the vagus nerve (Fig. 8-72).

17. EMBRYOLOGY

Brain Development

The cranial end of the neural tube begins to expand into definitive swellings and characteristic flexures during the fourth week of development, giving rise to the **forebrain, midbrain,** and **hindbrain** (Fig. 8-73). By the fifth week, these three divisions subdivide into five regions that ultimately give rise to the definitive brain structures.

Cranial Nerve Development

The 12 pairs of cranial nerves develop from cranial to caudal (except for CN XI, which arises from the upper cervical spinal cord) as direct extensions of the neural tube (CN I and II), or as peripheral nerve outgrowths to surface placodes,

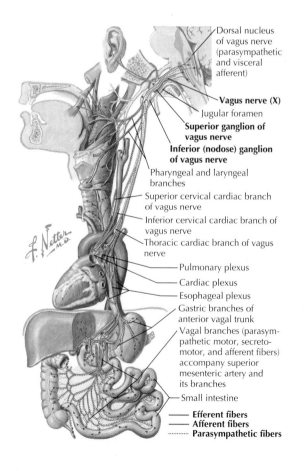

Dorsal nucleus of vagus nerve (parasympathetic and visceral afferent)
Vagus nerve (X)
Jugular foramen
Superior ganglion of vagus nerve
Inferior (nodose) ganglion of vagus nerve
Pharyngeal and laryngeal branches
Superior cervical cardiac branch of vagus nerve
Inferior cervical cardiac branch of vagus nerve
Thoracic cardiac branch of vagus nerve
Pulmonary plexus
Cardiac plexus
Esophageal plexus
Gastric branches of anterior vagal trunk
Vagal branches (parasympathetic motor, secretomotor, and afferent fibers) accompany superior mesenteric artery and its branches
Small intestine

Efferent fibers
Afferent fibers
Parasympathetic fibers

FIGURE 8-72 Pathway Summary for CN X. (From *Atlas of human anatomy*, ed 6, Plate 127.)

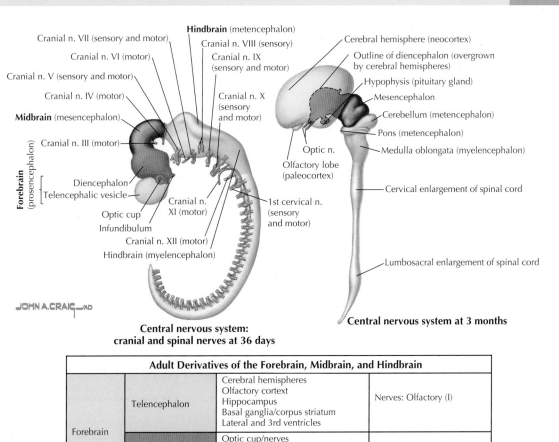

Central nervous system: cranial and spinal nerves at 36 days

Central nervous system at 3 months

		Adult Derivatives of the Forebrain, Midbrain, and Hindbrain		
Forebrain	Telencephalon	Cerebral hemispheres Olfactory cortex Hippocampus Basal ganglia/corpus striatum Lateral and 3rd ventricles		Nerves: Olfactory (I)
	Diencephalon	Optic cup/nerves Thalamus Hypothalamus Mammillary bodies Part of 3rd ventricle		Optic (II)
Midbrain	Mesencephalon	Tectum Cerebral aqueduct Red nucleus Substantia nigra Crus cerebelli		Oculomotor (III) Trochlear (IV)
Hindbrain	Metencephalon	Pons Cerebellum		Trigeminal (V) Abducent (VI)
	Myelencephalon		Medulla oblongata	Facial (VII) Vestibulocochlear (VIII) Glossopharyngeal (IX) Vagus (X) Hypoglossal (XI)

FIGURE 8-73 Brain Development at 5 Weeks and 3 Months.

somitomeres (head somites), and pharyngeal arches. Consequently, the cranial nerves innervate the structures and tissues derived from these targets (Fig. 8-74). The accessory nerve (CN XI) is unique in that it lacks a cranial root and innervates two muscles derived from cervical somites—the trapezius and sternocleidomastoid.

Pharyngeal Arch and Pouch Development

Pharyngeal arches develop from the human ancestral gill (branchial) arch system as an evolutionary adaptation to terrestrial life. The original six pairs of arches develop into four pairs, with a cranial nerve, the muscles it innervates, a cartilage/bone element, and an aortic arch associated with each arch (Fig. 8-75). The muscles associated with each pharyngeal arch include the following groups:

- **Arch 1:** muscles of mastication, mylohyoid, anterior belly of digastric, tensor tympani, and tensor veli palatini; all innervated by CN V_3.
- **Arch 2:** muscles of facial expression, posterior belly of digastric, stylohyoid, and stapedius; all innervated by CN VII.

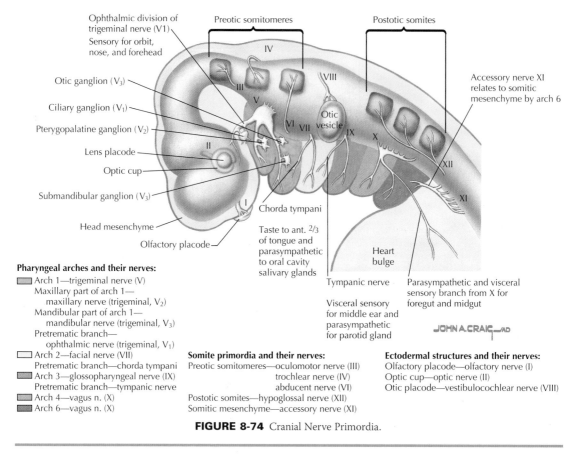

Ophthalmic division of trigeminal nerve (V1)
Sensory for orbit, nose, and forehead

Preotic somitomeres

Postotic somites

Accessory nerve XI relates to somitic mesenchyme by arch 6

Otic ganglion (V3)

Ciliary ganglion (V1)

Pterygopalatine ganglion (V2)

Lens placode

Optic cup

Submandibular ganglion (V3)

Head mesenchyme

Olfactory placode

Chorda tympani

Taste to ant. 2/3 of tongue and parasympathetic to oral cavity salivary glands

Heart bulge

Otic vesicle

Tympanic nerve

Visceral sensory for middle ear and parasympathetic for parotid gland

Parasympathetic and visceral sensory branch from X for foregut and midgut

JOHN A. CRAIG—AD

Pharyngeal arches and their nerves:
Arch 1—trigeminal nerve (V)
Maxillary part of arch 1— maxillary nerve (trigeminal, V2)
Mandibular part of arch 1— mandibular nerve (trigeminal, V3)
Pretrematic branch— ophthalmic nerve (trigeminal, V1)
Arch 2—facial nerve (VII)
Pretrematic branch—chorda tympani
Arch 3—glossopharyngeal nerve (IX)
Pretrematic branch—tympanic nerve
Arch 4—vagus n. (X)
Arch 6—vagus n. (X)

Somite primordia and their nerves:
Preotic somitomeres—oculomotor nerve (III)
trochlear nerve (IV)
abducent nerve (VI)
Postotic somites—hypoglossal nerve (XII)
Somitic mesenchyme—accessory nerve (XI)

Ectodermal structures and their nerves:
Olfactory placode—olfactory nerve (I)
Optic cup—optic nerve (II)
Otic placode—vestibulocochlear nerve (VIII)

FIGURE 8-74 Cranial Nerve Primordia.

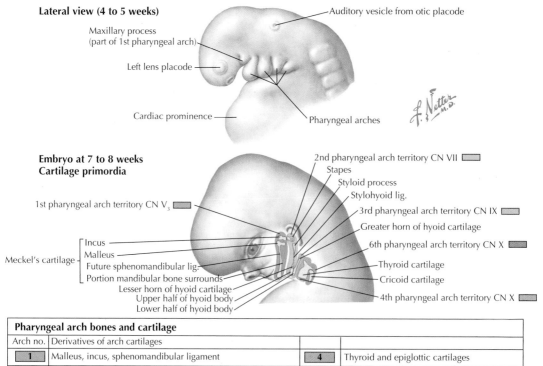

Lateral view (4 to 5 weeks)

Auditory vesicle from otic placode

Maxillary process (part of 1st pharyngeal arch)

Left lens placode

Cardiac prominence

Pharyngeal arches

Embryo at 7 to 8 weeks Cartilage primordia

2nd pharyngeal arch territory CN VII
Stapes
Styloid process
Stylohyoid lig.

1st pharyngeal arch territory CN V3

3rd pharyngeal arch territory CN IX
Greater horn of hyoid cartilage

6th pharyngeal arch territory CN X

Meckel's cartilage
- Incus
- Malleus
- Future sphenomandibular lig.
- Portion mandibular bone surrounds

Thyroid cartilage
Cricoid cartilage
4th pharyngeal arch territory CN X

Lesser horn of hyoid cartilage
Upper half of hyoid body
Lower half of hyoid body

Pharyngeal arch bones and cartilage			
Arch no.	Derivatives of arch cartilages		
1	Malleus, incus, sphenomandibular ligament	4	Thyroid and epiglottic cartilages
2	Stapes, styloid process, stylohyoid ligament, upper half of hyoid	6	Cricoid, arytenoid, and corniculate cartilages
3	Lower half and greater horns of hyoid		

FIGURE 8-75 Pharyngeal Arches.

- **Arch 3:** stylopharyngeus muscle; innervated by CN IX.
- **Arch 4:** muscles of the palate (except the tensor), pharyngeal constrictor muscles, and all the muscles of the larynx; all innervated by CN X.

Internally, each arch is also associated with an endoderm-derived **pharyngeal pouch,** an outpocketing of the foregut in the head and neck. Pharyngeal pouch development begins about the third to fourth week of embryonic development (Fig. 8-76) as an elaboration of bilateral endoderm-derived structures, which include the following:

- **Pouch 1:** auditory tube and middle ear.
- **Pouch 2:** tonsillar fossa and the epithelium of the palatine tonsils (the lymphoid tissue of the tonsil is derived from mesoderm).
- **Pouch 3:** inferior parathyroid glands and thymus gland.
- **Pouch 4:** superior parathyroid glands and C cells (parafollicular; calcitonin-secreting cells) of the thyroid gland.

Facial and Palatal Development

The face develops primarily from the neural crest by the fusion of an unpaired frontonasal prominence and paired **nasal placodes,** with bilateral maxillary and mandibular prominences that meet in the midline (Fig. 8-77). Initially, the eyes develop laterally, but as the face begins to grow, the eyes move medially to their definitive anterior position.

Internally, the common oral-nasal cavity becomes subdivided by a horizontal plate separating the oral cavity from the nasal cavity (Fig. 8-78). Fusion of the medial nasal processes gives rise to an intermaxillary segment called the **primary palate.** Swellings of the maxillary prominence of the face form **palatine shelves** that project medially and fuse along the midline to form the **secondary palate.** These primary and secondary palatal tissues fuse, and all meet at the site of the incisive foramen. As this occurs, a midline **nasal septum** that divides the nose into right and left halves extends downward from the roof of the nasal cavity and fuses with the palate below.

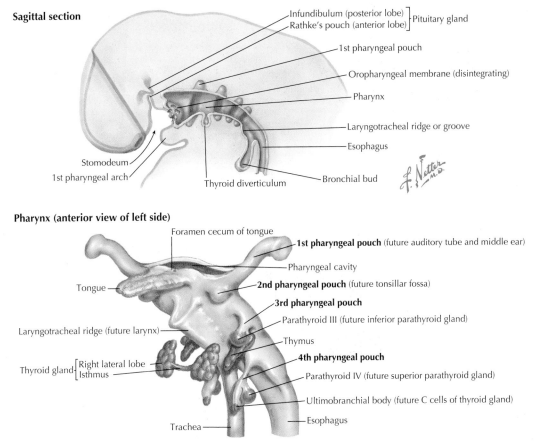

Sagittal section

Infundibulum (posterior lobe) ⎤
Rathke's pouch (anterior lobe) ⎦ Pituitary gland

1st pharyngeal pouch

Oropharyngeal membrane (disintegrating)

Pharynx

Laryngotracheal ridge or groove

Esophagus

Bronchial bud

Stomodeum

1st pharyngeal arch

Thyroid diverticulum

Pharynx (anterior view of left side)

Foramen cecum of tongue

1st pharyngeal pouch (future auditory tube and middle ear)

Pharyngeal cavity

Tongue

2nd pharyngeal pouch (future tonsillar fossa)

3rd pharyngeal pouch

Parathyroid III (future inferior parathyroid gland)

Laryngotracheal ridge (future larynx)

Thymus

4th pharyngeal pouch

Thyroid gland ⎡ Right lateral lobe
⎣ Isthmus

Parathyroid IV (future superior parathyroid gland)

Ultimobranchial body (future C cells of thyroid gland)

Esophagus

Trachea

FIGURE 8-76 Pharyngeal Pouch Derivatives.

Ventral view at 4 to 5 weeks

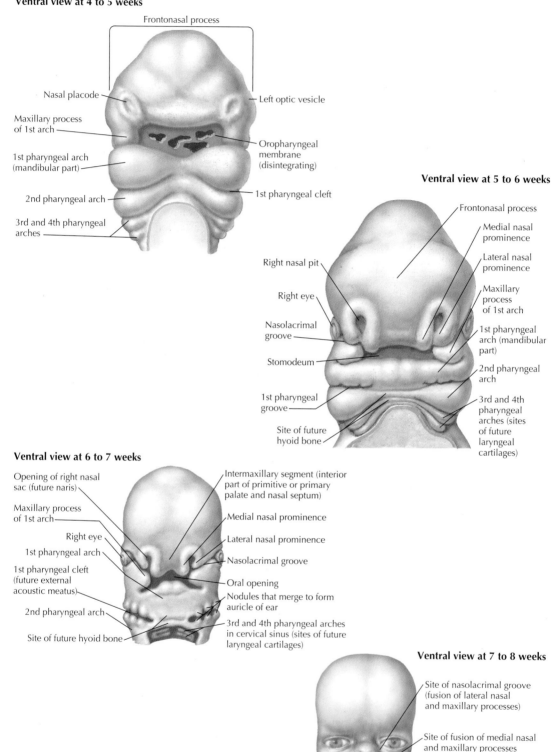

Frontonasal process

Nasal placode

Maxillary process of 1st arch

1st pharyngeal arch (mandibular part)

2nd pharyngeal arch

3rd and 4th pharyngeal arches

Left optic vesicle

Oropharyngeal membrane (disintegrating)

1st pharyngeal cleft

Ventral view at 5 to 6 weeks

Frontonasal process

Medial nasal prominence

Lateral nasal prominence

Maxillary process of 1st arch

1st pharyngeal arch (mandibular part)

2nd pharyngeal arch

3rd and 4th pharyngeal arches (sites of future laryngeal cartilages)

Right nasal pit

Right eye

Nasolacrimal groove

Stomodeum

1st pharyngeal groove

Site of future hyoid bone

Ventral view at 6 to 7 weeks

Opening of right nasal sac (future naris)

Maxillary process of 1st arch

Right eye

1st pharyngeal arch

1st pharyngeal cleft (future external acoustic meatus)

2nd pharyngeal arch

Site of future hyoid bone

Intermaxillary segment (interior part of primitive or primary palate and nasal septum)

Medial nasal prominence

Lateral nasal prominence

Nasolacrimal groove

Oral opening

Nodules that merge to form auricle of ear

3rd and 4th pharyngeal arches in cervical sinus (sites of future laryngeal cartilages)

Ventral view at 7 to 8 weeks

Site of nasolacrimal groove (fusion of lateral nasal and maxillary processes)

Site of fusion of medial nasal and maxillary processes (site of cleft lip)

Auricle of ear

Philtrum of upper lip (fusion of medial nasal processes)

FIGURE 8-77 Development of the Face.

Roof of stomodeum (inferior view; 6 to 7 weeks)

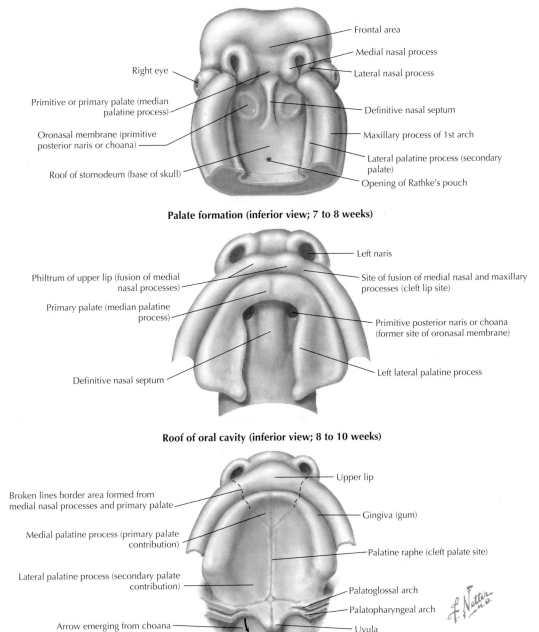

Frontal area

Medial nasal process

Right eye

Lateral nasal process

Primitive or primary palate (median palatine process)

Definitive nasal septum

Oronasal membrane (primitive posterior naris or choana)

Maxillary process of 1st arch

Lateral palatine process (secondary palate)

Roof of stomodeum (base of skull)

Opening of Rathke's pouch

Palate formation (inferior view; 7 to 8 weeks)

Left naris

Philtrum of upper lip (fusion of medial nasal processes)

Site of fusion of medial nasal and maxillary processes (cleft lip site)

Primary palate (median palatine process)

Primitive posterior naris or choana (former site of oronasal membrane)

Definitive nasal septum

Left lateral palatine process

Roof of oral cavity (inferior view; 8 to 10 weeks)

Upper lip

Broken lines border area formed from medial nasal processes and primary palate

Gingiva (gum)

Medial palatine process (primary palate contribution)

Palatine raphe (cleft palate site)

Lateral palatine process (secondary palate contribution)

Palatoglossal arch

Palatopharyngeal arch

Arrow emerging from choana

Uvula

FIGURE 8-78 Development of Hard Palate.

Salivary Gland and Tooth Development

The salivary glands develop as solid epithelial buds of the oral cavity that grow into the underlying mesenchyme (primitive mesoderm). The paired **parotid glands** develop first about the sixth week; they arise from oral ectoderm, differentiate and canalize, and then begin serous (watery) secretion of saliva at 18 weeks of development. The **submandibular glands** appear late in the sixth week

of development as endoderm-derived buds lateral to the tongue. They begin to secrete mixed serous and mucous saliva around the 16th week and continue to grow postnatally. The **sublingual glands** appear about the eighth week of development from multiple endodermal buds that differentiate into 10 to 12 ducts. These glands also secrete a seromucous saliva, but it is thicker because of a greater proportion of mucus.

Craniosynostosis

As the brain grows, so does the neurocranium, by bone deposition along suture lines. If this process is interrupted (because of unknown reasons or genetic factors), the cranium may compensate by depositing more bone along other sutures. If the sagittal suture closes prematurely, growth in width is altered, so growth occurs lengthwise and leads to a long, narrow cranium; coronal and lambdoid suture closure results in a short, wide cranium. The disorder occurs in about 1 in 2000 births and is more common in men than in women.

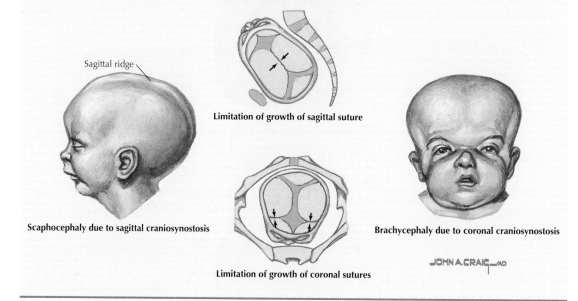

Sagittal ridge

Limitation of growth of sagittal suture

Scaphocephaly due to sagittal craniosynostosis

Limitation of growth of coronal sutures

Brachycephaly due to coronal craniosynostosis

JOHN A. CRAIG—AD

Congenital Anomalies of the Oral Cavity

Because the face and oral cavity develop largely by midline fusion of various prominences, incomplete or failed fusion can lead to cleft formation (lips and palate) or anomalous features (ankyloglossia, torus formations). The etiology is multifactorial, but genetics appears to play some role.

F. Netter M.D.

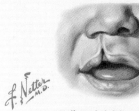

Unilateral cleft lip—partial

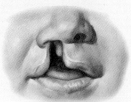

Unilateral cleft of primary palate—complete, involving lip and alveolar ridge

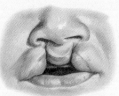

Bilateral cleft lip

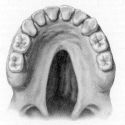

Partial cleft of palate

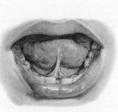

Ankyloglossia—restricted tongue movement from a short lingual frenulum

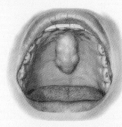

Torus palatinus—bone deposition on palate

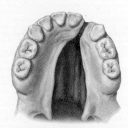

Complete cleft of secondary palate and unilateral cleft of primary palate

Pharyngeal Arch and Pouch Anomalies

Most anomalies of the pharyngeal apparatus involve fistulas, cysts, or ectopic glandular tissue. Some common anomalies and their sources from the associated pharyngeal pouch or wall are shown here in a composite illustration.

Source	
	Auditory tube
1st pharyngeal pouch	Tympanic cavity
	Eardrum
	Pharyngeal fistula
1st pharyngeal groove	External acoustic meatus
1st and 2nd pharyngeal arches	Auricle
	Nasopharynx
2nd pharyngeal pouch	Tonsillar fossa
	Epithelium of palatine tonsil
	Tongue (cut)
Ventral pharyngeal wall	Foramen cecum
	Persistent thyroglossal duct
3rd pharyngeal pouch	Aberrant parathyroid gland III
2nd pharyngeal pouch	Pharyngeal fistula
4th pharyngeal pouch	Parathyroid gland IV
	Ultimobranchial body
Ventral pharyngeal wall	Pyramidal and lateral lobes of thyroid gland
3rd pharyngeal pouch	Parathyroid gland III
	Persistent cord of thymus
3rd pharyngeal pouch	Pharyngeal fistula
3rd pharyngeal pouch	Aberrant parathyroid gland III
	Thymus gland

The **teeth** develop from oral ectoderm, mesoderm, and neural crest cells. The oral ectoderm gives rise to the **enamel,** the hardest substance in the human body. Mesenchyme, derived from the neural crest, and mesoderm gives rise to the other components of the tooth (dentine, pulp cavity). Development begins with the formation of tooth buds in the anterior mandibular region and then progresses posteriorly in both the maxilla and the mandible, under the regulation of *HOX* genes.

Cranial Nerve Summary

CRANIAL NERVE	FIBER TYPE	CRANIAL EXIT	LESION SITE	CLINICAL DEFICIT/ FINDINGS
Olfactory	Special sensory	Cribriform plate of ethmoid	Fracture of cribriform plate	Anosmia (loss of smell), cerebrospinal rhinorrhea
Optic	Special sensory	Optic canal	Fracture of optic canal, eye trauma, optic pathway lesion	Pupillary constriction, altered light reflex, visual field deficits, blindness
Oculomotor	Somatic motor Visceral motor	Superior orbital fissure	Pressure on nerve, cavernous sinus pathology, fracture	Dilated pupil, ptosis, absent pupillary reflex, eye directed down and out, diplopia, difficulty with lens accommodation
Trochlear	Somatic motor	Superior orbital fissure	Orbital fracture, cavernous sinus pathology, stretched	Cannot look down and in, diplopia
Trigeminal	General sensory (all 3 divisions) Branchial motor (V_3 only)	Superior orbital fissure (V_1) Foramen rotundum (V_2) Foramen ovale (V_3)	Fracture, herpes zoster, cavernous sinus pathology, orbital floor fracture, compression, mandibular fracture	Loss of sensation over face, jaws, anterior head, and most of the dura mater, loss of muscles of mastication and sensation over anterior two-thirds of tongue, (V_3), absent corneal reflex (V_1)
Abducent	Somatic motor	Superior orbital fissure	Fracture, cavernous sinus pathology	Cannot abduct eye, diplopia
Facial	General sensory Special sensory Branchial motor Visceral motor	Internal acoustic meatus, facial canal, stylomastoid foramen	Fracture of temporal bone, Bell's palsy, laceration over parotid region	Ipsilateral facial muscle paralysis (Bell's palsy), loss of taste at anterior two-thirds of tongue, dry eye (lacrimal gland), diminished salivation (submandibular and sublingual glands), dry nose and palate
Vestibulocochlear	Special Sensory	Internal acoustic meatus	Tumor fracture of temporal bone	Unilateral hearing loss, tinnitus, vertigo
Glossopharyngeal	Special sensory General sensory Visceral sensory Branchial motor Visceral motor	Jugular foramen	Brainstem lesion, neck laceration	Loss of taste at posterior one-third of tongue, diminished gag reflex, decreased pharynx sensation, diminished chemoreceptor reflex
Vagus	Special sensory General sensory Visceral sensory Branchial motor Visceral motor	Jugular foramen	Brainstem lesion, neck laceration	Hoarseness or loss of vocalization, deviated soft palate, uvula deviated to normal side, dysphagia, diminished baroreceptor and chemoreceptor reflexes, loss of sensation over occipital dura mater, cardiopulmonary disturbances, decreased bowel sounds, altered peristalsis
Accessory	Somatic motor	Jugular foramen	Neck laceration	Paralysis of sternocleidomastoid and trapezius muscles, drooping shoulder
Hypoglossal	Somatic motor	Hypoglossal canal	Basal skull fracture, neck laceration, trauma to floor of mouth	Ipsilateral atrophy of tongue, protruded tongue deviates to affected side, altered speech (dysarthria)

Challenge Yourself Questions

1. A 2-month-old infant presents with no evidence of a thymus and some uncertainty regarding the number and location of parathyroid tissue. Which of the following pharyngeal pouches may be responsible for these findings?

   A. First pouch
   B. Second and third pouches
   C. Third pouch
   D. Third and fourth pouches
   E. Fourth pouch

2. A 46-year-old woman presents with painful erythematous vesicular eruptions over the right upper eyelid and forehead and spreading into her hairline over the squamous portion of the temporal bone. She is diagnosed with herpes zoster (shingles). Which of the following nerves is most likely responsible for transmitting this virus?

   A. Auriculotemporal nerve
   B. Greater petrosal nerve
   C. Nasociliary nerve
   D. Supra-orbital nerve
   E. Zygomatic nerve

3. A 31-year-old man is diagnosed with a benign pituitary adenoma that has impinged on the right aspect of the cavernous sinus. Which of the following clinical signs is most likely to be evident in this patient?

   A. Bilateral painful ophthalmoplegia
   B. Left-sided diplopia
   C. Left-sided complete ptosis
   D. Right-sided pupillary dilation
   E. Right-sided dry eye

4. A teenage gang member receives a knife cut inferior to the angle of the mandible and receives emergency care for the repair of the vascular damage, cleansing of the wound, and closing of the incision. Unknown to the resident in the ER, the victim's hypoglossal nerve was completely severed. Which of the following muscles would mostly likely be affected?

   A. Anterior belly of the digastric
   B. Genioglossus
   C. Geniohyoid
   D. Mylohyoid
   E. Palatoglossus
   F. Stylohyoid

5. A 56-year-old woman presents in the clinic with diplopia of the left eye, complete left-sided ptosis, and an absent corneal reflex. Where is the most likely site of a lesion that would account for this presentation?

   A. Foramen ovale
   B. Foramen rotundum
   C. Inferior orbital fissure
   D. Optic canal
   E. Superior orbital fissure

6. A young child falls while sucking on a lollipop, and the stick lacerates the posterior wall of her oropharynx, stopped by a cervical vertebral body. As a precaution, the physician prescribes a broad-spectrum antibiotic. Which of the following spaces is most likely to harbor an infection after this type of puncture wound?

   A. Epidural space
   B. Mediastinum
   C. Pretracheal space
   D. Retropharyngeal space
   E. Subdural space

Multiple-choice and short-answer review questions available online; see inside front cover for details.

7. A baseball player is hit in his left eye and orbital region by a fastball that results in a blow-out fracture. The left orbital contents show evidence of an inferior herniation into which of the following spaces?

   A. Cavernous sinus
   B. Ethmoid sinus
   C. Frontal sinus
   D. Maxillary sinus
   E. Sphenoid sinus

8. An internist suspects a patient has an infection in the cavernous sinus. If the infection enters the infra-orbital veins, it can next pass directly into which of the following venous channels and endanger the inferior alveolar and lingual nerves?

   A. Facial
   B. Infra-orbital
   C. Pterygoid plexus
   D. Retromandibular
   E. Superficial temporal

9. A traumatic injury to the right side of the neck requires significant surgical attention. The patient has a hoarse voice, which will not resolve with time. Which of the following nerves was most likely damaged by this injury?

   A. Ansa cervicalis
   B. Hypoglossal
   C. Recurrent laryngeal
   D. Superior laryngeal
   E. Sympathetic trunk

10. An elderly woman stumbles while walking down her basement stairs but catches herself before falling. On examination by her physician, she presents with diplopia when looking inferiorly. Which of the following nerves is most likely affected?

    A. Abducent
    B. Oculomotor
    C. Ophthalmic (V_1)
    D. Optic
    E. Trochlear

11. A tumor compresses the sympathetic trunk in the lower neck. Which of the following muscles is most likely affected?

    A. Ciliary
    B. Geniohyoid
    C. Orbicularis oculi
    D. Pupillary constrictor
    E. Superior tarsal

12. The rupture of a berry aneurysm affecting the anterior communicating artery of the circle of Willis results in significant bleeding. Into which space will this bleeding occur?

    A. Cavernous sinus
    B. Epidural space
    C. Lateral ventricle
    D. Subarachnoid space
    E. Subdural space

13. A congenital malformation affecting the malleus and incus in the middle ear would be associated with the maldevelopment of which of the following structures?

    A. First pharyngeal arch
    B. Frontonasal process
    C. Pharyngotympanic tube
    D. Second pharyngeal arch
    E. Second pharyngeal pouch

14. A 56-year-old woman has had significant pain deep in her jaw, which has become localized to her temporomandibular joint (TMJ). Examination reveals that she has an inflamed TMJ. Which of the following muscles is most likely involved in this inflammatory process?

    A. Buccinator
    B. Lateral pterygoid
    C. Masseter
    D. Medial pterygoid
    E. Temporalis

For each condition described below (15-25), select the nerve from the list (A-Q) that is most likely responsible or affected.

(A)	Abducent	**(J)**	Nerve of pterygoid
(B)	Accessory		canal
(C)	Chorda tympani	**(K)**	Oculomotor
(D)	Deep petrosal	**(L)**	Olfactory
(E)	Facial	**(M)**	Optic
(F)	Glossopharyngeal	**(N)**	Trigeminal
(G)	Greater petrosal	**(O)**	Trochlear
(H)	Hypoglossal	**(P)**	Vagus
(I)	Lesser petrosal	**(Q)**	Vestibulocochlear

___ 15. A patient presents with diplopia and an inability to abduct the left eye.

___ 16. Trauma to the right middle cranial fossa results in ipsilateral pupillary constriction and partial ptosis.

___ 17. Sharp trauma to the left infratemporal fossa results in the ipsilateral loss of taste on the anterior two thirds of the tongue.

___ 18. In a patient with some hearing loss in one ear, the Rinne test confirms that the tuning fork is heard better when placed beside the affected ear than when placed on the mastoid process.

___ 19. During a routine examination, when the patient is asked to say "ah," the soft palate and uvula are elevated asymmetrically.

___ 20. A fracture of the middle cranial fossa, just along the anterior base of the petrous portion of the temporal bone, results in a decreased secretion of the ipsilateral parotid gland.

___ 21. You are talking and chewing gum at the same time and inadvertently bite your cheek. The site of injury is painful and begins to swell. You ask yourself, "What nerve mediates this pain?"

___ 22. During a routine tonsillectomy, a complication results in the loss of taste and sensation on the posterior third of the tongue.

___ 23. A severe bacterial infection of the left sphenoid sinus erodes into the bony floor of the sinus, resulting in an ipsilateral dry eye and dry nasal passage.

___ 24. A small child screams in pain following a bee sting on his upper lip.

___ 25. A blow to the head results in the rupture of the middle meningeal artery, causing an epidural hematoma, which is extremely painful.

Answers to Challenge Yourself Questions

1. **C.** The thyroid appears healthy, so we can assume that the C cells of the thyroid developed normally along with the superior parathyroid glands of the fourth pouch. The third pharyngeal pouch, however, gives rise to the thymus gland and the inferior parathyroids, so this is the pouch most likely affected.

2. **D.** The supra-orbital nerve is a branch of the ophthalmic division of the trigeminal nerve, and its distribution matches the description of the skin eruptions. The virus responsible for herpes resides in the sensory ganglia of nerves, in this case the semilunar ganglion of CN V.

3. **D.** The expansion to the right side will affect the right eye and orbit, and in this case it will affect the oculomotor nerve (CN III). The following nerves pass in close association with the cavernous sinus and can be affected by an expanding mass in this region: CN III, IV, V_1, V_2, and VI. The dilated pupil results from the unopposed sympathetic innervation of the dilator muscle; the constrictor of the pupil is affected by the compression on CN III, which carries the parasympathetics to the ciliary ganglion and this muscle.

4. **B.** Of the listed muscles, only the genioglossus is innervated by CN XII. The other two muscles innervated by CN XII are the hyoglossus and styloglossus.

5. **E.** These signs and symptoms are compatible with a lesion to CN III (denervation of four extra-ocular muscles and the levator palpebrae superioris muscle of the eyelid) and sensation over the cornea (ophthalmic division of the trigeminal nerve). Both these nerves enter the orbit via the superior orbital fissure.

6. **D.** The retropharyngeal space lies between the buccopharyngeal (visceral) fascia and the prevertebral fascia (specifically the alar layer) and extends from the base of the cranium to the posterior mediastinum. Infections in this space can easily spread superiorly or inferiorly via the contractions of the pharyngeal muscles and esophagus, which can "knead" the bacteria along the space.

7. **D.** The floor of the orbit is the roof of the underlying maxillary sinus. Fractures in this area can result in the partial herniation of the orbital contents inferiorly, especially the orbital fat (the eye may droop but is tethered by the optic nerve and extra-ocular muscles).

8. **C.** From the inferior ophthalmic veins, the infection could spread in several directions, but to involve the inferior alveolar and lingual nerves, it would need to spread to the pterygoid plexus of veins draining the infratemporal region.

9. **C.** The recurrent laryngeal (inferior laryngeal) nerve passes through the neck in the tracheo-esophageal groove as it ascends to innervate the muscles of the larynx. If injured, the only pair of abductors of the vocal folds would be compromised ipsilaterally (hemiparalysis of the posterior crico-arytenoids), leading to a hoarse voice.

10. E. The trochlear nerve (CN IV) innervates the superior oblique muscle, and the affected eye will be elevated and adducted. The patient will have difficulty looking inferiorly and medially as she steps down stairs or off curbs and will present with diplopia.

11. E. The superior tarsal muscle is the only muscle on the list innervated by the sympathetic fibers; when denervated, it will result in a partial ptosis ipsilaterally. This small smooth muscle connects to the superior tarsal plate. Complete ptosis is more often associated with denervation of the levator palpebrae superioris muscle by CN III. Compression of the sympathetic trunk would result in Horner's syndrome and present not only with partial ptosis but also miosis, anhidrosis, and flushed skin (vasodilation) ipsilaterally.

12. D. Bleeding from the cerebral arteries would occur in the subarachnoid space. Subdural hematomas usually occur from bleeding associated with the bridging veins passing to the superior sagittal dural venous sinus. Epidural bleeds are associated with bleeding from the middle meningeal artery or one of its many branches.

13. A. The first pharyngeal arch gives rise to Meckel's cartilage, and derivatives of this arch cartilage include the ossified mandible, malleus, incus, and sphenomandibular ligament. The sensory innervation comes from the mandibular division of the trigeminal nerve.

14. B. The lateral pterygoid muscle, in part, inserts into the articular disc of the TMJ and is the most likely muscle to be involved with this infection. Together, this pair of muscles help protrude the mandible and depress the chin in the initial act of opening the jaw.

15. A. Inability to abduct the eye without other movement impairment suggests that the lateral rectus muscle is affected, and it is innervated by the abducent nerve (CN VI).

16. D. Partial ptosis (denervation of the superior tarsal muscle) and pupillary constriction (absence of pupillary dilation) suggest an injury to the sympathetic system somewhere along its pathway to the head. Of the listed nerves, only the deep petrosal (postganglionic fibers from the superior cervical ganglion) nerve would show exclusively sympathetic involvement as it courses on the intracranial portion of the internal carotid artery.

17. C. If taste is the only sense affected, the answer is the chorda tympani nerve, which is damaged before joining the lingual nerve (apparently sensation on the anterior tongue is intact). One might also expect that some parasympathetics to the submandibular ganglion would also be affected, but this may not be immediately obvious. The chorda tympani carries taste fibers and preganglionic parasympathetic fibers.

18. Q. Normally, hearing by air conduction is better than by bone conduction. In an affected ear (decreased hearing), if the air conduction is still better than bone conduction, it suggests that the hearing loss is caused by sensorineural loss (inner ear problem vs. a middle or external ear problem) affecting the vestibulocochlear nerve (CN VIII).

19. P. An ipsilateral asymmetrical elevation of the soft palate and uvula suggests that the levator veli palatini muscle is affected, which is innervated by the vagus nerve.

20. I. The lesser petrosal nerve is found in this area and carries preganglionic parasympathetic secretory fibers to the otic ganglion, where the fibers synapse. Postganglionic fibers from the otic ganglion then join the auriculotemporal nerve to innervate the parotid gland. The lesser petrosal nerve arises from the tympanic plexus of CN IX (glossopharyngeal).

21. N. The pain is mediated by the large "sensory" nerve of the head, the trigeminal. Specifically, this buccal pain is mediated by the buccal branch of the mandibular division of CN V.

22. F. The glossopharyngeal nerve innervates one muscle (stylopharyngeus) and then passes into the posterior third of the tongue to provide general sensation and the special sense of taste to this portion of the tongue. As it does so, CN IX passes adjacent to the tonsillary fossa and may be damaged during a tonsillectomy.

23. J. The nerve of the pterygoid canal (vidian nerve) runs in the floor of the sphenoid sinus and conveys postganglionic sympathetic fibers (from the deep petrosal nerve) and preganglionic parasympathetic fibers (from the greater petrosal nerve). In this case, the parasympathetics to the pterygopalatine ganglion are affected, and the lacrimal gland and nasal mucous glands have been denervated by the infection to this nerve.

24. N. Sensation on the upper lip is conveyed by the trigeminal nerve. Specifically, it will be by a superior labial sensory branch of the maxillary division of CN V.

25. N. The great sensory nerve of the head is the trigeminal. CN V provides sensory innervation to most of the dura mater; the vagus nerve contributes some sensation to the posterior dura. The arachnoid and pia mater do not possess sensory innervation.

Index